CAWSON'S ESSENTIALS OF
ORAL PATHOLOGY
AND ORAL MEDICINE

Professor Roderick A. Cawson
BDS, FDSRCS, LMSSA, MB BS, MD, FRCPath

1921–2007

For Elsevier

Commissioning Editor: Michael Parkinson/Alison Taylor
Development Editor: Clive Hewat
Project Manager: Kerrie-Anne Jarvis
Design Direction: Erik Bigland
Illustrator: David Gardner
Illustrator Manager: Merlyn Harvey

CAWSON'S ESSENTIALS OF
ORAL PATHOLOGY AND ORAL MEDICINE

EIGHTH EDITION

R. A. Cawson MD FDSRCS FDSRCPS(Glas) FRCPath FAAOMP

Emeritus Professor of Oral Medicine and Pathology, Guy's, King's and St Thomas'
Dental Institute, King's College London
Visiting Professor in Oral Pathology, Baylor College of Dentistry, Texas A & M
University System, Dallas, Texas

and

E. W. Odell FDSRCS MSc PhD FRCPath

Professor of Oral Pathology and Medicine, King's College London
Honorary Consultant in Oral Pathology, Guy's and St Thomas' NHS
Foundation Trust, London

CHURCHILL
LIVINGSTONE

ELSEVIER

EDINBURGH LONDON NEW YORK OXFORD PHILADELPHIA ST LOUIS
SYDNEY TORONTO 2008

CHURCHILL
LIVINGSTONE
ELSEVIER

© Longman Group UK Limited 1991
Assigned to Pearson Professional 1995
© 1998, 2008, Elsevier Limited. All rights reserved.

First edition 1962
Second edition 1968
Third edition 1978
Fourth edition 1984
Fifth edition 1991
Sixth edition 1998
Seventh edition 2002

Main edition ISBN: 978-0443-10125-0
  Reprinted 2008
International edition ISBN: 978-0443-10365-0

British Library Cataloguing in Publication Data
A catalogue record for this book is available from the British Library

Library of Congress Cataloging in Publication Data
A catalog record for this book is available from the Library of Congress

ELSEVIER your source for books, journals and multimedia in the health sciences
www.elsevierhealth.com

Working together to grow
libraries in developing countries

www.elsevier.com | www.bookaid.org | www.sabre.org

ELSEVIER   **BOOK AID** International   **Sabre Foundation**

The Publisher's policy is to use **paper manufactured from sustainable forests**

Printed in China

Contents

v

Preface

Undergraduate students will never see many of the conditions discussed in this book. Despite this, on qualification they are expected to not only diagnose them, but also institute appropriate referral or treatment. This, the eighth edition of *Cawson's Essentials*, is therefore not only updated, but also designed to make clinical relevance immediately accessible to the learner.

We have used more colour illustrations and have introduced symbols to link the text to the diagnostic summary charts. The text has been updated with many new sections on cancer, premalignancy, osseointegration, sinusitis and disturbances of taste, as well as new diseases such as bisphosphonate-induced osteonecrosis. There is a new section on normal healing of tooth sockets, an important topic hardly covered elsewhere. Some chapters have changed relatively little, such as that on caries, but the importance of understanding the disease process is now more clearly linked to clinical practice in tables.

Self-directed learning is critical to develop understanding. New learning guides now follow each section, an attempt to help students direct their own learning from other sources, because no book can be comprehensive. References have been updated but remain largely unchanged. Often the older classic papers are those of most use to undergraduates and the retention of these older papers is deliberate.

Our thanks are due to Clive Hewat, Alison Taylor, Kerrie-Anne Jarvis, Erik Bigland, Mike Parkinson and all the team at Elsevier for maintaining the excellent production standards and rescuing many of the older, now almost irreplaceable, photomicrographs.

This edition of *Cawson's Essentials* is, sadly, the last to which Professor Cawson will contribute. He died shortly after the manuscript was completed. A dedicated teacher, he understood how students were often baffled by the complexity of our subjects. He was a master of succinct text and ruthless in editing out ideas without an 'evidence base', long before the expression had been invented. *Cawson's Essentials* has been published continuously since 1962 and it was the first textbook to integrate oral medicine, pathology and surgery in a practical, student-orientated fashion. The many students who have relied on it over the last nearly half-century give testimony to his breadth of knowledge, intellectual authority and the clarity of his writing.

E.W.O.
London 2008

Principles of investigation and diagnosis

The principles of patient investigation and diagnosis are summarised in Box 1.1.

Box 1.1   Principles of investigation and diagnosis

- A detailed history
- Clinical examination
  Extraoral
  Intraoral
- Special investigations (as appropriate)
  Testing vitality of teeth
  Radiography or other imaging techniques
  Biopsy for histopathology (including immunofluorescence, immunocytochemistry, electron microscopy, molecular biological tests)
  Specimen for microbial culture
  Haematological or biochemical tests

Table 1.1   Types of question

Type of question	Example
Open	Tell me about the pain?
Closed	What does the pain feel like?
Leading	Does the pain feel like an electric shock?

TAKING A HISTORY

History-taking needs to be tailored to suit the individual patient, but it is sometimes difficult to get a clear idea of the complaint. Many patients are nervous, some are inarticulate, others are confused.

Rapport is critical for eliciting useful information. Initial questions should allow patients to speak at some length and to gain confidence. It is usually best to start with an 'open' question (Tables 1.1 and 1.2). Medical jargon should be avoided and even regular hospital attenders who appear to understand medical terminology may use it wrongly and misunderstand. Leading questions, which suggest a particular answer, should be avoided because patients may feel compelled to agree with the clinician.

It is sometimes difficult to avoid interrupting patients when trying to structure the history for the records. Structure can only be given after the patient has had time to give the information. Constant note-taking while patients are speaking is undesirable.

Questioning technique is most critical when eliciting any relevant social or psychological history or dealing with embarrassing medical conditions. It may be appropriate to delay asking such questions until after rapport has been gained. Some patients do not consider medical questions to be the concern of the dentist and it is important to give reasons for such questions when necessary (Box 1.2).

Table 1.2   Advantages and disadvantages of types of question

Types of question	Advantages	Disadvantages
Open	Allows patients to use their own words and summarise their view of the problem Allows patients partly to direct the history-taking, gives them confidence and quickly generates rapport	Clinicians must listen carefully and avoid interruptions to extract the relevant information Patients tend to decide what information is relevant
Closed	Elicits specific information quickly Useful to fill gaps in the information given in response to open questions Prevents vague patients from rambling away from the complaint	Patients may infer that the clinician is not really interested in their problem if only closed questions are asked Important information may be lost if not specifically requested Restricts the patient's opportunities to talk

---

Box 1.2 Essential principles of history-taking

- Introduce yourself and greet the patient by name
- Put patients at their ease
- Start with an open question
- Mix open and closed questions
- Avoid leading questions
- Avoid jargon
- Explain the need for specific questions
- Assess the patient's mental state
- Assess the patient's expectations from treatment

During history-taking, the mental and emotional state of the patient should be assessed. This may have a bearing on psychosomatic disease and will also suggest what the patient expects to gain from the consultation and treatment. If the patient's expectations are unreasonable, it is important to try to modify them during the consultation, otherwise no treatment may be satisfactory.

Demographic details

The age, gender, ethnic group and occupation of the patient should be noted. Such information is occasionally critical. For instance, an elderly woman with arthritis and a dry mouth is likely to have Sjögren's syndrome (Ch. 18), but a young man with a parotid swelling due to similar lymphoproliferation is far more likely to have HIV infection (Ch. 24). Some diseases such as oral submucous fibrosis (Ch. 16) have a restricted ethnic distribution.

History of the present complaint

Frequently, a complaint, such as toothache, suggests the diagnosis. In many cases, a detailed history (Box 1.3) is required and sometimes, as in aphthous ulceration, a provisional diagnosis can be made on the history without examination or investigation.

Box 1.3 History of the present complaint

- Record the description of the complaint *in the patient's own words*
- Elicit the exact meaning of those words
- Record the duration and the time course of any changes in symptoms or signs
- Include any relevant facts in the patient's medical history
- Note any temporal relationship between them and the present complaint
- Consider any previous treatments and their effectiveness

If earlier treatment has been ineffective, the diagnosis should be reconsidered. Many patients' lives have been shortened by having malignant tumours treated with repeated courses of antibiotics.

Pain is completely subjective and, when physical signs are absent, special care must be taken to detail all its features (Table 1.3). Especially important are features suggesting a dental cause. A fractured tooth or cusp, dentinal hypersensitivity or pain on occlusion are easily misdiagnosed.

Factors triggering different causes of pain are discussed in detail in Chapter 34.

The medical history

A medical history is important as it aids the diagnosis of oral manifestations of systemic disease. It also ensures that medical conditions and medication which affect dental or surgical treatment are identified.

To ensure that nothing significant is forgotten, a printed questionnaire for patients to complete is valuable and saves time. It also helps to avoid medicolegal problems by providing a written record that the patient's medical background has been considered. However, a questionnaire does not constitute a medical history and the information must be checked verbally, verified and augmented as necessary. It is important to assess whether the patient's reading ability and

Table 1.3 Taking a pain history

Characteristic	Informative features
Type	Ache, tenderness, dull pain, throbbing, stabbing, electric shock. These terms are of limited use and the constancy of pain is more useful
Severity	Mild – managed with mild analgesics (e.g. aspirin/paracetamol) Moderate – unresponsive to mild analgesics Severe – disturbs sleep
Duration	Time since onset. Duration of pain or attacks
Nature	Continuous, periodic or paroxysmal If not continuous, is pain present between attacks?
Initiating factors	Any potential initiating factors Association with dental treatment or lack of it is especially important in eliminating dental causes
Exacerbating and relieving factors	Record all and note especially hot and cold sensitivity or pain on eating which suggest a dental cause
Localisation	The patient should map out the distribution of pain if possible. Is it well or poorly defined? Does it affect an area supplied by a particular nerve or artery?
Referred pain	Try to determine whether the pain could be referred

understanding are sufficient to provide valid answers to the questionnaire.

A sample medical history questionnaire is shown in Box 1.4.

If the history suggests, or examination reveals, any condition beyond the scope of the dentist's experience or clinical knowledge, referral for specialist medical examination may be necessary.

Box 1.4   An example of a medical history questionnaire

SURNAME   Address

Other names

Date of birth   Telephone number

The following questions are asked in the interests of your safety and any particular precautions that may need to be taken as a result of thorough knowledge of any previous illnesses or medications. Please, therefore, answer these questions as accurately as you can.

If you are in any doubt about how to answer them, please do not hesitate to ask.

1. Are you undergoing any medical   Yes   No
   treatment at present?
2. Do you have, or have you had any of the following:
   a. Heart disease?   Yes   No
   b. Rheumatic fever?   Yes   No
   c. Hepatitis?   Yes   No
   d. Jaundice?   Yes   No
   e. Epilepsy   Yes   No
   f. Diabetes?   Yes   No
   g. Raised blood pressure?   Yes   No
   h. Anaemia?   Yes   No
   i. Asthma, hay fever or other allergies?   Yes   No
   j. Familial or acquired bleeding tendencies? Yes   No
   k. Any other serious illnesses?   Yes   No
3. Have you suffered allergy or other reactions (rash, itchiness etc) to:
   a. Penicillin?   Yes   No
   b. Other medicines or tablets?   Yes   No
   c. Substances or chemicals?   Yes   No
4. Have you ever had any adverse effects   Yes   No
   from local anaesthetics?
5. Have you ever experienced unusually prolonged
   bleeding after injury or tooth extraction?   Yes   No
6. Have you ever been given penicillin?   Yes   No
7. Are you taking any medicines, tablets,   Yes   No
   injections (etc.) at present?

If YES can you please indicate the nature of this medication?

8. Have you been treated with any of the following in the past 5 years:
   a. Cortisone (hydrocortisone, prednisone etc)? Yes   No
   b. Blood-thinning medication?   Yes   No
   c. Antidepressants?   Yes   No
9. Have you ever received radiotherapy?   Yes   No
10. Do you smoke?   Yes   No

If YES how much on average per day?
11. For female patients – are you pregnant?   Yes   No

PLEASE ADD ANY OTHER INFORMATION OR COMMENTS ON YOUR MEDICAL HISTORY, BELOW

Signature   Date

Address (if not the patient)

Medical warning cards may indicate that the patient is, for example, a haemophiliac, on long-term corticosteroid therapy or is allergic to penicillin. It is also worthwhile to leave a final section open for patients to supply any other information that they think might be relevant.

A detailed drug history is essential. Drugs can have oral effects or complicate dental management in important ways (Chs 13 & 35).

In some ethnic groups, enquiry should be made about habits such as betel quid (pan) or smokeless tobacco use (Ch. 16).

The dental history

A dental history and examination are obviously essential for the diagnosis of dental pain or to exclude teeth as cause of symptoms in the head and neck region.

Symptoms of toothache are very variable and may masquerade as a variety of conditions from trivial to sinister. The relationship between symptoms and any dental treatment, or lack of it, should be noted.

The family and social history

Whenever a symptom or sign suggests an inherited disorder, such as haemophilia, the family history should be elicited. Ideally, this is recorded as a pedigree diagram noting the proband (presenting case) and all family members for at least three generations. Even when no familial disease is suspected, questions about other family members often usefully lead naturally into questions about home circumstances, relatives and social history which can be revealing if, for example, psychosomatic factors are suspected.

Consent

It is imperative to obtain patients' consent for any procedure. At the very least, the procedure to be used should be explained to the patient and verbal consent obtained. If no more than this is done, the patients' consent should be noted in their records. However, it is better to obtain written consent.

Patients frequently ask for particular types of treatment, such as fillings or extractions. This implies consent and usually no written agreement is expected. However, with the growing risk of litigation, many dental hospitals now require clinicians to give precise descriptions of treatment plans, however routine, and to obtain written consent. Written treatment plans are also required in dental practice.

Patients have a legal right to refuse treatment. Any such refusals may sometimes be due to failure of the clinician to explain the need for a particular procedure, or failure to soothe the patient's fears about possible complications. Some of these fears may be irrational, such as the idea of an inherited allergy to local anaesthetics. In such cases, even prolonged explanations and persuasion may be unsuccessful.

When a biopsy is necessary, its purpose should be explained and that the biopsied area may be sore after the local anaesthetic has worn off. Also, it seems likely that when the patient's tissue is to be retained, even in a block for histological examination, it should be explained that this has to be done in case future reference to it is needed and consent obtained accordingly.

In the case of more major surgery, a consent form should state the nature of the operation and also the likelihood of any significant complications or risks. In the case of an ameloblastoma, for example, it would be necessary to point out that a further operation may be unavoidable and that the alternative might be a relatively massive excision. Also, in such circumstances or when sedation or a general anaesthetic is indicated, patients should be encouraged to ask whatever questions or express any concerns about the procedure and to have it explained fully.

Even greater difficulties may arise in the matter of consent for parotid gland surgery. Explanation of the possibility of permanently disfiguring facial palsy has to be balanced against the need for complete eradication of a tumour. Also, in the case of older patients, it may seem probable that a benign tumour may not cause significant trouble within the patient's lifetime and that the operative risks are not justified. On the other hand, such a patient may find the idea of living with a tumour emotionally unacceptable so that surgery with its possible complications has to be accepted.

For consent to be legally valid, patients should be given sufficient information, in understandable terms, about the proposed treatment for them to make their own decisions. It is not enough to get a patient, due to have major oral surgery, to sign a blanket consent form without any explanations. Though this has happened many times, the patient may later claim for assault, particularly if there have been unexpected complications.

When a drug has to be prescribed, the difficulties can sometimes be considerable. First, the level of risk of an adverse reaction from a drug is frequently unknown. Severe reactions to penicillin are rare, but it is difficult to explain to a patient that anaphylactic reactions in persons not known to be allergic to penicillin are exceedingly rare but, nevertheless, potentially fatal.

Misunderstandings are common. Many patients think that the word 'drug' means a drug of addiction so that the words 'a medicine' are preferable.

It is also essential to point out any precautions necessary when taking a particular drug. To take a common example, patients are frequently concerned about the risks of taking aspirin. But in view of the fact that it is estimated that 3000 *tons* of it are consumed every year, the chances of a reaction are almost infinitessimally small. Most people who complain that aspirin disagrees with them or that they are 'allergic' to it, have merely taken the tablets on an empty stomach or without a drink of milk. Obvious though they may seem, such precautions must be emphasised whenever aspirin or a non-steroidal anti-inflammatory drug is prescribed.

Even when the statistical risk of an adverse reaction to a drug is known, the level of risk may be difficult to explain. It may be known that the risk is 0.0001%, but the patient is

an individual not a statistic and this does not mean that he or she will be the ten-thousandth patient and will necessarily be affected.

Risks from drugs are also in many ways unpredictable. For example, ataxia caused by carbamazepine is a recognised risk. Thus, one patient became unsteady on her feet as soon as she started taking it. By contrast, another patient who had been taking carbamazepine intermittently for many years without any adverse effects, suddenly lost his balance completely and repeatedly collapsed on the floor without any warning.

Another problem is that many patients are unclear about the difference between risk and harm and think that these are the same thing. It may be necessary to say therefore, 'The chances of anything going wrong are probably less than one in ten thousand'. Or perhaps, 'The risk is probably less than when you cross the road'.

However carefully the risks from a drug are explained, it is absolutely essential that patients are warned to come back as soon as they think that there has been an adverse reaction.[1]

A Consent Form should therefore be used and should state:

1. The type of operation or investigation.
2. Possible risks and complications
3. A signed and dated statement by the clinician that he or she has explained these matters and any options that may be available in terms understandable to the patient, parent or guardian.
4. A section for the patient, parent or guardian to confirm:
   a. that the information was understandable
   b. that the person signing the form has a legal right to do so, i.e. is the patient, parent or guardian
   c. that the procedure has been explained and agreed
   d. that there are certain additional procedures that would be completely unacceptable and should not be carried out.

The form should be signed and dated by the clinician and patient, parent or guardian.

National standard consent forms are produced for use in the National Health Service and most users will have specific guidance as to how these are to be used. Many organisations require use of these forms and audit compliance.

CLINICAL EXAMINATION

Extraoral

First, look at the patient, before looking into the patient's mouth. Anaemia, thyroid disease, long-term corticosteroid treatment, parotid swellings, or significantly enlarged cervical nodes are a few conditions that can affect the facial appearance.

---

[1]This advice about consent may seem excessive, but the eagerness with which patients now turn to litigation is a serious problem and failure to follow prescribed procedures is considered culpable even if no patient harm results.

The parotid glands, temporomandibular joints (for clicks, crepitus or deviation), cervical and submandibular lymph nodes and thyroid gland should be palpated. Lymphadenopathy (Ch. 26) is a common manifestation of infection, but may also signify malignancy – the cervical lymph nodes are often the first affected by lymphomas. Note the character (site, shape, size, surface texture and consistency) of any enlargement. Press on the maxilla and frontal bone over the sinuses to elicit tenderness if sinusitis is suspected.

Oral examination

Examination of the oral cavity can only be performed adequately with good light, mirrors and compressed air or other means of drying the teeth. If viscid saliva prevents visualisation of the tissues and teeth, a rinse with sodium bicarbonate mouthwash will help.

Soft tissues

The soft tissues of the mouth should usually be inspected first. Examination should be systematic to include all areas of the mouth. Care should be taken that mirrors or retractors do not obscure lesions. To ensure complete examination of the lateral tongue and posterior floor of mouth, the tongue must be held in gauze and gently extended from side to side.

Abnormal-looking areas of mucosa should be palpated for scarring or induration indicating previous ulceration, inflammation or malignancy. Examination should include deeper tissues accessible to palpation, including the submandibular glands.

If lesions extend close to the gingiva, the gingival crevice or pockets should be probed for any communication. Mucosal nodules, especially those on the gingiva or alveolar mucosa, which suggest sinus openings, should be probed to identify any sinus or fistula. Check the openings of the salivary ducts while expressing saliva by gentle pressure. Check that saliva flows freely and equally from all glands and is clear in colour. Do not mistake anatomical variations (Table 1.4) for disease.

After examination of the oral mucosa try to visualise the oropharynx and tonsils.

Teeth

When undertaking a consultation for a complaint apparently unrelated to teeth, dental examination must still be thorough both for the patient's sake and for medicolegal reasons. As a minimum, the standing teeth with a summary of their periodontal health, caries and restorative state, should be recorded. Tooth wear should be checked for 'parafunction'. When dental pain is a possibility, full charting, assessment of mobility and percussion of teeth are necessary and further dental investigations will probably be required.

Testing vitality of teeth The vitality of teeth must be checked if they appear to be causing symptoms. It is also essential to determine the vitality of teeth in the region of cysts and other radiolucent lesions in the jaws at presentation. The information may be essential for diagnosis.

To be absolutely certain, several methods may have to be used. Checking hot and cold sensitivity and electric pulp testing are relatively easily performed (Box 1.5).

Table 1.4	Some anatomical variants and normal structures often misdiagnosed as lesions
Structure	**Description**
Fordyce's spots	Sebaceous glands lying superficially in the mucosa are visible as white or cream coloured spots up to 0.5 mm across. Usually labial mucosa and buccal mucosa. Occasionally prominent and very numerous (Fig. 15.4)
Lingual tonsils	Enlarge with viral infection and occasionally noted by patients. Sometimes large or ectopic and then mistaken for disease (Figs 1.1 and 1.2)
Circumvallate papillae	Readily identifiable but sometimes prominent and misinterpreted by patients or health care workers
Retrocuspid papilla	Firm pink nodule 0.5–4 mm diameter on the attached gingiva lingual to the lower canine and lateral incisor, usually bilateral but sometimes unilateral. Prominent in children but regress with age
Dorsal tongue fur	Furring of the dorsal tongue mucosa is very variable and is heavier when the diet is soft. Even light furring is regarded as pathological by many patients. When pigmented black by bacteria and with overgrowth of the filiform papillae, the condition is called black hairy tongue (Ch. 14)
Leukoedema	A milky white translucent whitening of the oral mucosa which disappears or fades on stretching. Commoner in black races (Ch. 15)
Tori	Exostoses in the midline of the palate or in the lingual alveolus in the premolar region are termed tori (Ch. 9). They also arise at other sites, particularly on the maxilla over premolar and canine roots

Fig. 1.1 Large foliate papilla or lingual tonsil that may be mistaken for a lesion on the side of the tongue.

Box 1.5   Precautions for electric pulp testing

- Isolate individual teeth with a small portion of rubber dam if necessary
- Always record electric pulp test values in the notes – a progressive change in reading over time may indicate declining vitality
- If results remain uncertain, cut a test cavity or remove suspect restorations without local anaesthetic
- Poorly localised pulp pain from teeth of dubious vitality can be difficult to ascribe to an individual tooth. In such circumstances, a diagnostic local anaesthetic injection on a suspect tooth may stop the pain and indicate its source
- Other sources of referred pain may sometimes be identified by the same means

Table 1.5   Possible causes of misleading electric pulp test results

Problem	Causes to consider
Pulp by-passed by electric current	Electrical contact with next tooth by touching amalgam restorations Electrical contact with gingival margin by amalgam restoration or saliva film
Electrical insulation of the pulp	Large composite or non-conducting restorations
Falsely low reading	Incompletely formed root apex
Partially vital pulps	Multiple canals
No check on validity of results	No normal teeth for comparison
Patient fails to report accurately	Failure to differentiate pulpal from soft tissue sensation

Unfortunately, it may not be apparent that a pulp test result is misleading. Care must always be taken to avoid causes of false-positive or false-negative results (Table 1.5).

MEDICAL EXAMINATION

In practice, it is usual for dental investigations to be performed first, but the dentist should be capable of performing simple medical examinations of the head and neck. Examination of the skin of the face, hair, scalp and neck may reveal unexpected foci of infection to account for cervical lymphadenopathy or even malignant neoplasms. The eye can readily be inspected for conjunctivitis or signs of mucous membrane pemphigoid, anaemia or jaundice. Examination of the hands may also reveal relevant information (Table 1.6). Dentists should be able to examine cranial nerve function, but more extensive medical examination by dentists is usually done in hospital.

Table 1.6	Useful diagnostic information from examination of the hands
Site	**Signs**
Flexor surface of wrist	Rash (or history of rash) consisting of purplish papules suggests lichen planus, especially if itchy
Finger morphology	Clubbing may be associated with some chronic respiratory and cardiac conditions (including infective endocarditis) and sometimes remote malignancy Joint changes may suggest rheumatoid arthritis (joint swelling, ulnar drift) or osteoarthritis (Heberden's nodes)
Abnormal nails	Koilonychia suggests long-standing anaemia. Hypoplastic nails may be associated with several inherited epithelial disorders of oral significance including ectodermal dysplasia and dyskeratosis congenita (see also Ch. 15)
Skin of fingers	May be thin, shiny and white in Raynaud's phenomenon (periodic ischaemia resulting from exposure to cold – often associated with autoimmune conditions particularly systemic sclerosis (Fig. 1.3) or Sjögren's syndrome) Note any tobacco staining. Is the degree commensurate with the patient's reported tobacco use?
Palmar-plantar keratosis	Associated with several syndromes including Papillon–Lefèvre syndrome (including juvenile periodontitis)

Fig. 1.3 Hands with taut shiny pale skin on the tapering fingers, a result of Raynaud's phenomenon, in this case in systemic sclerosis.

Fig. 1.2 Section showing the nodular surface, small tonsillar crypts and lymphoid follicles in a foliate papilla.

MAKING A CLINICAL DIFFERENTIAL DIAGNOSIS AND INVESTIGATION PLAN

The diagnosis and appropriate treatment may be obvious from the history and examination. More frequently, there are various possible diagnoses and a clinical differential diagnosis and plan of investigation should be worked out. Possible diagnoses should be recorded in order of probability, based on their prevalence and likelihood of causing the symptoms and signs. Even if only one diagnosis seems appropriate, it is worthwhile noting the next most likely possibility and any other causes which can be excluded. This ensures that all appropriate investigations are remembered and reduces the possibility of the patient having to return for further investigations. Drawing up such a written differential diagnosis helps even experienced clinicians to organise their thoughts. The list also forms the basis on which special investigations are selected. Precise diagnosis may depend on histological findings, so that a preliminary generic diagnosis, such as 'benign neoplasm' or 'odontogenic tumour', often has to be made.

SPECIAL INVESTIGATIONS

Innumerable types of investigation are possible and it may be difficult to refrain from asking for every conceivable investigation in the anxiety not to miss something unsuspected and to avoid medicolegal complications. Though it may be tempting to explore every possibility, however remote, this approach may prove counterproductive in that it can produce a plethora of reports that confuse rather than inform. Laboratory staff soon also become aware of, and may become less helpful to, those who overburden them.

Special investigations should only be requested to answer specific questions about a possible diagnosis, not as a routine. Some investigations have a high specificity and sensitivity for particular diseases, but few investigations provide a specific diagnosis. A few diseases, such as mumps, may be diagnosed on the basis of a single test, but others, such as Sjögren's syndrome, may require many tests. Therefore, the usefulness ('predictive value') of each investigation must be borne in mind when interpreting the results.

Any test will occasionally produce an erroneous result. Sometimes this is the result of inappropriate samples or delay in specimen transport. However, for many blood tests, a result may be flagged as 'out of normal range' because the value is in the highest or lowest 5% of the population. This is not necessarily an abnormal result. Unexpected or inexplicable test results are often best repeated before accepting the result, provided the test is easily performed.

Imaging

The most informative imaging techniques in the head and neck are radiography and computerised tomography (CT), magnetic resonance imaging (MRI) and ultrasound. Their advantages and disadvantages are shown in Table 1.7.

Table 1.7	Imaging techniques for lesions of the head and neck	
Technique	**Advantages**	**Limitations**
Conventional radiography	Widely available and inexpensive Simple, many common lesions may be identified with a high degree of accuracy Panoramic radiographs can show unsuspected lesions	Small X-ray dose unavoidable Difficult to interpret in some areas of the jaws because of the complex anatomy Little information about soft tissue lesions
Computerised tomography (CT)	Good definition of soft tissue structures in any plane Useful for areas of complex anatomy such as maxilla or base of skull Definition further improved by use of contrast media	Expensive Available only in hospitals Frightening for patients. Scanner tunnel can provoke claustrophobia Shadows of dental restorations can obscure part of the image Larger X-ray dose than plain radiographs
Cone beam CT	Low cost high resolution CT ideal for the head and neck	As CT but lower dose and higher resolution Likely to become the routine radiological investigation for head and neck diagnosis
Radiography or CT with contrast medium	Valuable for outlining extent of duct systems, hollow structures such as cysts or blood vessels (angiography) etc.	Requires more expertise than plain radiography
Magnetic resonance imaging (MRI)	Produces clear tomograms in any plane without superimposition Particularly good for soft tissue lesions. Better than CT No X-ray dose Clear definition of bones and teeth	Expensive and limited availability Frighteningly noisy. May be refused by claustrophobic patient as for CT Slow. Sometimes up to two hours Possible risk to the fetus (unconfirmed)
Ultrasound	No X-ray dose Shows soft tissue masses and cysts well Useful for salivary gland cysts, Sjögren's syndrome and stones, and for thyroid and neck lesions May be combined with Doppler flow analysis to measure blood flow through a lesion	Requires expertise in interpretation Overlying bone obscures soft tissue lesions
Scintigraphy	Uses a radioactive isotope to visualise particular types of cells With technetium 99^m provides an assessment of function in each salivary gland Can be used if sialography not possible Other isotopes are used for detection of bone metastases	Equipment not always available Small radiation dose but isotope rapidly cleared
Positron emission tomography (PET scanning)	Short-life radioactive isotope used to identify biochemical activity, usually glycolysis, to identify putative tumour size, location or metastasis Good for identifying unsuspected metastases Helps identify neoplasms when post-surgical artefact or inflammation obscure CT or MRI Also available as a combined PET-CT scan	Expensive and not widely available Intake of radioactive substance

Plain radiography is widely available, but the value of additional techniques should be understood (Box 1.6). Even simple manoeuvres, such as introducing a gutta percha point or probe into a sinus to trace its origins, may provide critical information. It is also advisable to request a formal radiologist's report on radiographic films, whenever the radiographic features appear unusual or beyond the experience of the clinician.

> **Box 1.6   Requirements for useful oral radiographic information**
>
> - Always take bitewings when dental pain is suspected. Small carious lesions may be missed in periapical films and poorly localised pain may originate in the opposing arch
> - When imaging bony swellings always take two views at right angles
> - Panoramic tomograms cannot provide high definition of bony lesions. Only a cross-section of the lesion is in the focal trough and if the bone is greatly expanded only a small portion will be in focus. For more information, oblique lateral views of the mandible or oblique occlusal films should be taken
> - Radiography of soft tissues is occasionally useful, for instance to detect a foreign body or calcification in lymph nodes

Histopathology

Value and limitations

Removal of a biopsy specimen for histopathological examination is the mainstay of diagnosis for diseases of the mucosa, soft tissues and bone. In the few conditions in which a biopsy is not helpful, it may still be valuable to exclude other possible causes (Box 1.7).

> **Box 1.7   Possible reasons for failures in histological diagnosis**
>
> - Specimen poorly fixed or damaged during removal (Figs 1.4 and 1.5)
> - Specimen unrepresentative of the lesion or too small
> - Plane of histological section does not include critical features
> - The disease does not have diagnostic histological features, e.g. aphthous ulcers
> - The histological features have several possible causes, e.g. granulomas (Chs 28 and 29)
> - The histological features are difficult to interpret, e.g. malignant tumours may be so poorly differentiated that their type cannot be determined
> - Inflammation may mask the correct diagnosis

As with all other investigations, biopsy must address a specific question. For instance, recurrent aphthae lack specific microscopic features and biopsy is rarely justified. Conversely, a major aphtha may mimic a carcinoma that only microscopy will exclude.

Biopsy

Biopsy is the removal and examination of a part or the whole of a lesion. There are several types of biopsy technique (Box 1.8).

Fig. 1.4   An artefactual polyp produced by grasping normal mucosa with forceps to steady it during biopsy.

Fig. 1.5   Stringy artefact. This appearance is due to breakage of cells and their nuclei when the specimen is stretched or crushed. It is particularly common in lymphoma and some types of carcinoma.

> **Box 1.8   Types of biopsy**
>
> - Surgical biopsy (incisional or excisional)
>   Fixed specimen for paraffin blocks
>   Frozen sections
> - Fine needle aspiration biopsy
> - Thick needle/core biopsy

The most important technique is surgical biopsy. The only important contraindication is incisional biopsy of parotid gland tumours. The most common type (pleomorphic adenoma) has an unusual tendency to seed its cells and recur in the incision wound. Such tumours should therefore be examined microscopically only after excision with a margin of surrounding normal tissue.

Surgical biopsy

Incisional biopsy (removal of part of a lesion) is used to determine the diagnosis before treatment. Excisional biopsy (removal of the whole lesion such as a mucocele) is used to confirm a clinical diagnosis. It is a simple procedure, but certain precautions must be observed (Box 1.9).

Box 1.9   Essential biopsy principles

- Choose most suspicious area, e.g. red area when premalignancy is suspected
- Avoid sloughs or necrotic areas
- Give regional or local anaesthetic – not into the lesion
- Include normal tissue margin
- Specimen should preferably be at least 1 × 0.6 cm and 2 mm deep for mucosal disease, larger for large lesions
- Specimen edges should be vertical, not bevelled
- Pass a suture through the specimen to control it and prevent it being swallowed or aspirated by the suction
- For large lesions, several areas may need to be sampled
- Include every fragment for histological examination
- Never open, incise or divide the specimen, always send it intact
- Suture and control any postoperative bleeding
- Label specimen bottle with patient's name and clinical details
- Warn patient of possible soreness afterwards. Give an analgesic
- Check the findings are consistent with the clinical diagnosis and investigations
- Discuss with pathologist or repeat biopsy if diagnosis is unclear or not understood

---

Occasionally, general anaesthesia is required for children or problem patients. For those that gag, a short-acting benzodiazepine is usually effective. The request form should contain all the clinical information used to reach the clinical diagnosis. The purpose is to ensure an accurate diagnosis – not (as some clinicians seem to think) to see if the pathologist can guess it without the relevant information. If appropriate, give the vitality of teeth associated with the lesion.

Frozen sections (Box 1.10)

Frozen section technique allows a stained slide to be examined within 10 minutes of taking the specimen. The tissue is sent fresh to the laboratory to be quickly frozen, preferably to

---

Box 1.10   Advantages and limitations of frozen sections

- Can establish, at operation, whether or not a tumour is malignant and whether excision needs to be extended
- Can confirm, at operation, that excision margins are free of tumour
- Appearances differ from those in fixed material
- Freezing artefacts due to poor technique can distort the cellular picture
- Definitive diagnosis sometimes impossible

---

about −70°C by, for example, immersion in liquid nitrogen or dry ice. A section is then cut on a refrigerated microtome and stained. The theatre suite often includes equipment for frozen sections to speed the process even further.

Frozen sections can only be justified if the rapidity of the result will make an immediate difference to the operation in progress because the technique is less accurate than routine histopathology. This low risk of misdiagnosis means that frozen section is used more frequently to assess whether excision margins are free of malignancy than to make a primary diagnosis. If a rapid diagnosis is required in other circumstances, techniques such as fine needle aspiration biopsy or a routine specimen with special laboratory processing may be used.

Fine needle aspiration (FNA) biopsy (Box 1.11)

Even if not completely conclusive, the information from fine needle aspiration (FNA) is often sufficient to distinguish benign from malignant neoplasms, to initiate treatment, or to indicate a need for further investigations.

Box 1.11   Principles and uses of fine needle aspiration biopsy

- A 21 gauge needle is inserted into the lesion and cells aspirated and smeared on a slide
- Rapid and usually effective aid to diagnosis of swellings in lymph nodes and parotid tumours especially
- Cells can be fixed, stained and examined within minutes
- Valuable when surgical biopsy could spread tumour cells (e.g. pleomorphic adenomas)
- For deep lesions ultrasound or radiological guidance may be used to ensure that the needle enters the lesion
- No significant complications
- Small size of the needle avoids damage to vital structures in the head and neck
- Cells may be pelleted and processed for sections to allow immunocytochemistry and other specialised stains
- Some sample may be sent for microbiological culture
- Disadvantages
  Experience required for interpretation
  Small specimen may be unrepresentative
  Definitive diagnosis not always possible (though a differential diagnosis may be very helpful)

Needle/core biopsy (Box 1.12)

Box 1.12   Advantages and limitations of needle/core biopsy

- Needle up to 2 mm diameter used to remove a core of tissue
- Specimen processed as for a surgical biopsy
- Larger sample than FNA, preserves tissue architecture in the specimen
- Definitive diagnosis more likely than with FNA
- Risk of seeding some types of neoplasms into the tissues
- Risk of damaging adjacent anatomical structures
- Useful for inaccessible tumours, e.g. in the pharynx
- Less used in the head and neck now that FNA is more widely available, but may be used if FNA fails

---

Exfoliative cytology

Exfoliative cytology is examination of cells scraped from the surface of a lesion or occasionally of material from aspirates of a cyst (Box 1.13).

> **Box 1.13 Uses and limitations of exfoliative cytology**
>
> - Quick, easy
> - Local anaesthetic not required
> - Special techniques, such as immunostaining, can be applied
> - Most useful for detecting virally-damaged cells, acantholytic cells of pemphigus or candidal hyphae
> - Unreliable for diagnosing cancer. Frequent false-positive or false-negative results

Biopsy is always more reliable and can be so readily carried out in the mouth that it is mandatory when cancer or premalignancy is suspected. Exfoliative cytology samples only surface cells and provides no information on deeper layers. To improve its value, exfoliative cytology has been supplemented by DNA cytometry and has been claimed to achieve a sensitivity of 100% for oral cancer. However, simple exfoliative cytology has largely been replaced by brush biopsy.

Brush biopsy

This technique uses a round stiff-bristle brush to collect cells from the surface and subsurface layers of a lesion by vigorous abrasion and is discussed more fully in Chapter 17.

Laboratory procedures

Although a clinician does not need to understand the details of laboratory procedures, it is necessary to understand the principles to enable the optimal results to be obtained.

Fixation

In the absence of proper fixative, it is better to delay the biopsy and obtain the correct solution. Specimens placed in alcohols, saline or other materials commonly available in dental surgeries are frequently useless for diagnosis (Box 1.14).

> **Box 1.14 Essential points about specimen fixation**
>
> - Fixation is necessary to prevent autolysis and destruction of microscopic features of the specimen
> - The usual, routine fixative is 10% formal saline (formaldehyde solution in normal saline or a neutral pH buffer)
> - Fixation must be complete before the specimen can be processed
> - Fixative must diffuse into the specimen – a slow process
> - Small surgical specimens fix overnight, but large specimens take 24 hours or longer

- The centre of large specimens can autolyse before fixative diffuses in. The pathologist can incise them to allow fixative to penetrate after the surface is fixed, but this should not be performed on the fresh specimen by the clinician
- Chemical reaction with the tissue causes the fixative to become weaker as fixation proceeds. Therefore specimens should generally be put in at least ten times their own volume of fixative
- Never fix specimens for microbiological culture or immunofluorescence; take these fresh to the laboratory immediately on removal

Special types of fixative are required for electron microscopy and for urgent specimens. Whenever microbiological culture is required, the specimen should be sent fresh to the laboratory or a separate specimen taken because fixation will kill any microorganisms.

Tissue processing

The fixed tissue is dehydrated by immersion in a series of solvents and impregnated with paraffin wax. The wax block is mounted on a microtome and sections, usually 4 µm thick, are cut and mounted on glass microscope slides for staining. It takes 24–48 hours to fix, process, section and stain a specimen before the pathologist can report on it.

Some common stains used for microscopy

The combination of haematoxylin and eosin (H&E) is the most common routine histological stain. Haematoxylin is a blue-black basic dye; eosin is a red acid dye. Their typical staining patterns are shown in Table 1.8.

Periodic acid–Schiff (PAS) stain is probably the second most frequently used stain. It stains sugar residues in carbohydrates and glycosaminoglycans pink. This is useful to identify salivary and other mucins, glycogen and candidal hyphae in sections. Alcian Blue is a turquoise stain for proteoglycans with negatively charged sugars, such as the sialic acid containing salivary mucins. Salivary mucins therefore stain with both PAS

Table 1.8 Examples of haematoxylin and eosin staining of various tissues

Eosin (acidic, red)	Haematoxylin (basic, blue)
Cytoplasm of most cells*	Nuclei (DNA and RNA)
Keratin	Mucopolysaccharide-rich ground
Muscle cytoplasm	substance
Bone (decalcified only)	Reversal lines in decalcified bone
Collagen	

*The cytoplasm of some cells (such as oncocytes in some salivary gland tumours) is intensely eosinophilic. In others such as plasma cells it is basophilic or intermediate (amphophilic).

and Alcian Blue, whereas ground substance in myxoid connective tissue stains only with Alcian Blue.

Silver staining is also useful for identifying fungi in sections, but Gram-staining is quicker and more useful for smears. Silver stains also stain reticulin fibres black.

Decalcified and ground (undecalcified) sections

Specimens containing bone and teeth need to be softened by decalcifying in acid to enable a thin section to be cut. This delays the diagnosis by days or weeks according to the size of the specimen.

Decalcification must be avoided if examination of dental enamel is required, for instance to aid diagnosis of amelogenesis imperfecta, because the heavily mineralised enamel is almost completely dissolved. In such cases, a ground section is prepared by sawing and grinding using special saws and abrasives.

Immunofluorescent and immunohistochemical staining

Immunostaining methods make use of the highly specific binding between antibodies and antigens to stain specific molecules within the tissues. Fresh (unfixed) tissue is sometimes required.

Immunostaining has revolutionised histological diagnosis and has made some more complex techniques, such as electron microscopy, almost redundant. It is time-consuming and must be meticulously carried out with adequate controls to avoid both false-positive and false-negative results. In larger laboratories, immunostaining is automated.

The main circumstances where diagnosis depends on immunostaining are shown in Table 1.9.

Antibodies, often monoclonal, that recognise specific antigens of interest can be purchased. They bind extremely specifically to the target molecule and the combination is labelled, either by being coupled to fluorescein or an enzyme such as peroxidase. The antibody is incubated on the section where it binds specifically to the target molecule. Surplus reagent is washed off and any binding (a positive reaction) is visible by its fluorescence in an ultraviolet light microscope or by reacting the enzyme with synthetic substrate to produce a coloured product (Figs 1.6–1.8).

Molecular biological tests

Molecular biological diagnostic tests have revolutionised diagnosis, particularly in screening for and identification of genetic abnormalities and rapid identification of bacteria and viruses. Some malignant neoplasms have characteristic genetic abnormalities, mostly chromosomal translocations, which can be detected by cytogenetics, polymerase chain reaction (PCR) or fluorescent in situ hybridisation. Molecular techniques are also the method of choice for the diagnosis of some lymphomas which cannot be accurately categorised by routine histological methods.

Identification of many bacteria and viruses is now often undertaken using PCR. In this test, the clinical sample is

Table 1.9 Important uses of immunostaining techniques

Disease	Molecule detected	Significance
Pemphigus	Autoantibody binds to epithelial 'cement substance' (desmoglein 3)	Indicates pemphigus
Pemphigoid	Autoantibody and/or complement C3 binds to basement membrane	Indicates pemphigoid
Myeloma or B-cell lymphoma	Monoclonal production of kappa or lambda light chains of immunoglobulin	Monoclonal production (production of only one isotype of light chain) indicates a neoplastic process. Production of both types indicates a polyclonal infiltrate that is inflammatory in nature
Lymphomas	Cell surface markers specific for different types of T and B cells	Indicate whether a lymphoma is of B- or T-cell origin
Undifferentiated tumours	Intermediate filaments (components of the cytoskeleton)	Presence of keratins indicates an epithelial neoplasm, vimentin a mesenchymal neoplasm and desmin or myogenin a muscle neoplasm

NB Positive reactions, in themselves, are not necessarily diagnostic of disease and must be interpreted in the light of other histological and clinical findings.

solubilised and the nucleic acids hybridised with complementary probes which are specific for known pathogens. If the pathogen is present in the sample, PCR will copy the nucleic acid repeatedly until enough is synthesised to be seen in an electrophoresis gel (Fig. 1.9). If no pathogen is present no nucleic acid is synthesised. Identification of mycobacteria is a good example of the value of this type of test. Previously, identification of mycobacterial infection required approximately 6 weeks to culture the sample. PCR can be performed in 48 hours, is more sensitive and differentiates different types of mycobacteria with a high degree of precision. This test is therefore ideal for investigation of enlarged lymph nodes in the neck. A more recent application of PCR to detect micrometastases of tumours is potentially also of enormous value.

Such methods have yet to become widespread in dentistry, though they are available in most large hospitals. However, when confronted with a difficult diagnosis, it is sensible to discuss the case with the pathologist or microbiologist before biopsy, to ensure that appropriate samples are available for these specialised tests.

Fig. 1.6 **Method and application of direct immunofluorescence.** (A) Example: diagnosis of pemphigus and pemphigoid. Aim: to detect the site of the IgG autoantibody already bound to the tissues in a biopsy. Green fluorescence indicates site of antibody binding, red fluorescence is a stain for cell nuclei to make the tissue structure more easily interpreted. (B) In pemphigus, green fluorescence reveals IgG autoantibody bound around the surface of the prickle cells in the epithelium (see Fig. 13.24). (C) In pemphigoid, green fluorescence reveals IgG autoantibody bound along the basement membrane (see Fig. 13.29). Images courtesy Dr Balbir Bhogal.

Haematology, clinical chemistry and serology

Blood investigations are clearly essential for the diagnosis of diseases such as leukaemias, myelomas or leukopenias which have oral manifestations, or for defects of haemostasis which can greatly affect management. Blood investigations are also helpful in the diagnosis of other conditions such as some infections, and sore tongues or recurrent aphthae which are sometimes associated with anaemia.

There are many different types of haematological examinations but, despite the frequent use of the term 'routine blood test', no test should ever be requested as a routine, only to answer a specific question (Table 1.10). The request form should always be completed with sufficient clinical detail to

allow the haematologist or clinical chemist to check that the appropriate tests have been ordered and to allow the interpretation of the results. It is important to include details of any drug treatment on blood test request forms. Always put the blood into the appropriate tube because some anticoagulants are incompatible with certain tests. A haematologist will not be impressed with a request for assessment of clotting function on a specimen of coagulated blood.

Microbiology

Despite the fact that the most common oral diseases are infective, microbiology is surprisingly rarely of practical diagnostic

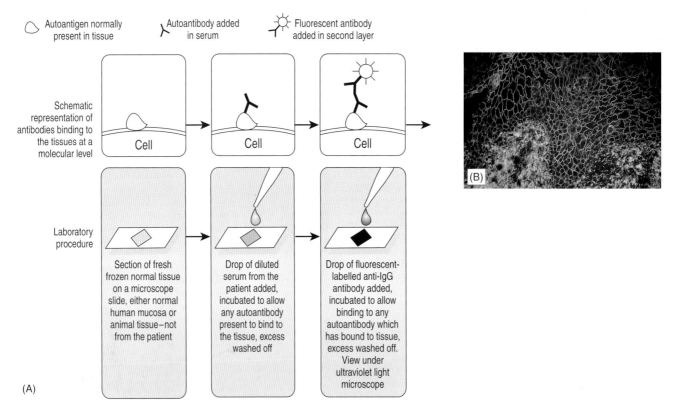

Fig. 1.7 **Method and application of indirect immunofluorescence.** (A) Example: control of treatment for pemphigus. Aim: to detect circulating autoantibody in the serum of patients with pemphigus. (B) If present, serum autoantibody binds around the surface of the prickle cells in the epithelium and is revealed by the binding to it of the green fluorescent antibody. In this example the nuclei are not counterstained red.

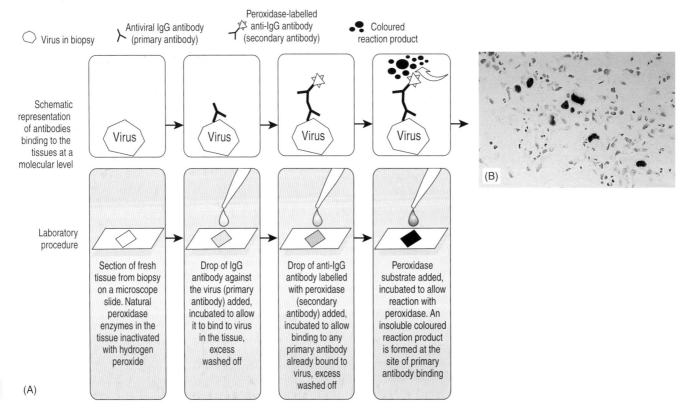

Fig. 1.8 **Method and application of immunocytochemistry.** (A) Example: diagnosis of viral infection. Aim: to detect viral antigens in infected cells. (B) In this example, brown reaction product identifies cells infected with cytomegalovirus

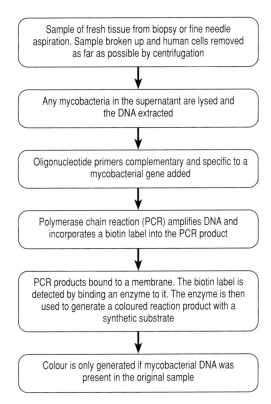

Sample of fresh tissue from biopsy or fine needle aspiration. Sample broken up and human cells removed as far as possible by centrifugation

↓

Any mycobacteria in the supernatant are lysed and the DNA extracted

↓

Oligonucleotide primers complementary and specific to a mycobacterial gene added

↓

Polymerase chain reaction (PCR) amplifies DNA and incorporates a biotin label into the PCR product

↓

PCR products bound to a membrane. The biotin label is detected by binding an enzyme to it. The enzyme is then used to generate a coloured reaction product with a synthetic substrate

↓

Colour is only generated if mycobacterial DNA was present in the original sample

Fig. 1.9 Example application for the technique of polymerase chain reaction for identification of mycobacterial infection.

value in dentistry (Table 1.11). Direct Gram-stained smears will quickly confirm the diagnosis of thrush or acute ulcerative gingivitis, and H&E-stained smears can show the distorted, virally infected epithelial cells in herpetic infections more easily than microbiological tests for the organisms themselves.

A key microbiological investigation is culture and sensitivity of pus organisms. Whenever pus is obtained from a soft tissue or bone infection it should be sent for culture and determination of antibiotic sensitivity of the causative microbes. Those of osteomyelitis, cellulitis, acute parotitis, systemic mycoses

Table 1.11 Microbiological tests useful in oral diagnosis

Test	Main uses
Culture and antibiotic sensitivity	Detect unusual pathogens, e.g. actinomycosis in soft tissue infection Antibiotic sensitivity for all infections, particularly osteomyelitis and acute facial soft tissue infection
Smear for candida	Candidosis
Viral culture or antigen screen	Viral culture identifies many viruses but requires considerable time Screening for viral antigen is faster but of more limited diagnostic value

Table 1.10 Types of blood test useful in oral diagnosis (see also Appendix 1.1)

Test	Main uses
'Full blood picture' usually includes erythrocyte number, size and haemoglobin indices and differential white cell count	Anaemia and the effects of sideropaenia and vitamin B_{12} deficiency associated with several common oral disorders. Leukaemias
Blood film	Leukaemias, infectious mononucleosis, anaemias
Erythrocyte sedimentation rate	Raised in systemic inflammatory and autoimmune disorders. Particularly important in giant cell arteritis and Wegener's granulomatosis
Serum iron and total iron binding capacity	Iron deficiency associated with several common oral disorders
Serum ferritin	A more sensitive indicator of body stores of iron than serum iron and total iron binding capacity but not available in all laboratories
Red cell folate level	Folic acid deficiency is sometimes associated with recurrent aphthous ulceration and recurrent candidosis
Vitamin B_{12} level	Vitamin B_{12} deficiency is sometimes associated with recurrent aphthous ulceration and recurrent candidosis
Autoantibodies (e.g. rheumatoid factor, antinuclear factor, DNA binding antibodies, SS-A, SS-B)	Raised in autoimmune diseases. Specific autoantibody levels suggest certain diseases
Viral antibody titres (e.g. Herpes simplex, Varicella zoster, mumps virus)	A rising titre of specific antibody indicates active infection by the virus
Paul–Bunnell or monospot test	Infectious mononucleosis
Syphilis serology	Syphilis
Complement component levels	Occasionally useful in diagnosis of SLE or familial angio-oedema.
Serum angiotensin converting enzyme	Sarcoidosis
Serum calcium, phosphate and parathormone levels	Paget's disease and hyperparathyroidism
HIV test	HIV infection (testing only possible under particular circumstances)
Skeletal serum alkaline phosphatase	Raised in conditions with increased bone turnover, e.g. Paget's disease and hyperparathyroidism Lowered in hypophoshatasia

(frequently mistaken for tumours), or other severe infections need to be identified if appropriate antimicrobial treatment is to be given. However, such treatment has usually to be started empirically without this information, but the sensitivity test may dictate a change.

Viral identification is rarely required for oral diseases as many oral viral infections are clinically typical and indicate the causative virus. A smear alone may show the nuclear changes of herpetic infection in epithelial cells from the margins of mucosal ulcers. A more sensitive and almost as rapid result may be obtained by sending a swab for virus detection using ELISA (enzyme-linked immunosorbent assay) or electron microscopy.

Box 1.15 Practical points

- Always take a sample of pus for culture and antibiotic sensitivity from bone and soft tissue infections *before* giving an antibiotic
- Always take the temperature of any patient with a swollen face, enlarged lymph nodes, malaise or other symptom or sign which might indicate infection
- Good clinical record keeping is essential for good patient management as well as for medicolegal reasons

---

Other clinical tests

Urine tests are valuable for the diagnosis of diabetes (suggested by repeated candidal or periodontal infection), kidney damage which can have resulted from autoimmune disorders such as Wegener's granulomatosis (Ch. 28) and for the detection of Bence-Jones protein in myeloma.

Taking the patient's temperature is an easily forgotten investigation. The temperature should be noted whenever bone or soft tissue infections are suspected. It helps distinguish facial inflammatory oedema from cellulitis and indicates systemic effects of infections and the need for more aggressive therapy.

Interpreting special investigations and making a diagnosis and treatment plan

Check that the results of each investigation are compatible with the preliminary diagnosis and do not indicate any need to avoid a particular treatment.

If a result appears at odds with other information, take into account the normal variation, perhaps with age or diurnal variation, and consider the possibility of false-positive and false-negative results. A common cause of unusual blood test results is a delay in taking blood samples to the laboratory.

Further advice and specialised tests may be appropriate. General medicine, ear, nose and throat surgery, neurology,

cardiology and psychiatry are among the specialties to whom dental patients may be referred. In referrals, it is important to state whether the dentist is requesting the medical specialist to exclude a condition and refer the patient back, or to take over investigation. If the latter, it is essential that dental causes have been completely eliminated as the cause of the problem.

Finally, ensure that the patient's notes include a complete record of the consultation and investigation results. This must be correctly dated, legible, limited to relevant facts and include a clear complaint history, list of clinical findings, test results and plan of treatment organised in a suitable form for quick reappraisal. It must be signed by the clinician and, in addition, the name should be printed below if the signature is anything less than perfectly legible. It should be possible for another person to continue to investigate or treat the patient without difficulty on the basis of the clinical record.

Photography or computerised video imaging is a very valuable adjunct to the clinical record. Pictures are especially useful in monitoring lesions which may vary in the course of a long follow-up, for instance white patches. It is useful to include teeth or a scale in the frame to allow accurate assessment of small changes in size. Photographs may also be helpful in explaining to patients about their condition and to show the effects of treatment, but consent for the intended uses of the photographs must be obtained first.

SUGGESTED FURTHER READING

Arends MJ, Bird CC 1992 Recombinant DNA technology and its diagnostic applications. Histopathology 21:303–313

Ghossein RA, Rosai J 1996 Polymerase chain reaction in the detection of micrometastases and circulating tumor cells. Cancer 78:10–16

Heatley MK 1996 Cytokeratins and cytokeratin staining in diagnostic histopathology. Histopathology 28:479–483

Kabala J, Goddard P, Cook P 1992 Magnetic resonance imaging of extracranial head and neck tumours. Br J Radiol 65:375–383

Komoroski RA, Pappas A, Hough A 1992 Nuclear magnetic resonance imaging in pathology. I. Principles and general aspects. Hum Pathol 22:1077–1084

Layton S, Korsen J 1994 Informed consent in oral and maxillofacial surgery: a study of the value of written warnings. Br J Oral Maxillofac Surg 32:34–36

Leong AS-Y, Leong TY-M 2006 Newer developments in immunohistology. J Clin Pathol 59:1117–1126.

Minden NJ, Fast TB 1994 Evaluation of health history forms used in U.S. dental schools. Oral Surg Oral Med Oral Pathol 77:105–109

Nathan AW, Havard CWH 1979 The face in diagnosis. Br J Hosp Med 21:104–111

O'Connor N 1995 Laboratory diagnosis in haematology. Medicine UK 23:489–494

Stanley MW 1995 False-positive diagnoses in exfoliative cytology (editorial). Am J Clin Pathol 104:117–119

Thibodeau EA, Rossomondo KJ 1992 Survey of the medical history questionnaire. Oral Surg Oral Med Oral Pathol 74:400–403

Whaites E 2006 Essentials of dental radiography and radiology, 4th edn. Churchill Livingstone, Edinburgh

**APPENDIX
1.1**

Normal haematological values

Red cells	
Haemoglobin	Males 13–17 g/dl. Females 11.5–16 g/dl (adults)
Haematocrit (packed cell volume – PCV)	Males 40–50%. Females 36–47%
Mean corpuscular volume (MCV)	78–98 fl
Mean corpuscular haemoglobin concentration (MCHC)	30–35 g/dl
Red cell count	Males 4–6 $\times$ 10^{12}/l. Females 4–5 $\times$ 10^{12}/l
Eythrocyte sedimentation rate (ESR)	0–15 mm/h
White cells	
Total count	4–10 $\times$ 10^9/l
Neutrophils	2–7.5 $\times$ 10^9/l
Lymphocytes	1–3 $\times$ 10^9/l
Monocytes	0.15–0.8 $\times$ 10^9/l
Eosinophils	0.05–0.4 $\times$ 10^9/l
Platelets	150–400 $\times$ 10^9/l

Note. These reference ranges are calculated assuming a normal distribution of results and excluding the upper and lower 2.5% of the range as abnormal. Therefore, approximately 5% of normal persons have values outside the figures quoted above. These are average values and may vary slightly between laboratories and you should always check normal values with the testing laboratory.

HARD TISSUE PATHOLOGY

Disorders of development of the teeth and related tissues

Development of an ideal dentition depends on many factors (Box 2.1).

Significant structural defects of teeth are uncommon, but disorders of occlusion due to irregularities of the teeth in the arch or abnormal relationship of the arches to each other are so common that their treatment has become a specialty in its own right. The main groups of disorders affecting development of the dentition are summarised in Box 2.2 and Summary chart 2.1 and Summary chart 2.2.

ABNORMALITIES IN THE NUMBER OF TEETH

Isolated hypodontia or anodontia

Failure of development of one or two teeth is relatively common and often hereditary. The teeth most frequently missing are third molars, second premolars or maxillary second incisors (Fig. 2.1). Absence of third molars can be a disadvantage if first or second molars, or both, have been lost. The absence of lower premolars worsens malocclusion if there is already

Fig. 2.1 Congenital absence of lateral incisors with spacing of the anterior teeth.

disparity between an underdeveloped mandible and a normal upper arch. Otherwise, absence of these teeth may have little or no noticeable effect.

Absence of lateral incisors can sometimes be conspicuous because the large, pointed canines erupt in the front of the mouth beside the central incisors. It is usually impossible to prevent the canine from erupting into this empty space, even if the patient is seen early. It is also very difficult to make room between the centrals and canines by orthodontic means to replace the laterals. An attempt has often therefore to be made to disguise the shape of the canines.

Total failure of development of a complete dentition (anodontia) is exceedingly rare. If the permanent dentition fails to form, the deciduous dentition is retained for many years but, when these deciduous teeth become excessively worn or too much damaged by caries, then they must be replaced by dentures or implants.

Hypodontia or anodontia with systemic defects

Anhidrotic (hereditary) ectodermal dysplasia

The main features are summarised in Box 2.3. In severe cases no teeth form. More often, most of the deciduous teeth form, but there are few or no permanent teeth. The teeth are usually peg-shaped or conical (Fig. 2.2).

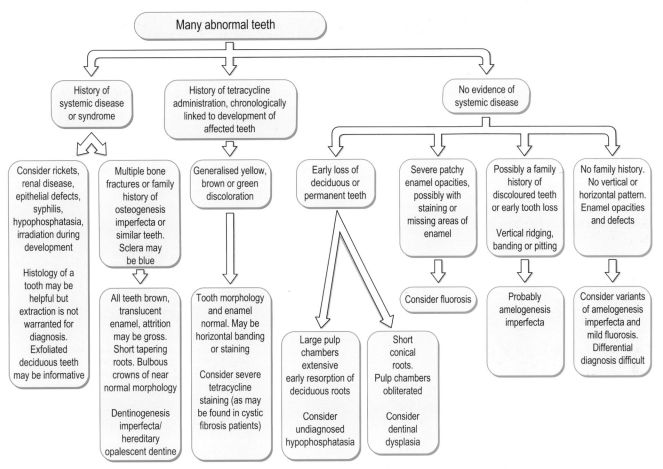

Summary chart 2.1 Differential diagnosis of developmental defects of the teeth.

Box 2.3   Anhidrotic ectodermal dyplasia: major features

- Usually a sex-linked recessive trait
- Hypodontia
- Hypotrichosis (scanty hair)
- Anhidrosis (inability to sweat)

When there is anodontia, the alveolar process, without teeth to support, fails to develop and has too little bone to support implants. The profile then resembles that of an elderly person because of the gross loss of vertical dimension. The hair is fine and sparse (Fig. 2.3), particularly in the tonsural region. The skin is smooth, shiny and dry due to absence of sweat glands. Heat is therefore poorly tolerated. The finger nails are usually also defective. All that can be done to improve the patient's appearance and mastication is to fit dentures, which are usually well tolerated by children.

Other conditions associated with hypodontia

There are many rare syndromes where hypodontia is a feature, but the only common one is Down's syndrome (Ch. 33). One or more third molars are absent in over 90% of these patients, while absence of individual teeth scattered about the arch is

Fig. 2.2 Anhidrotic ectodermal dysplasia showing conical teeth, giving an undesirable, Dracula-like appearance.

also common. Anodontia is rare. Palatal clefts may be associated, though this is also rare.

Additional teeth: hyperdontia

Additional teeth are relatively common. They are usually of simple conical shape (supernumerary teeth) but, less frequently, resemble teeth of the normal series (supplemental

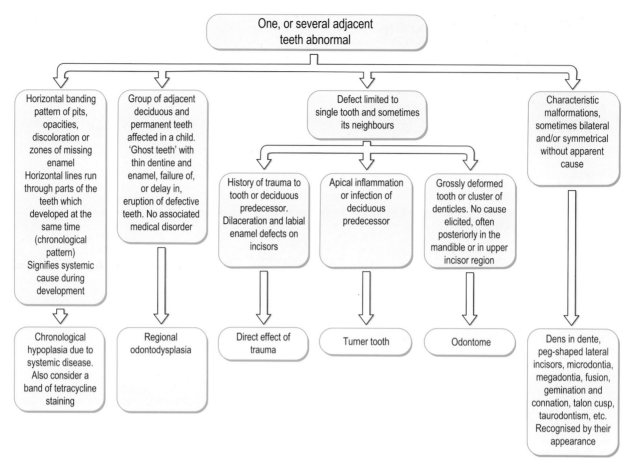

Summary chart 2.2 Differential diagnosis of developmental and acquired abnormalities of one or a group of teeth.

Fig. 2.3 Another case showing typical fine and scanty hair and loss of support for the facial soft tissues.

teeth). These are the results of excessive but organised growth of the dental lamina of unknown cause.

Supernumerary teeth → Summary p. 157. Conical or more seriously malformed additional teeth most frequently form in the incisor or molar region (Fig. 2.4) and very occasionally, in the midline (mesiodens, Fig. 2.5).

Supplemental teeth. Occasionally an additional maxillary incisor, premolar or, rarely, a fourth molar develops (also seen in Fig. 2.5).

Effects and treatment

Additional teeth usually erupt in abnormal positions, labial or buccal to the arch, creating stagnation areas and greater susceptibility to caries, gingivitis and periodontitis. Alternatively, a supernumerary tooth may prevent a normal tooth from erupting. These additional teeth should usually be extracted.

Syndromes associated with hyperdontia

These syndromes are all rare but probably the best known is cleidocranial dysplasia (Ch. 10) where many additional teeth develop but fail to erupt.

Fig. 2.4 A paramolar, a buccally placed supernumerary molar tooth.

Fig. 2.5 Maleruption of a midline tuberculate supernumerary and two supplemental premolars.

DISORDERS OF ERUPTION

Eighteenth-century parish registers are replete with the names of infants who had died as a result of teething. Nevertheless, the idea that teething, the normal eruption of infants' teeth, can cause systemic symptoms or serious illness is of course a myth. The time of teething coincides with a period of naturally low resistance to infection and declining maternal passive immunity so that infection during the period of teething is merely coincidental. As might be expected, several studies have shown that teething does not cause systemic disorders. Nevertheless, so resistant is this traditional belief to rational explanation, that yet another study was carried out in 2000, confirming yet again that teething was harmless.

However, an ingenious neuropathologist has suggested that the minute wounds left by the shedding of deciduous teeth could provide a means of entry for the BSE ('mad cow disease')

prion to cause variant CJD. In view of an incubation period of many years, this suggestion is consistent with the onset of the disease in adolescence. However, this theory is as yet unproven.

Eruption of deciduous teeth starts at about 6 months, usually with the appearance of the lower incisors, and is complete by about 2 years. Mass failure of eruption is very rare. More often eruption of a single tooth is prevented by local obstruction. In the permanent dentition, delay in eruption of a tooth or, more frequently, too early loss of a deciduous predecessor tends to cause irregularities because movement of adjacent teeth closes the available space.

Delayed eruption associated with skeletal disorders

Metabolic diseases, particularly cretinism and rickets, are now uncommon causes of delayed eruption of teeth. Cleidocranial dysplasia, in which there are typically many additional teeth but failure of most of them to erupt, has been mentioned earlier. In severe hereditary gingival fibromatosis, eruption may apparently fail merely because the teeth are buried in the excessive fibrous gingival tissue and only their tips show in the mouth (pseudoanodontia). In cherubism (Ch. 10), several teeth may be displaced by the proliferating connective tissue masses containing giant cells and are prevented from erupting.

Local factors affecting eruption of deciduous teeth

Having no predecessors, deciduous teeth usually erupt unobstructed. Occasionally, an eruption cyst may overlie a tooth but is unlikely to block eruption.

Local factors affecting eruption of permanent teeth

A permanent tooth may be prevented from erupting or misplaced by various causes (Box 2.4).

Box 2.4   **Local causes of failure of eruption of permanent teeth**

- Loss of space, crowding
- Abnormal position of the crypt
- Supernumerary and supplemental teeth
- Displacement in a dentigerous cyst or by other lesion
- Retention of a deciduous predecessor

Treatment depends on the circumstances, but room may be made for the unerupted tooth by orthodontic means or extractions. A retained deciduous tooth should be extracted if radiographs show a normal permanent successor. If a buried tooth partially erupts and becomes infected, it may have to be removed – mandibular third molars are the main source of this complication.

Changes affecting buried teeth

Teeth may occasionally remain buried in the jaws for many years without complications. The roots of these teeth may undergo varying degrees of hypercementosis or resorption. Alternatively, the teeth may become enveloped in dentigerous cysts, as in cleidocranial dysplasia for example.

DEFECTS OF STRUCTURE: HYPOPLASIA AND HYPOCALCIFICATION

Minor structural defects of the teeth, such as pitting or discoloration or, occasionally, more serious defects, may be markers of past disease, but only rarely is the disease still active. Hypoplasia of the teeth is not an important contributory cause of dental caries; indeed, hypoplasia due to fluorosis is associated

with enhanced resistance. The main clinical requirement is usually cosmetic improvement.

Defects of deciduous teeth

Calcification of deciduous teeth begins about the fourth month of intrauterine life. Disturbances of metabolism or infections that affect the fetus at this early stage without causing abortion are rare. Defective structure of the deciduous teeth is therefore uncommon but, in a few places, such as parts of India, where the fluoride content of the water is excessively high, the deciduous teeth may be mottled.

The deciduous teeth may be discoloured by abnormal pigments circulating in the blood. Severe neonatal jaundice may cause the teeth to become yellow, or there may be bands of greenish discoloration. In congenital porphyria, a rare disorder of haemoglobin metabolism, the teeth are red or purple. Tetracycline given during dental development is the main cause of permanent discoloration.

Defects of permanent teeth

Single permanent teeth may be malformed as a result of local causes such as periapical infection of a predecessor (Turner teeth – Fig. 2.6), damage, for instance by intubation while a preterm neonate (Fig. 2.7) or multiple teeth by systemic diseases as summarised in Box 2.5.

Amelogenesis imperfecta → Summary p. 21

Amelogenesis imperfecta is a group of conditions caused by defects in the genes encoding enamel matrix proteins. Classification is complex and based on pattern of inheritance, enamel hypoplasia, hypomineralisation or hypomaturation and appearance; smooth, rough or pitted. At least 16 forms are recognised on clinical grounds but some are accounted for by differing severity and the classification is contentious.

Inheritance can be autosomal dominant, recessive or X-linked. However, the most common types have an autosomal inheritance and are thought to be caused by mutations in the AMEL X gene, which codes for ameloblastin (C4), enamelin (C4) or tuftelin (C1). In the case of the autosomal dominant type of amelogenesis imperfecta, the locus of the defective gene is on chromosome 4q21 to which enamelin maps.

The less common X-linked types are caused by a variety of defects in the amelogenin genes and, confusingly, it seems the same mutation can sometimes cause hypoplasia, hypomineralisation or hypomaturation in different patients.

Genetic factors act throughout the whole duration of amelogenesis. Characteristically therefore, all teeth are affected and defects involve the whole, or are randomly distributed in the enamel. By contrast, exogenous factors affecting enamel formation (with the important exception of fluorosis) tend to act for a relatively brief period and produce defects related to that period of enamel formation.

Hypoplastic amelogenesis imperfecta

The main defect is inadequate formation of the matrix. The enamel is randomly pitted, grooved or very thin, but hard and translucent (Fig. 2.8). The defects tend to become stained, but the teeth are not especially susceptible to caries unless the enamel is scanty and easily damaged.

The main patterns of inheritance are autosomal dominant and recessive, X-linked and (a genetic rarity) an X-linked dominant type. In the last, there is almost complete failure

Fig. 2.6 Turner tooth, a hypoplastic tooth resulting from periapical infection, usually of the deciduous predecessor.

Box 2.5	Multiple malformed permanent teeth: important causes

Genetic
- Amelogenesis imperfecta
  Hypoplastic (type 1)
  Hypomaturation (type 2)
  Hypocalcified (type 3)
- Dentinogenesis imperfecta
  Shell teeth
- Dentinal dysplasia
- Regional odontodysplasia
- Multisystem disorders with associated dental defects
- Hypophosphatasia

Infective
- Congenital syphilis

Metabolic
- Childhood infections, rickets, hypoparathyroidism

Drugs
- Tetracycline pigmentation
- Cytotoxic chemotherapy

Fluorosis

Other acquired developmental anomalies
- Fetal alcohol syndrome

of enamel formation in affected males, while in females the enamel is vertically ridged (Figs 2.9–2.11). Occasionally, cases are difficult to classify (Fig. 2.12).

Hypomaturation amelogenesis imperfecta

The enamel is normal in form on eruption but opaque, white to brownish-yellow. The teeth appear similar to mottled fluoride effects (Figs 2.13 and 2.14). However, they are soft and vulnerable to attrition, though not as severely as the hypocalcified type.

Fig. 2.7 Localised dental disturbance caused by prolonged intubation during tooth development. The upper left central incisor shows enamel pitting incisally and the upper right central incisor is deformed and has failed to erupt.

Fig. 2.8 **Amelogenesis imperfecta, hypoplastic pitted type.** Enamel between pits appears normal.

Fig. 2.9 **Close-up of X-linked dominant hypoplastic type amelogenesis imperfecta.** These teeth, from an affected female, show the typical vertical ridged pattern of normal and abnormal enamel as a result of Lyonisation.

Fig. 2.11 Amelogenesis imperfecta X-linked dominant hypoplastic type in a male showing a thin translucent layer of defective enamel on the dentine surface.

There are several variants of hypomaturation defects such as a more severe, autosomal dominant (type 4) of hypomaturation combined with hypoplasia, and milder forms limited to some surfaces.

Hypocalcified amelogenesis imperfecta

Enamel matrix is formed in normal quantity but poorly calcified. When newly erupted, the enamel is normal in thickness and form, but weak and opaque or chalky in appearance.

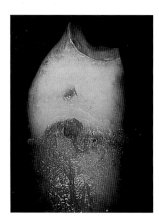

Fig. 2.10 **Amelogenesis imperfecta X-linked dominant hypoplastic form in a male.** This premolar has a cap of enamel so thin that the shape of the tooth is virtually that of the dentine core.

Fig. 2.12 Amelogenesis imperfecta, indeterminate type. Some cases, such as this, are difficult to classify but are clearly inherited, as shown by their long family history.

Fig. 2.14 Amelogenesis imperfecta, one of the several hypomaturation types. In this form there are opaque white flecks and patches affecting the occlusal half of the tooth surface.

Fig. 2.13 Amelogenesis imperfecta, hypomaturation type. Tooth morphology is normal but there are opaque white and discoloured patches.

Fig. 2.15 Amelogenesis imperfecta, hypocalcified type. The soft chalky enamel was virtually of normal thickness and form but has chipped away during mastication leaving a characteristic shoulder, seen best on the upper left central incisor.

The teeth tend to become stained and relatively rapidly worn away. The upper incisors may acquire a shouldered form due to the chipping away of the thin, soft enamel of the incisal edge (Fig. 2.15). There are dominant and recessive patterns of inheritance.

Dentinogenesis (odontogenesis) imperfecta →
Summary p. 21

This uncommon defect of collagen formation is transmitted as an autosomal dominant trait. The gene is closely related to that of osteogenesis imperfecta (Ch. 10) particularly type IV. Defects in the genes COL1A1 and COL1A2, for the procollagen alpha helix, prevent polymerisation into normal type 1 collagen.

In types III and IV osteogenesis imperfecta, dentinogenesis imperfecta is present in over 80% in the primary dentition. Tooth discoloration and attrition is less severe in the permanent teeth. Class III malocclusion is associated in over 70%. In type III disease, dental development is delayed in 20% but, in type IV disease, it is accelerated in over 20%. The dentine is soft and has an abnormally high water content.

Clinical features

The enamel appears normal but uniformly brownish or purplish and abnormally translucent (Fig. 2.16). The form of the teeth is essentially normal, but the crowns of the molars tend to be bulbous and the roots are usually short. Enamel is weakly attached and tends to chip away from the dentine abnormally easily. In severe cases, the teeth become rapidly worn down to the gingivae (Fig. 2.17). Early fitting of full dentures then becomes inevitable as the relatively soft dentine and short roots make crowning impractical.

In some patients, only a few teeth are severely affected, while the remainder appear normal. Radiographically, the main features are obliterated pulp chambers and stunted roots.

Pathology

The earliest-formed dentine under the amelodentinal junction usually appears normal. The deeper tissue is more defective,

27

Fig. 2.16 **Dentinogenesis imperfecta** showing the grey-brown translucent appearance of the teeth which are of normal morphology.

Fig. 2.17 **Dentinogenesis imperfecta.** In this 14-year-old, the teeth have worn down to gingival level but the pulp chambers have become obliterated as part of the disease process. Some enamel remains around the necks of the posterior teeth.

Fig. 2.18 Microscopic appearance of dentinogenesis imperfecta showing the grossly disorganised tubular structure with inclusions of pulp in the dentine and obliteration of the pulp cavity.

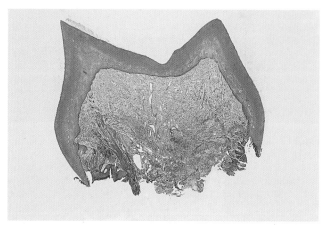

Fig. 2.19 **Shell tooth.** In this severe form of dentinogenesis imperfecta, only a thin mantle of dentine is formed and no root develops.

tubules become few, calcification is incomplete and the matrix is imperfectly formed. The pulp chamber becomes obliterated early and odontoblasts degenerate, but cellular inclusions in the dentine are common (Fig. 2.18). Scalloping of the amelo-dentinal junction is sometimes absent. The enamel tends to split from the dentine, but is otherwise normal in typical cases.

Shell teeth (dentinogenesis imperfecta type III) →
Summary p. 21

This rare anomaly is so called because only a thin shell of hard dental tissue surrounds overlarge pulp chambers. Like other types of dentinogenesis imperfecta there is normal, but thin, mantle dentine which covers irregular dentine (Fig. 2.19). The pulp lacks a normal odontoblast layer and consists of coarse connective tissue which becomes incorporated into the deep surface of the dentine.

Dentinal dysplasia ('rootless' teeth) → Summary p. 21

In dentinal dysplasia, the roots are very short and conical. The pulp chambers are obliterated by multiple nodules of poorly

organised dentine containing sheaves of tubules. Inevitably, these teeth tend to be lost early in life (Fig. 2.20).

Regional odontodysplasia (ghost teeth) → Summary p. 22

This localised disorder of development affects a group of teeth in which there are severe abnormalities of enamel, dentine and pulp.

The disorder is not hereditary and the aetiology is unknown. A few cases have been associated with facial vascular naevi or abnormalities such as hydrocephalus. There is no sex or racial predilection.

Clinically, regional odontodysplasia may be recognisable at the time of eruption of the deciduous teeth (2 to 4 years) or of the permanent teeth (7 to 11 years). The maxillary teeth

Fig. 2.20   Dentinal dysplasia. The pulp chamber in the short, broad root is obliterated by nodules of dentine.

Fig. 2.22   Regional odontodysplasia showing dysplastic dentine with a disorganised tubule structure, an irregular enamel space and mineralised enamel epithelium.

Fig. 2.21   Regional odontodysplasia. Both enamel and dentine are deformed and there is calcification of the reduced enamel epithelium.

Fig. 2.23   Radiographic appearance of regional odontodysplasia. On one side of the midline the deciduous incisors have poor root formation with thin radicular dentine and enamel. A poorly organised spotty calcification is present at the site of the permanent successors.

are most frequently affected. Either or both dentitions, and one or, at most, two quadrants may be affected. The abnormal teeth frequently fail to erupt, but if they do so, show yellowish deformed crowns, often with a rough surface.

Affected teeth have very thin enamel and dentine surrounding a greatly enlarged pulp chamber (Figs 2.21 and 2.22). In radiographs, the teeth appear crumpled and abnormally radiolucent or hazy, due to the paucity of dental hard tissues, to justify the term 'ghost teeth' (Fig. 2.23).

Histologically, the enamel thickness is highly irregular and lacks a well-defined prismatic structure. The dentine, which has a disorganised tubular structure, contains clefts and interglobular dentine mixed with amorphous tissue. The surrounding follicular tissue may contain small calcifications.

If they erupt, the teeth are susceptible to caries and fracture and their complications. If they can be preserved and restored, crown and root dentine continue to form and the teeth may survive long enough to allow normal development of the alveolar ridge and occlusion. However, extraction is often required, but this should not be done until it is certain that eruption has completely failed or the defects are too severe to be treatable, to allow for their replacement with a prothesis.

Segmental odontomaxillary dysplasia

This rare disorder may be a mild form of hemimaxillofacial dysplasia; it has been mistaken for fibrous dysplasia or regional odontodysplasia.

Segmental odontomaxillary dysplasia causes unilateral expansion of the alveolar process of the maxilla in a child in the stage of the primary or mixed dentition. The premolar and molar regions are most frequently affected. Enlargement is due to both fibrous enlargement of the gingiva and expansion of the alveolar bone. The antrum is small and the maxilla is distorted, sometimes to the extent of causing facial asymmetry. Eruption of teeth in the affected area is delayed and they are hypoplastic to varying degrees, often with enlargement of the pulps, an irregular pulp/dentine interface and many pseudoinclusions and pulp stones. There may also be defects in the tubular structure of the dentine. Permanent successors, particularly the premolars, may be absent.

Radiographically, there is a zone of sclerosis with a coarse trabecular pattern and loss of the cortex with missing and distorted teeth (Fig. 2.24). Histologically, the sclerotic zone consists of woven bone trabeculae in bland fibrous tissue and appears similar to the regressing stage of fibrous dysplasia. Both radiographs and histology are therefore necessary for diagnosis.

Multisystem disorders affecting the teeth

Ehlers–Danlos (floppy joint) syndromes

This group of collagen disorders is characterised (in varying degree) by hypermobile joints, loose hyperextensible skin, fragile oral mucosa and, in type VIII, early-onset periodontitis. There may also be temporomandibular joint symptoms such as recurrent dislocation.

Fig. 2.24 **Segmental odontomaxillary dysplasia** showing abnormal upper primary molars that are indistinct against a background of even, coarsely trabecular bone. Permanent successors are absent.

The main dental abnormalities are small teeth with short roots and multiple pulp stones (Fig. 2.25).

Gardner's syndrome (familial adenomatous polyposis)

Gardner's syndrome is characterised by multiple osteomas, especially of the jaws (Ch. 9), colonic polyps and skin tumours. The majority of patients have dental abnormalities. These include impacted teeth other than third molars, supernumerary or missing teeth and abnormal root formation. Both familial adenomatous polyposis and Gardner's syndrome are caused by mutations in the same gene, the APC tumour suppressor gene, but only some patients develop the extra-colonic manifestations such as the dental anomalies.

The colonic polyps have a 100% frequency of malignant change by middle age and the mortality is high. The dental abnormalities can be detected in childhood or adolescence and recognition of this syndrome may be life-saving by suggesting the need for colectomy.

Epidermolysis bullosa

Epidermolysis bullosa is a blistering disease of skin and mucosae (Ch. 13). Dental abnormalities include fine or coarse pitting defects, or thin and uneven enamel which may also lack prismatic structure. The amelodentinal junction may be smooth. Dental defects vary in the different subtypes of the disease, but are most frequent in the autosomal recessive, scarring type of epidermolysis bullosa in which there may be delayed, or failure of, eruption.

Infection

Congenital syphilis → Summary p. 21

Prenatal syphilis, the result of maternal infection, can cause a characteristic dental deformity, described by Hutchinson in 1858.

If the fetus becomes infected at a very early stage, abortion follows. Infants born with stigmata of congenital syphilis result from later fetal infection and the permanent teeth are affected. The characteristic defects are usually seen in the upper central incisors.

Fig. 2.25 Multiple pulp stones in a case of Ehlers–Danlos syndrome.

The incisors (Hutchinson's incisors) are small, barrel-shaped and taper towards the tip (Fig. 2.26). The incisal edge sometimes shows a crescentic notch or deep fissure which forms before eruption and can be seen radiographically. An anterior open bite is also characteristic. The first molars may be dome-shaped (Moon's molars) or may have a rough pitted occlusal surface with compressed nodules instead of cusps (mulberry molars). These defects are now largely of historical interest.

Pathology The effects are due to infection of the dental follicle by *Treponema pallidum*. The postulated consequences are chronic inflammation, fibrosis of the tooth sac, compression of the developing tooth and distortion of the ameloblast layer. *T. pallidum* causes proliferation of the odontogenic epithelium which bulges into the dentine papilla causing the characteristic central notch.

Metabolic disturbances → Summary p. 22

General disturbances of metabolism affecting the development of the teeth may be caused by the childhood fevers or severe infantile gastroenteritis.

Unlike inherited forms of hypoplasia, only a restricted area of enamel is defective, corresponding to the state of development at the time of the metabolic disturbance. Measles with severe secondary bacterial infection was the most common cause of this limited type of dental defect, but such defects have become uncommon because of more effective treatment.

Clinically, the typical effect is one or more rows of horizontally disposed pits or grooves across the crown of the incisors. These are usually in the incisal third, suggesting that the disorder had its effect during the first year or two of life, when such infections are most dangerous (Fig. 2.27). Metabolic disturbance in utero or around birth affects the primary teeth (Fig. 2.28).

Rickets can cause hypocalcification of the teeth, but only if unusually severe (see Ch. 10).

Early-onset idiopathic hypoparathyroidism is rare. Ectodermal effects are associated. The teeth may therefore be hypoplastic with ridged enamel, short blunt roots and persistently open apices (Fig. 2.29). The nails may be defective and there may be complete absence of hair. Patients with early-onset idiopathic hypoparathyroidism may later develop other endocrine deficiencies (polyendocrinopathy syndrome) but chronic candidosis may be the first sign (Ch. 15).

Hypophosphatasia → Summary p. 21. This rare genetic disorder can have severe skeletal effects as a result of failure of development of mature bone. There may also be failure of cementum formation causing loosening or early loss of teeth (Fig. 2.30).

Drugs

Tetracycline pigmentation → Summaries pp. 21, 22

Tetracycline is taken up by calcifying tissues and the band of tetracycline-stained bone or tooth substance fluoresces bright yellow under ultraviolet light.

The teeth become stained only when tetracycline is given during their development and it can cross the placenta to stain the developing teeth of the fetus. More frequently, permanent teeth are stained by tetracycline given during infancy. Tetracycline is deposited along the incremental lines of the dentine and, to a lesser extent, of the enamel.

Fig. 2.27 Chronological hypoplasia due to metabolic upset. Unlike the hereditary types of amelogenesis imperfecta, defects are linear and thought to correspond to a short period of amelogenesis disturbed by a concurrent severe illness.

Fig. 2.26 Congenital syphilis: Hutchinson's teeth. The characteristics are the notched incisal edge and the peg shape tapering from neck to tip. (Taken before the advent of colour photography.)

Fig. 2.28 Chronological hypoplasia with loss of primary molar occlusal enamel and a horizontal ridge on the upper canine.

The more prolonged the course of treatment the broader the band of stain and the deeper the discoloration. The teeth are at first bright yellow, but become a dirty brown or grey (Fig. 2.31). The stain is permanent and when the permanent incisors are affected the ugly appearance can only be disguised. When the history is vague, the brownish colour of tetracycline-stained teeth must be distinguished from dentinogenesis imperfecta. In dentinogenesis imperfecta, the teeth are obviously more translucent than normal and, in many cases, chipping of the enamel from the dentine can be seen. In tetracycline-induced defects, the enamel is not abnormally translucent and is firmly attached to dentine. In very severe cases, intact teeth may fluoresce under ultraviolet light. Otherwise, the diagnosis can only be confirmed after a tooth has been extracted. In an undecalcified section, the yellow fluorescence of the tetracycline deposited along the incremental lines can be easily seen (Fig. 2.32).

It is no longer necessary to give tetracycline during dental development. There are equally effective alternatives and it should be avoided from approximately the fourth month to at least the 12th year of childhood, ideally the 16th year. Nevertheless, tetracycline pigmentation is still seen.

Cytotoxic chemotherapy

Growing numbers of children are surviving malignant disease, particularly acute leukaemia, as a result of cytotoxic chemotherapy.

Among survivors, teeth developing during treatment may have short roots, hypoplasia of the crowns and enamel defects. Microscopically, incremental lines may be more prominent, corresponding with the period of chemotherapy but, in extreme cases, tooth formation may be aborted.

Fluorosis → Summary p. 21

Mottled enamel is the most frequently seen and most reliable sign of excess fluoride in the drinking water. It has distinctive features (Box 2.6).

Fig. 2.29 Teeth in childhood hypoparathyroidism with short blunt roots, open apices and large pulp chambers.

Fig. 2.30 Tooth in hypophosphatasia showing the enlarged pulp chamber and absence of cementum.

Fig. 2.31 Tetracycline staining. Note the chronological distribution of the dark-brown intrinsic stain.

Fig. 2.32 Tetracycline pigmentation. Ground (undecalcified) section (left) shows the broad bands of tetracycline deposited along the incremental lines of the dentine; (right) same section viewed under ultraviolet light shows fluorescence of the bands of tetracycline.

Box 2.6 Dental fluorosis: distinctive features

- Geographical distribution, endemic in areas where water-borne fluorides exceed about 2 parts per million
- Neighbouring communities with fluoride-free water do not suffer from the disorder
- Only those who have lived in a high-fluoride area during dental development show mottling. The defect is not acquired by older visitors to the area
- Permanent teeth are affected; mottling of deciduous teeth is rare
- Mottled teeth are less susceptible to caries than normal teeth from low-fluoride areas
- A typical effect is paper-white enamel opacities
- Brown staining of these patches may be acquired after eruption

Clinical features

Mottling ranges from paper-white patches to opaque, brown, pitted and brittle enamel. Clinically, it may be difficult to distinguish fluorotic defects from amelogenesis imperfecta when the degree of exposure to fluoride is unknown (Figs 2.33–2.35).

Fig. 2.33 Fluoride mottling. In this case, from an area of endemic fluorosis, there is generalised opaque white mottling with patchy enamel hypoplasia. Note the resemblance to the hypomaturation type of amelogenesis imperfecta.

Fig. 2.34 Fluorosis. Moderate effects from an area of endemic fluorosis. Irregular patchy discoloration.

There is considerable individual variation in the effects of fluorides. A few patients acquire mottling after exposure to relatively low concentrations (Fig. 2.36), while others exposed to higher concentrations appear unaffected.

Changes due to mottling are graded as shown in Box 2.7.

Box 2.7 Grading of mottled enamel

- Very mild. Small paper-white areas involve less than 25% of surface
- Mild. Opaque areas involve up to 50% of surface
- Moderate. The whole of the enamel surface may be affected with paper-white or brownish areas or both (Fig. 2.34)
- Severe. The enamel is grossly defective, opaque, pitted, stained brown and brittle (Fig. 2.35)

Pathology

Fluoride combines to form calcium fluorapatite in place of part of the hydroxyapatite. Damage to ameloblasts, leading to defective matrix formation, is seen only when the concentrations of fluorides are exceptionally high. At intermediate levels (2 to 6 ppm), the matrix is normal in structure and quantity. The form of the tooth is unaffected, but there are patches of incomplete calcification beneath the surface layer. These appear as opacities because of high organic and water content. Where there are high concentrations of fluorides (over 6 ppm), the enamel is pitted and brittle, with severe and widespread staining. Deciduous

Fig. 2.35 Fluorosis. Severe effects from an area of endemic fluorosis. Closer view showing irregular depressions caused by hypoplasia and white opaque flecks and patches.

Fig. 2.36 Fluorosis from an area of endemic natural fluorosis in Gloucestershire.

teeth are rarely mottled because excess fluoride is taken up by the maternal skeleton. However, when fluoride levels are excessively high (over 8 ppm), as in parts of India, mottling of deciduous teeth may be seen.

With severe mottling of the enamel, other effects of excessive fluoride intake, especially sclerosis of the skeleton, may develop. Radiographically, increased density of the skeleton may be seen in areas where the fluoride content of the water exceeds 8 ppm.

The severity of defects in relation to fluoride concentrations is shown in Table 2.1 and its relationship to caries prevalence in Figure 2.37.

Mild dental fluorosis is not readily distinguishable from non-fluoride defects and non-specific defects are more common in areas where the water contains less than 1 ppm of fluorine.

Other acquired developmental anomalies → Summary p. 22

Dilaceration

Trauma to a developing tooth can cause the root to form at an angle to the normal axis of the tooth – a rare deformity known as dilaceration. The sudden disturbance to odontogenesis may cause the formation of highly irregular dentine in the coronal part of the pulp chamber, but the angulated root may consist of normal tubular dentine. The hook-shaped tooth is likely to be difficult to extract (Figs 2.38 and 2.39).

Fig. 2.38 A dilacerated upper central incisor. There has been an abrupt change in the direction of root growth after approximately one-third of the root was formed.

Table 2.1 Effects on enamel of raised fluoride levels

Fluoride concentration	Effects	Clinical appearance
Less than 0.5 ppm	Very mild or mild defects in up to 6% of patients	Inconspicuous
0.5 to 1.5 ppm	At the upper limit, 22% show very mild defects	
2.5 ppm	Very mild or mild defects in over 50% Moderate or severe defects in nearly 10%	Noticeable
4.5 ppm	Nearly all patients affected to some degree; 46% have 'moderate' and 18% 'severe' defects	Disfiguring
6.0 ppm and more	All patients affected; 50% severely disfiguring	

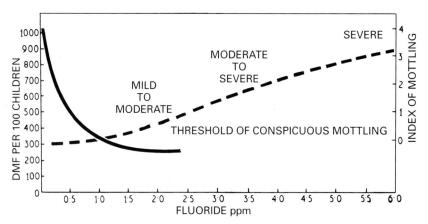

Fig. 2.37 Caries prevalence and mottling. The general relationship between the prevalence of caries (continuous line) and the severity of mottling (broken line) in persons continuously exposed to various levels of fluoride in the water during dental development. The optimum level of fluoride can be seen to be about 1 part per million. Higher concentrations of fluoride cause increasing incidence and severity of mottling without a comparable improvement in resistance to caries. The index of mottling is obtained by giving an arbitrary value for each degree of mottling and relating the numbers of patients with each grade to the total number examined.

Fig. 2.39 Another dilacerated tooth showing, in addition to the deflected root, a change in enamel contour and disorganised coronal dentine formed after the causative trauma.

Fig. 2.40 **Dens in dente or mild invaginated odontome.** In this radiograph, the enamel-lined invagination and its communication with the exterior at the incisal tip are clearly seen. The pulp is compressed to the periphery.

Fetal alcohol syndrome

Maternal alcoholism may cause developmental defects in the fetus. The eyes typically slant laterally, the lower half of the face is elongated and there is mental deficiency. Dental development may be delayed and there may be enamel defects, such as mottled opacities in the enamel near the incisal margins, but elsewhere abnormal enamel translucency.

Treatment of hypoplastic defects

Hypoplastic teeth can be disguised by restorative procedures such as bleaching, microabrasion, veneers of various types or full-coverage restorations. The more conservative procedures that are required at a young age, such as crown preparation, must be delayed until pulps become smaller. Techniques that were previously considered only as temporary solutions are frequently used as semipermanent or even permanent restorations in adult life now that adhesive materials are so durable.

ODONTOMAS → Summaries pp. 22, 157, 172

Odontomas result from aberrant development of the dental lamina. The most minor examples, though they are not usually called odontomas, are slight malformations, such as an exaggerated cingulum or extra roots or cusps on otherwise normal teeth. All gradations exist between these anomalies and composite odontomas where the dental tissues have developed in a completely irregular and haphazard manner bearing no resemblance to a tooth and occasionally forming a large mass (Ch. 8).

Dens invaginatus is an exaggeration of the process of formation of a cingular pit. Dentine and enamel-forming tissue invaginate the whole length of a tooth to appear radiographically as a tooth-within-a-tooth (*dens in dente* Fig. 2.40). Extension of this process causes the formation of an invaginated or dilated odontome (Fig. 2.41). Food debris lodges in the cavity to cause caries which rapidly penetrates the distorted pulp chamber. *Dens evaginatus* is the opposite, an enamel and dentine covered spur from the occlusal surface of a premolar or molar (Fig. 2.42). Fracture exposes the pulp.

Geminated teeth are most common in the maxillary incisor region. The pulp chambers may be entirely separate, joined in the middle of the tooth, or branched, with the pulp chambers of separated crowns sharing a common root canal. The crowns may be entirely separate or divided only by a shallow groove. The roots may be single or double.

These malformed teeth usually need to be removed before they obstruct the eruption of other teeth or become infected, or for cosmetic reasons.

Enamel pearls are uncommon, minor abnormalities, which are formed on otherwise normal teeth by ameloblasts displaced below the amelocemental junction. The pearls are usually round, a few millimetres in diameter, and often form at the bifurcation of upper permanent molars (Figs 2.43 and 2.44).

Fig. 2.41 **A dilated and invaginated odontome in a lateral incisor, sectioned vertically.** The central cavity communicates with the exterior through an invagination in the cusp tip.

Fig. 2.42 Dens evaginatus from a lower premolar, occlusal surface inset.

Fig. 2.43 **Enamel pearl.** There is a small mass of enamel at the root bifurcation.

Fig. 2.44 Enamel pearl associated with a spur of enamel joining the crown to the pearl.

Enamel pearls may consist of only a nodule of enamel attached to the dentine, or may have a core of dentine containing a horn of the pulp. They may cause a stagnation area at the gingival margin but, if they contain pulp, this will be exposed when the pearl is removed. The enamel and dentine are normal histologically (Fig. 2.45).

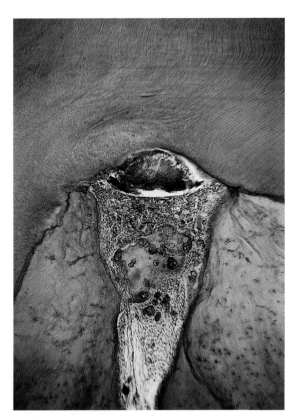

Fig. 2.45 Histological appearance of an enamel pearl showing a small isolated zone of enamel matrix on the root dentine.

GENETIC DISORDERS OF THE JAWS

Important developmental defects of the jaws are summarised in Box 2.8 and discussed more fully in subsequent chapters.

Box 2.8 Developmental defects of the jaws

- Hereditary prognathism
- Clefts of the palate and/or lip
- Craniofacial anomalies
- Cleidocranial dysplasia (Ch. 10)
- Cherubism (Ch. 10)
- Basal cell naevus syndrome (Ch. 7)
- Gardner's syndrome (Ch. 9)
- Osteogenesis imperfecta (Ch. 10)

Hereditary prognathism

Historically, hereditary prognathism is best known in the Spanish branch of the Hapsburg royal family. The defect is seen in striking form in contemporaneous portraits and persisted for 300 years.

CLEFTS OF THE LIP AND PALATE

Clefts can form in the lip or palate alone or in both (Figs 2.46 and 2.47). The aetiology is unknown but there is a genetic component in approximately 40%. The risk of having such defects is considerably greater if one, and particularly if both, of the parents are affected. No single gene appears to be responsible, but investigations in many countries suggest that possible candidates include MSX-1, PVRL1, RARA, GAD, PAX9, TGFB3, TCN2, RYK genes and PTCH gene variants.

Cleft lip (with or without a palatal cleft) is more common in males, while cleft palate alone is approximately twice as common in females. The incidence of cleft lip is about 1 per 1000 live births, while that of isolated palatal clefts is about 1 per 2000 live births. In terms of relative frequencies, cleft lips form about 22%, combined defects of lip and palate form about 58% and isolated palatal clefts form about 20% of this group of defects. The reasons for the variations in the sites of clefts is that the lip and anterior palate (the primary palate) develop before the hard and soft palates (the secondary palate). Fusion of the secondary palate is from behind forwards. Isolated cleft lip is therefore the result of an early developmental disorder, while isolated cleft palate results from influences acting later, after the primary palate has closed. By contrast, a prolonged disorder of development can prevent both primary and secondary palates from closing and leaves a severe combined defect.

Developmental disorders associated with clefting

In Down's syndrome, cleft lip or palate is present in approximately 1 in 200 patients (Ch. 33). In the less common trisomy 13 (Patau's syndrome), cleft lip or palate or both is present in up to 70% of cases, but multiple defects of the brain and other organs lead to early death. Clefts are also a feature of many other genetic craniofacial syndromes such as cleidocranial dysplasia.

Classification

The main types of cleft are summarised in Box 2.9.

Box 2.9 Clefts of lip and/or palate

Cleft lip
- Unilateral (usually on the left side), with or without an anterior alveolar ridge cleft
- Bilateral, with or without alveolar ridge clefts, complete or incomplete

Palatal clefts
- Bifid uvula
- Soft palate only
- Both hard and soft palate

Combined lip and palatal defects
- Unilateral, complete or incomplete
- Cleft palate with bilateral cleft lip, complete or incomplete

---

In the worst cases, there is complete separation of the anterior palate, which projects forward with the centre section of the lip and is attached only by the nasal septum.

Fig. 2.46 **Cleft palate.** A broad midline defect is present. (By kind permission of Mrs E Horrocks.)

Fig. 2.47 **Cleft lip and palate.** Complete unilateral cleft of palate, alveolar bone and lip joining the oral and nasal cavities. (By kind permission of Mrs E Horrocks.)

Fig. 2.48 **Collapsed maxilla resulting from traditional surgical repair of cleft palate.** Scarring and growth disturbance produce a distorted narrow maxilla. (By kind permission of Mrs E Horrocks.)

Associated defects

1. *Local*. Teeth in the region of the defect are typically absent or malformed.
2. *Systemic*. Major congenital defects, particularly heart disease, limb defects, spina bifida or mental defects are associated in about 50% of these patients and can seriously affect their management. This is particularly so in the case of Down's syndrome.

Management

Important considerations are summarised in Box 2.10. Clefts are sometimes repaired a few months or even a few days after birth to improve appearance and feeding. Nevertheless, early operation can severely inhibit growth both by damaging the delicate growing tissues and, particularly, by consequent scarring. Severe malocclusion can result and re-operation may be necessary to lessen the deformity (Fig. 2.48).

Box 2.10 **Management of clefts: important considerations**

- Provision for feeding in infancy when palatal clefts are severe
- Prevention of movement of the two halves of the maxilla or premaxilla
- Measures to counteract speech defects
- Cosmetic repair of cleft lips

Between the ages of 1 and 5 years, attention needs to be paid to hearing for which ear grommets may be necessary. Occlusion can be improved by orthodontic treatment and, if necessary, bone grafting between the ages of 5 and 12 years. At this time, measures may need to be taken to improve speech. Thereafter, up to late teenage, final measures to improve appearance include excision of scars, rhinoplasty and orthognathic surgery.

More recently, observation of untreated clefts has shown that the growth potential of these tissues is virtually normal. In some centres, therefore, a soft palate cleft is repaired early but hard palate repair is delayed until 8 or 9 years after temporary closure with an obturator. The results are good facial growth and occlusion, but speech may be impaired to some degree.

The prominent premaxilla in bilateral clefts can be managed by repositioning of this segment with bilateral bone grafts. Bilateral complete clefts of lip and palate in older children has been successfully managed by means of synchronous palatal closure and premaxillary set back.

Severe maxillary deficiency may be managed by Le Fort I internal distraction to remedy malocclusion and speech defects, without relapse.

Despite the Eurocleft project, controversies remain about the timing of these operations.

However effective the treatment, patients with clefts tend to have poorer hygiene, more gingivitis and more dental caries necessitating regular preventive care.

Submucous cleft palate

Submucous clefts are clefts in the bone or muscle covered by intact mucosa. The result is an abnormality of the attachment of the muscles of the soft palate. They are present in approximately 1 in 1200 births but are frequently missed. The chief effects are slowness in feeding and nasal regurgitation. Middle ear infections and speech defects result from the defective muscle attachments as frequently as in those with overt clefts. Symptoms are absent in only 10% of cases.

Clinically, a submucous cleft is visible as a translucent area along the midline of the soft palate and frequently a bifid uvula. On palpation, a notched posterior nasal spine may be felt. The diagnosis can be confirmed by imaging techniques, such as videofluoroscopy. Operation to repair the muscle attachments is usually delayed for about 2½ years, to enable the speech and degree of the defect to be assessed.

DEVELOPMENTAL DEFECTS OF THE ORAL SOFT TISSUES

These defects (Box 2.11) are discussed in more detail in later chapters.

Box 2.11   Important developmental defects of oral soft tissues

The gingivae and periodontium (Ch. 5)
- Hereditary gingival fibromatosis
- Ehlers–Danlos syndrome type VIII

The oral mucosa (Ch. 15)
- White sponge naevus
- Epidermolysis bullosa
- Ehlers–Danlos syndrome

Other genetic diseases relevant to dentistry

There are many rare hereditary disorders which can affect the mouth or jaws, but from the practical clinical viewpoint, haemophilia is the most important (Ch. 23).

SUGGESTED FURTHER READING

Aine L, Mäki M, Collin P et al 1990 Dental enamel defects in celiac disease. J Oral Pathol Med 19:241–245

Aldred MJ 1992 Unusual dentinal changes in dentinogenesis imperfecta associated with osteogenesis imperfecta. A case report. Oral Surg Oral Med Oral Pathol 73:461–464

Bhat M, Nelson KB, Cummins SK, Grether JK 1992 Prevalence of developmental enamel defects in children with cerebral palsy. J Oral Pathol Med 21:241–244

Chapple ILC 1993 Hypophosphatasia: dental aspects and mode of inhertittance. J Clin Periodontal 20:615–622

Crawford PJM, Aldred MJ 1989 Regional odontodysplasia: a bibliography. J Oral Pathol Med 18:251–263

Dong J, Gu TT, Simmons D et al 2000 Enamelin maps to human chromosome 4q21 within the autosomal dominant amelogenesis imperfecta locus. Eur J Oral Sci 108:353–359

Fanibunda KB, Soames JV 1996 Odontodysplasia, gingival manifestations, and accompanying abnormalities. Oral Surg Oral Med Oral Pathol Radiol Endod 81:84–88

Mäki M, Aine L, Lipsanen V et al 1991 Dental enamel defects in first degree relatives of celiac disease patients. Lancet 337:763–764

Markus AF, Smith WP, Delaire J 1993 Primary closure of cleft palate: a functional approach. Br J Oral Maxillofac Surg 31:71–77

O'Connell AC, Marini JC 1999 Evaluation of oral problems in an osteogenesis imperfecta population. Oral Surg Oral Med Oral Pathol Radiol Endod 87:189–196

Peyritz RE 2000 Ehlers–Danlos syndrome. N Engl J Med 342:730–732

Precious DS, Delaire J 1993 Clinical observations of cleft lip and palate. Oral Surg Oral Med Oral Pathol 75:141–151

Van der Wal JE, Rittersma J, Baart JA, van der Waal I 1993 Odontodysplasia: report of three cases. Int J Oral Maxillofac Surg 22:356–358

Wolff G, Wienker TF, Sander H 1993 On the genetics of mandibular prognathism: analysis of large European noble families. J Med Genet 30:112–116

Dental caries

> Quote: For sweetness and decay are of one root and sweetness ever riots to decay   *Author, regrettably, unknown*

Dental caries is progressive and, initially, subsurface demineralistion of teeth by bacterial acid. Caries is one of the most common of all diseases and still a major cause of loss of teeth.

The ultimate effect of caries is to break down enamel and dentine and thus open a path for bacteria to reach the pulp. The consequences are inflammation of the pulp and, later, of the periapical tissues. Acute pulpitis and apical periodontitis caused in this way are the most common causes of toothache. Infection can spread from the periapical region to the jaw and beyond. Though this is rare in Britain, people in other countries occasionally die from this cause.

AETIOLOGY

In 1890, W. D. Miller showed that lesions similar to dental caries could be produced by incubating teeth in saliva when carbohydrates were added. Miller concluded that caries could result from decalcification caused by bacterial acid production followed by invasion and destruction of any remaining tissue. Though he took a laudably cautious view as to how these findings should be interpreted, Miller's basic hypothesis has been upheld, even though the infective nature of the disease was not confirmed until 1954 when Orland and his associates in the USA showed that caries did not develop in germ-free animals. However, dental caries develops only in the presence of several interacting variables (Fig. 3.1 and Box 3.1).

Box 3.1   Essential requirements for development of dental caries

1. Cariogenic (acidogenic) bacteria
2. Bacterial plaque
3. Stagnation areas
4. Fermentable bacterial substrate (sugar)
5. Susceptible tooth surfaces
6. Time

Possible interventions
Reduce intake of cariogenic sugars, particularly sucrose

Possible interventions
Reduce *Strep. mutans* numbers by:
• treduction in sugar intake
• active or passive immunization

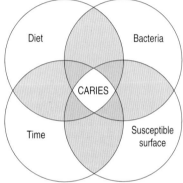

Possible interventions
Avoid frequent sucrose intake ('snacking')
Stimulate salivary flow and sugar clearance

Possible interventions
Water and other types of fluoridation
Prevention during post-eruptive maturation
Fissure sealing
Remineralising solutions
Properly contoured restorations

Fig. 3.1   The four major factors in the aetiology of dental caries.

MICROBIOLOGY

Substantial evidence indicates that streptococci are essential for development of caries, particularly of smooth (interstitial) surfaces. These are viridans streptococci which are a heterogeneous group including *Streptococcus mutans, S. sobrinus, S. salivarius, S. mitior* and *S. sanguis*.

Viridans streptococci vary in their ability to attach to different types of tissues, their ability to ferment sugars (particularly sucrose) and the concentrations of acid thus produced. They also differ in the types of polysaccharides that they form.

Certain strains of *S. mutans* are strongly acidogenic; at low pH, with freely available sucrose, they also store an intracellular, glycogen-like, reserve polysaccharide. When the supply of substrate dries up, this reserve is metabolised to continue acid production for a time. Drastic reduction in dietary sucrose intake is followed by virtual elimination of *S. mutans* from plaque and reduces or abolishes caries activity. When sucrose is made freely available again *S. mutans* rapidly recolonises the plaque.

Germ-free animals do not develop dental caries when fed a sucrose-rich diet which causes caries in animals with a normal oral flora. Experiments using gnotobiotes have shown that the most potent causes of dental caries are a limited number of strains of the *S. mutans* group which are able to form cariogenic plaque.

S. mutans strains are a major component of plaque in human mouths, particularly in persons with a high dietary sucrose intake and high caries activity (Fig. 3.2). *S. mutans* isolated from such mouths are virulently cariogenic when introduced into the mouths of animals.

However, simple clinical observation of the sites (interstitially and in pits and fissures) where dental caries is active,

Fig. 3.2 Extensive caries of decidous incisors and canines. This pattern of caries is particularly associated with the use of sweetened dummies and sweetened infant drinks.

Fig. 3.3 The stagnation area in an occlusal pit. A ground section of a molar showing the size of the stagnation area in comparison with a toothbrush bristle placed above it. The complete inaccessibility of the stagnation area to cleaning is obvious.

shows that the bacteria responsible are not those floating free in the saliva. Dental caries develops only at the interface between tooth surface and dental plaque in stagnation areas, particularly in occlusal fissures and approximally (Fig. 3.3).

Bacterial polysaccharides

The ability of *S. mutans* to initiate smooth surface caries and form large amounts of adherent plaque depends on its ability to polymerise sucrose into high-molecular-weight, dextran-like, extracellular polysaccharides (glucans) (Box 3.2). The cariogenicity of *S. mutans* depends as much on its ability to form large amounts of insoluble extracellular glucans as on its ability to produce acid.

Box 3.2 Essential properties of cariogenic bacteria

- Acidogenic
- Able to produce a pH low enough (usually pH <5) to decalcify tooth substance
- Able to survive and continue to produce acid at low levels of pH
- Possess attachment mechanisms for firm adhesion to smooth tooth surfaces
- Able to produce adhesive, insoluble plaque polysaccharides (glucans)

Glucans enable streptococci to adhere to one another and to the tooth surface, probably via specific receptors. In this way, *S. mutans* and its glucans may initiate their attachment to the teeth and enable critical masses of plaque to be built up. Production of sticky, insoluble, extracellular glucan produced by strains of *S. mutans* is strongly related to their cariogenicity.

The importance of sucrose in this activity depends on the high energy of its glucose–fructose bond which allows the synthesis of polysaccharides by glucosyltransferase without any other source of energy. Sucrose is thus the main substrate for such polysaccharides. Other sugars are, to a variable degree, less cariogenic (in the absence of preformed plaque), partly because they are less readily formed into cariogenic glucans.

Plaque polysaccharides, synthesised by bacteria, play an essential role in the pathogenesis of dental caries. The proportions of the different types of polysaccharide, and the overall amounts formed, depend both on the kinds of bacteria present and the different sugars in the diet.

On a sucrose-rich diet, the main extracellular polysaccharides are glucans. Fructans formed from fructose are produced in smaller amounts. They are more soluble than glucans and less important in caries. Acid-producing microorganisms that do not produce insoluble polysaccharides do not appear to be able to cause caries of smooth surfaces. Even mutant strains of *S. mutans* which produce more soluble polysaccharides seem not to be cariogenic. Polysaccharides thus contribute to the adhesiveness, bulk and resistance to solution of plaque.

In the past, lactobacilli were thought to be the main cause of dental caries because they are numerous in the saliva and can be isolated from carious cavities. They are also acidogenic. However, they are present only in relatively small numbers in dental plaque until after caries has developed.

In gnotobiotic animals, lactobacilli are weakly cariogenic but some can produce fissure caries where adherent plaque formation is less important. Overall, there is little evidence that lactobacilli are clinically important in initiating dental caries, but they may contribute to tooth destruction after the process has started.

Many other microorganisms can also be found in plaque. The role of the many filamentous forms is not known. Strains of actinomyces are also found, particularly when caries is rampant, but appear capable only of causing root surface lesions.

Though bacteria are responsible for acid production, bacterial plaque (Fig. 3.4) enables large concentrations of them to adhere to the teeth and, in stagnation areas, prevents effective buffering of bacterial acids by saliva. Important points about microbiological aspects of dental caries are summarised in Box 3.3.

Fig. 3.4 Bacterial plaque. A decalcified section showing darkly staining plaque lying on enamel and within a carious cavity. The plaque has remained intact and adherent to the enamel throughout the processes to which the specimen was subjected in preparation for sectioning.

Box 3.3   Microbiological aspects of dental caries

- Dental caries is a bacterial disease
- The organisms mainly responsible are specific strains of *Streptococcus mutans*
- The cariogenicity of *S. mutans* has been established by inoculating it into the mouths of otherwise germ-free animals (gnotobiotes)
- The presence of *S. mutans* in the human mouth is associated with caries activity
- Other bacteria including lactobacilli and other strains of streptococci are only weakly cariogenic or are non-cariogenic despite being able to produce acid

---

The cariogenicity of *S. mutans* depends on properties summarised in Box 3.4.

Box 3.4   Cariogenic properties of *Streptococcus mutans*

- It produces lactic acid from sucrose
- It can live at a pH as low as 4.2
- It forms large amounts of extracellular, sticky and insoluble glucan plaque matrix
- It adheres to pellicle and contributes to plaque formation

BACTERIAL PLAQUE

Plaque is a tenaciously adherent deposit that forms on tooth surfaces. It consists of an organic matrix containing a dense concentration of bacteria (Figs 3.4–3.6).

In microbiological terms, plaque is a biofilm. Biofilms consist of a hydrated viscous phase formed from bacteria and their extracellular polysaccharide matrices. In such a film, molecules and ions exist in concentrations that can be widely different from those of the surrounding fluid phase (saliva). Bacteria in biofilms can also exhibit cooperative activity and behave

Fig. 3.5 This scanning electronmicrograph of plaque shows the large number of filamentous organisms and, in addition, many cocci clustered amongst them. (By kind permission of Dr Sheila J Jones.)

differently from the same species in isolation in a culture medium. As a consequence, a biofilm may be resistant to antimicrobials or to immunological defences to which the individual bacteria are normally sensitive. Bacterial plaque must therefore be regarded as a living entity and not as a mere collection of bacteria. In particular, the ability of dental plaque to concentrate and retain acid was recognised long before the special properties of biofilms were discovered.

Fig. 3.6 This scanning electronmicrograph at higher power shows cocci attached to filamentous organisms to produce the corn-cob type of arrangement sometimes seen in plaque. (By kind permission of Dr Sheila J Jones.)

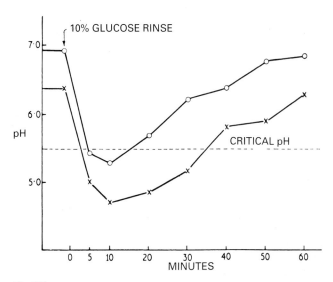

Fig. 3.7 **Stephan curves.** This is the usual form of curves obtained when changes in reaction to bacterial plaque are measured directly. When the pH falls below the critical level, enamel may become demineralised. Patients with active caries tend to show a lower fall in pH, as in the lower curve. Noteworthy features are the very rapid fall in pH and the slow recovery to the normal level in spite of the very short time the sugar is in the mouth. Carbohydrates which are retained on the teeth have a more prolonged effect still.

Box 3.5   **Stages of plaque formation**

- Deposition of structureless cell-free, pellicle of salivary glycoprotein
- Further deposition of pellicle enhanced by bacterial action precipitating salivary proteins
- Colonisation of the cell-free layer by bacteria, particularly by *S. sanguis* and *S. mutans* strains within 24 hours
- Progressive build-up of plaque substance by bacterial polysaccharides
- Proliferation of filamentous and other bacteria as the plaque matures

---

Clinically, bacterial plaque is a tenaciously adherent deposit on the teeth. It resists the friction of food during mastication and can only be readily removed by toothbrushing. However, neither toothbrushing nor fibrous foods will remove plaque from inaccessible surfaces or pits (stagnation areas – see Fig. 3.3).

Plaque becomes visible, particularly on the labial surfaces of the incisors, when toothbrushing is stopped for 12–24 hours. It appears as a translucent film with a matt surface that dulls the otherwise smooth and shiny enamel. It can be made obvious when stained with disclosing agents. Little plaque forms under conditions of starvation, but it forms rapidly and abundantly on a high-sucrose diet.

In stagnation areas where they are undisturbed, plaque bacteria can form acid from sugars over sufficiently long periods as to attack tooth surfaces.

Adhesion of bacteria to the teeth from which they would otherwise be washed away is an essential requirement for the colonisation of enamel. Attachment depends on complex mechanisms and depends on such molecules as glucans and/or glucosyltransferase. Components of plaque, which act as adhesion receptors, include a group of proline-rich proteins (PRPs) from the saliva.

Stages of formation of bacterial plaque

If teeth are thoroughly cleaned by polishing with an abrasive, plaque quickly re-forms (Box 3.5).

Acid production in plaque

Sucrose diffuses rapidly into plaque and acid production quickly follows. These changes have been measured directly in the human mouth using microelectrodes in direct contact with plaque. It has been shown by this means that, after rinsing the mouth with a 10% glucose solution, the pH falls within 2–5 minutes, often to a level sufficient to decalcify enamel. Even though no more sucrose may be taken and the surplus is washed away by the saliva, the pH level remains at a low level for about 15–20 minutes; it returns only gradually to the resting level after about an hour. These changes (the so-called Stephan curve) are shown diagramatically in Figure 3.7. The rapidity with which the pH falls is a reflection of the speed with which sucrose can diffuse into plaque and the activity of the concentration of enzymes produced by the great numbers of bacteria in the plaque. The slow rate of recovery to the resting pH – a critical factor in caries production – depends mainly on factors summarised in Box 3.6.

Box 3.6   Factors contributing to maintenance of low plaque pH

- Rapid production of a high concentration of acid within the plaque temporarily overcomes local buffering
- Escape of acid into the saliva is delayed by the diffusion-limiting properties of plaque and its thickness
- Diffusion of salivary buffers into plaque hampered by the diffusion-limiting properties of plaque and its thickness
- Continued acid production from bacterial intracellular storage polysaccharides after dietary sugar is exhausted

---

As discussed in relation to the pathology of dental caries, it is clear that acid production is responsible for the carious attack. Lactic acid is mainly responsible. When plaque is sampled after exposure to sucrose, lactic acid is the quantitatively predominant acid during plaque activity, particularly during the trough of the Stephan curve. Lactic acid has a lower pK constant and causes a greater fall in pH than equimolar solutions of acetic or propionic acids that may also be detected in plaque.

Plaque minerals

In addition to bacteria and their polysaccharides, salivary components also contribute to the plaque matrix. Calcium, phosphorus and, often, fluorides are present in significant amounts. There is some evidence of an inverse relationship between calcium and phosphate levels in plaque and caries activity or sucrose intake. The ability of plaque to concentrate calcium and phosphorus is used in mineralising mouthwashes. The level of fluoride in plaque may be high, ranging from 15 to 75 ppm or more, and is largely dependent on the fluoride level in the drinking water and diet. This fluoride is probably mostly bound to organic material in the plaque but, at low pH levels, may become available and active in ionic form.

SUCROSE AS A PLAQUE SUBSTRATE

Direct measurement of pH changes in the mouth shows that there is intermittent acid production on the surface of the teeth and this follows the pattern shown earlier in the Stephan curves. Ingestion of sucrose leads to a burst of activity in the plaque so that the pH may fall low enough to attack enamel before slowly returning to the resting level. The frequency with which substrate is made available to the plaque is therefore important. When sucrose is taken as a sweet drink, any surplus beyond the capacity of the organisms in the plaque to metabolise at the time is washed away. If sucrose-containing drinks are taken repeatedly at short intervals, the supply of substrate to the bacteria can be sufficiently frequently renewed to cause acid in the plaque to remain persistently at a destructive level.

A similar effect may be caused by carbohydrate in sticky form, such as a caramel, which clings to the teeth and is slowly dissolved, releasing substrate over a long period. The effects of maintaining plaque activity by repeated administration of small quantities of sucrose have been demonstrated by the use of animal feeding devices to dispense metered quantities of sucrose in diets at fixed intervals. These show that a given amount of sucrose is more cariogenic when fed in small increments, but at intervals to maintain maximal plaque activity, than the same amount fed as a single dose.

Effects of sucrose on plaque polysaccharide production

As discussed earlier, the cariogenicity of plaque depends on its ability to adhere to the teeth, to resist dissolution by saliva and its protection of bacterial acids from salivary buffering. These properties depend on the formation of insoluble polysaccharides produced particularly by cariogenic strains of *S. mutans*.

Effects of sucrose on the oral microbial flora

Colonisation by cariogenic bacteria, especially *S. mutans*, is highly dependent on the sucrose content of the diet. In the absence of sucrose, *S. mutans* cannot usually be made to colonise the mouths of experimental animals. In humans, the plaque counts of *S. mutans* also appear to depend on the sucrose content of the diet. Severe reduction in dietary sucrose causes *S. mutans* to decline in numbers or disappear from plaque.

Experimental evidence for the essential contribution of sucrose to caries activity is summarised in Box 3.7.

Box 3.7   Experimental evidence for the critical contribution of sucrose to caries activity

- In caries-susceptible animals a sucrose-rich diet promotes caries production
- Caries is not induced in susceptible animals if sucrose is fed only by stomach-tube – its effect is entirely local
- Sucrose in sticky form clings to the teeth and remains available to bacteria for a longer period and is more cariogenic
- Sucrose-containing fluids are quickly cleared from the mouth and less cariogenic
- Frequent feeds of small quantities of sucrose are more cariogenic than the same total amount fed on a single occasion
- Desalivation, by delaying clearance of sugars, enhances caries activity

---

The importance of sucrose in human caries depends mainly on epidemiological studies and a few interventional studies. The findings of epidemiological studies are summarised in Box 3.8.

Box 3.8   Epidemiological evidence for sucrose as the cause of dental caries

- Low caries prevalence in populations with low sucrose intakes
- The decline in caries prevalence during wartime sucrose shortages
- The rise of caries prevalence with increasing availability of sucrose
- Archaeological evidence of low caries prevalence in eras before sucrose became freely available
- Low caries prevalence in disorders of sucrose metabolism (hereditary fructose intolerance)

Dental caries has been most prevalent in well-nourished, westernised communities, such as Britain, the USA and others with similar lifestyles where large quantities of sucrose, particularly in the form of sweets or snack bars, are eaten. In the past particularly, there have been many studies of poor communities living on traditional diets with little or no sucrose content. A low prevalence of caries has been shown (for example) in parts of China and of Africa, the Seychelles, Tristan da Cunha, Alaska and Greenland. Many studies were carried out on Eskimo races who were caries-free when consuming their traditional diet of seal or whale meat, and fish. Similarly, in South African races, despite a high-starch carbohydrate diet, caries was found in fewer than 9% of those examined, but greatly increased when there was access to a modern sucrose-rich diet.

In such studies, no association has been found between malnutrition and caries. Generally, the reverse is true and, when nutrition is poor, caries is infrequent. These diets also vary widely in content, from rice as the staple in China or coarsely ground cereals in Africa to a mainly meat and fish diet among Eskimos. The common feature of these diets, and one differentiating them sharply from westernised diets, is low or negligible consumption of refined sugar, particularly sucrose.

Britain is an example of a country where consumption of sucrose is exceptionally high and where the rest of the diet is more than adequate. A survey in England and Wales in 1973 showed, for example, that (in spite of the benefits of a National Health Service) 78% of 8-year-old children had active decay and many teeth which had been filled or lost from this cause. A survey in 1978 showed that dentate adults had on average only 13 sound and unfilled teeth. Though there has been dramatic improvement nationally, such consequences are still found in some populations.

In Britain and other countries, the incidence of caries has risen roughly parallel with rising consumption of sucrose. The incidence of caries has risen in spite of the much greater consumption of so-called 'protective' foods, namely dairy products, meat and fruit, in recent years. As a consequence of this more varied diet, carbohydrates overall have formed a smaller proportion of the diet. Nevertheless, sucrose forms a higher proportion of the carbohydrate component.

Where there has been a change from simple natural diets to a westernised diet, as in Alaska, caries has increased sharply and Inuit children now have a caries incidence at least as high as other American children. A similar state of affairs is developing in Africa as sweet eating and sweet between-meals 'snacks' have become popular. In Nigeria, many of the older adults are still totally caries-free, but the prevalence of dental caries among children and young people who have picked up sweet-eating habits is rising rapidly. This effect has also been strikingly well documented in the population of Tristan da Cunha who, up to the late 1930s, lived on a simple meat, fish and vegetable diet with a minimal sucrose content and had a very low caries prevalence. With the adoption of westernised diet, the caries prevalence had risen up to eightfold in some age groups by the mid-1960s. Even in Europe, in the 1930s and 1940s there were isolated communities, such as the Outer Hebrides or the Lötschental in Switzerland, where dental caries prevalence rose 20-fold or more when sucrose and sweets became widely consumed.

The effect of limiting sucrose consumption was shown on a vast scale during the Second World War. Those countries which suffered food shortages during the 1939–45 war had severe restrictions, mainly of meat, fats and sucrose. To maintain an adequate caloric intake, overall consumption of starchy carbohydrates rose considerably. In occupied Norway, where shortages were particularly severe, the pattern of dental caries during and after the war is shown diagrammatically in Figure 3.8. As sucrose became more plentiful at the end of the war, caries prevalence progressively rose.

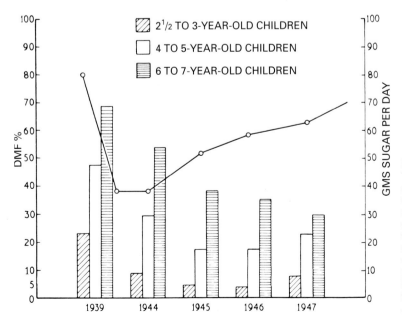

Fig. 3.8 The wartime restrictions on diet and caries in Norway. The continuous line shows an estimate of the individual daily sugar consumption during and after the war. The heights of the columns show the incidence of caries in children of various ages. Rationing of sugar started in 1938, but it is apparent that the incidence of caries declined slowly and continued for a short time after sugar became freely available. The greatest reduction in caries was in the youngest group of children whose teeth were exposed to the wartime diet for the shortest periods; the mothers of these children, on the other hand, had been exposed to the wartime diet throughout pregnancy and for a long period before that. (Mainly after Toverud G 1949 Journal of the American Dental Association 39:127.)

In Japan also, rising caries prevalence has been associated with rising sucrose consumption. Towards the end of the Second World War, sugar consumption and caries levels were very low. More recently, Japan is one of the few countries where sucrose consumption, from 16.5 kg per head in 1961, nearly doubled in 1970. Caries prevalence has risen in parallel. Unlike most other countries, this picture has not been significantly masked by use of fluoride toothpastes where the market share of fluoride toothpastes is only 15%.

Caries has become epidemic only in relatively recent years as sucrose became cheaper and widely available. In Britain, there was a sudden, widespread rise in sucrose consumption in the middle of the 19th century. This resulted both from the falling cost of production and, in 1861, the abolition of a tax on sugar. Evidence from exhumed skulls confirms the low prevalence of caries before sucrose became widely available and the steady rise in prevalence thereafter.

Patients unable to metabolise fructose as a result of an enzyme deficiency cannot tolerate fructose-containing foods including disaccharides such as sucrose where fructose forms part of the molecule. These children therefore learn to avoid all sucrose-containing foods and have an unusually low incidence of caries.

Experimental studies on humans

In the Vipeholm study, over 400 adult patients were studied in a closed institution. They received a basic low-carbohydrate diet to establish a baseline of caries activity for each group.

Fig. 3.9   The Vipeholm dental caries study. A simplified diagram showing the results in some of the groups of patients and, in particular, the striking effect on caries activity of sticky sweets eaten between meals when compared with the eating of sweet stuffs at mealtimes. The broken lines indicate those who consumed sugar only at meals, the continuous line shows those who consumed sugar both at and between meals. (After Gustafsson et al. 1954 Acta Odontologica Scandinavica 11:232.)

They were then divided into seven groups which were each allocated different diets. A control group received the basic diet made up to an adequate calorie intake with margarine. Two groups received supplements of sucrose at mealtimes, either in solution or as sweetened bread. The four remaining groups received sweets (toffees, caramels, or chocolate) which were eaten between meals.

The effects of sucrose in different quantities and of different degrees of adhesiveness, and of eating sucrose at different times were thus tested over a period of 5 years. Caries activity was greatly enhanced by the eating, between meals, of sticky sweets (toffees and caramels) that were retained on the teeth. Sucrose at mealtimes only had little effect (Fig. 3.9). The incidence of caries fell to its original low level when toffees or caramels were no longer given and caries activity was very slight in the control group having the low-carbohydrate diet.

In another large-scale clinical experiment in Turku (Finland), an experimental group was allowed a wide range of foods sweetened with xylitol (a sugar alcohol) but no sucrose. The control group was allowed as much sugary (sucrose-containing) foods as desired. After 2 years, the experimental group showed 90% less caries than those who had been allowed sucrose.

Essential features of sucrose incriminating it as the most cariogenic substrate are summarised in Box 3.9.

Box 3.9   Factors determining the cariogenicity of sucrose

- Sucrose forms up to a third of the carbohydrate content of many persons' diets
- It promotes colonisation of teeth by *Streptococcus mutans*
- Its disaccharide bond alone contains enough energy to react with bacterial enzymes to form extracellular dextran matrix
- Its small molecular size allows it to diffuse readily into plaque
- Bacterial metabolism of sucrose is rapid

Use of sugar substitutes (artificial sweeteners) in place of sucrose greatly reduces caries activity. The cariogenicity of sugars and artificial sweeteners are summarised in Table 3.1.

SUSCEPTIBILITY OF TEETH TO CARIES

Teeth may be resistant to decay because of factors affecting the structure of the tooth during formation. Serious efforts were made in the past to confirm the misguided belief that dental caries was due to hypocalcification of the teeth and was essentially a vitamin deficiency disease. This simplistic view of course ignored the extensive epidemiological findings that the best-nourished populations had the worst record for dental disease, while poverty-stricken communities on deficient diets had a low caries prevalence, as discussed earlier.

Hereditary hypoplasia or hypocalcification of the teeth, in which there are severe disturbances of structure, are also not particularly susceptible to caries and there is no evidence that the degree of calcification of the teeth affects their resistance

Table 3.1 Sugars and non-sugar sweeteners

Compound	Nature and uses	Cariogenicity
Sucrose	A disaccharide sugar (ß1–4-linked glucose–fructose)	Highest of all sugars
Glucose, fructose	Monosaccharide sugars	Less cariogenic than sucrose
Lactose and galactose	Monosaccharide (lactose) and disaccharide (galactose) sugars	Less cariogenic than sucrose
Glucose syrups and maltodextrins	Hydrolysis products of starch used as bulk sweeteners	Less cariogenic than sugars
Hydrogenated glucose syrup and lycasins	Hydrolysis products of starch which are then hydrogenated, used as bulk sweeteners	Less cariogenic than sugars
Isomalt	Mixture of two unusual 12-carbon sugars	Low cariogenicity
Xylitol, sorbitol, mannitol, lactitol etc.	Sugar alcohols (polyols) sometimes used as bulk sweeteners	Non-cariogenic
Saccharin, aspartame, thaumatin, acesulfame K and cyclamate	Non-sugar intense sweeteners	Non-cariogenic

to caries. However, newly erupted teeth are generally caries susceptible, apparently because of a hypomineralised enamel structure which is made progressively less vulnerable by deposition of materials from saliva ('post-eruptive maturation').

Effects of fluorides

Fluorides from drinking water and other sources are taken up by calcifying tissues during development. When the fluoride content of the water is 1 ppm or more, the incidence of caries declines substantially. Fluoride may affect caries activity by a variety of mechanisms (Box 3.10). Exposure to fluoride during dental development affects the structure of the developing teeth. This is shown by mottling of the enamel produced by excessive levels of fluoride. However, it is believed that the lower incidence of dental caries where water is fluoridated is due to its continued environmental effect on the teeth to reduce solubility of the enamel and promote remineralisation. These effects are more important than the effect of fluoride on the initial structure of the enamel.

Box 3.10 Actions of fluoride on dental caries

- Fluoride is incorporated into the teeth during development
- Fluoride acts mainly after eruption in early lesions by reducing enamel solubility and favouring remineralisation
- A constant supply of small amounts of fluoride is most effective in reducing dental caries
- Fluoride may reduce acid generation in plaque

Fluoride is the only nutrient that has been proven to have this protective action. Despite the difficulties in distinguishing the degree of resistance of the teeth from the virulence of their cariogenic environment, it has become clear that fluorides have had a major impact on caries prevalence. There has undoubtedly been a significant decline in the prevalence of dental caries in countries where drinking water has been fluoridated. In Britain, as a result of widespread use of fluoridised dentifrices, there has also been so great a decline in the disease as significantly to affect the nature of dental practice. These changes cannot be related to any comparable decline in sucrose consumption.

SALIVA AND DENTAL CARIES

The immediate environment of the teeth is bacterial plaque, but saliva is the medium in which plaque develops and works. Though saliva inevitably plays some part in the process of caries, it is a complex secretion whose rates of flow, composition and properties are not easy to determine.

Effects of desalivation

Salivary flow is highly important in clearing cariogenic foods from the mouth. In animals, removal or inactivation of major salivary glands leads to increased caries activity roughly in proportion to the reduction in saliva production. Dental caries may also become rampant in humans with xerostomia due to salivary gland disease (Ch. 18).

Rate of flow and buffering power

The buffering power of saliva depends mainly on its bicarbonate content and is increased at high rates of flow. The buffering power of the saliva affects the buffering power of dental plaque to some degree and helps to prevent the pH from falling to very low levels. A rapid flow rate, with the greater salivary buffering power that is associated, has been found to be associated with low caries activity. In Down's syndrome, caries activity is low in spite of gross accumulation of plaque and immunodeficiencies, possibly because of the high rate of salivation with greater buffering power. While a rapid flow of saliva of low viscosity assists clearance of foodstuffs from the mouth, other physical properties of different salivas have not been shown to have a significant relationship to caries activity.

Other factors

Inorganic components and enamel maturation

Radioactive isotope studies suggest that there is some exchange of calcium and phosphate ions between enamel surface and saliva. In particular, enamel undergoes post-eruptive changes. Clinical observations suggest that newly erupted teeth are more susceptible to caries than adult teeth and radioactive tracer studies show that newly erupted teeth can incorporate 10 to 20 times as much inorganic material in ionic form as adult teeth. More important is that saliva is a vehicle for fluoride which can enter plaque from the saliva and affect caries activity.

Enzymic activity

Salivary amylase breaks down polysaccharides such as starch. This contribution to digestion is small and its main value is to make food residues on the teeth more soluble to assist their clearance. The breakdown of polysaccharides leads to production of sugars, but the amounts and their contribution to caries are small and are only likely to be seen with experimental sucrose-deficient diets. Usually, the amount of sucrose present in the diet overwhelms that produced by amylase activity. In general, therefore, amylase activity and caries prevalence are not closely related.

Antibacterial activities

Saliva contains thiocyanates, a lysozyme-like substance and other theoretically antibacterial substances. Nevertheless, the mouth teems with bacteria and there is no evidence that non-specific antibacterial substances in saliva have any significant effect on caries activity.

Immunological defences

IgA is secreted in saliva but small amounts of IgG enter the mouth from the gingival crevice. Persons who suffer from defects in non-specific host defences (complement and neutrophils) or specific immunological defences (IgA deficiency, Down's syndrome or AIDS) do not appear to suffer an excess of dental caries. Nevertheless, an immunological host resistance to dental caries is detectable experimentally in man and appears to act by reducing the number of *S. mutans* in plaque. The effect does not appear to be very potent and is easily overwhelmed if the diet is high in sucrose or if low levels of the relevant antibody are produced.

Immunological defences against *S. mutans* could be mediated by salivary IgA or serum IgG from the crevicular fluid. Although salivary IgA is capable of preventing caries in experimental animals, it appears to play no significant role in humans. Immunisation of monkeys against *S. mutans* generates specific serum IgG which protects them against caries. Serum IgG also

appears to protect against *S. mutans* in humans, but the response varies widely between individuals.

It has been shown that dripping a solution of monoclonal antibody against *S. mutans* onto the teeth prevents recolonisation by *S. mutans* in humans. For this to be effective, plaque must be removed before treatment by using chlorhexidine and effective oral hygiene. This effect of antibody lasts for several months after applications and this 'passive immunisation' has the potential to reduce caries activity significantly. The effects are probably not mediated by traditional immune mechanisms but rather by binding to the bacteria and preventing adhesion to the forming new plaque. Once new plaque is established without *S. mutans,* the stable biofilm ecosystem prevents colonisation long after the antibody has been washed away.

Key facts about the effects of saliva on plaque activity are summarised in Box 3.11.

Box 3.11   Key facts about the effects of saliva on plaque activity

- Salivary components contribute to plaque formation and form much of its matrix
- Sucrose dissolves in saliva and is actively taken up by plaque
- The buffering power of saliva may limit the fall in pH caused by acid formed in plaque
- The buffering power of saliva is related to the rate of secretion. High flow rates may be associated with lower caries activity
- Gross reduction in salivary secretion leads to increased caries activity when a cariogenic diet is eaten
- IgA is present in saliva but has little effect on caries activity; it may prevent bacterial species from colonizing plaque

---

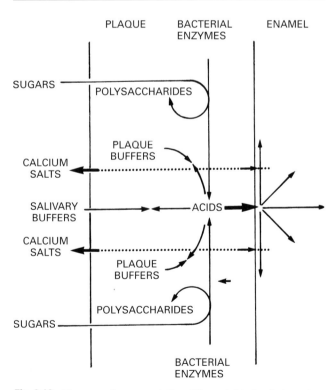

Fig. 3.10 Diagrammatic representation of the main biochemical events in dental plaque, initiating caries. (From McCracken AW, Cawson RA 1983 Clinical and oral microbiology. McGraw-Hill.)

The main biochemical events in dental plaque in the development of dental caries are summarised diagrammatically in Figure 3.10.

PATHOLOGY OF ENAMEL CARIES

Enamel is the usual site of the initial lesion unless dentine or cementum becomes exposed by gingival recession. Enamel, the hardest and densest tissue in the body, consists almost entirely of calcium apatite with only a minute organic content. It therefore forms a formidable barrier to bacterial attack. However, once enamel has been breached, infection of dentine can spread with relatively little obstruction. Preventive measures must therefore be aimed primarily at stopping the attack or at making enamel more resistant.

The essential nature of the carious attack on enamel is permeation of acid into its substance. The crystalline lattice of calcium apatite crystals is relatively impermeable, but part of the organic matrix of enamel which envelops the apatite crystals has a relatively high water content and is permeable to hydrogen ions. Permeation of enamel by acid causes a series of submicroscopic changes. This process of enamel caries is a dynamic one and, initially at least, consists of alternating phases of demineralisation and remineralisation, rather than a continuous process of dissolution.

Enamel caries develops in four main phases (Box 3.12). These stages of enamel caries are distinguishable microscopically and are also clinically significant. In particular, the early (white spot) lesion is potentially reversible, but cavity formation is irreversible and requires restorative measures to substitute for the lost tissue.

Box 3.12 Stages of enamel caries

- The early (submicroscopic) lesion
- Phase of non-bacterial enamel crystal destruction
- Cavity formation
- Bacterial invasion of enamel
- Undermining of enamel from below after spread into dentine

The early lesion

The earliest visible changes are seen as a white opaque spot that forms just adjacent to a contact point. Despite the chalky appearance, the enamel is hard and smooth to the probe (Fig. 3.11). The microscopic changes under this early white spot lesion may be seen in undecalcified sections but more readily when polarised light is used. Microradiography indicates the degree of demineralisation seen in the different zones.

The initial lesion is conical in shape with its apex towards the dentine and a series of four zones of differing translucency can be discerned. Working back from the deepest, advancing edge of the lesion, these zones consist first of a translucent zone most deeply; immediately within this is a second dark zone; the third consists of the body of the lesion and the fourth consists of the surface zone (Fig. 3.12).

These initial changes are not due to bacterial invasion, but due to bacterial lactic or other acids causing varying degrees of demineralisation and remineralisation in the enamel. The features of these zones are summarised in Table 3.2.

The translucent zone is the first observable change. The appearance of the translucent zone results from formation of submicroscopic spaces or pores apparently located at prism boundaries and other junctional sites such as the striae of Retzius. When the section is mounted in quinoline, it fills the pores and, since it has the same refractive index as enamel, the normal structural features disappear and the appearance of the pores is enhanced (Fig. 3.13). Microradiography confirms that the changes in the translucent zone are due to demineralisation.

Fig. 3.11 Early enamel caries, a white spot lesion, in a deciduous molar. The lesion forms below the contact point and in consequence is much larger than an interproximal lesion in a permanent tooth (see Fig. 3.19).

Fig. 3.12 Early interproximal caries. Ground section in water viewed by polarised light. The body of the lesion and the intact surface layer are visible. The translucent and dark zones are not seen until the section is viewed immersed in quinoline.

Table 3.2 Key features of the enamel zones preceding cavity formation

Zone	Key features	Comments
Translucent zone	1% mineral loss. Earliest and deepest demineralisation	Broader in progressing caries, narrow or absent in arrested or remineralised lesions
Dark zone	2–4% mineral loss overall but a zone of remineralisation just behind the advancing front	Broader in arrested or remineralised lesions, narrow in advancing lesions
Body	5–25% mineral loss	Broader in progressing caries, replaced by a broad dark zone in arrested or remineralised lesions
Surface zone	1% mineral loss. A zone of remineralisation resulting from the diffusion barrier and mineral content of plaque. Cavitation is loss of this layer, allowing bacteria to enter the lesion	Relatively constant width, a little thicker in arrested or remineralising lesions

Fig. 3.13 **Early interproximal caries.** Ground section viewed by polarised light after immersion in quinoline. Quinoline has filled the larger pores, causing most of the fine detail in the body of the lesion to disappear (Fig. 3.12), but the dark zone with its smaller pores is accentuated.

Fig. 3.14 The same lesion (Figs 3.12 and 3.13) viewed dry under polarised light to show the full extent of demineralisation. (Figs 3.12–3.14 by kind permission of Professor Leon Silverstone and the Editor of Dental Update 1989;10:262.)

The dark zone is fractionally superficial to the translucent zone. Polarised light microscopy shows that the volume of the pores in this zone has increased to 2–4% of the enamel volume. This change is due mainly to formation of additional small pores. Two different-size pores thus coexist in the dark zone. The small ones are so minute that molecules of quinoline are unable to enter and the tissue has become transformed into a molecular sieve. The small pores therefore remain filled with air – this appears to produce the zone's dark appearance.

Microradiography confirms that the dark zone has suffered a greater degree of demineralisation. However, when the lesion is exposed to saliva or synthetic calcifying solutions in vitro, the dark zone actually extends further. This may indicate that the formation of the dark zone may be due not merely to creation of new porosities but possibly also to remineralisation of the large pores of the translucent zone so that they become micropores impermeable to quinoline. It is widely believed therefore that these changes in the dark zone are evidence of remineralisation, as discussed later.

The body of the lesion forms the bulk of the lesion and extends from just beneath the surface zone to the dark zone. By transmitted light, the body of the lesion is comparatively translucent compared with normal enamel and sharply demarcated from the dark zone. Within the body of the lesion, the striae of Retzius appear enhanced, particularly when mounted in quinoline and viewed under polarised light. Polarised light examination (Fig. 3.14) also shows that the pore volume is 5% at the periphery but increases to at least 25% in the centre.

Fig. 3.16 Undecalcified section showing early enamel lesions in the enamel surrounding and deep to an occlusal pit.

Fig. 3.15 **Early interproximal caries.** A microradiograph of the same section as in Figures 3.12–3.14, showing radiolucency following the same pattern, the intact surface zone and accentuation of the striae of Retzius. (By kind permission of the late Professor Al Darling.)

Microradiography, which will detect demineralisation in excess of 5%, shows that the area of radiolucency corresponds closely with the size and shape of the body of the lesion, in contrast to the surface zone which appears relatively radiopaque (Fig. 3.15). Alternating radiopaque and radiolucent lines, about 30 μm apart, can also be seen passing obliquely through the subsurface region. The radiolucent lines show an apparently preferential demineralisation and probably represent the striae of Retzius. At higher magnifications, still finer lines running at right angles to the enamel surface, and others parallel to the surface, may be discerned. These lines may represent preferential demineralisation along the junctional sites mentioned earlier and represent the prism boundaries and the cross-striations, respectively.

The surface zone represents one of the most important changes in enamel caries in terms of prevention and management of the disease. It shows the paradoxical feature that it has not merely remained intact during this stage of the attack but remains more heavily mineralised and radiopaque than the deeper zones. It has a pore volume of only 1%.

When the surface zone is removed and the enamel is exposed to an acid buffer, the more highly mineralised surface zone reappears over the deeper changes described earlier. The surface zone therefore appears to form partly by remineralisation. The remineralising salts may come either from those concentrated in the plaque or from precipitation of calcium and phosphate ions diffusing outwards as the deeper zones are demineralised.

In pit and fissure caries, the same changes take place but, as acid diffuses out from the pit, the lesion forms a ring round it. However, in a two-dimensional view, the same zones as in smooth surface caries are seen on either side of the fissure (Fig. 3.16).

As noted earlier, the initial attack on enamel appears to be by highly mobile hydrogen ions permeating the organic matrix enabling them to attack the surface of the apatite crystals. The apatite crystals become progressively smaller. Microdissection of the translucent zone has shown that the apatite crystals have declined in diameter from the normal of 35–40 nm to 25–30 nm and in the body of the lesion to 10–30 nm. In the dark zone, by contrast, enamel crystals appeared to have grown to 50–100 nm and in the surface zone to 35–40 nm. These findings also suggest that demineralisation and remineralisation are alternating processes. However, as the lesion progresses and cavitation develops, demineralisation comes to dominate the process.

In broad general terms, therefore, enamel crystallites are progressively dissolved until disintegration becomes visible microscopically. Defects eventually become large enough to allow bacteria to enter.

There is evidence of preferential destruction of the prism cores and, experimentally, a similar effect is seen when enamel is exposed to dilute acid (Figs 3.17 and 3.18). Whatever the precise nature of these changes, bacteria do not physically penetrate enamel until acid destruction of the tissue has provided pathways large enough for them to enter, the stage of cavitation (Figs 3.19 and 3.20).

Cavity formation

Once bacteria have penetrated the enamel they reach the amelodentinal junction and spread laterally to undermine the enamel (Fig. 3.21). This has three major effects. First, the enamel loses the support of the dentine and is therefore greatly weakened. Second, it is attacked from beneath (Fig. 3.22). Third, spread of bacteria along the amelodentinal junction allows them to attack the dentine over a wide area (Fig. 3.23). Thus, the primary lesion provides the bridgehead for the attack on enamel, but undermining of the enamel determines the area of a cavity.

Clinically, this is frequently evident when there is no more than a pinhole lesion in an occlusal pit, but cutting away the surrounding enamel shows it to be widely undermined.

As undermining of the enamel continues, it starts to collapse under the stress of mastication and to fragment around the edge of the (clinically obvious) cavity. By this stage, bacterial damage to the dentine is extensive.

The process of enamel caries is summarised in Box 3.13.

Fig. 3.17 Chalky enamel. An electronphotomicrograph of chalky enamel produced by the action of very dilute acid. The crystallites of calcium salts remain intact in the prism sheaths, while the prism cores and some of the interprismatic substance have been destroyed. The same appearance is seen in chalky enamel caused by early caries. (By kind permission of Dr K Little.)

Fig. 3.18 The organic matrix of developing enamel. An electronphotomicrograph of a section across the lines of the prisms before calcification showing the matrix to be more dense in the region of the prism sheaths than in the prism cores or interprismatic substance. (By kind permission of Dr K Little.)

Box 3.13 Process of enamel caries

- Permeation of the organic matrix by hydrogen ions causes submicroscopic changes
- The early damage is submicroscopic and seen as a series of zones of differing translucency
- Microradiography confirms that these changes represent areas of increasing demineralisation
- The surface zone is largely formed by remineralisation
- There is alternating demineralisation and remineralisation, but demineralisation is predominant as cavity formation progresses
- Bacteria cannot invade enamel until demineralisation provides pathways large enough for them to enter (cavitation)

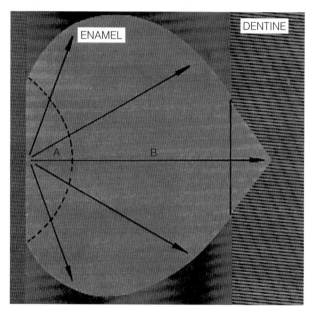

Fig. 3.19 Diagram summarising the main features of the precavitation phase of enamel caries as indicated here in this final stage of acid attack on enamel before bacterial invasion, decalcification of dentine has begun. The area (A) would be radiolucent in a bite-wing film but the area (B) could be visualised only in a section by polarised light microscopy or microradiography. Clinically, the enamel would appear solid and intact but the surface would be marked by an opaque white spot over the area (A) as seen in Figure 3.11 (From McCracken AW, Cawson RA 1983 Clinical and oral microbiology. McGraw-Hill.)

Fig. 3.20 Early cavitation in enamel caries. The surface layer of the white spot lesion has broken down, allowing plaque bacteria into the enamel.

Fig. 3.21 **Low-power view of caries spreading along the amelodentinal junction.** Note how it spreads only a small distance in advance of caries in dentine. The amelodentinal junction is only a little more susceptible to carious spread than dentine.

Fig. 3.22 Caries spread along the amelodentinal junction at higher power showing how enamel is undermined and invaded from below. The terminations of the dentinal tubules are also infected but destruction, at this stage, is mainly at the expense of the enamel because of its higher mineral content.

Fig. 3.23 Bite-wing radiograph showing interproximal caries below many of the contact points.

PATHOLOGY OF DENTINE CARIES

The initial (non-bacterial) lesion forms deep to carious enamel before a cavity has formed. Diffusion of acid into the dentine leaves its collagenous matrix intact at this stage. However, once bacteria have penetrated the enamel, they spread along the amelodentinal junction to attack the dentine over a wide area. The lesion is therefore conical with its apex towards the pulp (Fig. 3.24).

Infection of the lesion is facilitated by the dentinal tubules which form a pathway open to bacteria (Fig. 3.25). After demineralisation, the dentine matrix is progressively destroyed by proteolysis.

Streptococci play the major role in the attack on enamel, but lactobacilli may be as important in dentine caries. As the lesion progresses, the bacterial population becomes increasingly mixed and their relative contributions to dentine destruction become more difficult to disentangle.

At first, the decalcified dentine retains its normal morphology and no bacteria can be seen. Once bacteria have reached the amelodentinal junction they extend down the tubules, soon fill them and spread along any lateral branches. The tubules become distended into spindle shapes by the expanding masses of bacteria and their products, which the softened matrix cannot confine. As a result, adjacent less heavily infected tubules become bent. Later still, the intervening tubule walls are destroyed and collections of bacteria in adjacent tubules coalesce to form irregular liquefaction foci. These, in turn, coalesce to form progressively more widespread tissue destruction (Figs 3.26 and 3.27).

In some areas, bacteria also spread laterally and, occasionally, large bacteria-filled clefts form at right angles to the general direction of the tubules. Clinically, these clefts may allow carious dentine sometimes to be excavated in flakes in a plane parallel to the surface (Fig. 3.28).

The main events in dentine caries are summarised in Box 3.14.

Box 3.14 **Key events in the development of dentine caries**

- Non-bacterial, precavitation, acid softening of matrix
- Widening of tubules by demineralisation
- Migration of pioneer bacteria along tubules
- Distortion of tubules by expanding masses of bacteria
- Breakdown of intervening matrix forming liquefaction foci
- Progressive disintegration of remaining matrix tissue

Protective reactions of dentine and pulp under caries

The reactions in dentine are mainly due to odontoblast activity, so that dentine and pulp should be considered as one tissue. These reactions are not specific and may be provoked by other irritants such as attrition, erosion, abrasion and restorative procedures. Reactionary changes in dentine start even before cavity formation in enamel, but are more likely to develop significantly under slowly progressing caries.

HISTOPATHOLOGY   ENAMEL CARES

1   2   3a   3b   4a   4b   5   6

NAKED EYE

BITEWING X4

PROBE

NAKED EYE

CLINICAL X4

WHITE ▨CAVITY ■
SPOT

KEY TO HISTOPATHOLOGY:		SPACES	DECALCIFICATION	ORGANIC CHANGE
☐	TRANSLUCENT ZONE	1%	–	–
▦	DARK ZONE	2–4%	+	–
☐	BODY OF LESION	5–25%	+ + OR + + +	–
▨	ORGANIC CHANGE	25%	+ + + +	+

Fig. 3.24 This diagram summarises the sequential changes in enamel from the stage of the initial lesion to early cavity formation and relates the different stages in the development of the lesion with the radiographic appearances and clinical findings. (Diagram kindly lent by the late Professor Al Darling and reproduced by courtesy of the Editor of the British Dental Journal 1959; 107:27–30.)

Fig. 3.25 **Infection of the dentinal tubules.** This electronphotomicrograph shows bacteria in the lumen of the tubules. Between the tubules is the collagenous matrix of the dentine. (By kind permission of K Little.)

Reactionary changes in dentine are summarised in Table 3.3. These reactionary changes start to develop early but at best can only slow the advance of dental caries. Even sclerotic dentine is vulnerable to bacterial acid and proteolysis and once bacteria have penetrated the normal dentine they can invade any reactionary dentine to reach the pulp (Figs 3.29–3.32).

Root surface caries

When the neck of the tooth becomes exposed by recession of the gingival margin in later life, a stagnation area may be formed and the cementum attacked. Cementum is readily

Fig. 3.26 **Caries of dentine.** Infected tubules and fusiform masses of bacteria have expanded into the softened tissue. Adjacent tubules in the demineralised dentine have been bent and pushed aside by these masses.

decalcified and presents little barrier to infection. The cementum therefore softens beneath the plaque over a wide area, producing a saucer-shaped cavity and the underlying dentine is soon involved. Cementum is invaded along the direction of Sharpey's fibres. Infection spreads between the lamellae along the incremental lines, with the result that the dentine becomes split up and progressively destroyed by a combination of

Fig. 3.27 **Advanced dentine caries.** The dentine is disintegrating (left). To the right is a large liquefaction focus and tubules packed with bacteria.

Fig. 3.28 **Clefts in carious dentine.** Infection is tracking along the tubules but has also spread across the tubules, forming heavily infected clefts. The appearances suggest that there are lines of weakness in the dentine, along which infection spreads easily.

Fig. 3.29 **A translucent zone.** The dentinal tubules are seen in cross-section. Those in the centre of the picture have become obliterated by calcification of their contents; only the original outline of the tubules remains visible and the zone appears translucent to transmitted light. On either side are patent tubules filled with stain. (Kindly lent by Dr GC Blake, and reproduced by courtesy of the Honorary Editors, Proceedings of the Royal Society of Medicine 1958; 51:678.)

Arrested caries and remineralisation

Precavity (white spot) interstitial caries may become arrested when the adjacent tooth is lost so that the stagnation area is removed. The lesion may become remineralised by minerals from the saliva.

Dentine caries may occasionally be arrested as a result of destruction of so much enamel that a wide area of dentine becomes exposed. If this surface is then subjected to attrition, plaque deposition may be prevented and saliva in contact with

demineralisation and proteolysis. The further progress of caries in the underlying dentine is essentially similar to that in other parts of the tooth.

Table 3.3	Reactionary changes in dentine
Response	**Key facts**
Tubular sclerosis	Peritubular dentine reduces the size of the dentinal tubules, preventing bacterial penetration and generating a more heavily mineralised dentine. Tubular sclerosis usually forms in a band about halfway between the pulp and amelodentinal junction. It forms a translucent zone which may be visible radiographically and is detectable with hand instruments when excavating caries
Regular reactionary dentine	Forms at the pulp–dentine interface and retains the tubular structure of dentine. Forms in response to mild stimuli and may obliterate pulp horns, increasing the dentine thickness between caries and pulp. Unfortunately, it often forms most on the floor and sides of the pulp chamber where it is of little value in defence against caries
Irregular reactionary dentine	Forms in response to moderate or severe insult by caries and correspondingly ranges from dentine with irregular tubules to a disorganized bone-like mineralised tissue ('eburnoid')
Dead tracts	Formed when odontoblasts die and their tubules become sealed off. If peritubular dentine formation was extensive before odontoblast death, the dead tract may be sclerotic and inhibit advance of caries. If not, it may allow more rapid progress

Fig. 3.30 **Regular reactionary dentine below occlusal caries.** Bacteria extend more than half the distance from the amelodentinal junction to the pulp and the underlying pulp horn has been obliterated by reactionary dentine. The reactionary dentine bulges into the pulp. Note the lack of inflammation in the pulp.

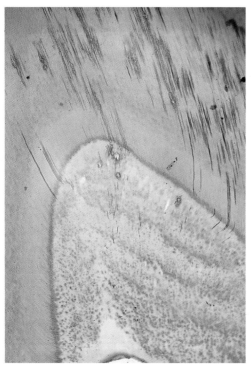

Fig. 3.31 **Secondary (reactionary) dentine and caries.** Regular, tubular, secondary dentine has formed under a carious cavity. A line marks the junction of the primary and secondary dentine where the tubules change direction. Bacteria spreading down the tubules of the primary tissue have extended along the junction and into the tubules of the reactionary dentine.

Fig. 3.32 **A dead tract.** The empty tubules below the worn incisal edge have been filled with a stain to which they are permeable from the surface, so that the whole zone appears black. At the proximal end of the tubules the dead tract has been sealed off by impermeable reactionary dentine through which the stain cannot penetrate. The pulp is thus protected from irritants penetrating along the dentinal tubules.

Under favourable conditions, carious demineralisation can be reversed and early lesions can remineralise. Use of fluorides and consumption of a less cariogenic diet may cause a surface lesion in enamel to heal entirely. Even under natural conditions, approximately 50% of interproximal enamel lesions may show no radiographic evidence of progression for 3 years. Similarly, in some patients, secondary caries may not necessarily develop at the margins of restorations overhanging the enamel.

Adult and childhood caries

In adults, caries usually progresses slowly and a small cavity may take several months to develop. By contrast, childhood

the lesion can contribute to remineralisation. More frequently, but still uncommonly, dentine is exposed by attrition and remains caries-free for the same reason. It becomes smooth, polished and stained (see Fig. 4.36).

Table 3.4 **The pathology of dental caries and its relevance to caries progression and treatment**

Feature	Significance
Plaque flora is a stable ecosystem	The bacterial flora is influenced by its environment but the ecosystem will resist change in the short term. Denial of cariogenic substrate by dietary control will reduce the number of cariogenic species but dietary change must be maintained to be effective
The early carious lesion is a subsurface process	Bacteria cannot enter the enamel until the surface layer is destroyed and until then can be removed by cleaning. Until cavitation, complete repair by remineralisation is possible and prevention of cavitation is critical
Enamel is permeable, pores between crystallites account for 0.1% of its volume. Odontoblast processes extend to the enamel–dentine junction	Enamel is porous, acids diffuse in readily to initiate caries and diffuse to dentine to trigger pulp defence reactions early in the lesion's lifespan, well before a lesion cavitates
The translucent zone in enamel caries is present in only approximately half of carious lesions examined	The translucent zone indicates progression. Many lesions are not active much of the time
The dark zone of enamel caries is seen in almost all lesions	The dark zone indicates remineralisation. Therefore, almost all lesions undergo periodic phases of remineralisation. In a remineralised or arrested lesion, the dark zone extends to replace much of the body of the lesion
Carious lesions undergo rapid phases of demineralisation and remineralisation. Activity or arrest may be the outcome depending on the relative proportion of each	Caries may remineralise, arrest or progress only very slowly so that, initially, observation or preventive intervention rather than restoration is appropriate for most enamel lesions
The surface zone of an enamel lesion is only 30 µm thick and porous	Pressure from probing may cavitate lesions, converting an arrested or slowly progressing lesion into an active lesion. Diagnosis should not attempt to indent the surface to judge 'stickiness', only to remove plaque and feel the surface texture Fluoride and other remineralising agents may enter the lesion easily Porous enamel takes up exogenous pigments so that long-standing lesions become 'brown spot' lesions
Fissure caries spreads laterally into the walls of a fissure, not into its base	The surface layer of occlusal enamel becomes undermined but is not initially directly involved. It may not fracture or appear abnormal until the underlying lesion is large (occult caries)
The shape of the enlarging occlusal lesion is guided inwards and laterally by the prism direction	An occlusal lesion involves a much greater area of dentine than a comparably-sized smooth surface lesion
The shape of the advancing front of a carious lesion in dentine is smooth and rounded	To conserve tooth structure, cavities should have smooth rounded outlines and no sharp internal angles
Caries spreads laterally along the amelodentinal junction	Lateral extension of a cavity is often determined by clearing caries from the amelodentinal junction (ADJ). However, caries usually only spreads laterally to approximately the extent of the lesion at the surface and in underlying dentine. Although leaving caries at the junction is undesirable because it leaves enamel poorly supported, removal of ADJ caries can be undertaken conservatively
Cavitation develops unpredictably in relation to the size and extent of an approximal lesion on a radiograph	Some assessment of the patient's caries risk involving dietary analysis, fluoride and other factors is required before deciding that any lesion requires operative intervention. Lesions in a high-risk patient cavitate earlier than in a low-risk patient
The pulp–dentine complex responds to caries. The dentine just before the advancing front of a carious lesion is relatively impermeable as a result of remineralisation and tubular sclerosis	The pulp–dentine defence reactions should be preserved and this is best achieved by non-operative intervention rather than restoration. Minimal dentine should be removed in cavity preparation. In deep lesions, removal of all softened dentine over the pulp should be avoided
Dentine caries may be divided into zones of demineralisation, penetration	Traditionally, cavity preparation involved removal of infected dentine. However, it is not necessary to remove all infected dentine to provide a successful restoration. The correct amount to remove is

(continued)

57

Table 3.4 *(continued)*

Feature	Significance
and destruction or into zones of infected and affected dentine	usually judged by the degree of softening. Discoloration is a less effective indicator. Discoloured but 'reasonably firm' (not hard) dentine may be left in situ. These zones are of little significance beyond understanding the disease process and none can be reliably identified clinically
Peritubular dentine and remineralisation form a sclerotic zone that walls off the lesion	Lateral spread is slowed as caries penetrates dentine. When removing softened dentine with hand instruments or a slowly revolving bur, sclerotic dentine may be felt to be harder than adjacent dentine and should be preserved
Peritubular dentine forms slowly	Only slowly advancing lesions are delayed by this defence reaction. A sclerotic zone visible radiographically indicates a slowly progressing or arrested lesion
Dentinal tubules in mature teeth are slightly smaller than bacterial cocci	Bacterial penetration of dentine towards the pulp can only take place after some dentine demineralisation
Demineralisation precedes bacterial invasion in dentine by a small and variable distance	Not all softened dentine must be removed during cavity preparation
The advancing front of bacterial penetration into dentine is irregular at a microscopic level	The relatively large mechanical instruments used to remove softened dentine will always leave some infected dentine behind. However, if sealed effectively below restorations, these bacteria will be rendered inert
Superficial infected dentine is denatured and cannot remineralise. Deeper dentine will remineralise even though it contains bacteria	It is not necessary to remove all infected dentine to place a restoration, only the dentine that cannot remineralise if sealed below the restoration. Therefore, caries removal may be more conservative below a well-sealed adhesive restoration than below an amalgam
Dentine matrix is denatured by bacteria in the superficial layers of the zone of destruction	This renders the dentine susceptible to chemomechanical caries removal using proprietary mixtures of sodium hypochlorite. This procedure removes only the most damaged carious dentine, a conservative approach that preserves the deeper layers that can remineralise
Dentine splits transversely along incremental lines of growth in the zone of destruction	Dentine caries in the outer zone of destruction is easily removed in large flakes with hand instruments
Caries indicator dyes stain softened as well as infected dentine	Adhering strictly to the dye protocol will remove remineralisable dentine that should be left in situ. Caries indicator dyes promote overcutting
Reactionary dentine forms slowly and varies markedly in amount, quality and permeability and is found below only half the lesions in permanent teeth (more frequent in primary teeth)	Reactionary dentine provides little protection below rapidly progressing lesions
Formation of reactionary dentine requires a good blood supply and healthy pulp	Less is formed in older individuals. Once the pulp is inflamed the quality of any reactionary dentine is poor and it is unlikely to be of much benefit
Symptoms of pulpitis do not correlate well with caries activity, lesion size, pulpal inflammation or even direct pulp involvement	Pulp vitality may be lost without symptoms, or with only mild symptoms. An assessment of the state of a pulp is desirable to plan restoration of a deep carious lesion but, if based on symptoms, is unlikely to be accurate
Lesions of root caries also have a surface remineralised layer	Avoid hard probing of apparently intact though discoloured surfaces, as for enamel caries
Bacteria penetrate dentine early in root caries lesions but are accessible to preventive measures	Removal of infected dentine is not always necessary to treat early root caries
Primary teeth have approximately half the thickness of enamel of permanent teeth, larger pulps, longer pulp horns and, at least initially, larger dentinal tubules	Caries progresses faster in primary teeth than in permanent teeth

caries, particularly of deciduous teeth, may be so rapid that the pulp becomes exposed long before the tooth is due to be shed.

Pulpitis

Pulpitis follows penetration of dentine by bacteria or their metabolites and represents the breakdown of the protective hard dental tissues and opening of the soft tissues to infection.

Clinical aspects of reactions to caries

The reactive changes described above render the dentine immediately under a carious cavity more or less impermeable, unless caries is advancing very rapidly.

A good knowledge of all phases of the carious process is essential to understand the rationale of modern preventive and restorative treatment. The clinical relevance of caries pathology is shown in Table 3.4.

SUGGESTED FURTHER READING

Bowen WH 1999 Wither or whither caries research? Caries Res 33:1–3

Brathall D 1992 Caries, views and perspectives. Scand J Dent Res 100:47–51

Carlsson J 1989 Microbial aspects of frequent intake of products with high sugar concentrations. Scand J Dent Res 97:110–114

Costerton JW et al 1987 Bacterial biofilms in nature and disease. Ann Rev Microbiol 41:435–464

Frank MJ 1990 Structural events in the caries process in enamel, cementum and dentine. J Dent Res 69(Spec Iss):559–566

Gibbons RJ 1989 Bacterial adhesion to oral tissues: a model for infectious diseases. J Dent Res 68:750–760

Hardie JM, Whiley RA 1999 Plaque microbiology of crown caries. In: Newman HN, Wilson M (eds). Dental plaque revisited. Bioline, Cardiff

Kishimoto D, Hay DI, Gibbons RJ 1989 A human salivary protein which promotes adhesion of *Streptococcus mutans* serotype c strains to hydroxyapatite. Infect Immun 57:3702–3707

Levine RS 1989 Saliva: 2. Saliva and dental caries. Dental Update 14:158–165

Liang L, Drake D, Doyle RJ 1989 Stability of the glucan-binding lectin of oral streptococci. J Dent Res 68(Spec Iss):1677

McHugh WD 1999 Dental plaque: thirty years on. In: Newman HN, Wilson M (eds). Dental plaque revisited. Bioline, Cardiff

Mergenhagen SE et al 1987 Molecular basis of bacterial adhesion in the oral cavity. Rev Infect Dis 9(Suppl 5):S467–475

Moller H, Scroder U 1986 Early natural subsurface caries. A SEM study of the enamel surface before and after remineralisation. Caries Res 20:97–102

Newbrun E 1989 Frequent sugar intake – then and now: interpretation of the main results. Scand J Dent Res 97:103–109

Roberts MW, Li S-H 1987 Oral findings in anorexia nervosa and bulimia nervosa: a study of 47 cases. JADA 115:407–410

Rugg-Gunn AJ, Hackett AF, Appleton DR 1987 Relative cariogenicity of starch and sugars in a 2-year longitudinal study of 405 English schoolchildren. Caries Res 21:464–473

Russell MW, Hajishengallis G, Childers NK et al 1999 Secretory immunity in defense against cariogenic *mutans* streptococci. Caries Res 33:4–15

Shaw JH 1987 Causes and control of dental caries. N Engl J Med 317:996–1003

Shellis RP, Dibdin GH 1988 Analysis of the buffer systems in dental plaque. J Dent Res 67:438–446

Tabak LA, Bowen WH 1989 Role of saliva (pellicle), diet and nutrition on plaque formation. J Dent Res 68(Spec Iss):1560–1566

Van Houte J 1994 Role of micro-organisms in caries etiology. J Dent Res 73:672–681

Woodward M, Walker ARP 1994 Sugar consumption and dental caries: evidence from 90 countries. Br Dent J 176:297–302

Pulpitis, apical periodontitis, resorption and hypercementosis

PULPITIS → Summaries pp. 66, 448

Pulpitis is the most common cause of dental pain and loss of teeth in younger persons. The usual cause is caries penetrating the dentine, but there are other possibilities (Box 4.1). Pulpitis, if untreated, is followed by death of the pulp and spread of infection through the apical foramina into the periapical tissues. This in turn causes periapical periodontitis.

Box 4.1   Causes of pulpitis

- Dental caries
- Traumatic exposure of the pulp
- Fracture of a crown or cusp
- Cracked tooth syndrome
- Thermal or chemical irritation

Dental caries is by far the most common cause and is usually obvious unless it is concealed beneath a restoration.

Exposure during cavity preparation allows bacteria to enter the pulp and also damages it mechanically (Fig. 4.1).

Fracture may either open the pulp chamber or leave so thin a covering of dentine that bacteria can enter.

A tooth, particularly a restored premolar, may split, usually under masticatory stress (Fig. 4.2). These minute cracks are often invisible, but allow bacteria into the pulp chamber. The affected tooth may sometimes be identified by applying pressure to the occlusal fissure with a ball-ended burnisher to open up the crack. Pulp pain usually then results. Alternatively, the crack may be made visible with oblique transillumination or, possibly more easily, by wetting the crown of the tooth with a dye such as fluorescein and visualising it with ultraviolet light.

Insufficient cooling during cavity cutting, especially of deep cavities, can cause immediate damage to the pulp. Large unlined metal restorations may also allow continuous low-grade thermal stimuli to damage the pulp over a longer period. Some restorations without a protective lining, particularly in the past, were sufficiently irritant to kill the pulp.

Clinical features

The pulps of individual teeth are not precisely represented on the sensory cortex. The pulp pain is therefore poorly localised

Fig. 4.1   Traumatic exposure. The pulp has been exposed during cavity preparation and dentine chippings and larger fragments have been driven into the pulp. The tooth was extracted before a strong inflammatory reaction has had time to develop, but it is clear that some inflammatory cells have already localised around the debris which will have introduced many bacteria to the pulp.

and may be felt in any of the teeth of the upper or lower jaw of the affected side. Rarely, pain may be referred to a more distant site such as the ear. Pulp pain is not provoked by pressure on the tooth. The patient can chew in comfort unless there is a large open cavity allowing fragments of food to press on the pulp through the softened dentine.

Acute pulpitis   In the early stages the tooth is hypersensitive. Very cold or hot food causes a stab of pain which stops as soon as the irritant is removed. As inflammation progresses, pain becomes more persistent and there may be prolonged attacks of toothache. The pain may start spontaneously, often when the patient is trying to get to sleep.

The pain is partly due to the pressure on the irritated nerve endings by inflammatory infiltrate within the rigid pulp chamber and partly due to release of pain-producing substances

Fig. 4.4   Acute pulpitis. Low-power view showing occlusal caries penetrating to the pulp through a layer of reactionary dentine. There is acute inflammation localised to the pulp horn.

Fig. 4.2   Cracked tooth. The pulp died beneath this crack which was undetected clinically but which has opened up after decalcification of the tooth.

Fig. 4.5   Acute pulpitis. Beneath the carious exposure (top right) a dense inflammatory infiltrate is accumulating. More deeply, the pulp is intensely hyperaemic.

Fig. 4.3   Pulpal hyperaemia. While bacteria are still some distance from the pulp, acid permeating along the dentinal tubules gives rise to hyperaemia, oedema and a light cellular inflammatory infiltrate in the pulp.

from the damaged tissue. The pain at its worst is excruciatingly severe, sharp and stabbing in character. It is little affected by simple analgesics.

The outcome of acute pulpitis is unpredictable. Acute pulpitis may be deemed irreversible on the basis of constant severe pain or the persistence of pain after a hot or cold stimulus but, even then, the pulp may survive. Though pulp death is the likely outcome, acute pulpitis may progress to chronic pulpitis and treatment can still preserve pulp vitality. Diagnosis of irreversible pulpitis is considered an indication for extirpation of the pulp, but it must be recognized that the criteria are poorly defined.

Chronic pulpitis   Chronic pulpitis may develop with or without episodes of acute pulpitis. However, many pulps under large carious cavities die painlessly. The first indication is then development of periapical periodontitis, either with pain or seen by chance in a radiograph. In other cases, there are bouts of dull pain, brought on by hot or cold stimuli or coming on spontaneously. There are often prolonged remissions and there may be recurrent acute exacerbations.

61

Fig. 4.6   Acute pulpitis. Infection has penetrated the reactionary dentine causing inflammation to spread down the pulp and pus to form in the corner.

Fig. 4.8   Acute pulpitis – terminal stage. The entire pulp has been destroyed and replaced by inflammatory cells and dilated vessels.

Fig. 4.7   Acute caries and pulpitis. Infection has penetrated to the pulp. Part of the pulp has been destroyed and an abscess has formed, containing a bead of pus.

Pathology

Pulpitis may result from a variety of causes (see Box 4.1). Pulpitis caused by caries results from penetration of acid and bacterial products through the dentine and, later, from a mixed bacterial infection penetrating to the pulp.

Acute closed pulpitis   Histologically, there is initial hyperaemia limited to the area immediately beneth the irritant (Fig. 4.3). Infiltration by inflammatory cells and destruction of odontoblasts and adjacent mesenchyme follow. A limited area of necrosis may result in formation of a minute abscess, localised by granulation tissue (Figs 4.4–4.7). Later, inflammation spreads until the pulp is obliterated by dilated blood vessels and acute inflammatory cells (Fig. 4.8). Necrosis follows.

Chronic closed pulpitis   The main features are a predominantly mononuclear cell infiltrate and a more vigorous connective tissue reaction. A small area of pulpal necrosis and pus formation may be localised by a well-defined wall of granulation tissue and a minute abscess may thus form. The remainder of the pulp may then appear normal.

Rarely, inflammation may be well localised beneath an exposure so that a partial calcific barrier forms beneath the lesion, or considerable amounts of reactionary dentine continue to form round the opening. Such changes are particularly likely to follow pulp capping. Calcific barriers (seen radiographically as 'dentine bridges') are frequently poorly formed and inflammation progresses beneath them (Figs 4.9 and 4.10). However, in successful cases, formation of a complete barrier of tubular reactionary dentine may allow preservation of the remainder of the pulp.

The chief factor hampering pulpal survival is its enclosure within the rigid walls of the pulp chamber and, in fully formed teeth, the limited aperture for the apical vessels. In acute inflammation, these vessels can readily be compressed by inflammatory oedema and thrombose. The blood supply of the pulp is thus cut off and it dies. This may be rapid in the case of acute pulpitis, or delayed in chronic lesions. The relatively

Fig. 4.9 **Calcific barriers.** (A) Another pulpitis and formation of a thick calcific barrier, but with an abscess immediately below it. The rest of the pulp is inflamed. (B) This higher-power view of another barrier induced by pulp capping shows the calcific barrier in more detail, in particular its irregular structure and failure to hold back the infection.

Fig. 4.11 **Open pulpitis.** Beneath the wide exposure the pulp has survived in the form of granulation tissue with the most dense inflammatory infiltrate beneath the open surface.

Fig. 4.10 **Pulp capping.** The procedure has allowed the pulp to survive until reactionary dentine has proliferated greatly beside the exposure. Failure of the procedure is indicated by the inflammatory cells concentrated below the opening.

prolonged survival of chronically inflamed pulps is shown by the persistence of symptoms over a long period. However, pulp death is the end result unless treatment is successful.

Open pulpitis Occasionally the pulp survives but is chronically inflamed, beneath a wide exposure, despite the heavy infection (Fig. 4.11). This is traditionally believed to be associated with open apices which allow an adequate blood supply.

Chronic hyperplastic pulpitis (pulp polyp) Rarely, despite wide exposure and heavy infection, the pulp not merely survives but proliferates through the opening. This may even happen in fully formed teeth.

Clinically, a pulp polyp appears as a dusky red or pinkish soft nodule protruding into the cavity. It is painless but may be tender and bleed on probing. It should be distinguished from proliferating gingival tissue extending over the edge of the cavity by tracing its attachment (Fig. 4.12).

Histologically, few odontoblasts survive and the pulp becomes replaced by granulation tissue (Fig. 4.13). As this mass grows out into the cavity in the tooth it can become epithelialised and covered by a layer of well-formed stratified

Fig. 4.12 **Pulp polyp.** An inflamed nodule of granulation tissue can be seen growing from the pulp chamber of this broken down first permanent molar.

Fig. 4.14 **Pulp polyp.** In this broken down molar, granulation tissue is proliferating from the pulp cavity and has acquired an epithelial covering over much of its surface. Note also the internal resorption (left) as a result of pulpal inflammation.

Box 4.2 **Treatment options for pulpitis**

- If fractured or cracked, stabilise fracture and seal pulp temporarily
- Removal of caries, obtundent or steroid dressing
- Removal of caries and pulp capping
- Pulpotomy in deciduous teeth
- Endodontic treatment
- Extraction
- Analgesics are largely ineffective

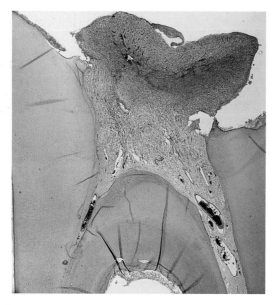

Fig. 4.13 **Pulp polyp.** A hyperplastic nodule of tissue is growing out through a wide exposure of the pulp. The masses of inflammatory cells and the many new vessels are characteristic of granulation tissue.

Open pulpitis is usually associated with gross cavity formation and it is rarely possible to save the tooth, despite the vitality of the pulp.

Key features of pulpitis are summarised in Box 4.3 and the sequelae of pulpitis are shown in Summary chart 4.1.

Box 4.3 **Key features of pulpitis**

- Pulpitis is caused by infection or irritation of the pulp, usually by caries
- Severe stabbing pain in a tooth, triggered by hot or cold food or starting spontaneously, indicates acute irreversible pulpitis
- Pulp pain is poorly localised
- Chronic pulpitis is often symptomless
- Untreated pulpitis usually leads to death of the pulp and spread of infection to the periapical tissues

---

squamous epithelium. This protects the mass and allows inflammation under it to subside and fibrous tissue to replace the granulation tissue. This degree of pulpal proliferation can occasionally be seen in teeth with fully formed roots (Fig. 4.14).

Management

The chances of survival of an inflamed pulp are poor and treatment options are limited (Box 4.2).

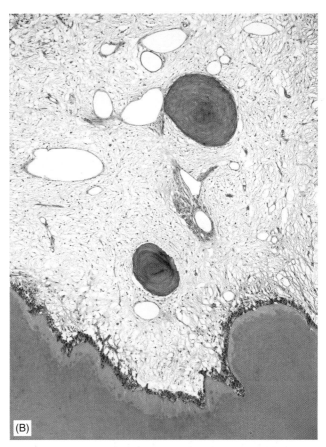

Fig. 4.15 **Pulp stones.** (A) The dystrophic pulp mineralisations often found as an age change. (B) Rounded nodules of calcified tissue, in this case resembling bone rather than dentine.

PULP CALCIFICATIONS

Pulp stones

Rounded masses of dentine may form within the pulp and can be seen in radiographs as small opacities. In the past, they were thought to cause symptoms but are developmental anomalies. For unknown reasons, they are common in the teeth of patients with Ehlers–Danlos (floppy joint) syndrome, a genetic defect of collagen formation.

Histologically, pulp stones consist of dentine which may show complete or incomplete tubule formation (Fig. 4.15). A distinction used to be drawn between free and attached pulp stones. However, this is frequently an illusion caused by a plane of section which fails to pass through the connection between the pulp stone and the pulp wall.

Diffuse calcification

Amorphous dystrophic calcifications may sometimes be seen histologically in the pulp and are thought to be an age-related degenerative change.

Pulp stones and diffuse calcification are of no clinical significance except insofar as they may obstruct endodontic treatment. Otherwise they can be ignored.

PERIAPICAL PERIODONTITIS → Summary p. 66

Periapical inflammation is usually due to spread of infection following death of the pulp (Box 4.4). It characteristically causes tenderness of the tooth in its socket. Local (periapical) periodontitis must be distinguished from chronic (marginal) periodontitis in which infection and destruction of the supporting tissues spread from chronic infection of the gingival margins (Ch. 5).

Box 4.4 **Causes of apical periodontitis**

- Infection
- Trauma
- Chemical irritation

Infection is by far the most common cause. The usual sequence of events is caries, pulpitis, death of the pulp and periodontitis (see Summary chart 4.1).

The pulp sometimes dies from a blow which damages the apical vessels. The necrotic pulp probably becomes infected by bacteria from the gingival margins, leading to apical periodontitis. A high filling or biting suddenly on a hard object sometimes cause an acute but usually transient periodontitis.

During endodontic treatment, instruments may be pushed through the apex or side of the root, damaging the periodontal membrane and carrying infected debris from the pulp chamber into the wound.

Irritant antiseptics used to sterilise a root canal can escape through the apex and damage the surrounding tissues. A root-canal filling may also extend beyond the apex with similar effect.

ACUTE APICAL PERIODONTITIS → Summaries pp. 66, 409

Clinical features

The patient may give a history of pain due to previous pulpitis. When periodontitis develops, escape of exudate into the periodontal ligament causes the tooth to be extruded by a minute amount and the bite to fall more heavily on it. The tooth is at

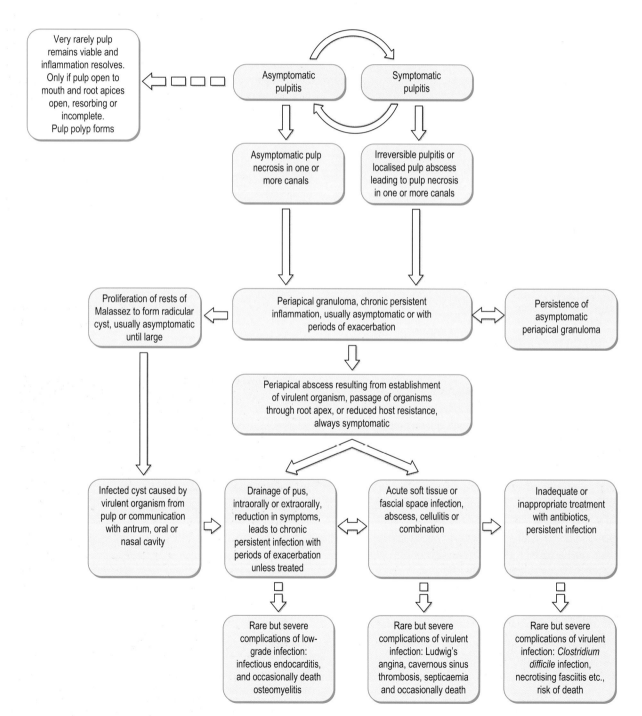

Summary chart 4.1 Sequelae of pulpitis.

first uncomfortable, then increasingly tender, even to mere touch. Hot or cold substances do not cause pain in the tooth unless some viable pulp remains, as it may in multirooted teeth. As inflammation becomes more severe and pus starts to form, pain becomes intense and throbbing in character. There is often a large carious cavity or filling in the affected tooth, or it may be discoloured due to death of the pulp earlier. At this stage, the gingiva over the root is red and tender, but there is no swelling while inflammation is confined within the bone. Unlike pulpitis, the pain of apical periodontitis is accurately localized by the patient because periodontal ligament receptors are triggered.

Radiographs give little information because bony changes have had too short a time to develop. Immediately round the apex, the lamina dura may appear slightly hazy and the periodontal space may be slightly widened. When acute periodontitis is due to exacerbation of a chronic infection, the original lesion can be seen as an area of radiolucency at the apex.

Exudate may penetrate overlying bone and periosteum a day or so after the onset of pain, allowing relief of the pressure. Pain quickly abates but exudate, if it cannot escape, distends the soft tissues to form a swelling. When an upper canine is affected, the swelling quickly spreads to the face and eyelid and may close the eye on that side (Fig. 4.16). In spite of the alarming appearance, the swelling is due initially only to oedema. It subsides when the tooth is extracted or the infection is drained.

The regional lymph nodes may be enlarged and tender, but general symptoms are usually slight or absent.

Inflammation typically remains localised. Further spread of infection can cause inflammation of the surrounding bone (osteomyelitis) or cellulitis (Ch. 6), but only exceedingly rarely.

Pathology

Acute apical periodontitis is a typical acute inflammatory reaction with engorged blood vessels and packing of the tissue with neutrophils (Fig. 4.17). These changes are initially localised to the immediate vicinity of the apex as a consequence of the rich blood supply to this area. The immediately adjacent lamina dura becomes resorbed and an abscess cavity may form if not aborted by treatment (Box 4.5).

Box 4.5   **Possible complications of acute apical periodontitis**

- Suppuration
- Regional lymphadenopathy
- Spreading infection

Treatment

Extraction of the diseased tooth removes the source of infection and drains the exudate. This is the simplest and most

Fig. 4.16   **Oedema due to acute apical periodontitis.** An acute periapical infection of a canine has perforated the buccal plate of bone causing oedema of the face; this quickly subsided when the infection was treated.

Fig. 4.17   **Acute apical periodontitis.** In this early acute lesion, inflammatory cells, mainly neutrophil polymorphonuclear leucocytes, are seen clustered around the apex of a non-vital tooth. The inflammatory cells are spreading around and into bone and there has not yet been time for significant bone resorption to develop.

effective treatment. Antibiotics should not be given for simple acute periodontitis if immediate dental treatment is available. Alternative treatment is to retain the tooth by endodontic treatment, which should also serve to drain the infection.

CHRONIC APICAL PERIODONTITIS → Summary p. 66

Clinical features

Chronic periodontitis is a low-grade infection. It may follow an acute infection that has been inadequately drained and incompletely resolved. The tooth is non-vital and may be slightly tender to percussion but, otherwise, symptoms may be minimal. Frequently, chronic periodontitis is first recognised as a rounded area of radiolucency at the apex of a tooth (an 'apical granuloma') in a routine radiograph (Fig. 4.18). The area is usually about 5mm in diameter and has well-defined margins. A distinct cortex is sometimes interpreted as early cyst formation, but this is partly a radiological artefact dependent on the size of the lesion. Cyst formation cannot be confirmed without a biopsy.

Pathology

Chronic periodontitis is a typical chronic inflammatory reaction characterised by lymphocytes, macrophages and plasma cells. Infection is confined by inflammatory cells and granulation tissue surrounds the area. The granulation tissue grows into a rounded mass (a 'granuloma') and osteoclasts resorb the bone to accommodate it (Figs 4.19 and 4.20).

Despite absence of symptoms, there is no spontaneous healing because of the persistent reservoir of infection in the root canal. Instead, granulation tissue proliferates round the focus of irritation at the tooth apex and surrounding bone is resorbed to leave a round area of radiolucency. Healing only follows extraction, effective endodontic treatment or apicectomy (Fig. 4.21).

Fig. 4.18 Chronic apical abscess. Periapical bone resorption has developed as a result of inflammation. The area of radiolucency corresponds with the histological changes seen in the next figure.

Variable degrees of proliferation of the epithelial rests of Malassez in a periapical granuloma at the apex of a dead tooth are common (Fig. 4.22). Epithelial proliferation may be sufficient to lead ultimately to cyst formation and is the most common cause of jaw cysts (Box 4.6).

Box 4.6   Possible complications of chronic apical periodontitis
• Periapical granuloma formation • Radicular cyst formation • Suppuration and sinus formation • Acute exacerbations

Fig. 4.19 Chronic periapical abscess. At the apex of the non-vital tooth is an abscess cavity surrounded by a thick fibrous wall densely infiltrated by inflammatory cells, predominantly neutrophils. Periapical bone has been resorbed and the trabeculae reorientated around the mass.

Fig. 4.20 High-power view of an apical granuloma showing neutrophils, lymphocytes and plasma cells in loose oedematous fibrous tissue.

This epithelium forms irregular strands or loops. Sometimes a microscopic cyst cavity, with a lining of hyperplastic epithelium, forms and represents the earliest stage of radicular cyst. In other cases, the epithelium is scanty or destroyed by the inflammation.

Periapical granulomas usually remain localised within the bone. Occasionally, there is abscess formation and pus may reach the surface by resorption of the bone (usually on the buccal surface of the gingiva) immediately over the apex of the tooth. A nodule of granulation tissue forms in response to the irritation by pus and marks the opening of the sinus.

An uncommon complication, but sometimes the first sign of periapical periodontitis, is the tracking of a sinus onto the skin surface. This most frequently happens on or near the chin as a result of a long-forgotten blow and death of a lower incisor (Fig. 4.23). In such cases, the crown of the damaged tooth is usually discoloured (Fig. 4.24) and may be chipped. A radiograph shows the periapical area of bone destruction. Many patients fail to associate the sinus with dental infection, but competent endodontic treatment causes the sinus to heal remarkably quickly.

Fig. 4.21 **Low-power detail shows the effects of apicectomy.** The chronic inflammatory reaction has entirely cleared. New bone has formed to replace the excised apex and there is a condensation of connective tissue across the deep end of the root canal filling.

Fig. 4.23 **A persistent skin sinus from a lower incisor rendered non-vital by a blow some time previously.** This young woman was seen and treated unsuccessfully for 2 years by her doctor, surgeons and dermatologists before anyone looked at her teeth.

Fig. 4.22 **Epithelial proliferation in an apical granuloma.** Inflammation induces proliferation of odontogenic epithelium in rests of Malassez. This change may lead to cyst formation (Ch. 7).

Fig. 4.24 **Non-vital incisor teeth, in this case as a result of trauma.** Haemorrhage and products of autolysis of the pulp discolour the dentine and darken the teeth.

Toothache or pain felt in teeth or alveolus							
Pain of pulpal origin Sensitivity to sweet, hot or cold, poorly localised			Pain of periodontal ligament origin Pain on biting or pressure on tooth, usually well localised to one or more teeth			Neurological or vascular pain	Psychogenic pain
Dentine hypersentivity	Pulpitis Tooth is vital or partially vital and may be hypersensitive to testing		Cracked tooth or cusp	Periapical periodontitis	Periodontal abscess	Sinusitis		
Pain of short duration more or less limited to period of stimulus, particularly cold Confirm diagnosis by identifying exposed dentine or toothwear and applying appropriate treatment	Reversible pulpitis Symptoms may be limited to duration of stimulus or persist for varying period afterwards, caries or other cause may be evident May resolve on treating cause but once established may progress to irreversible pulpitis, even after an asymptomatic period	Irreversible pulpitis Poorly defined entity, usually identified by severe continuous or spontaneous pain Responds most reliably to extirpation of pulp or extraction	Shooting or electric shock-like pain on biting, often only on one cusp or in one direction, also when a fracture line involves periodontal ligament Confirm by identifying crack	Pain on pressure to single tooth, caries or other cause of pre-existing pulpitis may be present, periapical, lateral canal or furcation radiolucency only in long-standing cases Resolves on drainage or extirpation of pulp or extraction	Pain on pressure to single tooth, tooth vital, abscess in ligament visible or revealed by probing furcation or deep pocket Resolves on drainage and local treatment or extraction	Tenderness on pressure to teeth with apices near sinus, usually concurrent or recent nasal or sinus symptoms, not usually severe pain Resolves on treatment of sinusitis	Teeth vital unless previously devitalised for other reasons Consider mimics of pulpitis such as trigeminal neuralgia and the prodromal symptoms of facial Herpes zoster infection	Unusual localisation trigger or perceived cause, associated with depression, anxiety or delusional states, teeth vital unless previously devitalised for other reasons Consider atypical odontalgia, atypical facial pain, 'phantom tooth' etc, but only after excluding organic causes

Summary chart 4.2   Diagnosis of pulpal, periodontal and other pain in the teeth and alveolus.

Treatment

According to the state of the rest of the dentition, extraction or endodontic treatment are the main options. Competent endodontic treatment leads to healing even if cystic change has started. Persistence of chronic periodontitis after root canal treatment is usually due to technical faults and apicectomy may be required (see Fig. 4.21).

The diagnosis of pulpal, periodontal and other pain in the teeth and alveolus is summarized in Summary chart 4.2.

RESORPTION OF TEETH

The deciduous teeth are progressively loosened and ultimately shed as a result of progressive resorption of the roots as a physiological process arising from the pressure of the underlying successors. Resorption of permanent teeth is always pathological.

Whenever resorption takes place, there is usually some attempt at repair by apposition of cementum or bone. During resorption of deciduous teeth, a period of resorption is followed by one of repair, so that, clinically, the looseness of these teeth varies before they are shed.

Resorption is rarely important but, very occasionally, results from some destructive disease such as a tumour. Hypercementosis is also rarely important but may occasionally be a cause of difficult extractions.

Pathology

Pressure is probably the main factor. However, in some cases no cause is apparent. Resorption is mainly carried out by osteoclasts which, during active phases, may be seen in lacunae in the hard tissue with which their cytoplasm appears to merge (Fig. 4.25). When resorption is very slow, osteoclasts may not be seen and, being intermittent in their action, disappear during inactive periods. Humoral mediators, such as prostaglandins, may also contribute to bone resorption.

Resorption of deciduous teeth

Resorption of deciduous teeth occasionally leads to a few minor complications.

Ankylosis

In the resting stages of resorption, excessive repair tissue may be deposited until the root becomes fused to the adjacent bone.

Fig. 4.25 **Resorption during periapical periodontitis.** Active osteoclastic resorption of dentine is continuing in the presence of inflammatory exudate. This is a common change but usually minor in extent.

Fig. 4.26 Inflammatory resorption of the root apex induced by periapical periodontitis resulting from the non-vital pulp.

Box 4.7 **Important causes of resorption of permanent teeth**

- Periapical periodontitis. The most common cause, but is usually slight
- Impacted teeth pressing on the root of an adjacent tooth
- Unerupted teeth. Over the course of years these may undergo resorption or hypercementosis, or both
- Replanted teeth. These are sometimes rapidly and grossly resorbed
- Neoplasms. Resorption of related teeth is a typical sign of an intraosseous neoplasm such as an ameloblastoma
- Idiopathic. Peripheral and internal

This may prevent the tooth from being shed and the permanent successor from erupting. If not removed, the ankylosed tooth becomes partially submerged by the continued growth of the surrounding alveolar ridge. The tooth should be removed, surgically if necessary, to allow the successor to erupt.

Separation of an apex

Resorption may be irregular so that part of the tooth is cut off. The fragment remains buried or eventually appears on the surface.

Failure of resorption

Absence or misplacement of a permanent successor is the usual cause. The deciduous tooth may then remain in the arch for many years.

Resorption of permanent teeth

Resorption of permanent teeth is usually limited in extent, but may rarely destroy a large part of them. There are various causes (Box 4.7).

Cementum is most readily resorbed while enamel is the most resistant. When an impacted tooth presses on the roots of another, these are resorbed, but sometimes the crown of the impacted tooth may be destroyed.

Inflammation is a common cause and a minor degree of resorption is common on teeth associated with periapical

granulomas. Occasionally, this is a prominent feature leading to concern over the diagnosis (Fig. 4.26).

Idiopathic resorption

Internal resorption ('pink spot') is a curious and uncommon condition in which dentine is resorbed from within the pulp. Resorption tends to be localised, producing the characteristic sign of a well-defined rounded area of radiolucency in the crown (Fig. 4.27). This may affect an incisor tooth and a rounded pink area appears where the vascular pulp has become visible through the attenuated hard tissue. The cause is unknown, but it may possibly be a late result of damage to the blood supply of the pulp by a blow.

Idiopathic internal resorption can also affect any part of other teeth but causes no signs until the pulp is opened and allows access to infection. Alternatively, resorption may be detected by chance in a routine radiograph.

External resorption may be localised or generalized, the latter often affecting a group of teeth but, sometimes, the whole dentition. Both are of unknown cause, though a mild degree of inflammation is often suspected. Usually, a limited area of the root is attacked from its external surface near the

Fig. 4.27 Idiopathic internal resorption ('pink spot'). In this unusually severe example, resorption has progressed into the roots of three lower incisors.

Fig. 4.29 Idiopathic external resorption. A localised area of destruction of dentine produced by osteoclastic activity. The cavity is filled with proliferating connective tissue. The pulp shows no reaction and the sparing of the circumpulpal dentine until a late stage is a characteristic feature of external resorption.

Pathology

Vascular granulation tissue replaces the part of the periodontal ligament or pulp. Osteoclasts border the affected dentine or enamel. Inflammatory changes may be superimposed if the pulp chamber has been opened by destruction of its walls. Irregular repair with bone or cementum may take place (Figs 4.29 and 4.30).

Treatment

Idiopathic resorption is usually untreatable. However, if a pink spot in an incisor tooth is noticed at an early stage, endodontic treatment should be carried out before the pulp chamber becomes widely exposed.

Resorption of teeth may result from pressure exerted by impacted teeth (Fig. 4.31) and this is an indication for removal of the unerupted tooth.

Fig 4.28 Idiopathic external resorption. Resorption frequently starts at the amelocemental junction. In this case, the pulp is exposed.

amelocemental junction (Fig. 4.28) and resorption goes on until the pulp is reached. External resorption often preferentially destroys the root before penetrating to the pulp (Fig. 4.29). Accessible defects may be amenable to restoration with mineral trioxide or other materials, but long-term success is infrequent and unpredictable.

Generalised resorption may also start at the amelodentinal junction or near the apex. Over the course of years, the root may be destroyed. The lost tissue is partially repaired by bone-like tissue. Devitalising teeth does not slow progress and no treatment is effective.

HYPERCEMENTOSIS → Summary p. 173

Apposition of excessive amounts of cementum is not uncommon and due to several possible causes (Box 4.8), of which inflammation is probably the commonest pathological cause (Fig. 4.32).

Fig. 4.32 Hypercementosis as a result of apical inflammation.

Fig. 4.30 **Idiopathic resorption.** A grossly resorbed central incisor with a widely perforated pulp wall. The pulp has been replaced by granulation tissue and bony repair tissue has been laid down more deeply.

Fig. 4.31 Gross root resorption of two upper central incisors induced by an unerupted canine that has migrated across the midline.

Fig. 4.33 **Hypercementosis in Paget's disease.** An irregular craggy mass of bone-like cementum has been formed over thickened regular and acellular cementum.

Increased thickness of cementum is not itself a disease and no treatment is necessary. If hypercementosis is gross, as in Paget's disease, extractions become difficult (Fig. 4.33).

Concrescence

Rarely, hypercementosis causes fusion of the roots of adjacent teeth (Figs 4.34 and 4.35). It is rarely noticed until an attempt is made to extract one of the teeth. The two teeth are then found to move in unison and surgical intervention becomes necessary.

Box 4.8 **Causes of hypercementosis**

- Ageing
- Periapical periodontitis. A common cause but minor in amount. Close to the apex there is usually a little resorption, but coronally, cementum is laid down, forming a shoulder
- Functionless and unerupted teeth. Hypercementosis and resorption may alternate
- Paget's disease. Alternating, irregular apposition and resorption, with apposition predominating, produce an irregular mass of cementum on the root with a histological 'mosaic' pattern
- Cementoblastoma and cemento-osseous dysplasia (Ch. 8)

73

Fig. 4.34 **Concrescence.** Two upper molars fused together by cementum.

Fig. 4.35 **Concrescence.** Histological section of fused teeth reveals that the teeth are joined by cementum and not dentine.

CHRONIC (NON-CARIOUS) INJURIES TO TEETH

Non-carious chronic damage to the teeth may be referred to as *tooth-wear*. The latter may be caused by attrition, abrasion or erosion, or combinations of these influences.

Fig. 4.36 **Attrition.** Excessive wear of the occlusal surfaces of the teeth, as a result of an abrasive diet. The site of the pulp of several teeth is marked by reactionary dentine which is porous and stained. Teeth remain vital.

Attrition

Attrition is tooth-to-tooth wear and results more rapidly from a gritty diet and may be seen in immigrants from developing countries or in ancient skulls. Attrition may also be seen in the elderly and can result from a subconscious tooth grinding habit which may be nocturnal and is termed bruxism.

Attrition can eventually flatten the masticatory surfaces and expose the dentine. Reactionary dentine formation in response to this slow process protects the pulp (Fig. 4.36).

Bruxism

Bruxism is the term given to periodic repetitive clenching or rhythmic forceful grinding of the teeth. Some 10–20% of the population report the habit, but the incidence rises to 90% when mild subconcious grinding is included. It has an equal sex incidence, is commoner in children and young adults and uncommon after middle age. The aetiology is unknown but probably multifactorial. Bruxism is performed during light sleep and some consider it primarily a sleep disorder. Bruxism is also common in those with disability (Ch. 33). Grinding the teeth is often also a subconscious response to frustration and though usually then brief, may be acquired as a more prolonged habit and damage the teeth.

Bruxism is divided into nocturnal and daytime types. In nocturnal bruxism, the teeth are clenched or ground many times each night but for only a few seconds at a time. Even so, the forces exerted and the total time of occlusal contact is much longer than normal. Bruxism is often performed in a protrusive or lateral excursion so that the forces are borne on few teeth and in an unfavourable direction. The resulting attrition can be deeply destructive, particularly in a Class II division 2 occlusion. The signs of bruxism are shown in Box 4.9.

Only the grinding itself is diagnostic. Attrition may also be seen in the elderly, particularly as a result of physiological wear (see above). The muscle pain of bruxism is felt in the morning

---

Box 4.9 Features and effects of bruxism

- Noise during grinding
- Attrition, wear facets and occasionally sensitivity
- Fracture of cusps and restorations
- Mobility of teeth
- Hypertrophy of masseter and anterior temporalis muscles
- Sometimes, though rarely, myalgia and limitation of jaw movement
- Sometimes, though rarely, tenderness on palpation of masticatory muscles

---

Fig. 4.37 Attrition and abrasion. Chronic physical trauma to the teeth produced by chewing and overvigorous use of a toothbrush. The incisal edges of the teeth have worn into polished facets, in the centres of which the yellowish dentine is visible. The necks of the two nearest teeth have been deeply incised by tooth brushing, also exposing dentine. The pulp has been obliterated by secondary dentine formation, but its original site can be seen in the centre of the exposed dentine.

and is the same as muscle pain after exercise. However, most 'bruxists' experience no pain and pain does not correlate with the severity of the grinding or clenching.

Bruxism is often considered to be linked to pain dysfunction syndrome, but the association is not strong (Ch. 11). It has also been suggested that bruxism may result from occlusal interference, but bruxism may even be carried out with complete dentures.

Management

Bruxism should be treated conservatively and any intervention should be reversible. Reassurance and explanation are often all that are required and stress management such as relaxation, hypnosis or sleep advice may be tried.

Appliances are widely prescribed, but there is no firm evidence to support their use. Claims that appliances act by changing the vertical dimension, relieving occlusal interference, repositioning the condyles, changing mandibular posture or preventing periodontal ligament proprioception are unproven and their mechanisms of action are unknown. Nevertheless, appliances frequently appear to be effective and they are useful to protect against severe attrition. Appliances may be attached to upper and lower arches, including flat bite planes and various types of occlusal splints. All should be worn at night only and initially for one month. If there is no improvement, treatment should be discontinued to prevent adverse effects on the soft tissues and occlusion. If effective, the appliances may be worn intermittently during exacerbations. Soft vacuum-formed appliances are cheap and readily fitted as a short-term diagnostic aid but are quickly worn out by determined bruxism. Any type of appliance occasionally worsens bruxism. If bruxism appears related to anxiety, a short course of an anxiolytic, such as diazepam, may help break the habit. Occlusal adjustment has been shown to be ineffective and should be avoided.

Those who indulge in bruxism during the day may grind, clench, or perform other parafunctional habits such as cheek, tongue or nail biting or tongue thrusting. Appliances probably do not help daytime bruxism.

Abrasion

Abrasion of the necks of the teeth is seen mainly in the elderly as a consequence of overvigorous tooth brushing or use of an

Fig. 4.38 Mixed pattern tooth loss. In this case, an element of erosion may be present. Note the shiny polished surface produced by abrasion.

abrasive dentifrice. The exposed dentine is shiny and smooth. Eventually, grooves worn into the necks of the teeth can be so deep as to extend into the pulp chamber, but reactionary dentine protects the pulp (Figs 4.37 and 4.38). The crown of the tooth may even break off without exposing the pulp.

Fig. 4.39 Localised abrasion caused by opening hair grips.

A variety of abrasive habits may also caused localized abrasion such as pipe smoking and opening hairpins or holding pins (Fig. 4.39).

Erosion

Erosion is progressive dissolution of tooth substance by exposure to acids. It appears to be a growing problem as a result of overconsumption of soft drinks or fruit juices, or both (Fig. 4.40). To emphasise that abrasion, erosion and attrition all contribute to most lesions, the term tooth-wear is often used. However, in most cases, erosion is the primary cause and dietary acid is the commonest aetiological factor.

Chronic regurgitation of gastric secretions, typically as a consequence of chronic pyloric stenosis, can cause a characteristic erosion particularly of the palatal surfaces of the upper teeth (see Fig. 29.1). Similar damage can result from self-induced vomiting. The latter is characteristic of bulimia, a psychological disorder in which there are episodes of binge gorging followed by self-induced vomiting to maintain a thin figure.

Fig. 4.40 **Erosion.** Saucer-shaped defects on the labial enamel resulting from acid drinks being trapped between the upper lip and teeth.

In the past, industrial exposure to corrosive chemicals was a significant cause of dental erosion. This is now of only historical interest, but exposure to wine in wine tasters and acid swimming pool water can all induce erosion as an occupational hazard.

SUGGESTED FURTHER READING

Bergenholtz G 1981 Inflammatory response of the dental pulp to bacterial irritation. J Endod 7:100–104

Brook I, Frazier EH, Gher ME 1996 Microbiology of periapical abscesses and associated maxillary sinusitis. J Periodontol 67:608–610

Currie WJR, Ho V 1993 An unexpected death associated with an acute dentoalveolar abscess. Br J Oral Maxillofac Surg 31:296–298

Kuc I, Peters E, Pan J 2000 Comparison of clinical and histologic diagnoses in periapical lesions. Oral Surg Oral Med Oral Pathol Radiol Endod 89:333–337

Lewis MAO, MacFarlane TW, McGowan DA 1986 Quantitative bacteriology of acute dentoalveolar abscesses. J Med Microbiol 21:101–104

Morse DR, Furst ML, Belot RM et al 1987 Infectious flare-ups and serious sequelae following endodontic treatment: a prospective randomised trial on antibiotic prophylaxis in cases of asymptomatic pulpal-periapical lesions. Oral Surg Oral Med Oral Pathol 64:96–109

Trowbridge HO 1981 Pathogenesis of pulpitis resulting from dental caries. J Endod 7:52–60

Wright EF, Gullickson DC 1996 Identifying acute pulpalgia as a factor in TMD pain. JADA 127:773–780

Gingivitis and periodontitis

THE NORMAL PERIODONTAL TISSUES

The gingival tissues comprise a series of anatomical regions (Box 5.1).

Histologically, gingival epithelium is stratified squamous: the free and attached gingiva are parakeratinised. The *epithelial attachment* consists of flattened stratified squamous epithelium adhering to enamel (Fig. 5.1). The attachment apparatus consists of a basal lamina and hemidesmosomes. The attachment to the enamel appears histologically as a clear cuticle (Fig. 5.2). It forms an effective seal, protecting the underlying connective tissues. The epithelial attachment is so firmly adherent to the tooth surface that mechanical damage, which would otherwise pull the epithelium from the tooth, tears apart

> **Box 5.1 Anatomical regions of normal healthy gingival tissue**
>
> - *Junctional epithelium*. Extends from the amelocemental junction to the floor of the gingival sulcus and forms the epithelial attachment to the tooth surface
> - *Sulcular epithelium*. Lines the gingival sulcus and joins the epithelial attachment to the free gingiva
> - *Free gingiva*. Coronal to the amelocemental junction and attached gingiva and includes the tips of the interdental papillae
> - *Attached gingiva*. Extends apically from the free gingiva to the mucogingival junction and is bound down to the superficial periodontal fibres and periosteum.

the epithelial cells (Fig. 5.2). This epithelium has a relatively high turnover rate and the epithelial attachment is probably actively maintained and reformed. This enables the attachment

Fig. 5.1 Gingival sulcus and epithelial attachment. This sagittal section of a specimen from a woman of 27 shows the normal appearances. Enamel removed by decalcification of the specimen has left the triangular space. The epithelial attachment forms a line from the top of the papilla to the amelocemental junction; its enamel surface, the actual line of attachment, is sharply defined. The gingival sulcus, minute in extent, is formed where the papilla curves away from the line of the enamel surface. There is hardly any inflammatory infiltrate.

Fig. 5.2 The strength of the epithelial attachment. On this tooth the epithelial attachment has migrated on to the surface of the cementum as a result of periodontal disease. The epithelium has been torn away from the tooth but the tear is within the junctional epithelium, leaving some of its cells still adherent to the cementum and attached by a clear cuticle. A similar strength is seen when the junctional epithelium is attached to enamel.

to migrate apically until it becomes attached to cementum when periodontitis develops.

The *attached gingiva* is firmly bound down to the underlying bone to form a tough mucoperiosteum. Its stippled appearance is due to the intersections of its underlying epithelial ridges at the junction with the connective tissue.

The alveolar mucosa is continuous with the attached gingiva, but is sharply demarcated by its smooth surface, darker colour and increasing separation from the bone.

Gingival and periodontal fibres

The principal fibres of the periodontal ligament form fibrous bundles interspersed by loose connective tissue containing blood vessels and nerves. These components provide a viscoelastic supportive mechanism resisting both compressive and tensile forces on the teeth. The normal thickness of the periodontal ligament is about 0.1–0.3 mm.

The principal fibres are arranged in a series of fairly well-defined groups (Box 5.2).

Box 5.2   Principal fibres of the periodontal ligament

- *Oblique fibres* form a suspensory ligament from socket to root in coronal to apical directions
- *Horizontal fibres* form a dense group attaching neck of tooth to rim of socket
- *Transeptal fibres* of the horizontal group are not attached to alveolar bone but pass superficially to it and join adjacent teeth together. They protect the interdental gingiva by resisting forces that would otherwise separate the teeth and open the contact points
- *Gingival fibres* form a cuff round the neck of the tooth supporting the soft tissues. They resist separation of the gingivae from the tooth and help to prevent formation of pockets

---

The periodontal ligament fibres are embedded in cementum at their inner ends and in the lamina dura at their outer ends. New fibres replacing those which have aged, or forming in response to new functional stresses, are attached by apposition of further layers of cementum which becomes thicker with age. The lamina dura is a layer of compact bone continuous, at the mouths of the sockets, with the cortical bone of the jaw. The radiographic appearance of the lamina dura has limited diagnostic value in periodontics as its presence largely depends on the alignment of the beam.

Gingival crevicular fluid (exudate)

In health, a minute amount of fluid can be collected from the gingival margins. It differs in composition from saliva, which contains IgA, while gingival fluid has a variable but significant content of IgG, IgM and leucocytes. Unlike saliva, gingival fluid is not a secretion (there are no glands in this region), but is inflammatory exudate. It therefore increases greatly with the degree of inflammation.

NOMENCLATURE AND CLASSIFICATION OF PERIODONTAL DISEASE

The term *periodontal disease* usually refers only to plaque-related inflammatory disease of the dental supporting tissues. A wide variety of diseases of the oral mucosa can also affect the gingivae occasionally, so that conditions as diverse as tuberculosis or lichen planus can produce lesions in this area. Such conditions do not play any significant part in the development of periodontal disease in its commonly accepted sense.

Chronic gingivitis is, with few exceptions, the preliminary stage to the development of chronic periodontitis, but clinically no sharp dividing line can be drawn between chronic gingivitis and the onset of periodontitis. Nevertheless, the distinction is important in that chronic gingivitis can generally be cured by plaque control. By contrast, loss of bone and tooth support due to chronic periodontitis are largely irreversible.

The main *clinical* types of periodontal disease are grouped together on the basis of what seems to be the predominant pathological process (Box 5.3).

CHRONIC GINGIVITIS

Clinical features

Chronic gingivitis is asymptomatic, low-grade inflammation of the gingivae. The latter become red and slightly swollen with oedema (Fig. 5.3). Plaque, deposited along the gingival margins, is readily detectable. In most patients, chronic gingivitis is due to local factors and, in particular, ineffective toothbrushing. It should be curable by effective oral hygiene.

Chronic hyperplastic gingivitis is a term sometimes given to chronic gingivitis in which inflammtory oedema is prominent. However, there is no soft tissue hyperplasia. Maintenance of strict oral hygiene brings resolution.

Systemic disorders can exacerbate chronic gingivitis but rarely play a significant role (Box 5.4).

Pathology

Fig. 5.3   Gingivitis. A florid, bright-red band of gingival inflammation results from very poor oral hygiene. Thick accumulations of plaque are visible on all tooth surfaces.

Box 5.3 Types of periodontal disease

I. **Gingivitis and periodontitis**
- Chronic gingivitis (common plaque-related type)
- Chronic adult periodontitis (common, plaque-related type)

II. **Less common types of gingivitis**
- Acute necrotising ulcerative gingivitis
- HIV-associated gingivitis
- Herpetic gingivostomatitis (Ch. 12)
- Wegener's granulomatosis (Ch. 28)
- HIV-associated periodontitis

III. **Uncommon types of periodontitis**
- Prepubertal periodontitis
- Juvenile periodontitis
- Rapidly progressive periodontitis
- Acute leukaemic periodontal destruction

IV. **Miscellaneous periodontal disorders**
- Gingival hyperplasia
  Familial
  Drug-related
- Periodontal atrophy recession
- Periodontal (lateral) abscess
- Pericoronitis

Box 5.4 Factors contributing to or exacerbating chronic gingivitis

Local
- Poor tooth cleaning technique
- Dental irregularities providing stagnation areas
- Restorations or appliances causing stagnation areas

Systemic
- Pregnancy
- Down's syndrome
- Poorly-controlled diabetes mellitus

Fig. 5.4 Chronic gingivitis. The epithelial attachment remains at the level of the amelocemental junction and inflammatory cells are concentrated below the junctional epithelium and extend into the deeper gingiva, around the interradicular fibres. The alveolar crest is not resorbed.

Gingivitis is an inflammatory response to plaque bacteria. By definition, inflammation is restricted to the gingival margins and does not affect the periodontal ligament or bone (Fig. 5.4).

The development of gingivitis has been arbitrarily divided into three histological stages (Boxes 5.5 and 5.6), while the fourth stage refers to chronic periodontitis. It must be appreciated that these stages are artificially distinguished, being largely based on animal studies.

Box 5.5 'Initial stage' chronic gingivitis

- Develops within 24–48 hours of exposure to plaque
- Plaque related to gingival sulcus
- Vasodilatation
- Infiltration predominantly of neutrophils
- Leakage of exudate into gingival sulcus

Box 5.6 Established chronic gingivitis

- Dense, predominantly plasmacytic infiltrate
- Infiltrate fills but limited to interdental papillae
- Destruction of superficial connective tissue fibres
- Deepened gingival crevice
- Epithelial attachment remains at or near amelocemental junction
- Alveolar bone and periodontal ligament remain intact

Variations in plaque bacteria with stage of disease *Healthy (uninflamed) gingivae.* The plaque is supragingival and thin (10 to 20 cells thick). Gram-positive bacteria predominate and include *Actinomyces* species, *Rothia*, viridans streptococci and *S. epidermidis*. In elderly patients in periodontal health, Gram-positive bacteria, particularly streptococci, form the largest single group (50% of the predominant cultivable flora), while Gram-negative bacteria only account for 30%. The latter include porphyromonas and fusobacterium species.

Early (and experimental) gingivitis. If toothbrushing is neglected for several days, plaque grows in thickness and is typically 100 to 300 cells thick. In the earliest stages, bacteria proliferate but the plaque remains Gram-positive in character and *Actinomyces* species become predominant.

Chronic gingivitis. With the passage of time, persistence of plaque leads to chronic inflammation and Gram-negative organisms become increasingly prominent. *Veillonella*, *Fusobacterium* and *Campylobacter* species become conspicuous.

Calculus Calculus is calcified plaque. The calcification is less significant than the bacterial content which induces inflammation and, later, tissue destruction. However, calculus distorts the gingival crevice and, by extending the stagnation area, probably promotes even greater bacterial proliferation (Fig. 5.5). Supragingival calculus mainly forms opposite the orifices of the major salivary glands in the lower incisor and upper first molar areas. It cannot be removed by the patient and provides a rough, plaque-retentive surface.

Several compounds, such as pyrophosphates, added to dentifrices have been shown to reduce calculus formation to variable degrees. However, any clinical benefit has not been unequivocally established.

Management

Chronic gingivitis is readily recognisable from the clinical features already described. Gentle probing shows absence of pocketing and radiographs show intact crestal alveolar bone. The diagnosis is confirmed by resolution of gingivitis when effective oral hygiene measures (including calculus removal, effective toothbrushing and interdental cleaning habits) become established (Figs 5.6 and 5.7). Any exacerbating factors must be dealt with if possible.

Pregnancy gingivitis

Pre-existing gingivitis may become more severe in the first two months of pregnancy (see Fig. 31.9). Inflammatory erythema and oedema typically become more severe and a localised vascular lesion (a pregnancy tumour) may develop. The latter has the same structure as a pyogenic granuloma (Ch. 19).

Pregnancy gingivitis can be much ameliorated or abolished by a strict oral hygiene regimen and improves after parturition. However, if a pregnancy tumour persists, it should be excised.

Fig. 5.5 Subgingival calculus showing the layered structure resulting from incremental deposition. The calculus has a brown colour as a result of blood and bacterial pigment within it. A thick layer of plaque adheres to the deep surface.

Down's syndrome

In Down's syndrome, gingivitis is exacerbated by excessive plaque formation and difficulties in establishing effective toothbrushing habits. The multiple immunodeficiencies typical of this disorder contribute. Progress to periodontitis and early tooth loss are frequent consequences (see Figs 33.3 and 33.4).

Diabetes mellitus

In poorly-controlled diabetes, periodontal health may deteriorate sharply. In well-controlled diabetes, acceleration of gingivitis may not be noticeable. However, it appears that, overall, diabetics suffer somewhat more severe periodontal disease and slightly earlier tooth loss than healthy, control populations. The neutrophil defect typical of this disease is probably the main factor involved.

CHRONIC ADULT PERIODONTITIS

Clinical features

Chronic periodontitis (the 'advanced lesion') is the chief cause of tooth loss in later adult life, but symptoms are typically

Fig. 5.6 Accumulation of plaque stained after 24 hours by disclosing solution.

Fig. 5.7 **The effects of tooth brushing in the same patient.** Plaque remains interdentally in most areas, explaining why gingivitis is often localised here.

minimal. Many patients remain unaware of the disease until teeth become loose.

Gingivitis persists and patients may complain of gingival bleeding or an unpleasant taste. Later, gingival recession or loosening of the teeth may become conspicuous. Periodontitis is a potent and common cause of foul-smelling breath (halitosis). The congested gingival margins become purplish-red, flabby and swollen. The interdental papillae 'split' and can be separated from the teeth. Later, the papillae are destroyed and the gingival margin tends to become straight with a swollen, rounded edge.

Pressure on the gingival margins causes bleeding and sometimes pus can be expressed from round the necks of the teeth. Bacterial plaque and calculus are widespread.

Loss of attachment leads to pocketing which allows a probe to be passed down between teeth and gingiva. In pockets, the rough surface of subgingival calculus can be felt. Eventually, teeth become increasingly loose and dull to percussion.

Radiography

The earliest change is loss of definition and blunting of the tips of the alveolar crests. Bone resorption usually progresses in a regular manner and its level remains the same along a row of teeth. A straight line can be drawn along the crest of the alveolar bone (horizontal bone loss – Fig. 5.8). Complex patterns of bone loss may also be seen, probably due to the effects of variable degrees of loss of attachment superimposed upon the underlying anatomical features. Thus, in areas where bone is thin, destruction results in horizontal bone loss, but where alveolar bone is thicker, partial destruction gives rise to vertical or angular bone defects.

Aetiology and pathology

Conditions promoting stagnation and maintenance of infection at the gingival margins have been discussed earlier. Persistence of infection at the gingival margins leads to progressive inflammation and destruction of the supporting tissues. Usually, local factors are most important in the progress of chronic periodontitis but, for reasons which are unclear, there is wide individual response.

The main features of the pathology of chronic periodontitis are summarised in Box 5.7.

Plaque Bacterial plaque, a dense mat of bacteria (Box 5.8), extends from the gingival margins into pockets.

Fig. 5.8 Early and severe horizontal bone loss in advanced chronic adult periodontitis.

Box 5.8   Important bacteria associated with periodontal disease

- Actinobacillus actinomycetemcomitans
- Actinomyces viscosus
- Capnocytophaga species*
- Eikenella corrodens
- Fusobacterium nucleatum*
- Porphyromonas gingivalis*
- Prevotella intermedia*
- Treponemas and other spirochaetes*
- Wolinella recta

(*anaerobes)

Subgingival calculus Extension and calcification of plaque leads to formation of subgingival calculus within periodontal pockets. The deposits are thin, more widely distributed, harder, darker and more firmly attached than supragingival calculus. Calculus appears laminated histologically, with altered staining, probably due to breakdown products from blood cells oozing into the pockets. Subgingival calculus helps to perpetuate chronic periodontitis. It forms a reservoir of bacteria, helping to sustain inflammation, and acts as a barrier to healing.

Box 5.7   Pathological processes in chronic periodontitis

- Chronic inflammation
- Destruction of periodontal ligament fibres
- Resorption of alveolar bone
- Migration of the epithelial attachment towards the apex
- Formation of pockets around the teeth
- Formation of subgingival plaque and calculus

Fig. 5.9 Transition from chronic gingivitis to periodontitis. No pocket has yet formed but the epithelial attachment has extended on to the cementum and inflammation has induced epithelial hyperplasia, as evidenced by rete hyperplasia.

Fig. 5.10 Established chronic periodontitis. In this woman of 33, periodontal pockets have extended well beyond the amelocemental junction and inflammatory cells fill the interdental gingiva.

Chronic inflammation Plasma cells typically predominate but are accompanied by lymphocytes and neutrophils which migrate into pockets. Inflammatory cells infiltrate the connective tissue and spread between the principal fibres (Figs 5.9 and 5.10). Dense masses of these cells accumulate, especially under the epithelium in the connective tissue apposed to plaque and calculus.

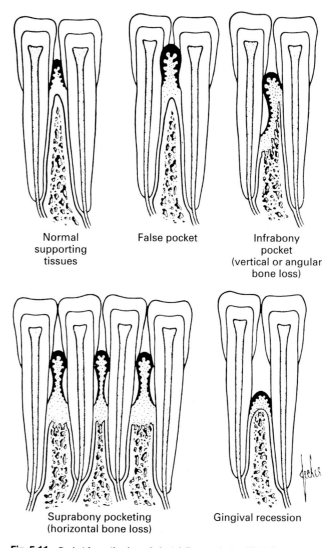

Normal supporting tissues   False pocket   Infrabony pocket (vertical or angular bone loss)

Suprabony pocketing (horizontal bone loss)   Gingival recession

Fig. 5.11 Pocket formation in periodontal disease. A simplified diagram to show the relationship between periodontal soft tissues and alveolar bone in the different presentations of periodontal disease.

Pocketing Pocketing, a characteristic feature of chronic periodontitis, is due to the slower destruction of gingival soft tissues than of periodontal ligament and bone (Fig. 5.11). Less frequently, where gingival tissue is thin, it may be lost at the same rate as the supporting tissues and gingival recession results. Pockets round the teeth provide a protected environment in which bacteria grow more freely. There is no effective drainage and the wall of the pocket presents a large area where bacteria or their products can irritate the tissues. Pockets also favour the growth of anaerobes which probably contribute greatly to tissue destruction.

Pockets surround the teeth. One wall is formed by cementum, the other soft tissue replacing the destroyed bone and periodontal fibres. The outer wall consists of connective tissue infiltrated by chronic inflammatory cells and lined by epithelium continuous with the gingival epithelium at the pocket mouth. The epithelial attachment forms the deep boundary.

The epithelium is often hyperplastic, but blood vessels may extend through it almost to its surface.

'Ulceration' of the lining is often described but rarely seen histologically.

Epithelial migration The epithelial attachment migrates from enamel on to cementum, forming the floor of the pocket (Figs 5.12 and 5.13). The attachment to cementum is strong and a clear refractile cuticle (see Fig. 5.2) can sometimes be seen joining the epithelium to the root surface. The length of the epithelial attachment is variable but may extend several millimetres.

Destruction of periodontal fibres Periodontal fibres are destroyed progressively from the gingival margin down to the level of the floor of the pocket. More deeply, the fibres retain their normal appearance.

Destruction of alveolar bone Bone destruction starts at the alveolar crest. The usual level of the remaining bone is just

deep to the floor of the pocket where the superficial fibres of the periodontal ligament are attached. The zone of inflammation is separated from the underlying bone by a zone of fibrous tissue. This so-called fibrous walling-off is typical of chronic periodontitis and invariably present (see Fig. 5.12). It has been suggested that the inflammatory lesion may extend beyond this to affect the alveolar bone and remaining periodontal ligament during periods of active disease, but histological evidence of this is lacking. Osteoclasts are rarely seen, probably because their action is intermittent and the rate of bone destruction extremely slow.

Osteoporosis and premature alveolar bone loss Confirmation that osteoporosis may be related to premature alveolar bone loss has been handicapped by the difficulties in measuring bone mineral density (BMD) accurately. However, it has been confirmed that diminished bone mineral density, measured by dual X-ray absorptiometry in several parts of the skeleton, showed a highly significant correlation with the thickness of the mandibular alveolar process in the first premolar region.

Other studies have also shown that age-related bone loss is greater in women than men after the age of 50 years. There is also a significant increase in mandibular cortical porosity and concomittant decline in bone mass, with an estimated loss of bone mineral content of 1.5% per year in women, but only 0.9% in men.

Role of specific bacteria in destructive periodontitis With formation of pockets and subgingival plaque there is enormous proliferation of bacteria of all kinds. Subgingival plaque appears to have a dense zone attached to the tooth surface where the bacteria are mainly Gram-positive. By contrast, plaque

Fig. 5.12 **Chronic periodontitis.** The amelocemental junction lies at the top of the picture covered by plaque and calculus that extends into the upper pocket. The epithelium of the pocket is hyperplastic and irregular but the epithelial attachment is tightly apposed to the cementum. The alveolar crest shows resting and reversal lines indicating remodelling. A broad band of uninflamed densely fibrous tissue, almost scar tissue, separates the bone from the inflamed tissue.

Fig. 5.13 **Chronic periodontitis.** Higher-power view showing the epithelial attachment lying against cementum. Note how collagen has been lost from the areas containing inflammatory cells.

related to the pocket wall is less densely packed but involves many Gram-negative bacteria, including anaerobes and spirochaetes. Bacteria particularly associated with destructive disease include *Porphyromonas gingivalis*, *Actinobacillus actinomycetemcomitans*, *B. intermedius*, *Wolinella recta*, spirochaetes with axial filaments, or in other cases *Eikenella corrodens*, and other corroding bacteria. The latter's colonies cause pitting ('corrosion') of the surface of culture media.

Also present are *Fusobacterium nucleatum* and as yet unidentified anaerobic vibrios and spirochaetes. Where there is severe and relatively acute bone loss associated with severe inflammation, in young adults, for example, *Actinobacillus actinomycetemcomitans* and *Porphyromonas gingivalis* appear to be particularly important. Where inflammation is minimal in spite of extensive bone loss there may be greater numbers of *Prevotella melaninogenica* and *Eikenella corrodens*. Many of the bacteria implicated in destructive periodontitis are dangerous pathogens and in other body sites can cause severe or lethal systemic infections. For example, *Capnocytophaga ochraceus*, *Selenomonas sputigena* and *Eikenella corrodens* have been implicated in life-threatening infections, particularly in patients with granulocytopenia.

In human periodontal disease, it remains unclear which particular types of bacteria are responsible for tissue destruction. However, inoculation of specific bacteria into the mouths of germ-free animals has yielded somewhat unexpected results. Thus, various Gram-positive bacteria typically produce large amounts of plaque, but Gram-negative bacteria do not. Certain bacteria of either group can induce or accelerate periodontal tissue damage, but there is typically little inflammation or lymphocytic infiltration of the tissues. In Gram-positive infections also, few osteoclasts are seen. However, *A. viscosus* in particular produces a bone-resorbing factor. Gram-negative bacteria also stimulate osteoclastic activity and numerous osteoclasts are seen at the sites of tissue destruction.

That individual species of bacteria may be responsible for periodontal tissue destruction is also suggested by the finding in monkeys that the severity of periodontal damage correlates well with the numbers of *Porphyromonas gingivalis* which can be isolated. Further, antimicrobial treatment that suppressed *P. gingivalis* led to healing and bone regeneration. Greater numbers of *P. gingivalis* also appear to be associated with enhanced periodontal disease activity in humans.

Bacterial mediators of tissue damage Periodontal destruction may result from the actions of bacterial products or indirectly from immunologically mediated processes or both in varying degree. Bacterial products (virulence factors) that may contribute to tissue damage include enzymes, toxins and bone-resorbing factors.

Enzymes. Destruction of periodontal fibres may be due to collagenases. *Prevotella* species, for example, produce collagenase, trypsin, fibrinolysin, hyaluronidase, chondroitin sulphatase, heparinase, aribonuclease and deoxyribonuclease. Cytotoxic metabolic products such as indole, ammonia and hydrogen sulphide may also contribute. *Porphyromonas*

species, especially *P. gingivalis*, are regularly associated with human destructive periodontitis.

Toxins. Certain strains of *A. actinomycetemcomitans* produce a powerful leukotoxin, while *P. gingivalis* and *P. intermedius* produce an epitheliotoxin.

Endotoxin, a lipopolysaccharide (LPS) component of Gram-negative bacteria cell walls, is released after cell lysis. It can liberate lysosomal enzymes from phagocytes and activate complement via the alternative pathway. Endotoxins can therefore mediate an inflammatory response. Endotoxins from some bacteria can enhance osteoclastic resorption to variable degrees and, in this respect, endotoxin from *P. gingivalis* is ten times more potent than that from *A. actinomycetemcomitans*. The Gram-positive cell wall component, lipoteichoic acid (LTA) is also a potent mediator of inflammation and enhances bone resorption.

Bone resorbing factors. *A. viscosus* produces factors which induce decalcification of bone in vitro. Lipopolysaccharide can also induce bone resorption under experimental conditions, as can crude soluble extracts of human supragingival plaque and some other bacterial products. Bacterial factors can also cause bone resorption by stimulating release of, or acting synergistically with lymphokines, osteoclast activating factors and prostaglandin E_2.

Interference with host defence mechanisms Other virulence factors act by interfering with host defences. Substances cytotoxic for human leucocytes (leukotoxins) are produced by *A. actinomycetemcomitans* in particular. This bacterium is involved in juvenile periodontitis and can also cause osteomyelitis and infective endocarditis in humans. Other bacterial factors potentially capable of damaging host defences are immunoglobulin proteases. *Neisseria gonorrhoeae* can produce IgA proteases which help it overcome mucosal defences and contributes to the inability of infected persons to develop protective immunity. Several of the oral viridans streptococci have also been shown to produce IgA proteases. Lipopolysaccharides, dextran and levan may also be immunosuppressive, but under different circumstances may be immunopotentiating.

Smoking

Smokers have greater susceptibility to periodontitis but, paradoxically, less inflammation evident clinically. The reasons for this are not understood but smoking is known to interfere with inflammatory and immune reactions probably by activating endothelial and inflammatory cells inappropriately in the lungs and circulation, and by inducing them to secrete cytokines and other compounds. Also, nicotine is a vasoconstrictor, though its effects on the gingiva have proved difficult to measure. Overall, smokers have greater loss of attachment, early tooth loss and respond less well to treatment.

Immunological processes in periodontal disease

Immunological mechanisms are involved in periodontal disease, as they are in every microbial disease. Antibodies are produced against plaque bacterial antigens. These may, for example, mediate opsonisation and killing of bacteria by neutrophils and macrophages. Complement is also activated by antigen/antibody complexes and contributes to the inflammatory reaction. In the process of inflammation, microbes are killed but there may also be some damage to host tissues in so-called innocent bystander damage.

Many T lymphocytes are also present and may be involved in cell-mediated reactions to plaque pathogens. Other hypersensitivity reactions may also participate.

However, it must be appreciated that the immunological reactions in chronic periodontitis are essentially protective. With loss of normal immune competence, as in conditions of neutropenia for example, periodontal destruction may be greatly accelerated. Severely destructive periodontitis may also be seen in AIDS.

The remarkable feature of periodontal disease is that, despite the presence of innumerable major pathogens in periodontal pockets, tissue destruction is so slow. In an otherwise healthy person, it is not uncommon for half a century to pass before 1 cm of alveolar bone is lost. This represents a loss of an average of 0.2 mm of bone a year.

Progress of chronic periodontitis

Chronic periodontitis, once established, is self-perpetuating. Pockets cannot drain effectively and favour proliferation of bacteria. The epithelial lining, plaque and subgingival calculus effectively obstruct healing. Further destruction of periodontal fibres and alveolar bone causes the pockets to deepen. The natural termination of the process is loosening and exfoliation of the teeth.

General principles of management of chronic periodontitis

The main components of the management of periodontal disease are summarised in Box 5.9.

> **Box 5.9** **General principles of management of periodontal disease**
>
> - Control of bacterial plaque
> - Establishment of healthy gingiva accessible to plaque control
> - Minimisation of periodontal tissue loss
> - Use of antibiotics in selected cases
> - Mucogingival surgery in selected cases

It may be depressing for readers who have steeped themselves in the complexities of the immunology of periodontal disease to find that its management largely depends on time-honoured, manual methods of plaque control.

Effective daily plaque removal by the patient is imperative for success. Conscientious toothbrushing and interdental cleaning with aids such as floss, wooden sticks, or small brushes, as necessary, are required. These simple measures will bring about complete resolution of simple gingivitis as mentioned earlier.

Anything hampering plaque control, particularly calculus and faulty restorations, should be dealt with. Other conditions promoting stagnation (Box 5.10) may be more difficult to eliminate.

> **Box 5.10** **Factors promoting stagnation and persistence of plaque**
>
> - Calculus
> - Overhanging restorations
> - Food packing due to faulty contact points
> - Irregularities of the teeth
> - Mouthbreathing
> - Pocketing

Treatment of periodontal pockets

Successful treatment depends upon thorough supragingival and subgingival plaque removal. The latter may be achieved by subgingival scaling or root planning, which also removes some cementum to ensure plaque elimination from surface irregularities. The aim is to produce a root surface to which the detached gingival tissue may adhere. Such methods should result in resolution of inflammation in the pocket wall. The junctional epithelial attachment to the root surface may extend in length coronally and there is usually shrinkage of the gingival margin, thus exposing more root surface. The clinical result is greater recession, shallower probing depth and less bleeding on probing. Failure to achieve clinical improvement is due to either a lapse in plaque control by the patient or failure to remove subgingival plaque (Box 5.11).

> **Box 5.11** **Factors compromising subgingival plaque removal**
>
> - Excessive pocket depth
> - Distorted root morphology and furcations
> - Inaccessible root surfaces (e.g. distal surfaces of posterior teeth)
> - Operator competence
>   Failure of benefit from root planing is shown by:
> - Bleeding or exudation of pus on probing the depth of pocket
> - Increasing probing depths
> - Deterioration of bone levels seen radiologically

Subgingival scaling or root planing will not remove subgingival plaque entirely and may force pocket bacteria into the tissues. However, competent performance of these procedures reduces bacterial bulk, changes the composition of the flora and frequently produces clinical improvement.

When root planing fails, mucogingival surgery may be used to excise pockets to enable the patient to keep the root surfaces clean. The earliest form of resective surgery was gingivectomy.[1] This is still a useful procedure, particularly in patients with false pockets due to fibrous gingival hyperplasia and unresponsive to non-surgical treatment. However, gingivectomy is

---

[1]Gingivectomy dates back at least 800 years. Crusaders' gums were so swollen by scurvy that they had to have them cut away to enable them to eat.

unsuitable for (1) pockets extending beyond the mucogingival junction such that excision would remove all the keratinised gingiva and (2) when the base of the pocket is apical to the bone crest. Gingivectomy for deep pocketing also exposes the necks of the teeth and produces a 'horse-tooth' appearance unacceptable to most patients.

Flap operations Surgical approaches usually depend on elevation of flaps and are designed to facilitate cleaning of the root. Inflamed tissue is curetted away and the root surfaces are cleaned. The flaps are then sutured back around the necks of the teeth. The flap can be replaced at or near the preoperative level or it can be repositioned apically so that it just covers the alveolar crest. The former approach requires that the flap must reattach to the denuded root surface, whereas the latter aims to eliminate the pocket. Apical placement of the flap may produce an aesthetically undesirable result and exposure of complex root forms may not facilitate plaque control by the patient.

Reattachment surgery The ultimate goal of this technique is the promotion of new cementum apposition to anchor periodontal fibres to a healthier root surface. This ideal result ('new attachment') would obviously be the most satisfactory method of treatment. Unfortunately, it has been largely unsuccessful, mainly as a consequence of rapid re-epithelialisation of the root surface and production of a long junctional epithelium. Until recently, methods designed to retard or redirect epithelial migration at the healing dentogingival junction have not been successful. A new connective tissue attachment will only form if cells from the remaining healthy periodontal ligament repopulate the root surface. Insertion of a barrier membrane between the flap and root surface may prevent epithelial and gingival connective tissue ingrowth ('guided tissue regeneration'). Histological evidence suggests that new attachment that forms after this procedure is only in relatively small amounts.

Limitations of periodontal surgery Periodontal surgery may be of little benefit when multirooted teeth have furcation involvement. When one root is more severely affected than another, resection of the affected root or half the tooth (hemisection) may be successful.

Overall, however, clinical trials comparing gingivectomy and various flap procedures have shown minimal differences in results under conditions where the standard of plaque control is high. If plaque control is poor they are equally ineffective and may lead to greater loss of periodontal support. Most patients with periodontal disease can be successfully treated by a non-surgical approach and, when surgical and non-surgical treatment have been compared, similar results have been obtained. Surgery may have advantages when treating deep pockets, while the non-surgical approach is better for shallower pockets.

Antibiotics for control of plaque bacteria

Antibiotics reaching periodontal plaque cause considerable disturbance of the bacterial flora and have the potential for destroying important pathogens. It might be suspected that this effect would be transient, but it must be borne in mind that the complex interdependent ecosystem of plaque bacteria associated with periodontal disease is built up over many years. Although plaque bacteria can undoubtedly develop resistance, anaerobes generally do not lose antibiotic sensitivity as readily as many aerobes.

Antibiotics have been used particularly for the management of periodontal disease responding poorly to conventional treatment. Overall, tetracyclines seem to be the most effective. They have the widest spectrum of activity of all antibiotics, and the side-effects, particularly of topical applications, are minimal. Even when given systemically, tetracyclines may reach concentrations in the gingival sulcus several times greater than serum levels. They also bind to calcified tissues such as cementum. In various studies, tetracyclines appear to have produced significant changes in the composition of plaque. They have brought clinical improvement, particularly when combined with conventional treatment such as root planing.

Tetracycline-containing plastic fibres have also been placed in the gingival sulcus for direct delivery of a high local concentration. Putative plaque pathogens, such as *Porphyromonas* species and other anaerobes, were found not to have repopulated the plaque within the period of follow-up. Though the use of antibiotics in the management of periodontal disease is not universally accepted, it seems likely that they can produce long-term reduction in plaque pathogenicity. By interfering with complex bacterial ecosystems, less harmful species may proliferate. With the small doses used in topical applications, significant adverse effects seem unlikely to be troublesome.

However, some long-term studies have shown little or no benefit from the use of tetracyclines over scaling and root-planing alone.

Treatment of advanced periodontal disease

Once pocketing has extended beyond the point where treatment can be beneficial, the teeth should be extracted. Deep pockets are a source of sepsis which may have remote effects such as infective endocarditis. Deep pockets are most frequent in elderly patients, who have the highest susceptibility to and mortality from infective endocarditis. At the local level, if infection is allowed to persist, excessive resorption of the alveolar bone may cause difficulties in retaining dentures.

Prognosis in periodontal disease

Reliable predictions about the results of treatment cannot always be made, but some factors obviously affect the outcome (Box 5.12).

Box 5.12 Factors affecting prognosis of periodontal disease
• Oral hygiene status and motivation • Degree of bone loss • Age • Tooth factors • Host resistance

Much depends on the level of oral hygiene maintained by patients and whether they are sufficiently strongly motivated to cooperate in a long regimen of treatment. The degree of attachment loss, as shown by pocket depth and radiographic assessment, clearly determines whether teeth can be saved. However, in patients with the same amount of destruction of supporting tissues, the older the patient the better the prognosis, as the disease is of slower progress. Dental factors such as tooth type, root length, root anatomy and degree of furcation involvement can significantly affect the response to periodontal surgery. If also the teeth are heavily restored or have had faulty endodontic treatment, extensive periodontal treatment may be inappropriate (Figs 5.15 and 5.16).

Despite intensive investigation, there remains, for no clear reasons, a 'high-risk' group for periodontitis who suffer more extensive bone loss than others of similar age.

Complications of chronic periodontitis

Complications can be local or systemic (Box 5.13).

Of the systemic complications, infective endocarditis is discussed in Chapter 27. It only needs to be emphasised here that bacteraemias resulting from movement of teeth in their sockets are most severe and most likely to lead to infective endocarditis in the elderly with advanced chronic periodontitis.

More controversial is the role of chronic periodontitis in contributing to atherosclerosis and its consequences, myocardial infarction or stroke.

Fig. 5.15 A neglected dentition such as this, despite the buried root and advanced bone loss round the other tooth, might nevertheless be suitable for expert periodontal care.

Fig. 5.14 **Advanced chronic periodontitis.** The cementum on the pocket walls is covered with a thin layer of plaque. The epithelium of the pocket lining is hyperplastic and the pocket extends beyond the lower edge of the picture.

Fig. 5.16 Attempts at periodontal surgery to preserve teeth such as these are hopeless. With so little supporting bone it is surprising that they have remained in place at all.

Box 5.13   Complications of chronic periodontitis

Local
- Periodontal abscess
- Tooth mobility
- Tooth loss through exfoliation

Systemic
- Infective endocarditis
- Atherosclerosis and cardiovascular disease (?)

It has been suggested that chronic infection contributes to the development of atherosclerosis and coronary heart disease; several large surveys have shown an association between the latter and chronic periodontitis. This concern has persisted, but evidence for the role of chronic periodontitis in this disease remains inconclusive.

PERIODONTAL (LATERAL) ABSCESS

A periodontal abscess results from acute infection of a periodontal pocket. It sometimes follows treatment such as root planing when trauma to the pocket lining implants bacteria into the tissues. Otherwise the causes are uncertain, but an abscess may result from some change in the pocket flora or damage by a foreign body, such as a fish bone driven through the floor of a pocket. Food packing down between the teeth with poor contact points may also contribute. Drainage through the pocket mouth is poor and made worse by inflammatory oedema and soft tissue swelling. Pericoronitis is a form of periodontal abscess in a false pocket.

Clinical features

The onset is rapid. Gingival tenderness progresses to throbbing pain. The tooth affected is vital and tender to percussion. The overlying gingiva is red and swollen. Pus may exude from the pocket, but a deep periodontal abscess may point on the alveolar mucosa, forming a sinus. More generalised chronic periodontitis is usually associated. The vitality of the tooth and its less severe tenderness usually distinguish a lateral abscess from acute apical periodontitis. The great depth of the pocket from which pus may exude helps to make the diagnosis clear (Fig. 5.17).

Radiographic changes are not visible until after about a week. A radiolucent area may then be seen beside the tooth.

Pathology

The bony wall of the pocket is actively resorbed by many osteoclasts. There is dense infiltration by neutrophils and pus formation (Figs 5.18 and 5.19). The pocket deepens rapidly by destruction of periodontal fibres, sometimes to the apex of the tooth. Alveolar bone in the floor of the original pocket is destroyed and the pocket extends between the tooth and alveolar bone. An intrabony pocket may thus form. Occasionally, pus tracks apically or from a deeply sited pocket so that a facial abscess or cellulitis results.

Treatment

A periodontal abscess should be drained, ideally through the pocket. Infected tissue can be removed by subgingival curettage and the root surfaces thoroughly debrided. Occasionally, incision through the overlying gingiva is needed, but is best avoided as a permanent soft tissue fenestration may result. However, if periodontal disease is severe and widespread, it may be more appropriate to extract the affected tooth.

JUVENILE PERIODONTITIS

Juvenile periodontitis is uncommon, having a prevalence of about 1:1000, with males and females equally affected. Its

Fig. 5.17   Periodontal abscess. The abscess is pointing on the alveolar mucosa well above the attached gingiva. The probe is inserted deeply in the pocket communicating with the abscess.

Fig. 5.18 **Acute periodontal abscess.** There is well-advanced chronic peri-odontitis, but acute inflammatory changes have developed in this pocket with destruction of periodontal ligament and alveolar bone with formation of an abscess and a deep intrabony pocket (from a man of 55).

Fig. 5.19 **Periodontal abscess.** Higher-power view of the floor of the pocket shows the purulent inflammation and gross resorption of alveolar bone extending to the apex.

Fig. 5.20 **Localised juvenile periodontitis.** Drifting of upper central incisors due to gross loss of attachment. There is some marginal inflammation but oral hygiene is good and the clinical appearance belies the periodontal destruction.

rare, more generalised form which appears to be a less clearly definable disease entity. Several systemic diseases can cause premature periodontal destruction, but the term 'juvenile peri-odontitis' is usually reserved for cases in which clinically sig-nificant systemic disease is absent.

Aetiology

There is a familial predisposition, but the immediate cause may be a specific bacterial infection and an associated neutrophil defect. The bacterium commonly found in the diseased sites is *Actinobacillus actinomycetemcomitans*, strains of which produce a potent leukotoxin. Antibodies to this bacterium and the leukotoxin are found in the serum and gingival fluid. Neutrophils from many patients have a defect of chemotaxis and poor surface receptor binding capacity. The defect may be genetically determined, while acquisition of the organism is probably from other family members.

Clinical features

The incisor and first molar teeth are usually the most severely affected. Gingivitis is minimal or absent and the main feature is drifting and loosening of teeth, most noticeably in the front of the mouth. The teeth may also tilt or become extruded (Fig. 5.20).

Radiography

Deep, angular bone loss and displacement of the anterior teeth are typical findings (Fig. 5.21). The remarkable symmetry seen in this condition is often such as to make the sides of the mouth appear almost as mirror images of each other.

Pathology

Little material has become available for histological examina-tion, but there is degeneration of principal periodontal fibres,

onset may be around puberty or earlier. It appears to comprise a spectrum of disorders and only generalisations can be made about it here.

The main features are rapid breakdown of the periodontal tissues of permanent first molars and incisors. There is also a which become replaced by a loose oedematous network of connective tissue, without significant inflammatory infiltration. Alveolar bone is resorbed. These features are largely the same as those of chronic adult periodontitis and biopsy is of no value in diagnosis.

Treatment

Severely affected teeth may require extraction. Currently, early surgical treatment and tetracycline administration are advised. Surgical excision of the pocket lining may help to eradicate bacteria colonising the epithelial lining and possibly bacteria within the diseased tissue. Tetracycline is effective against *A. actinomycetemcomitans* and given for 2–3 weeks. This treatment may be dramatically successful in the early stages of the disease.

There is a tendency for the condition to slow down or burn out in some individuals in their twenties. The residual disease is referred to as post-juvenile periodontitis.

Other causes of early-onset periodontal destruction

Very rarely, severe periodontal destruction may affect the deciduous and permanent dentition in a condition termed *prepubertal periodontitis*. These children have profound neutrophil or monocyte dysfunction, or both, and suffer from other infections such as otitis media. Another form of generalised severe periodontitis, which affects young individuals in their twenties and early thirties, may also be associated with a phagocyte defect and is referred to as 'rapidly progressive periodontitis' or 'aggressive periodontitis'. Recognised causes of premature periodontal destruction are summarised in Box 5.14.

Box 5.14   Systemic causes of premature periodontal tissue destruction

Immunodeficiencies
- Down's syndrome (Ch. 33)
- Leucopenia (Ch. 24)
- Severe, uncontrolled diabetes mellitus
- HIV infection
- Papillon–Lefèvre syndrome

Genetic syndromes
- Hypophosphatasia
- Ehlers–Danlos syndrome (type VIII)

Others
- Eosinophilic granuloma (Langerhans cell histiocytosis – Ch. 9)

It should be noted that the pathological mechanisms of these different types of premature periodontal tissue destruction are diverse. In the immunodeficiencies, there is acceleration of the usual bacterial processes of tissue destruction. By contrast, in the genetic syndromes mentioned above, there are structural defects in the periodontal tissues, while in Langerhans cell histiocytosis (see below) there is tumour-like destruction of the periodontal tissues.

Fig. 5.21   **Juvenile periodontitis.** Young adult patient aged 20, showing severe bone destruction around three first permanent molars and upper and lower incisors. Probing depths exceeded 10 mm. Courtesy Dr R Saravanamuttu.

All (except Down's syndrome) are uncommon or rare, but are important to distinguish from early-onset periodontitis in that the underlying disorder may threaten the patient's health or life.

Immunodeficiencies

Some types of immunodeficiency disease are associated with premature destructive periodontitis. Down's syndrome, in which there are multiple immunodeficiencies, is the most common example. Agranulocytosis and acute leukaemia may also be associated with necrotising gingivitis and periodontal tissue destruction. Agranulocytosis is mainly a disease of adults, while the common childhood type of acute leukaemia (acute lymphocytic leukaemia) typically does not show periodontal destruction. The importance of cyclic neutropenia has been greatly exaggerated. It is little more than a pathological curiosity and early-onset periodontitis is by no means always associated. It should be emphasised that early-onset periodontitis in patients with immunodeficiency disorders (unlike 'idiopathic' juvenile periodontitis) is typically associated with abnormal susceptibility to non-oral infections. Currently, the development of necrotising ulcerative gingivitis/periodontitis in the absence of disorders described above should lead to suspicion of HIV infection.

Papillon–Lefèvre syndrome

Papillon–Lefèvre syndrome is an exceedingly rare autosomal recessive disorder. The main features are, typically, hyperkeratosis of palms and soles starting in infancy and early-onset periodontal destruction. As a cause of the latter, *A. actinomycetemcomitans* has frequently been implicated. However, it has been shown that there is loss-of-function mutation in the cathepsin C gene. Those with the disease are homozygous for the mutation and completely lack cathepsin C activity. Carriers are heterozygous, have low cathepsin C activity but suffer no ill-effects. Parents of children with Papillon–Lefèvre syndrome have low cathepsin C activity, but do not seem to have premature periodontal destruction.

Cathepsin C, a lysosomal protease, plays an essential role in activating granule serine proteases in bone marrow-derived effector cells, particularly neutrophils. Lack of activation of these enzymes impairs host responses to bacteria in periodontal pockets. The possibility that depressed cathepsin C activity may be responsible for common types of periodontitis seems unlikely.

There is also speculation that cathepsin C might also have a role in the abnormal keratosis in Papillon–Lefèvre syndrome.

Ehlers–Danlos syndrome (type VIII)

Ehlers–Danlos syndrome is an important cause of floppy joint syndromes and its main oral effects are on the temporomandibular joint, where it can be responsible for recurrent dislocations. However, in the type VIII variant, which is inherited as an autosomal dominant, there is bruising, soft and hyperextensible skin and hypermobile joints. Early-onset periodontal disease is related to a defect in collagen formation and low levels of collagen 1. This is usually the result of mutations in the COL1A2 gene. Teeth are commonly lost by the age of 30 years.

Langerhans cell histiocytosis (eosinophilic granuloma)

Eosinophilic granuloma is a tumour or tumour-like disease (Ch. 9). A typical effect is destruction of the bone of the jaw with formation of a tumour-like mass. It can also cause a distinctive type of periodontal tissue destruction which exposes the roots of the teeth. Radiographically, this gives an appearance described as 'teeth floating on air'.

Hypophosphatasia

Hypophosphatasia is a rare genetic disorder which can have severe skeletal effects as a result of failure of development of mature bone. There may also be failure of cementum formation causing loosening or exfoliation of the teeth without signs of gingivitis or periodontitis. Premature loss of the deciduous teeth, especially the incisors, is characteristic and occasionally the only overt manifestation of the disease.

ACUTE PERICORONITIS

Incomplete eruption of a wisdom tooth produces a large stagnation area under the gum flap. It can easily become infected, causing pericoronitis. Several factors (Box 5.15) may contribute.

Box 5.15   Factors contributing to pericoronitis
• Impaction of food and plaque accumulation under the gum flap • An upper tooth biting on the gum flap • Acute ulcerative gingivitis (rarely)

Pericoronitis is caused by a mixed infection and various pathogens of dental plaque, particularly anaerobes, can be causative.

Clinical features

Young adults are affected. The main symptoms are soreness and tenderness around the partially erupted tooth (Figs 5.22 and 5.23). There is pain, swelling, difficulty in opening the mouth, lymphadenopathy, sometimes slight fever and, in severe cases, suppuration and abscess formation. Swelling and difficulty in opening the mouth may be severe enough to prevent examination of the area.

Management

Food debris should be removed from under the gum flap by irrigation. The position of the affected tooth, its relationship to the second molar and any complicating factors should be determined by radiography.

Fig. 5.22 **Pericoronitis.** A pocket has formed between the gingiva and the crown of a partially erupted third molar, which is overlaid by the operculum.

Fig. 5.23 **Pericoronitis.** Section through the operculum shows the heavy deposits of microbial plaque beneath it and along its anterior edge (left) (Gram stain).

In mild cases, it may be enough for patients to keep the mouth clean and to use hot mouth rinses whenever symptoms develop, until the inflammation subsides. This may happen naturally by further eruption or by extraction of the tooth after the infection has been overcome.

If radiographs show that the third molar is badly misplaced, impacted or carious, it should be extracted after inflammation has subsided. Spread of infection (cellulitis or osteomyelitis) may follow extraction of the tooth while infection is still acute, but is rare.

When an upper tooth is biting on the flap, it is often preferable to extract it, especially if the lower tooth is ultimately to be removed. If there are strong reasons for retaining the upper tooth, the cusps should be ground away sufficiently to prevent it from traumatising the flap. In the past, caustic agents such as trichloracetic acid were commonly used to reduce the operculum. This was very effective but carries a risk of accidental burns to adjacent mucosa or skin. Electrocautery may also be used. In severe cases, particularly when there is fever and lymphadenopathy, penicillin or penicillin and metronidazole should be given.

Pus may track posteriorly from the operculum to cause serious fascial space infection as described in the next chapter. In the pre-antibiotic era, acute infection from pericoronitis was a relatively common cause of death in young adults.

Both treated and untreated acute pericoronitis may become chronic if the operculum remains. In the absence of further acute episodes there is extensive bone loss around the partially erupted tooth and its neighbours.

ACUTE NECROTISING ULCERATIVE GINGIVITIS

Acute ulcerative gingivitis is a distinct and specific disease which can cause significant periodontal tissue damage but does not often contribute to chronic periodontal disease. The following account describes the disease in HIV-negative persons.

Clinical features

The incidence of ulcerative gingivitis has declined sharply in the Western world since the Second World War. It typically affects apparently healthy young adults, usually those with neglected mouths.

Typical features are summarised in Box 5.16.

Box 5.16 Typical features of acute necrotizing ulcerative gingivitis

- Young adult males mainly affected
- Often cigarette smokers and/or with minor respiratory infection
- Cratered ulcers starting at the tips of the interdental papillae
- Ulcers spread along gingival margins
- Gingival soreness and bleeding
- Foul breath
- No significant lymphadenopathy
- No fever or systemic upset
- Smears from ulcers dominated by Gram-negative spirochaetes and fusiform bacteria
- Responds to oral hygiene and metronidazole in immunocompetent patients

---

Crater-shaped or punched-out ulcers form initially at the tips of the interdental papillae. Ulcers are sharply defined by erythema and oedema; their surface is covered by a greyish or yellowish tenacious slough. Removal of the slough causes free bleeding. The severe halitosis, likened to rotting hay, is characteristic.

Lesions remain restricted to the gingivae and supporting tissues. They mainly spread along the gingival margins and deeply, destroying interdental soft and hard tissues, but rarely across the attached gingiva. Deep spread can cause rapid destruction of both soft tissues and bone, producing triangular spaces between the teeth (Fig. 5.24).

If treatment is delayed, the end result can be considered distortion of the normal gingival contours, promoting stagnation and possibly recurrences or chronic periodontal disease.

In the past particularly, localised spread to immediately adjacent oral mucosa was occasionally seen but acute ulcerative gingivitis does not spread over the oral mucosa.

Aetiology

The bacteria responsible are a complex of spirochaetes and fusiforms (Fig. 5.25). These organisms may be present in small numbers in the healthy gingival flora. With the onset of ulcerative gingivitis, both bacteria proliferate until they dominate the bacterial picture in smears from the lesions. This overwhelming proliferation of the spirochaete and fusobacterium at the site of tissue destruction, invasion of the tissues by spirochaetes seen by electron microscopy, and the sharp fall in their numbers with effective treatment indicate that they are the responsible agents. Nevertheless, it is still uncertain whether this spirochaetal complex is the sole cause of ulcerative gingivitis and other bacteria have been implicated (Box 5.17).

Despite doubts about the precise identity of the bacterial cause of acute ulcerative gingivitis, it is clearly an anaerobic infection and responds rapidly to metronidazole.

Fig. 5.24 Acute necrotising ulcerative gingivitis. The characteristic features of the lesion, the crater-shaped ulcers starting at the tips of the interdental papillae, are covered by a slough, as shown here.

Fig. 5.25 A smear from an ulcer of acute necrotising ulcerative gingivitis shows the dense proliferation of *Treponema vincentii* and *Fusobacterium nucleatum*.

Box 5.17   Bacteria implicated in acute ulcerative gingivitis

- *Treponema vincentii*
- *Fusobacterium fusiformis*
- *Prevotella intermedia*
- *Porphyromonas gingivalis*
- *Selenomonas sputigena*
- *Leptotrichia buccalis*

Host factors Ulcerative gingivitis is a disease of otherwise healthy young adults usually with neglected, dirty mouths. However, ulcerative gingivitis may also develop in children having immunosuppressive treatment and in patients with HIV infection (see below).

Local factors appear to be important and ulcerative gingivitis does not appear to be transmissible. Ulcerative gingivitis ('trench mouth') was almost epidemic among soldiers in the 1914–1918 war and civilians subjected to bombing in the 1939–1945 war. Malnutrition has been excluded as a factor during these periods but being shelled or bombed can (reasonably enough) be regarded as stressful. Other evidence also suggests that chronic anxiety may be a predisposing factor in this infection. Smoking and upper respiratory infections have also been implicated. However, ulcerative gingivitis is relatively rarely seen in the UK now (Box 5.18) and its aetiology remains uncertain.

Box 5.18   Differential diagnosis of acute necrotising ulcerative gingivitis

- Primary herpetic gingivostomatitis
- HIV-associated acute ulcerative gingivitis (see below)
- Gingival ulceration in acute leukaemia or aplastic anaemia

Treatment

Oral hygiene (debridement) is essential. Metronidazole (200 mg by mouth, taken after food three times a day for three days) greatly accelerates resolution. Side-effects are few, apart from interaction with alcohol, and rarely significant.

Follow-up treatment and rehabilitation of the mouth Once the acute phase has subsided, the state of oral hygiene should be brought to as high a standard as possible to lessen the risk of recurrence.

HIV-ASSOCIATED GINGIVITIS

HIV-positive persons can suffer severe necrotising ulcerative gingivitis as their immune function declines. Clinically, it resembles ulcerative gingivitis in HIV-negative persons, but rapidly progresses to HIV-associated periodontitis.

Another distinctive HIV-associated gingivitis can be an early sign and precede other opportunistic infections. It appears as a distinct erythematous band extending along the free and attached gingiva. Clinically, it resembles so-called desquamative gingivitis (Ch. 13) rather than common chronic gingivitis, but profuse bleeding is characteristic (Box 5.19).

Box 5.19   Typical features of HIV-associated gingivitis

- Well-demarcated band of erythema along free and attached gingiva
- Resembles 'desquamative gingivitis' clinically
- Profuse bleeding
- Bacteria similar to those from periodontal pockets

The precise aetiology of HIV-associated gingivitis is unclear, especially as the bacteria isolated from it are similar to those from advanced chronic periodontitis.

HIV-ASSOCIATED PERIODONTITIS

HIV-associated ulcerative gingivitis, as described earlier, is associated with soft-tissue necrosis and rapid destruction of the periodontal tissues. It is typically intensely painful. There is little deep pocketing because soft tissue and bone are lost virtually simultaneously. More than 90% of the attachment can be lost within 3–6 months and the soft-tissue necrosis can lead to exposure of bone and sequestration.

The pain of HIV-associated periodontitis is usually aching in character and felt within the jaw rather than in the gingivae. It may be felt before tissue destruction becomes obvious. HIV-associated gingivitis and periodontitis are usually generalised but are sometimes localised to one or more discrete areas.

Bacteriologically, HIV-associated periodontitis resembles that of classical periodontitis in HIV-negative persons. It is typically associated with a low CD4 count and a poor prognosis for the patient.

Management

Debridement and removal of any sequestra under local anaesthesia, chlorhexidine mouth rinses, systemic metronidazole and analgesics may be effective. Additional broad-spectrum antibiotics have been recommended by some, but increase the risk of thrush to which these patients are particularly susceptible. If thrush is present or develops, antifungal treatment is required. For persistent pain, oral analgesics are indicated.

HERPETIC GINGIVOSTOMATITIS

In children particularly, primary herpetic stomatitis is associated with acute gingivitis. The gingivae are conspicuously erythematous and oedematous (Fig. 5.26). Herpetic ulcers may form on the tips of the interdental papillae or on any other anatomical regions of the gingivae, but are not an essential feature. Unlike ulcerative gingivitis, herpetic vesicles and ulcers extend widely over the oral mucosa. Lymphadenopathy is associated and systemic upset may be severe.

Smears from the lesions show typical viral damaged cells and the gingivitis resolves with control of the virus. This may be hastened by use of aciclovir (Ch. 12).

MISCELLANEOUS PERIODONTAL DISORDERS

Gingival swelling

Gingival swelling may be due to fibrous hyperplasia or to nonfibrous inflammatory or other infiltrations (Box 5.20).

Hereditary gingival fibromatosis

Gingival fibromatosis is a feature of several heritable syndromes and may also develop as an isolated condition. All are rare, but the most common type is an autosomal dominant

syndrome in which gingival fibromatosis may be associated with hypertrichosis and mental retardation.

Gingival enlargement may precede eruption of the teeth or may not develop until later in childhood. The gingivae may be so grossly enlarged as completely to bury the teeth and are

---

Box 5.20   Causes of gingival enlargement

Fibrous gingival hyperplasia
- Genetic
- Drug-associated
  Phenytoin
  Calcium-channel blockers
  Cyclosporin

Inflammatory gingival swelling
- Chronic 'hyperplastic' gingivitis
- Pregnancy gingivitis
- Leukaemia infiltration
- Wegener's granulomatosis
- Sarcoidosis
- Orofacial granulomatosis
- Scurvy

---

pale, firm and smooth or stippled in texture (Fig. 5.27). The facial features may also be coarse and thickened, simulating acromegaly, and there may be excessive hairiness (hypertrichosis). Epilepsy or mental retardation are rare features.

Histologically, the gingival tissue consists of thick bundles of collagenous connective tissue with little or no inflammatory exudate (Fig. 5.28).

The excess gingival tissue can only be removed surgically but is likely to re-form. Gingivectomy should be delayed as long as possible, preferably until after puberty, when the rate of growth of the tissues is slower. Maintenance of oral hygiene is important to prevent infection becoming established in the deep false pockets. However, inflammation is frequently insignificant.

Fig. 5.26   **Acute herpetic gingivostomatitis.** There is diffuse reddening of the attached gingiva with ulceration in the lower incisor region extending beyond the attached gingiva (see also Ch. 12).

Fig. 5.27   **Hereditary gingival fibromatosis.** Fibrous overgrowth of the gingiva has covered the crowns of the teeth and almost buried them (pseudo-anodontia).

Fig. 5.28 **Gingival fibromatosis.** Both the genetic and drug-induced types share this histological picture of gross fibrous proliferation (red) and (frequently, as here) absence of inflammation.

Fig. 5.29 **Gingival hyperplasia due to phenytoin.** Characteristically (unlike Fig. 5.27), the fibrous overgrowth has originated in the interdental papillae, which become bulbous but remain firm and pale. Localised gross enlargement such as that around the upper central incisor may result and can form a plaque trap.

Drug-induced hyperplasia

Long-term use of the anti-epileptic drug phenytoin (Epanutin[2]) can cause gingival hyperplasia. The overgrowth principally involves the interdental papillae, which become bulbous and overlap the teeth (Fig. 5.29). Typically, the gingivae are firm and pale and the stippled texture is exaggerated, producing an orange-peel appearance.

Infection appears to contribute and overgrowth of the gingivae can sometimes be kept under control by rigorous oral hygiene. Frequently, however, gingivectomy becomes necessary or is demanded by patients who are embarrassed by what they regard as a stigma of their disease.

Clinically, similar changes are seen with use of calcium-channel blockers such as nifedipine and diltiazem (for hypertension or angina) and with the immunosuppressive drug cyclosporin. Clinically, they all cause preferential enlargement of the interdental papillae and histologically they all resemble the genetic type of gingival hyperplasia.

INFLAMMATORY GINGIVAL SWELLINGS

Chronic 'hyperplastic' and pregnancy gingivitis have been discussed earlier.

Wegener's granulomatosis → Summary p. 324

Wegener's granulomatosis (Ch. 28) is an uncommon, frequently lethal disease of which the typical features are granulomatous ulceration of the nasopharynx, pulmonary cavitation and renal damage. Occasionally, the first sign is a characteristic form of proliferative gingivitis, bright or dusky red in colour and with a granular surface, to which the term 'strawberry gums' has been applied. Recognition of this type of gingivitis and confirmation of the diagnosis by biopsy, which shows the characteristic giant cells, may be life-saving by enabling treatment to start exceptionally early.

Sarcoidosis and orofacial granulomatosis

As discussed in Chapters 28 and 29, these diseases can give rise to gingival swelling in which granuloma formation is seen histologically. They cannot be distinguished by gingival biopsy alone.

Acute leukaemia

Gingival swelling is most frequently seen in acute myelomonocytic leukaemia. The abnormal white cells are unable to perform their normal defensive function and cannot control infection at the gingival margins. The abnormal leucocytes pack the area until the gingivae become swollen with leukaemic cells (Fig. 5.30). These cells are so defective that infection progresses, leading to ulceration and breakdown of the tissues.

Clinically, the gingivae are swollen, shiny, pale or purplish in colour and frequently ulcerated (Fig. 5.31). Other signs of leukaemia (pallor, purpura or lassitude) may also be seen.

Topical antibiotics or chlorhexidine and improved oral hygiene may lead to regression of the swelling (Fig. 5.32), but the patient's general prognosis is poor.

[2]Dilantin is an American proprietary name for phenytoin that has not been used in the UK.

Fig. 5.30 **Acute myelomonocytic leukaemia.** The gingival swelling can be seen to be due to packing of the gingivae with leukaemic cells. The periodontal tissues have broken down as a result of the poor resistance to infection.

Fig. 5.31 **Acute myelomonocytic leukaemia.** The gingival margins are swollen and soft due to the leukaemic infiltrate.

Scurvy

Grossly swollen and congested gingivae are a classical sign of scurvy but, though the disease is largely of historical interest, occasional cases are reported even now.

The gingival swelling is due to a combination of chronic inflammation and an exaggeration of the inflammatory congestion due to scorbutic purpura. The diagnosis should only be made on clear evidence of dietary deficiency and of purpura. In these cases, treatment with vitamin C and adequate oral hygiene relieves the gingival condition.

Fig. 5.32 **Acute leukaemia.** (A) Gross leukaemic infiltration has caused the gingival margins to reach the incisal edges of the teeth. (B) The benefits of plaque control with an antibiotic mouth rinse and oral hygiene have restored the normal appearance.

GINGIVAL RECESSION

Recession of the gingivae and eventual exposure of the roots is common (Figs 5.33 and 5.34). It is usually, but not invariably, associated with ageing, as susceptibility to it varies. The major predisposing factor is thinness of the gingival tissue. This is readily damaged by trauma from forceful toothbrushing and plaque-induced inflammation. One hypothesis suggests that epithelial proliferation of the junctional epithelium in inflammation results in an epithelial 'bridge' extending to the external gingival epithelium across the narrow band of inflamed connective tissue. This is followed by remodelling of the gingival margin. It seems likely that plaque-induced loss of attachment in areas of thick tissue can lead to pocket formation, whereas thin tissue is destroyed entirely. The resulting receded gingival margins often appear relatively uninflamed.

Gingival abrasion

Abrasion causes recession of the gingivae and damage to the teeth. Early changes may be seen in some young adults and severe examples in later life. Forceful toothbrushing with a stiff brush used with a sawing motion across the teeth and use of an

Fig. 5.33 **Advanced periodontitis with recession.** In this neglected mouth, deposits of plaque and supragingival calculus adhere to the exposed roots, which are vulnerable to caries.

Fig. 5.34 **Periodontitis with recession.** In this case, gingival destruction is almost as great as the degree of bone resorption so that excessively long clinical crowns have been produced. Supragingival calculus and a dense inflammatory infiltrate in the gingiva can be seen.

abrasive dentifrice is the usual cause. Grooves are worn into the necks of the teeth and reactionary dentine forms beneath. Eventually, the necks of teeth may be cut so deeply that the crowns break off, but the pulp remains covered by reactionary dentine (see Fig. 4.37). The gingival margins recede but they remain conspicuously firm, pale and healthy. Nearby, there may be chronic gingivitis where the toothbrush cannot reach.

Treatment of gingival recession

Recession of the gingivae sometimes causes patients to fear that they will soon lose their teeth. In older patients, where enough alveolar bone remains, the teeth can remain in useful function for many years and patients can be reassured. The main requirement is to keep the gingival margins plaque-free, especially in the enlarged interstitial spaces. In the case of abrasive gingival recession, the patient must also be shown how to keep the teeth clean without causing further damage.

Various surgical procedures have been devised to correct localised areas of gingival recession or to produce thicker zones of gingiva which, it is hoped, are more resistant to recession. Their long-term results are disappointing.

An early result of abrasion is exposure of the dentine, which may be hypersensitive. Many treatments for it have been introduced, but their number betrays their limitations. Traditional remedies are topical applications of strong astringents such as zinc chloride or silver nitrate. Proprietary preparations such as Tresiolan and Durophat may be more effective.

SUGGESTED FURTHER READING

Armitage GC 1999 Development of a classification system for periodontal diseases and conditions. Ann Periodontol 4:1–6

Bozzo L, Almeida OP, Scully C, Aldred MJ 1994 Hereditary gingival fibromatosis. Report of an extensive four-generation pedigree. Oral Surg Oral Med Oral Pathol 78:452–454

Corbet EF, Davies WIR 1993 The role of supragingival plaque in the control of progressive periodontal disease. J Clin Periodontol 20:307–313

De Vree J, Steenackers K, De Boever JA 2000 Periodontal treatment of rapid progression periodontitis in 2 siblings with Papillon-Lefevre syndrome: 15-year follow-up. J Clin Periodontol 27:354–360

Fairbrother KJ, Heasman PF 2000 Anticalulus agents. Clin Periodontol 27:285–301

Feres M, Haffajee AD, Goncalves C et al 1999 Systemic doxycycline administration in the treatment of periodontal infections (1). Effect on the subgingival microflora. J Clin Periodontal 26:775–783

Fine DH 1994 Microbial identification and antibiotic sensitivity testing, an aid for patients refractory to periodontal therapy. J Clin Periodontol 21:98–106

Grossi SG, Zambon JJ, Ho AW et al 1994 Assessment of risk for periodontal disease. I. Risk indicators for attachment loss. J Periodontol 65:260–267

Grossi SG, Genco RJ, Machtei EE et al 1995 Assessment of risk for periodontal disease. II. Risk factors for alveolar bone loss. J Periodontol 66: 23–29

Hildebolt CF 1997 Osteoporosis and oral bone loss. Dentomaxillofacial Radiol 36:3–15

Holmstrup P, Westergaard J 1994 Periodontal disease in HIV-infected patients. J Clin Periodontol 21:270–280

Hornung GM, Cohen ME 1995 Necrotizing ulcerative gingivitis, periodontitis, and stomatitis: clinical staging and predisposing factors. J Periodontol 66:990–998

Ishikawa I, Umeda M, Laosrisin N 1994 Clinical, bacteriological and immunological examinations and the treatment process of two Papillon-Lefèvre patients. J Clin Periodontol 65:364–371

Jeffcoat MK, Chestnut CH 1993 Systemic osteoporosis and oral bone loss. Evidence shows increased risk. J Am Dent Assoc 124:49–56

Johnson BD, Engel D 1986 Acute necrotising ulcerative gingivitis: a review of diagnosis, etiology and treatment. J Periodontol 57:155–161

Johnson NW, Bain CA 2000 Tobacco and oral disease. EU-Working Group on Tobacco and Oral Health. Br Dent J 189:200-206

Jonasson G, Kiliaridis S, Gunnarsson R 1999 Cervical thickness of the mandibular alveolar process and skeletal bone mineral density. Acta Odontol Scand 57:155–161

Liede KE, Haukka JK, Hietanen JHP et al 1999 The association between smoking cessation and periodontal status and salivary proteinase levels. J Periodontol 70:1361–1368

Liljenberg B, Lindhe J, Berglundh T et al 1994 Some microbiological, histopathological and immunohistochemical characteristics of progressive periodontal disease. J Clin Periodontol 21:720–727

Linden GJ, Mullaly BH 1994 Cigarette smoking and periodontal destruction in young adults. J Periodontol 65:718–723

Löe H, Brown J 1991 Early onset periodontitis in the United States of America. J Periodontol 62:608–616

Luke DA 1992 The structure and function of the dentogingival junction and periodontal ligament. Br Dent J 172:187–190

Margiotta V, Pizza I, Pizza G, Barbaro A 1996 Cyclosporin- and nifedepine-induced gingival overgrowth in renal transplant patients: correlations with periodontal and pharmacological parameters, and HLA-antigens. Oral Pathol Med 25:128–134

Nery EB, Eson RG, Lee KK et al 1995 Prevalence of nifedipine-induced gingival hyperplasia. J Periodontol 66:572–578

Palmer RM, Scott DA, Meeking TN et al 1999 Potential mechanisms of susceptibility to periodontitis in tobacco smokers. J Periodont Res 34:363–369

Plagmann H-C, Kocher T, Kuhrau N, Caliebe A 1994 Periodontal manifestation of hypophosphatasia. A family case report. J Clin Periodontol 21:710–716

Praytino SW, Addy M, Wade WG 1993 Does gingivitis lead to periodontitis in young adults? Lancet 342:471–472

Renvert S, Dahlén G, Wikström M 1996 Treatment of periodontal disease based on microbiological diagnosis. Relation between microbiological and clinical parameters during 5 years. J Periodontol 67:562–571

Robinson PG, Winkler JR, Palmer G et al 1994 The diagnosis of periodontal conditions associated with HIV infection. J Periodontol 65:236–243

Ronderos M, Jacobs DR, Himes JH et al 2000 Associations of periodontal disease with femoral bone mineral density and estrogen therapy: cross-sectional evaluation of US adults from NANES III. J Clin Periodontol 27:778–786

Smith GLF 1994 Diagnosis of periodontal disease activity by detection of key mocrobial antigens. J Clin Periodontol 21:615–620

Socransky SS, Haffajee AD 1991 Microbial mechanisms in the pathogenesis of destructive periodontal disease: a critical assessment. J Periodontol 26:322–331

Socransky SS, Haffajee AD 1992 The bacteriology of destructive periodontal disease: current concepts. J Periodontol 63:195–212

Thakker N 2000 Genetic analysis of Papillon-Lefèvre syndrome. Oral Dis 6:263

Timmerman MF, van der Weijden GA, van Steenbergen TJM et al 1996 Evaluation of the long-term efficacy and safety of locally applied minocycline in adult periontitis patients. J Clin Periodontol 23:707–716

Williams DM, Hughes FJ, Odell EW, Farthing PM 1992 Pathology of periodontal disease. Oxford University Press, Oxford

Major infections of the mouth, jaws and perioral tissues

Severe oral and perioral infections are uncommon. It is hardly surprising, however, in view of the vast number of bacteria in the mouth, that oral and perioral infections are of local origin. Periodontal pockets, in particular, contain great concentrations of bacteria, many of which are potent pathogens. Moreover, these bacteria can give rise to serious systemic infections, such as infective endocarditis. Also, in the past particularly, but occasionally today, they can be life-threatening or fatal by direct spread.

Syphilitic, actinomycotic and tuberculous osteomyelitis of the jaws are recognised entities, but largely of historical interest.

ACUTE OSTEOMYELITIS OF THE JAWS → Summaries pp. 66, 190, 448

Osteomyelitis of the jaws is mainly a disease of adults with several potential sources of infection (Box 6.1).

> **Box 6.1   Acute osteomyelitis of the jaws: potential sources of infection**
>
> - Periapical infection
> - A periodontal pocket involved in a fracture
> - Acute necrotising gingivitis or pericoronitis (even more rarely)
> - Penetrating, contaminated injuries (open fractures or gunshot wounds)

Many patients have a predisposing cause and the most important are summarised in Box 6.2. Rare causes include osteopetrosis (Ch.10). The effect of immunodeficiency is variable and acute osteomyelitis of the jaw is uncommon in HIV infection.

Clinical features

Most patients with osteomyelitis are adult males with infection of the mandible. Osteomyelitis of the maxilla is a rare disease of neonates or infants after either birth injuries or uncontrolled middle ear infection.

Early complaints are severe, throbbing, deep-seated pain and swelling with external swelling due to inflammatory oedema. Later, distension of the periosteum with pus and, finally,

---

> **Box 6.2   Important predisposing conditions for osteomyelitis**
>
> **Local damage to or disease of the jaws**
> - Fractures including gunshot wounds
> - Radiation damage
> - Causes of osteosclerosis
>
>   Paget's disease
>   Late stages of fibro-osseous lesions
>   Osteopetrosis
>
> **Impaired immune defences**
> - Acute leukaemia
> - Poorly controlled diabetes mellitus
> - Sickle cell anaemia
> - Chronic alcoholism or malnutrition

---

subperiosteal bone formation cause the swelling to become firm. The overlying gingiva is red, swollen and tender.

Associated teeth are tender. They may become loose and pus may exude from an open socket or gingival margins. Muscle oedema causes difficulty in opening the mouth and swallowing. Regional lymph nodes are enlarged and tender and anaesthesia or paraesthesia of the lower lip is characteristic.

Frequently, the patient remains surprisingly well but, in the acute phase, there may be fever and leucocytosis. A severely ill or very pale patient suggests underlying disease which requires investigation.

Radiographic changes do not appear until after at least 10 days. Loss of trabecular pattern and areas of radiolucency indicate bone destruction. These areas have ill-defined margins and have a fluffy or moth-eaten appearance (Fig. 6.1). Areas of dead bone appear as relatively dense areas which become more sharply defined as they are progressively separated as sequestra. Later, in young persons particularly, subperiosteal new bone formation causes a buccal swelling and appears as a thin, curved strip of new bone below the lower border of the jaw in lateral radiographs.

Pathology

Oral bacteria, particularly anaerobes such as *Bacteroides*, *Porphyromonas* or *Prevotella* species are important causes, but

Fig. 6.1 **Osteomyelitis of the mandible following dental extractions.** The outlines of the extraction sockets can be seen, together with dense sequestra of bone lying in a poorly circumscribed radiolucency.

Fig. 6.2 High-power view of a sequestrum showing non-vital bone (the osteocyte lacunae are empty) and eroded outline with superficial lacunae produced by osteoclastic resorption and a dense surface growth of bacteria.

Fig. 6.3 **Late-stage chronic osteomyelitis.** A sequestrum trapped in a cavity within the bone. It is surrounded by fibrous tissue containing an infiltrate of inflammatory cells. Surgical intervention is needed to remove an infected sequestrum such as this.

At the boundaries between infected and healthy tissue, osteoclasts resorb the periphery of the dead bone which eventually becomes separated as a sequestrum (Fig. 6.3). Once infection starts to localise, new bone forms around it, particularly subperiosteally.

Where bone has died and been removed, healing is by granulation with formation of coarse fibrous bone in the proliferating connective tissue. After resolution, woven bone is gradually replaced by compact bone and remodelled to restore normal morphology.

Management

The main requirements are summarised in Box 6.3.

Box 6.3 **Summary of management of osteomyelitis**

Essential measures
- Bacterial sampling and culture
- Vigorous (empirical) antibiotic treatment
- Drainage
- Analgesics
- Give specific antibiotics based on culture and sensitivities
- Debridement
- Remove source of infection, if possible

Adjunctive treatment
- Sequestrectomy
- Decortication if necessary
- Hyperbaric oxygen*
- Resection and reconstruction for extensive bone destruction

*Mainly of value for osteoradionecrosis and, possibly, anaerobic infections.

---

the infection is often mixed. Staphylococci may be responsible when they enter from the skin via an open fracture.

The mandible has a relatively limited blood supply and dense bone with thick cortical plates. Infection causes acute inflammation in the medullary soft tissues and inflammatory exudate spreads infection through the marrow spaces. It also compresses blood vessels confined within the rigid boundaries of the vascular canals. Thrombosis and obstruction then lead to further bone necrosis. Dead bone is recognisable microscopically by lacunae empty of osteocytes but filled with neutrophils and colonies of bacteria which proliferate in the dead tissue (Fig. 6.2).

Pus, formed by liquefaction of necrotic soft tissue and inflammatory cells, is forced along the medulla and eventually reaches the subperiosteal region by resorption of bone. Distension of the periosteum by pus stimulates subperiosteal bone formation, but perforation of the periosteum by pus and formation of sinuses on the skin or oral mucosa are rarely seen now.

Bacteriological diagnosis A specimen of pus or a swab from the depths of the lesion must first be taken for culture and sensitivity testing.

Antimicrobial treatment Immediately a specimen has been obtained, vigorous antibiotic treatment should be started.

Initially, penicillin, 600–1200 mg daily can be given by injection (if the patient is not allergic), with metronidazole 200–400 mg 8-hourly. Clindamycin penetrates avascular tissue better and is frequently effective. The regimen is adjusted later in the light of the bacteriological findings.

Debridement   Removal of foreign or necrotic material and immobilisation of any fracture are necessary if there has been a gunshot wound or other contaminating injury.

Drainage   Pressure should be relieved by tooth extraction, bur holes or decortication, as necessary, and exudate drained into the mouth or externally.

Removal of sequestra   Dead bone should not be forcibly separated and vigorous curetting is inadvisable but, in the late stages, a loosened sequestrum may have to be removed. Teeth should be extracted only if loosened by tissue destruction.

Adjunctive treatment   Decortication or hyperbaric oxygen therapy, or both, may be attempted, particularly in radiation-associated osteomyelitis, though the effectiveness of hyperbaric oxygen is unproven.

Complications

Anaesthesia of the lower lip usually recovers with elimination of the infection. Rare complications include pathological fracture caused by extensive bone destruction, chronic osteomyelitis after inadequate treatment, cellulitis due to spread of exceptionally virulent bacteria or septicaemia in an immunodeficient patient.

Key features of acute osteomyelitis of the jaws are summarised in Box 6.4.

> **Box 6.4   Acute osteomyelitis of the jaws: key features**
>
> - Mandible mainly affected, usually in adult males
> - Infection of dental origin – anaerobes are important
> - Pain and swelling of jaw
> - Teeth in the area are tender: gingivae are red and swollen
> - Sometimes paraesthesia of the lip
> - Minimal systemic upset
> - After about 10 days, radiographs show moth-eaten pattern of bone destruction
> - Good response to prompt antibiotic treatment and debridement

CHRONIC OSTEOMYELITIS → Summaries pp. 66, 190, 448

Rarely, inadequately treated acute osteomyelitis may lead to chronic suppurative osteomyelitis, which may also be a complication of irradiation (Fig. 6.4). Persistent low-grade infection is associated with bone destruction and granulation tissue formation, but little suppuration.

Chronic osteomyelitis more frequently arises de novo as a result of infection by weakly virulent bacteria or in avascular bone.

Chronic osteomyelitis is commoner than acute osteomyelitis. Like the acute condition, there are usually predisposing factors

Fig. 6.4   Chronic osteomyelitis secondary to radiotherapy. Part of the necrotic portion of the mandible is visible, having ulcerated through the skin.

Fig. 6.5   Chronic osteomyelitis. The extent of destruction is much more readily apparent than in acute osteomyelitis. Note the sequestra lying close to the lower border and the peripheral sclerosis. Subperiosteal new bone formation is evident below the lower border.

such as those in Box 6.2. However, local bone sclerosis is a much more likely predisposing factor for chronic osteomyelitis than acute.

Clinically, the picture is often dominated by persistent ache or pain with exposed bone and radiographic changes rather than florid infection. Radiographic appearances are variable but sometimes distinctive (Fig. 6.5). Sequestra will usually separate spontaneously or may occasionally reincorporate into healing bone after effective antibiotic treatment. Chronic osteomyelitis must be treated aggressively. Infection may spread widely through abnormal bone or in a debilitated host (Fig. 6.6). Low-virulence organisms or repeated inadequate antibiotic treatment may lead to longstanding osteomyelitis with extensive

Fig. 6.6 Sequestration of the entire mandible following chronic osteomyelitis of odontogenic origin.

sclerosis of the remaining viable bone, in so-called diffuse sclerosing osteomyelitis (Box 6.5).

Box 6.5   Diffuse sclerosing osteomyelitis: key features

- Adults
- No sex predilection
- Sclerosis round site of periapical or periodontal chronic inflammation
- Persistent ache or pain but no swelling
- Radiographically resembles but is distinct from florid cemento-osseous dysplasia

Pathology
- Bone sclerosis and remodelling
- Scanty marrow spaces and little or no inflammatory infiltrate, though adjacent to areas of inflammation

Treatment
- Elimination of originating source of inflammation, but sclerotic areas remain radiographically

---

CHRONIC LOW-GRADE OSTEOMYELITIS AND OSTEITIS → Summaries pp. 173, 190

In some cases, a focus of osteomyelitis is so small or caused by such low-virulence organisms that the clinical presentation is dominated by the local bone reaction to the infection rather than the infection itself. Suppuration and infiltration of marrow spaces by inflammatory cells are absent and bacteria are not readily cultivable. Diffuse sclerosing osteomyelitis (see Box 6.5) was noted above. Other examples of such conditions are focal sclerosing osteomyelitis and proliferative periostitis.

Focal sclerosing osteomyelitis (Box 6.6) is characterised by sclerosis of the surrounding bone and is commoner in the young and in very longstanding infection.

Box 6.6   Focal sclerosing osteomyelitis: key features

- Bony reaction to low-grade periapical infection or unusually strong host defensive response
- Children and young adults affected
- Premolar or molar region of mandible affected
- Bone sclerosis associated with a non-vital or pulpitic tooth
- Localised but uniform radiodensity related to tooth with widened periodontal ligament space or periapical area
- No expansion of the jaw

Pathology
- Dense sclerotic bone with scanty connective tissue or inflammatory cells

Treatment
- Elimination of the source of inflammation by extraction or endodontic treatment

---

Chronic osteomyelitis in children and adolescents is unusual, but often elicits florid proliferative periostitis as a healing response (Box 6.7). Layers of periosteal new bone formation may expand the cortex by up to a centimetre or more in thickness. Vague pain and prominent bony enlargement are the main features and computerised tomography is useful to identify a small focus of chronic infection or sequestration in the expanded bone.

Box 6.7   Proliferative periostitis ('Garrè's osteomyelitis'*): key features

- Adolescents mainly affected
- Usually associated with periapical but sometimes other inflammatory foci
- Periosteal reaction affecting lower border of mandible causing 'onion skin' thickening and swelling of bone

Pathology
- Parallel layers of highly cellular woven bone interspersed with scantily inflamed connective tissue
- Small sequestra if present

Treatment
- Eliminate focus of infection
- Bone gradually remodels after 6 to 12 months

*Garrè's osteomyelitis is a misnomer. In his original description he made no mention of proliferative changes in the lesion, X-rays had not then been invented and he provided no histological back-up.

Sclerosing osteitis is a term given to a localised area of sclerosis without evidence of infection. These are probably a reaction to inflammation rather than infection and are frequently seen around the roots of non-vital teeth (Fig. 6.7) resembling lesions of cemento-osseous dysplasia. No treatment is required other than to remove the causative tooth.

BISPHOSPHONATE-INDUCED OSTEONECROSIS

Bisphosphonates inhibit bone resorption by suppressing osteoclast activity and are frequently used to lessen bone destruction by metastases to bone, particularly from multiple myeloma,

Fig. 6.7 Sclerosing osteitis, a focal zone of sclerosis associated with periapical inflammation from a non-vital lower first molar. Courtesy of Mr EJ Whaites.

Fig. 6.8 Exposed necrotic bone in bisphosphonate-induced osteonecrosis, **(A)** following extraction and **(B)** apparently spontaneous. Despite exposure of large areas of necrotic bone there is no overt infection in these early lesions. Courtesy Dr J Fantasia. Published in *Oral Surgery, Oral Medicine, Oral Pathology, Oral Radiology and Endontology*, Vol 102, Ruggiero SL et al, Bisphosphonate-related osteonecrosis of the jaw, pp 433–41, © Elsevier, 2006.

breast and prostate carcinoma. This is highly effective, constraining growth of metastases and inhibiting pathological fractures and their consequences, particularly nerve injury from spinal collapse.

However, treatment with high-potency bisphosphonates such as alendronate, pamidronate and zoledronate, especially when administered long term and in high doses intravenously, can lead to osteonecrosis.[1] Occasional cases have also been reported following oral administration. Osteonecrosis affects primarily the jaws, usually the mandible.

The mechanisms of necrosis are unclear, but bisphosphonates reduce vascularity as well as inhibiting oseoclasts. It is not known whether the bone becomes necrotic before infection is introduced or whether necrosis results from infection. Typical presenting lesions are either non-healing extraction sockets or exposed bone; they are refractory to conservative treatment and antibiotic therapy. In many patients, dental surgery, particularly extractions, within the previous year appeared to be the precipitating factor. A striking presentation is also painless exposed bone; some patients may develop no acute symptoms or infection for prolonged periods.

Once infection is introduced, the condition develops into acute or chronic osteomyelitis depending on the virulence of the organism and resistance of the patient. The drugs cause reduced bone turnover so that sequestra of necrotic bone separate very slowly and large areas of exposed bone result (Figs 6.8 and 6.9). Later complications can include oroantral and cutaneous fistulas with suppuration. Surgical treatment is often not possible; the whole bone is involved.

Bisphosphonate osteonecrosis is a recently recognised condition and treatment guidelines are not yet evidence-based. Discontinuation of the bisphosphonates does not appear to help because their effects last at least a year after administration and may be permanent.

First principles dictate that prevention of infection is paramount. Potential problems should be eliminated before bisphosphonate treatment. After administration of bisphosphonates, patients at risk must be identified by medical history and additional predisposing factors sought (Box 6.8). Caries and periodontitis must be controlled. Ideally, all surgical dentistry should be avoided for as long as possible after drug administration and there is a role for temporary restorations and interim endodontics. If extractions cannot be delayed, they are probably best followed by postoperative antibiotics and chlorhexidine rinses until the sockets are fully epithelialised. Unfortunately, these precautions are not always successful.

Box 6.8   Risk factors for bisphosphonate-induced osteonecrosis

- Intravenous high-dose bisphosphonate treatment usually for bone metastases or hypercalcaemia of malignancy
- Radiotherapy to head and neck
- Immunosuppression from chemotherapy or steroids
- Anaemia
- Dental surgery or sepsis, ill-fitting dentures and poor oral hygiene
- Female patients
- Elderly patients
- Smoking

When bone is exposed but symptoms are minimal, chlorhexidine mouth rinses reduce pain and the risk of infection. If there is infection or soft tissue swelling, aggressive and long-term antibiotic therapy based on the results of antibiotic culture and sensitivity is required. Severe complications including

---

[1]Bisphosphonate-induced osteonecrosis resembles the toxic necrosis of bone called *phossy jaw*, a scourge of match factory workers in Victorian times who ingested white phosphorus (P_4). They frequently died or lost a whole jaw from osteonecrosis. Public outrage and a famous strike in East London forced improvements in factory conditions and the introduction of the (slightly) safer red phosphorus match.

Fig. 6.9 **Bisphosphonate-induced osteonecrosis.** Non-healing extraction sockets in a breast cancer patient receiving bisphosphonate treatment. (A) There are minimal changes initially but 12 months later, (B) there is a large sequestrum still incompletely separated extending from the premolar region, just above the lower border cortex and involving most of the ramus. Courtesy Dr J Fantasia. Published in *Oral Surgery, Oral Medicine, Oral Pathology, Oral Radiology and Endontology*, Vol 102, Ruggiero SL et al, Bisphosphonate-related osteonecrosis of the jaw, pp 433–41, © Elsevier, 2006.

extraoral sinuses and pathological fractures may require surgical intervention. Managing pain is difficult and may require potent analgesics.

Osteonecrosis only develops in a very small proportion of those treated with bisphosphonates. It is not yet clear whether the placement of implants in apparently unaffected patients carries significant risk.

OSTEORADIONECROSIS

Osteoradionecrosis is osteomyelitis with radiotherapy as its predisposing cause (see Fig. 6.4). Radiotherapy induces endarteritis of vessels, compromising the already tenuous blood supply to bones. The complication has declined in incidence with the advent of modern radiotherapy techniques that, tumour site allowing, lower the dose to bone. Diagnosis is based on the history of radiotherapy.

Once infection develops, the features are no different from those of conventional osteomyelitis except that the low resistance of the bone favours more extensive infection and delayed sequestration.

Prevention by identifying patients at risk is critical. Extractions and other potential causes of infection must be carried out atraumatically and postoperative anbiotic treatment provided.

ALVEOLAR OSTEITIS

Alveolar osteitis (dry socket) can hardly be termed a major infection but can be mistaken clinically for osteomyelitis which can rarely follow. It is by far the most frequent painful complication of extractions. Nevertheless, it is uncommon overall.

The normal healing of a tooth socket is described in Appendix 6.1.

Aetiology

Alveolar osteitis is frequently unpredictable and without any obvious predisposing cause, but numerous possible aetiological factors exist (Box 6.9).

Box 6.9 **Possible aetiological factors for alveolar osteitis**

- Excessive extraction trauma
- Limited local blood supply
- Local anaesthesia
- Oral contraceptives
- Osteosclerotic disease
- Radiotherapy

Difficult disimpactions of third molars frequently lead to painful alveolar osteitis. However, the blood supply to the area often appears to be critical. In healthy persons, alveolar osteitis virtually only affects the lower molar region where the bone is more dense and less vascular than elsewhere. Alveolar osteitis is also an expected complication of extractions in Paget's disease and, particularly, after radiotherapy where endarteritis causes ischaemia of the bone. Alveolar osteitis is also more frequent in susceptible patients when local anaesthesia is used.

Loss of clot from the extraction socket was traditionally ascribed to bacterial proteolytic enzymes. However, it appears frequently to be due to excessive local fibrinolytic activity. The alveolar bone and other oral tissues have a high content

Fig. 6.10 **Dry socket.** Typical appearances of chronic alveolar osteitis; the socket is empty and the bony lamina dura is visible.

Fig. 6.11 **Sequestration in a severe dry socket.** Almost the whole of the lamina dura and attached trabeculae have become necrotic, forming a sequestrum. Healing is delayed while the sequestrum remains in place. Most dry socketrs are not associated with sequestration, or with only small sequestra.

of fibrinolysin activators (plasmin) which are released when the bone is traumatised. Nevertheless, once the clot has been destroyed, infection from the mouth is inevitable and anaerobes are likely to play a major role.

The oestrogen component of oral contraceptives apparently enhances serum fibrinolytic activity and, reportedly, is also associated with a higher incidence of alveolar osteitis.

Clinical features

Women are more frequently affected. Pain usually starts a few days after the extraction, but sometimes may be delayed for a week or more. It is deep-seated, severe and aching or throbbing.

The mucosa around the socket is red and tender. There is no clot in the socket, which contains, instead, saliva and often decomposing food debris (Fig. 6.10). When debris is washed away, whitish, dead bone may be seen or may be felt with a probe as a rough area. Sometimes the socket becomes concealed by granulations growing in from the gingival margins. Pain often continues for a week or two, or occasionally longer. Sequestration of the socket wall may sometimes be seen radiograpically (Fig. 6.11).

Pathology

The initial event is destruction of the clot which normally fills the socket. This leaves an open socket in which infected food and other debris accumulates in direct contact with the bone. Bone damaged during the extraction, particularly the dense bone of the lamina dura, dies. The necrotic bone lodges bacteria which proliferate freely, protected from leucocytes unable to reach them through this avascular material. In the surrounding tissue, inflammation usually localises infection to the socket walls. Dead bone is gradually separated by osteoclasts and sequestra are usually shed in tiny fragments. Healing is by granulation from the base and walls of the socket.

Prevention

Since damage to bone appears to be an important predisposing factor, extractions should obviously be carried out with minimal trauma. Immediately after the extraction the socket edges should be squeezed firmly together and held for a few minutes until the clot has formed. In the case of disimpactions of third molars, where alveolar osteitis is more common, prophylactic antibiotics are often given. Their value is unproven and there is no indication for using antibiotics for routine dental extractions. However, in patients who have had irradiation for oral cancer or osteosclerotic Paget's disease where there is extensive infection, antibiotic cover should be given and the tooth removed surgically, with as little damage as possible to surrounding bone.

There remain a few patients who otherwise appear to be well but are especially prone to alveolar osteitis which follows every extraction under local anaesthesia including regional blocks. In such patients, dry socket may be preventable if general anaesthesia is used.

Treatment

Local conditions strongly favour persistence of infection and it is more surprising that the infection is well localised than that it responds poorly to treatment. It is important to explain this to patients and to warn them that they may have a week or more of discomfort. It is also important to explain that the pain is not due, as patients usually think, to a broken root.

Treatment should aim to keep the open socket clean and to protect exposed bone. The socket should be irrigated with mild warm antiseptic or saline, then the opening filled with an obtundant dressing containing some non-irritant antiseptic to prevent food and debris from accumulating. This should be followed by frequent use of hot mouth rinses. Many socket dressings have been formulated, but a convenient proprietary preparation is Alvogel. It is easy to manipulate and patients report that it gives a sensation of warmth in place of the pain. Apart from being obtundant and antiseptic, the socket dressing should preferably be soft, adhere to the socket wall and be absorbable. Non-absorbable dressings must be removed as soon as possible to allow the socket to heal. Most cases become free from pain after one or two dressings. Dressing packed hard into the socket will delay healing.

Key features of alveolar osteitis are summarised in Box 6.10.

Box 6.10   Alveolar osteitis: key features

- The most common painful complication of dental extractions
- Loss of clot normally filling extraction socket
- Loss of clot may be due to excessive local fibrinolytic action or bacterial enzymes or both
- Bare, whitish lamina dura exposed in socket
- Pain relieved by irrigation and repeated dressing of socket
- Dead bone usually shed as crumb-like fragments
- Eventual healing of socket from its base by granulation

SCLEROTIC BONE ISLANDS

These areas of sclerosis, also known as dense bone islands, enostoses or idiopathic osteosclerosis, are found in all endochondral bones including the jaws. They are sometimes seen by chance in routine, particularly panoramic, radiographs (Fig. 6.12). They appear to be a normal anatomical variant and should not be mistaken for a low-grade bone infection (particularly if first noticed after a surgical procedure) as they have sometimes been. They resemble sclerosing osteitis but are not associated with a focus of infection or inflammation. Histologically, they comprise an island of normal cortical bone within the medullary cavity.

Operative interference should be avoided as it may lead to complications and medicolegal claims, without being beneficial.

Fig. 6.12   Sclerotic bone island in the posterior mandible, a relatively dense example. The periphery may be sharply or less well defined. Courtesy Mr EJ Whaites.

FASCIAL SPACE INFECTIONS (CERVICOFACIAL CELLULITIS) → Summaries pp. 66, 409

Usually, acute periapical infections result in abscess formation. In an abscess, bacteria cause localised tissue necrosis and pus forms by the action of neutrophil proteolytic enzymes. The process is localised by granulation tissue forming the abscess wall. However, the surrounding soft tissues may become swollen by diffusion of fluid (inflammatory exudate) into them.

Fascial space infections are a form of cellulitis in which, unlike an abscess, bacteria spread in the soft tissues. Fasciae covering muscle bundles are normally in close apposition. If these fasciae are forced apart, avascular spaces are created. If localisation of an infection by virulent bacteria fails, inflammatory exudate opens up the fascial spaces carrying bacteria with it into the tissue planes. The latter extend from the base of the skull to the mediastinum. Unlike simple inflammatory oedema therefore, the exudate in cellulitis forms the vehicle for the spread of the infection.

Deep fascial space infections cause gross inflammatory exudate and tissue oedema, associated with fever and toxaemia. Before the advent of antibiotics the mortality was high and the disease is still life-threatening if treatment is delayed. The main types are sublingual, submandibular (Fig. 6.13) and parapharyngeal. *Ludwig's angina* involves several of these regions.

Fig. 6.13   Paths of infection spread from lower molars. By penetrating the lingual plate of the jaw below the attachment of mylohyoid (C) infection immediately enters the submandibular space (A). Below the mylohyoid is the main body of the submandibular salivary gland with its deep process curving around the posterior border of the muscle: infection from the third molar can follow the same route to enter the sublingual space (B).

Fig. 6.14 Paths of infection from the third molar. The diagram shows the lingual aspect of the jaw and indicates how infection penetrating from the lingual plate of bone can enter the sublingual space above, or the submandible space below, the mylohyoid muscle which forms the major structure of the floor of the mouth. Moreover, since this point is at the junction of the oral cavity and pharynx, infection can also spread backwards to reach the lateral surface of superior constrictor, i.e. the lateral pharyngeal space.

Fig. 6.16 Ludwig's angina. Incision and drainage of the front of the neck to relieve the pressure of exudate which compromises the airway. The neck is grossly swollen, shiny and dusky in hue; the edges of the wound have pulled apart, indicating the distension of these normally lax tissues.

Fig. 6.15 Cellulitis. Infection spreading through the tissues is accompanied by a dense infiltrate of neutrophils, here separating muscle bundles in a facial muscle.

Fig. 6.17 Facial cellulitis arising from an infected upper tooth. The tissues are red, tense and shiny and the patient is incapacitated by the systemic effects of infection. (By kind permission of Professor JD Langdon.)

The characteristic features are diffuse swelling, pain, fever and malaise. The swelling is tense and tender, with a characteristic board-like firmness. The overlying skin is taut and shiny. Pain and oedema limit opening the mouth and often cause dysphagia. Systemic upset is severe with worsening fever, toxaemia and leucocytosis. The regional lymph nodes are swollen and tender.

In Ludwig's angina particularly, airway obstruction can quickly result in asphyxia.

Pathology

Anaerobic bacteria are mainly responsible and infection mainly spreads from mandibular third molars whose apices are closely related to several fascial spaces (Figs 6.13 and 6.14). Fasciae covering muscles and other structures are normally adherent but can be spread apart by inflammatory exudate. Spaces created in this way are almost avascular and inflammatory exudate carries bacteria widely through them (Fig. 6.15).

Ludwig's angina is a severe form of cellulitis which usually arises from the lower second or third molars. It involves the sublingual and submandibular spaces bilaterally, almost simultaneously and readily spreads into the lateral pharyngeal and pterygoid spaces and can extend into the mediastinum.

The main features are rapidly spreading sublingual and submandibular cellulitis with painful, brawny swelling of the upper part of the neck and the floor of the mouth on both sides (Fig. 6.16). With involvement of the parapharyngeal space, the swelling tracks down the neck (Figs 6.17 and 6.18) and oedema can quickly spread to the glottis.

Swallowing and opening the mouth become difficult and the tongue may be pushed up against the soft palate. The latter or oedema of the glottis causes worsening respiratory obstruction. The patient soon becomes desperately ill, with fever, respiratory distress, headache and malaise.

Management

The main requirements are (1) immediate admission to hospital, (2) securing the airway by tracheostomy if necessary, (3) procurement of a sample for culture and sensitivity testing, (4)

Fig. 6.18 Ludwig's angina. There is cellulitis and gross oedema of the right submandibular and sublingual spaces extending on to the left side and into the neck and parapharyngeal space. (By kind permission of Professor JD Langdon.)

aggressive antibiotic treatment and (5) drainage of the swelling to reduce pressure.

Key features of fascial space infections are summarised in Box 6.11.

Box 6.11 Fascial space infections: key features

- Potentially life-threatening infections due to spread of bacteria into perioral fascial spaces
- Infection usually arises from lower second or third molars
- Ludwig's angina comprises bilateral involvement of sublingual and submandibular spaces and readily spreads into lateral pharyngeal and pterygoid spaces
- Affected tissues swollen and of board-like hardness
- Severe systemic upset
- Glottic oedema or spread into the mediastinum may be fatal

NECROTISING FASCIITIS → Summary p. 66

Necrotising fasciitis is an uncommon, rapidly spreading, potentially lethal infection causing necrosis of the subcutaneous tissues and loss of attachment of the overlying skin. Rarely, the infection can have a dental source and may threaten the airway. Many types of bacteria, both aerobic and non-aerobic can be responsible. Most patients are of middle age or older, but predisposing diseases are uncommon.

Clinically, there is initially a rapidly spreading area of erythema of the skin; the margins soon become ill-defined. Thrombosis and necrosis cause the skin to become painful and oedematous, dusky red then purplish and black. Undermining of the skin causes separation from the underlying connective tissue and accumulation of subcutaneous gas which may be visible on radiographs.

Aggressive surgery is required as soon as the condition is recognised. The extent of undermining of the skin should be explored and widely opened to drainage. Penicillin and metronidazole or clindamycin should be given empirically until bacteriological findings dictate alternatives.

CAVERNOUS SINUS THROMBOSIS → Summary p. 66

Cavernous sinus thrombosis is an uncommon life-threatening complication of infection that can sometimes originate from an upper anterior tooth. Blindness or death can result.

Clinically, gross oedema of the eyelid is associated with pulsatile exophthalmos due to venous obstruction. Cyanosis, proptosis, a fixed dilated pupil and limited eye movement rapidly develop. The patient is seriously ill with rigors, a high swinging fever and deteriorating sight.

Early recognition and treatment of cavernous sinus thrombosis is essential. The main measures are use of antibiotics, drainage of pus and possibly anticoagulant treatment. There is a 50% mortality and 50% of survivors may lose the sight of one or both eyes.

MAXILLOFACIAL GANGRENE (NOMA, CANCRUM ORIS)

Noma is an overwhelmingly severe oral infection, extending on to and destroying part of the face, and fatal if inadequately treated. It has been described as a 'severe scourge to mankind' as children are mainly affected.

The disease was first described in 1595 in Holland where, as in other parts of Europe, severe malnutrition and debilitating diseases were widespread. The term 'noma' was coined in 1680.

Since then, noma has virtually disappeared from Europe though there were many cases among starving prisoners, particularly children in Nazi concentration camps, in the 1940s and invariably fatal. Otherwise, noma is so widespread in sub-Saharan Africa as to have become a subject for a World Health Organization project to assess prevalence and preventive measures have been instituted. The overall prevalence in Africa has been variably estimated to be from 30 000 to over 100 000 cases. Smaller numbers of cases have been reported from South America and the Far East. Malnutrition due to poverty and climatic disasters is the major factor in the aetiology. Other factors are poor oral hygiene and other infections, particularly herpetic. In adults, the development of noma is likely to be secondary to HIV infection, but only rarely, despite the severity of the immune deficiency.

Apart from a few adults with AIDS, children under 10 years are affected. Aetiological factors include severe malnutrition, poor oral and general hygiene, and contributory infections such as measles which impair immunity. The main bacteria isolated are anaerobes including *Fusobacterium necrophorum*,

Fig. 6.19 Cancrum oris. In the maxilla there is extension of necrotising gingivitis into the alveolar process and in the lower arch anteriorly, resulting in destruction of much of the lower lip.

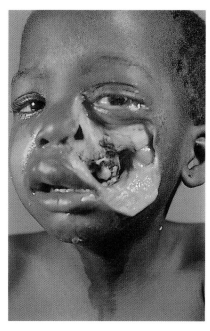

Fig. 6.21 Cancrum oris. Gross destruction and sloughing of facial tissues as a result of spread of infection from the maxillary gingivae. A molar tooth is visible centrally in the defect. (By kind permission of the late Professor RD Emslie.)

Fig. 6.20 Cancrum oris. Muscle has been invaded by spirochaetes and fusiforms. There is rapid necrosis and only a light inflammatory response of neutrophils.

Prevotella intermedia and spirochaetes. *F. necrophorum* is a commensal in the gut of herbivores and also a cause of necrotising infections in animals. It may play an important role in noma in Africa as a result of patients living in close proximity to and often sharing drinking water with cattle.

Noma starts within the oral cavity from an acute necrotising ulcerative gingivitis associated with extensive oedema, but extends outwards, rapidly destroying soft tissues and bone (Fig. 6.19). The gangrenous process starts as a painful, small, reddish-purple spot or indurated papule which ulcerates. The ulcer spreads to involve the labiogingival fold, adjacent mucosa and underlying bone. Diffuse oedema of the face, foetor and profuse salivation are associated. As the overlying tissues become ischaemic the skin turns blue-black.

The gangrenous area becomes increasingly sharply demarcated and ultimately sloughs away. Muscle, invaded by spirochaetes and fusiform bacteria, undergoes rapid necrosis associated with only a weak inflammatory response (Fig. 6.20). The slough is cone-shaped, with its apex superficially so that the

underlying destruction of hard and soft tissues is more extensive than external appearances suggest. As the slough separates, the bone dies: sequestration and exfoliation of teeth follow. A gaping facial defect is left (Fig. 6.21).

Management

Malnutrition and underlying infections must be treated. A combination of penicillin or an aminoglycoside and metronidazole will usually control the local infection, but debridement of necrotic soft tissue is also needed. After control of the infection and recovery of health, reconstructive surgery is usually required to prevent permanent mutilation. However, there is a significant mortality.

Remarkably, at the end of World War II, starving children with noma, who survived until release from Nazi concentration camps, responded rapidly to a high-calorie diet, nicotinic acid and injections of a sulphonamide.

ACTINOMYCOSIS

Actinomycosis is a chronic, suppurative infection caused by a filamentous bacterium, usually *Actinomyces israelii*. Though common in the past, it has become rare.

Bacteria causing actinomycosis are common in the normal mouth. Injuries, especially dental extractions or fractures of the jaw, can provide a pathway and sometimes precede infection but, in fact, rarely do so. Most patients were previously healthy and it is uncommon even in patients with AIDS. The pathogenesis is therefore unclear.

Fig. 6.22 **Actinomycosis.** This single, complete loculus was from an early case of actinomycosis that followed dental extraction. The colony of actinomyces with its paler staining periphery (a 'sulphur' granule) is in the centre; around it is a dense collection of inflammatory cells, surrounded in turn by proliferating fibrous tissue. It will be apparent that an antibiotic cannot readily penetrate such a fibrous mass and must be given in large doses to be effective.

Clinically, men are predominantly affected, typically between the ages of 30 and 60 years. A chronic soft tissue swelling near the angle of the jaw in the upper neck is the usual complaint. The swelling is dusky-red or purplish, firm and slightly tender. The skin eventually breaks down as discharging sinuses form. There is often difficulty in opening the mouth, but pain is minimal. Healing leads to scarring and puckering of the skin and, in the absence of treatment, a large fibrotic mass can form, covered by scarred and pigmented skin, on which several sinuses open. However, such a picture is rarely now seen. Currently, the usual clinical features are a persistent subcutaneous collection of pus or a sinus, unresponsive to conventional, short courses of antibiotics.

Pathology

A. israelii spreads by direct extension through the tissues and causes chronic suppurative inflammation. In the tissues, colonies of actinomyces form rounded masses of filaments with peripheral, radially-arranged club-shaped thickenings. Neutrophils mass round the colonies; pus forms centrally, chronic inflammatory cells surround the focus and an abscess wall of connective tissues forms (Fig. 6.22).

The abscess eventually points on the skin, discharging pus in which so-called sulphur granules (colonies of actinomyces) may be visible. The abscess continues to discharge and surrounding tissues become fibrotic. Nevertheless, infection spreads to cause further abscesses. Untreated, the area can become honeycombed with abscesses and sinuses, and widespread fibrosis.

Management

Actinomycosis should be suspected if a skin sinus fails to heal after a possible focus has been found and eliminated. A fresh specimen of pus is needed. A positive diagnosis can rarely be made without 'sulphur granules' which may be found by rinsing the pus with sterile saline. The laboratory should be warned that actinomycosis is suspected, to enable appropriate media to be used and the culture maintained long enough for these slow-growing organisms to develop.

Frequently, small amounts of penicillin have been given earlier. These are insufficient to control the infection but make bacteriological diagnosis difficult.

The mainstay of treatment is penicillin, which should be continued for 4–6 weeks or occasionally longer, as pockets of surviving organisms may persist in the depths of the lesion to cause relapse. Abscesses should be drained surgically as they form. For patients allergic to penicillin, erythromycin can be given.

The key features of actinomycosis are given in Box 6.12.

Box 6.12   Actinomycosis: key features

- Rare chronic infection by filamentous bacterium, usually *A. israelii*
- Infection spreads through the tissues to produce multiple abscesses and sinuses, in severe cases
- More usually now, there is only a localised subcutaneous collection of pus
- Microscopy shows colonies of actinomyces with peripheral, radially-arranged club-shaped thickenings
- Pus forms centrally and connective tissue forms an abscess wall
- Sulphur granules (colonies of actinomyces) from the pus, required for culture
- Responds to prolonged treatment with penicillin or tetracycline
- Surgical drainage of locules of pus may be needed

THE SYSTEMIC MYCOSES

The systemic mycoses are rare in Britain, but may be seen in immunocompromised patients or in those from endemic areas such as South America (Box 6.13). Though superficial candidosis is common, there are surprisingly few reports of oral lesions due to systemic mycoses in AIDS patients. Cryptococcosis is the most common mycosis in AIDS and is sometimes the presenting disease. Clinically, most of the systemic mycoses can cause oral lesions at some stage, and often then give rise to a nodular and ulcerated mass, which can be tumour-like in appearance (Fig. 6.26). Mulberry-like gingival ulcerations with bleeding and purulent foci have been described in paracoccidioidomycosis in a patient with AIDS.

Box 6.13   Some systemic mycoses that can affect the mouth

- Histoplasmosis
- Rhinocerebral mucormycosis
- Rhinocerebral aspergillosis
- Cryptococcosis
- Paracoccidioidomycosis (South American blastomycosis)

Fig. 6.23 **Histoplasmosis.** Part of an oral biopsy under high power, showing typical round yeast forms with their clear haloes (PAS stain).

Fig. 6.24 **Aspergillosis.** Tissue densely infiltrated by aspergillus hyphae. In this section, stained with PAS stain, the septate hyphae appear as tubes with a red PAS-positive wall.

Fig. 6.25 **Mucormycosis.** Necrotic tissue infiltrated by the broad, knobbly branching hyphae of *Mucor* spp.

Microscopically, most systemic mycoses give rise to granulomas similar to those of tuberculosis, but there may also be abscess formation. Characteristic yeast forms or hyphae may sometimes be seen with special stains such as PAS (Figs 6.23–6.25). However, microscopy may not be diagnostic and culture of unfixed material may be necessary.

Fig. 6.26 **Histoplasmosis.** The gross nodular swelling of the tongue and ulceration are typical of many of the systemic mycoses.

Treatment

Amphotericin remains the most generally effective drug for most systemic mycoses but, given intravenously, can cause renal damage and severe hypersensitivity reactions. Liposomal amphotericin is less toxic and as effective. Ketoconazole and its analogues have mainly been used for maintenance.

SYSTEMIC INFECTIONS BY ORAL BACTERIA →
Summary p. 66

The mouth harbours a great variety of microbes and virulent pathogens, particularly in periodontal pockets, but high levels of immunity keep the infection localised. Oral bacteria, even some such as *Leptotrichia buccalis* which were long thought to be harmless, once they reach the blood stream of immunocompromised patients, can cause septicaemias which can be fatal.

Infective endocarditis

A special example of a systemic infection of dental origin is infective endocarditis, which can occasionally follow dental operations, particularly extractions, and cause irreparable damage to heart valves (Ch. 27).

Lung and brain abscesses

Some of these abscesses are due to oral anaerobic bacteria which are probably aspirated during sleep to cause a lung abscess and a secondary brain abscess. Isolated brain abscesses caused by oral bacteria are recognised but difficult to explain.

Immunodeficiency states

In severe immunodeficiency states, such as AIDS, immunosuppression for organ transplants, lymphoreticular diseases, or neutropenia due to cytotoxic chemotherapy, bacteraemias of oral origin can sometimes cause septicaemias. Viridans streptococcal bacteraemia is a recognised complication of neutropenia, but is not due to dental manipulations. Mucosal ulceration due to cytotoxic drugs is believed to be the portal of entry.

If antibiotic cover is thought necessary for dental operations, particularly extractions or periodontal treatment, a combination of amoxycillin 3 g plus metronidazole 400 mg by mouth, one hour before operations may possibly offer some protection and can be repeated six hours later, if thought desirable. However, there is no definitive prophylactic regimen, as the causes are varied and unpredictable.

Prosthetic joint replacements

There is no evidence of a significant risk of infection of prosthetic joints from dental operations.

SUGGESTED FURTHER READING

Akula SK, Creticos CM, Weldon-Linne CM 1989 Gangrenous stomatitis in AIDS. Lancet 1:955

Aldesberger L 1946 Medical observations in Auschwitz concentration camp. Lancet 1:317

Barrios TJ, Aria AA, Brahay C 1995 Cancrum oris in an HIV-positive patient. J Oral Maxillofac Surg 53:851–855

Bochud P-Y,Clandra T, Francioli P 1994 Bacteremia due to viridans streptococci in neutropenic patients: a review. Am J Med 97:256

Cawson RA, Langdon JD, Eveson JW 1996 Surgical pathology of the mouth and jaws. Wright, Oxford

Cawson RA, Binnie WH, Barrett AW, Wright J 2001 Color atlas of oral disease, 3rd edn. Mosby-Wolfe, London

Chow AW 1992 Life-threatening infections of the head and neck. Clin Infect Dis 14:991–1004

Cohen ME, Simecek JW 1995 Effects of gender-related factors on the incidence of localized alveolar osteitis. Oral Surg Oral Med Oral Pathol Oral Radiol Endod 79:416–422

Denning DW 2000 Early diagnosis of invasive aspergillosis. Lancet 355:423

Diamond RD 1991 The growing problem of mycoses in patients infected with the human immunodeficiency virus. Rev Infect Dis 13:480–486

Emslie RD 1963 Cancrum oris. Dent Pract Dent Rec 13:481–494

Enwonwu CO, Falker WA, Idigbe EO, Savage KO 1999 Noma (cancrum oris): questions and answers. Oral Dis 5:144–149

Enwonu CO, Falker WA, Idigbe EO 2000 Oro-facial gangrene (noma/cancrum oris): pathogenetic mechanisms. Crit Rev Oral Biol Med 11:159–171

Geist JR, Katz JO 1990 The frequency and distribution of idiopathic osteosclerosis.Oral Surg Oral Med Oral Pathol 69:388–393

Giovani EM, Mantesso A, Locucca SVL et al 2000 Paracoccidioidomycosis in an HIV-positive patient: a case report with gingival aspects. Oral Dis 6:327–329

Glueck CJ, McMahon RE, Bouquot J et al 1996 Thrombophilia, hypofibrinolysis, and alveolar osteonecrosis of the jaws. Oral Surg Oral Med Oral Pathol Radiol Endod 81:557–566

Griffin JM, Bach DE, Nespeca JA, Marshall KJ 1983 Noma. Report of two cases. Oral Surg 56:605–607

Har-El G, Aroesty JH, Shaha A, Lucente FE 1992 Changing trends in deep neck abscess. A retrospective study of 110 patients. Oral Surg Oral Med Oral Pathol 77:446–450

Indresano AT, Haug RH, Hoffman MJ 1992 The third molar as cause of deep space infections. J Oral Maxillofac Surg 50:33–35

Jansma J, Vissink A, Spijkervet FKL et al 1992 Protocol for the prevention and treatment of oral sequelae resulting from head and neck radiation therapy. Cancer 70:2171

Koorbusch GF, Fotos P, Goll TK 1992 Retrospective study of osteomyelitis. Etiology, demographics, risk factors and management in 35 cases. Oral Surg Oral Med Oral Pathol 74:149–154

Kuriyama T, Karasawa T, Nakagawa K et al 2000 Bacteriologic features and antimicrobial susceptibility in isolates from orofacial odontogenic infections. Oral Surg Oral Med Oral Pathol Oral Radiol Endod 90:600–608

Larsen PE 1992 Alveolar osteitis after removal of impacted mandibular third molars. Identification of the patient at risk. Oral Surg Oral Med Oral Pathol 72:393–397

Lortholary O, Denning DW, Dupont B 1999 Endemic mycosis: a treatment update. J Antimicrob Chemother 43:321–331

McDonnell D 1993 Dense bone islands. A review of 107 patients. Oral Surg Oral Med Oral Pathol 76:124–128

Marple BF 1999 Ludwig angina. A review of current airway management. Arch Otolaryngol Head Neck Surg 125:596–600

Martinez D, Burgueno M, Forteza G et al 1992 Invasive maxillary aspergillosis after dental extraction. Oral Surg Oral Med Oral Pathol 74:466–468

Marx RE, Sawatari Y, Fortin M et al. 2005 Bisphosphonate-induced exposed bone osteonecrosis/osteopetrosis of the jaws: risk factors, recognition, prevention, and treatment. J Oral Maxillofac Surg 63:1567–1575

Maximew WG, Wood RE, Liu F-F 1991 Postradiation dental extractions without hyperbaric oxygen. Oral Surg Oral Med Oral Pathol 72:270–274

Notani K-I, Sato O,Hashimoto I et al 2000 Intracranial *Aspergillus* infection from the paranasal sinus. Oral Surg Oral Med Oral Pathol Radiol Endod 89:9–11

Ogundiya DA, Keith DA, Mirowski J 1989 Cavernous sinus thrombosis and blindness as a complication of an odontogenic infection. Report of a case and review of the literature. J Oral Maxillofac Surg 47:1317

Peterson LJ 1993 Contemporary management of deep neck infections. J Oral Maxillofac Surg 51:226–231

Richard P, Del Valle GA, Moreau P et al 1995 Viridans streptococcal bacteraemia in patients with neutropenia. Lancet 345:1607–1609

Ruggiero SL, Fantasia J, Carlson E 2006 Bisphosphonate-related osteonecrosis of the jaw: background and guidelines for diagnosis, staging and management. Oral Surg 102:433–441

Sakamoto H, Aoki T, Kise Y et al 2000 Descending necrotizing mediastinitis due to odontogenic infections. Oral Surg Oral Med Oral Pathol Radiol Endod 89:412–419

Schneider LC, Mesa ML 1990 Differences between florid osseous dysplasia and chronic diffuse sclerosing osteomyelitis. Oral Surg Oral Med Oral Pathol 70:308–312

Shroyer JV, Lew D, Abreo F, Unhold GP 1991 Osteomyelitis of the mandible as a result of sickle cell disease. Report and literature review. Oral Surg Oral Med Oral Pathol 72:25–28

Smithe OP, Prentice HG, Madden GM, Nazareth B 1990 Lingual cellulitis causing upper airways obstruction in neutropenic patients. BMJ 300:24

Sposto MR, Scully C, de Almeida OP et al 1993 Oral paracoccidioidomycosis. A study of 36 South American patients. Oral Surg Oral Med Oral Pathol 75:461–465

Sposto MR, Mendes-Giannini MJ, Moraes RA et al 1994 Paracoccidioidomycosis manifesting as oral lesions: clinical, cytological and serological investigation. J Oral Pathol Med 23:85–87

Tempest MN 1966 Cancrum oris. Br J Surg 53:949–969

Thorn JJ, Hansen HS, Specht L et al 2000 Osteoradionecrosis of the jaws: clinical characteristics and relation to the field of irradiation. J Oral Maxillofac Surg 58:1088–1093

Tibbles PM, Edelsberg JS 1996 Hyperbaric oxygen therapy. N Engl J Med 334:1642–1648

Tsumoda R, Suda S, Fukaya T et al 2000 Descending necrotizing mediastinitis caused by odontogenic infection: a case report. J Oral Maxillofac Surg 58:240–242

Van Merkensteyn JPR, Balm AJM, Bakker AJM, Borgmeyer-Hoelen AMMJ 1994 Hyperbaric oxygen treatment of osteoradionecrosis of the mandible with repeated pathological fracture. Report of a case. Oral Surg Oral Med Oral Pathol 77:461–464

Normal healing of an extraction socket

Stages in the normal healing of a single-rooted tooth extraction socket are shown in Figure 6.27.

The first stage of healing is the formation of a clot. Normal clotting mechanisms produce a loose clot that fills the bony and soft tissue socket. Platelets retract the clot, expressing fluid so that it becomes harder and shrinks below the level of the adjacent soft tissues, pulling any mobile soft tissue inwards to reduce the area of the clot exposed. Clot retraction is usually complete in 4 hours and the surface of the clot changes from shiny to matt. After retraction, the clot continues to stabilise by fibrin cross-linking so that avoiding rinsing is usually recommended for 24 hours. A socket containing early clot is shown at the top of Figure 6.27(A). Much of the clot (1) is bright red from trapped erythrocytes and the periodontal ligament can still be seen around the socket periphery (2).

Lysis of the clot begins within 2 days, caused primarily by the fibrinolytic enzyme plasmin, generated by activation of plasminogen in the clot. A 2-day-old socket is shown in (B) and (C). In (B), the section is stained with haematoxylin and eosin and in (C) with a stain that shows fibrin in yellow, bone in red and the periodontal ligament in turquoise. The ligament is still sharply defined but, at higher power, the emigration of inflammatory cells into the clot would be seen. It is at this stage, when fibrinolysis has started but the clot is not well anchored to the wall, that the risk of dry socket from clot lysis or loss is highest.

At 4 days, capillaries and fibroblasts (granulation tissue) are growing into the blood clot from the periphery so that it is now fixed to the socket wall. Macrophages migrate into the clot and start to demolish it ready for replacement by granulation tissue. The surface of the clot is white and porous clinically. Bacterial enzymes have lysed the surface fibrin and there are bacteria in the superficial fibrin, which gradually disintegrates. Epithelium at the gingival margin undergoes hyperplasia and starts to grow over the intact clot, below the surface debris.

At 8 days (D), the socket is filled by granulation tissue (3) and the superficial layers contain inflammatory cells (4). The granulation tissue is soft or gelatinous and contains little collagen. It appears red if exposed ('socket granulations'). The periodontal ligament is no longer clearly identifiable. The lamina dura of the socket (5) is intact but, at higher power, osteoclasts would be seen on its surface. There is early resorption. Depending on the surface area of the socket mouth, epithelial migration is complete between 7 and 10 days; in this socket it is delayed and there is inflammation at the surface.

At 18 days (E), the socket is filled by granulation tissue and the fibroblasts within it have laid down a collagen network. The outline of the lamina dura is still visible (6) and woven bone is forming around the periphery of the socket. On the left, there is a thick layer of woven bone trabeculae (7) and a blue rim of cellular osteogenic tissue at the bone-forming front (8).

By 6 weeks (F), the woven bone has filled the socket and is remodelling to lamellar bone (9). The outline of the lamina dura (10) persists for a very variable length of time, depending on the bone turnover rate. By 3 months, it is usually not detectable radiographically, but socket outlines may persist for years in the elderly.

Fig. 6.27 Stages in the normal healing of a single-rooted tooth extraction socket.

Cysts of the jaws

Cysts are the most common cause of chronic swellings of the jaws. They are more common in the jaws than in any other bone because of the many rests of odontogenic epithelium remaining in the tissues. Cysts formed from this epithelium (odontogenic cysts) account for most cysts of the jaws. By far the most common is the radicular (periodontal or 'dental') cyst.

> **Practical point** Cysts are pathological fluid-filled cavities lined by epithelium

TYPICAL FEATURES OF JAW CYSTS

Most jaw cysts behave similarly and usually grow slowly and expansively. They differ mainly in their relationship to a tooth and the radiographic features are usually a good guide as to their nature (Box 7.1). Even when it is not possible to decide the nature of a cyst, this affects treatment only with less common types. However, it is particularly important to distinguish odontogenic keratocysts and unicystic ameloblastomas from common types. These occasionally have identical radiographic appearances and diagnosis ultimately depends on histopathology.

Box 7.1 Key features of jaw cysts

- Form sharply-defined radiolucencies with smooth borders
- Fluid may be aspirated and thin-walled cysts may be transilluminated
- Grow slowly, displacing rather than resorbing teeth
- Symptomless unless infected and are frequently chance radiographic findings
- Rarely large enough to cause pathological fracture
- Form compressible and fluctuant swellings if extending into soft tissues
- Appear bluish when close to the mucosal surface

The classification of cysts is summarised in Box 7.2. There is not currently a complete classification of cysts that is accepted internationally.

Box 7.2 Classification of cysts of the jaws (WHO – modified)

Developmental cysts
- Odontogenic
  'Gingival cysts' of infants (Epstein pearls)
  Odontogenic keratocyst ('primordial' cyst)
  Orthokeratinised odontogenic cyst
  Dentigerous (follicular) cyst
  Eruption cyst
  Lateral periodontal cyst
  Gingival cyst of adults
  Glandular odontogenic; sialo-odontogenic cyst
- Non-odontogenic cysts
  Nasopalatine duct cyst
  Nasolabial cyst

Inflammatory odontogenic cysts
- Radicular
  Residual
  Lateral
- Paradental

OTHER CYSTIC OR CYST-LIKE LESIONS →
Summary p. 157

Cystic odontogenic tumours are not included in the above classification, but cystic ameloblastomas and calcifying odontogenic (ghost cell) cysts can be mistaken radiographically for radicular or other non-neoplastic cysts as discussed later.

Also excluded from the above classification are cysts (in bone cavities) without epithelial lining (pseudocysts), namely solitary (simple) bone cysts and aneurysmal bone cysts. These also are cystic only in their radiographic appearances. They are skeletal diseases and affect the jaws only occasionally, as discussed in Chapter 9.

Odontogenic cysts (not surprisingly) affect the tooth-bearing region of the jaws. Most non-odontogenic, true cysts are developmental and form in the region of the anterior maxilla. Their relative frequency is shown in Box 7.3, though figures in the different surveys vary as a result of differences in categorisation, what kinds of cysts are included and other factors.

Radicular cysts are discussed first as, being the most common type, their treatment forms the basis for that of most other jaw cysts.

Box 7.3	Relative frequency of different types of jaw cysts
Radicular	65–70%
Dentigerous	15–18%
Odontogenic keratocyst	3–5%
Nasopalatine	5–10%
Lateral periodontal	<1%
Paradental	<1%

RADICULAR CYSTS → Summaries pp. 135, 190

Clinical features

Radicular cysts are the most common cause of major, chronic swellings and the most common type of cyst of the jaws. They are rarely seen before the age of 10 and are most frequent between the ages of 20 and 60 years. They are more common in males than females, roughly in the proportion of 3 to 2. The maxilla is affected more than three times as frequently as the mandible.

Radicular cysts, like other cysts of the jaws, cause slowly progressive painless swellings, with no symptoms until they become large enough to be conspicuous (Fig. 7.1). If infection enters, the swelling becomes painful and may rapidly expand, partly due to inflammatory oedema. The swelling is rounded and at first hard. Later, when the bone has been reduced to eggshell thickness, a crackling sensation may be felt on pressure. Finally, part of the wall is resorbed entirely away, leaving a soft fluctuant swelling, bluish in colour, beneath the mucous membrane. The dead tooth from which the cyst has originated is (by definition) present and its relationship to the cyst will be apparent in a radiograph (Fig. 7.2).

Practical point Always determine the vitality of teeth associated with a jaw cyst

Pathogenesis and pathology

The main factors responsible for cyst development are summarised in Box 7.4.

Box 7.4	Major factors in the pathogenesis of cyst formation
• Proliferation of epithelial lining and fibrous capsule	
• Hydrostatic pressure of cyst fluid	
• Resorption of surrounding bone	

Epithelial proliferation Infection from the pulp chamber induces inflammation and proliferation of the epithelial rests of Malassez. If infection can be eliminated from the root canal, small radicular cysts (up to 1 or 2 cm diameter) may occasionally regress without surgery.

Hydrostatic effects of cyst fluids That radicular and many other cysts expand in balloon-like fashion, wherever the local anatomy permits, indicates that internal pressure is a factor in their growth. The hydrostatic pressure within cysts is about 70 cm of water and therefore higher than the capillary blood pressure.

Cyst fluid is largely inflammatory exudate and contains high concentrations of proteins, some of high molecular weight which can exert osmotic pressure. Consistent with the inflammation usually present in cyst walls, cyst fluid may contain cholesterol, breakdown products of blood cells, exfoliated epithelial cells and fibrin.

Fig. 7.1 Typical clinical appearance of a large cyst. This radicular cyst in the right maxillary alveolar process forms a rounded swelling with a bluish colour.

Fig. 7.2 A radicular cyst on a grossly carious and non-vital first permanent molar. A rounded and sharply defined area of radiolucency is associated with the apices of the roots.

The cyst wall does not seem to act entirely as a simple semi-permeable membrane.

Low-molecular-weight proteins are present in similar concentrations to those in the plasma, but there are smaller amounts of high-molecular-weight proteins. The capillaries in the cyst wall are more permeable as a result of inflammation and contribute varying amounts of immunoglobulins and other proteins. The net effect is that pressure is created by osmotic tension within the cyst cavity.

Bone-resorbing factors Experimentally, cyst tissues in culture release bone-resorbing factors. These are predominantly prostaglandins E2 and E3. Different types of cysts and tumours may produce different quantities of prostaglandins but, if so, it is unclear whether this affects the mode of growth of the cyst. Collagenases are present in the walls of keratocysts, but their contribution to cyst growth is also unclear.

Pathology

All stages can be seen from a periapical granuloma containing a few strands of proliferating epithelium derived from the epithelial rests of Malassez (Figs 7.3 and 7.4), to an enlarging cyst with a hyperplastic epithelial lining and dense inflammatory infiltrate. Epithelial proliferation results from irritant products leaking from an infected root canal to cause chronic periapical inflammation.

Epithelial lining The epithelial lining consists of stratified squamous epithelium of variable thickness. It lacks a well-defined basal cell layer and is sometimes incomplete. Early, active epithelial proliferation is associated with obvious chronic inflammation and may then be thick, irregular and hyperplastic or appear net-like (Fig. 7.5), forming rings and arcades (Fig. 7.6). Hyaline bodies may be seen in the epithelium (Fig. 7.7) and mucous cells may be present as a result of metaplasia (Fig. 7.8). Longstanding cysts typically have a thin flattened epithelial lining, a thick fibrous wall and minimal inflammatory infiltrate.

The cyst capsule and wall The capsule consists of collagenous fibrous connective tissue. During active growth the capsule is vascular and infiltrated by chronic inflammatory cells adjacent to the proliferating epithelium. Plasma cells are often prominent or predominant and are a response to antigens leaking through the tooth apex.

In the bony wall, there is osteoclastic activity and resorption. Beyond the zone of resorption there is usually active bone formation. The net effect is that a cyst expands but retains a bony wall, even after it has extended beyond the normal bony contours. This bony wall, nevertheless, becomes progressively thinner since repair is slower than resorption, until it forms a mere eggshell, then ultimately disappears altogether. The cyst then starts to distend the soft tissues and appears as a soft bluish swelling (see Fig. 7.1).

Fig. 7.4 **A developing radicular cyst.** An epithelium-lined cavity has formed in this large periapical granuloma. There is a thick fibrous capsule infiltrated by chronic inflammatory cells. The alveolar bone has been resorbed and remodelled to accommodate the slowly expanding swelling.

Fig. 7.3 **The earliest stages of formation of a radicular cyst.** Some periapical granulomas, such as this, contain proliferating strands of odontogenic epithelium. In places the epithelium has broken down centrally to form small epithelium-lined spaces.

Fig. 7.5 **Radicular cyst.** The epithelial lining often assumes this arcaded pattern with numerous inflammatory cells beneath its surface.

Clefts Within the cyst capsule there are often areas split up by fine needle-shaped clefts (Figs 7.9 and 7.10). These are left by cholesterol dissolved out during preparation for sectioning. The cholesterol is derived from breakdown of blood

Fig. 7.6   Higher power of the lining of a radicular cyst. The arcaded epithelium contains numerous neutrophils emigrating into the lumen and there are pale-staining areas of foamy macrophages in the inner wall.

Fig. 7.7   Hyaline or Rushton bodies. These translucent or pink-staining lamellar bodies are formed by the cyst lining epithelium and indicate the odontogenic origin of a cyst.

Fig. 7.8   Mucous metaplasia in a radicular cyst. The numerous goblet cells can be seen but are more typical of dentigerous cysts.

Fig. 7.9   Cholesterol clefts in a cyst wall. This low-power view shows the relationship of cholesterol clefts to the cyst. Cholesterol crystals are formed in the fibrous wall. The epithelium overlying this focus has broken down and the cholesterol has leaked into the cyst contents. Elsewhere the lumen is lined by a flattened layer of squamous epithelium.

Fig. 7.10   Cholesterol clefts. Cholesterol has been dissolved out during preparation of the section, leaving clefts. The crystals are treated as foreign bodies and flattened multinucleate foreign body giant cells are seen along the edges of several clefts.

Fig. 7.11 **Cholesterol crystals from a cyst aspirate indicating the presence of inflammation.** The rectangular shape with a notched corner is characteristic.

Fig. 7.12 **Residual cyst.** The causative tooth has been extracted leaving the cyst in situ. See also Figure 7.13.

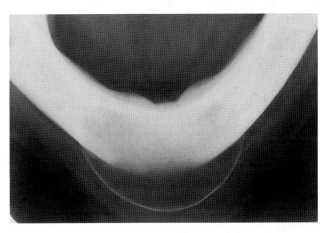

Fig. 7.13 **Radiographic appearance of the residual cyst shown in Figure 7.12.** Note the thin bulging periosteal new bone layer which can give rise to the clinical sign of eggshell crackling. (Figures 7.12 and 7.13 kindly lent by Mr P Robinson.)

cells. Small clefts are enclosed by foreign body giant cells and extravasated red cells and blood pigment are associated. Clefts may also be seen extending into the cyst contents but are formed in the cyst wall.

Cyst fluid The fluid is usually watery and opalescent but sometimes more viscid and yellowish, and sometimes shimmers with cholesterol crystals. A smear of this fluid may show typical notched cholesterol crystals microscopically (Fig. 7.11). Histologically, the protein content of the fluid is usually seen as amorphous eosinophilic material, often containing broken-down leucocytes and cells distended with fat globules.

Radiography

A radicular cyst appears as a rounded, radiolucent area with a sharply defined outline. A condensed radiopaque periphery is present only if growth is unusually slow and is usually more prominent in longstanding cysts. The dead tooth from which the cyst has arisen can be seen and often has a large carious cavity. Adjacent teeth may be tilted or displaced a little or occasionally become slightly mobile. Very large cysts in the maxilla may extend in any available direction and become irregular. Infection of a cyst causes the outline to become hazy as a result of greater vascularity and resorption of the surrounding bone.

Key features of radicular cysts are summarised in Box 7.5.

Box 7.5 **Radicular cyst: key features**

- Form in bone in relation to the root of a non-vital tooth
- Arise by epithelial proliferation in an apical granuloma
- Are usually asymptomatic unless infected
- Diagnosis is by the combination of radiographic appearances, a non-vital tooth and appropriate histological appearances
- Clinical and radiographic features are usually adequate for planning treatment
- Do not recur after competent enucleation
- Residual cysts can remain after the causative tooth has been extracted and diagnosis is then less obvious
- Cholesterol crystals often seen in the cyst fluid but not specific to radicular cysts

---

Residual and lateral radicular cysts → Summaries
pp. 135, 190

A radicular cyst may persist after extraction of the causative tooth. Residual cysts are a common cause of swelling of the edentulous jaw in older persons (Figs 7.12 and 7.13). Residual cysts may interfere with the fit of dentures, but may slowly regress spontaneously. This is suggested by the progressive thinning of the lining (Fig. 7.14).

Lateral radicular cysts can occasionally form at the side of a non-vital tooth as a result of the opening of a lateral branch of the root canal. They are rare and must be distinguished from lateral periodontal cysts which are another entity as discussed earlier.

Differential diagnosis

There are many causes of circumscribed areas of radiolucency in the jaws (Box 7.6).

Radicular cysts are usually readily recognised by their clinical and radiographic features. The cystic nature of a lesion can be confirmed by aspirating its contents through a needle inserted through the wall under aseptic conditions. The detection

Fig. 7.14 Lining of a residual cyst. There is only a minor degree of inflammation and the epithelium forms a thin regular layer.

Box 7.6 Differential diagnosis of cyst-like areas of radiolucency

- Anatomical structures (maxillary antrum and foramina)
- Solitary and aneurysmal bone 'cysts' (Ch. 10)
- Neoplasms, particularly ameloblastoma (Ch. 8)
- Giant cell granuloma of the jaws (Ch. 9)
- Hyperparathyroidism (Ch. 10)
- Cherubism (Ch. 10)

---

of fluid does not distinguish one cyst from another or a cystic neoplasm from a true cyst. The presence of cholesterol crystals is not of diagnostic significance.

Histologically, the lining of simple stratified squamous epithelium with an inflammatory infiltrate confirms the diagnosis. Distinguishing features of other types of cysts are discussed below.

Neoplasms Benign (odontogenic) tumours or, occasionally, an ameloblastoma may resemble a simple cyst radiographically. Resorption of adjacent teeth suggests a neoplasm rather than a cyst but is not diagnostic in itself. It is essential that the whole of a cyst lining be available for examination, since part of the lining, even though neoplastic, may appear as a thin layer of flattened stratified squamous epithelium like that of a simple cyst.

Rarely, a metastasis in the jaw may cause a sharply defined area of radiolucency. More often it causes a lesion with a hazy outline and irregular shape. Tumours also tend to be painful and to grow more rapidly than cysts. Nevertheless, it may be difficult or impossible to distinguish them from infected cysts radiographically, but at operation the solid nature of a tumour will be obvious and histological examination will confirm the diagnosis.

Treatment

Enucleation and primary closure Enucleation is the usual method and usually entirely effective (Box 7.7). The affected (dead) tooth may be extracted or root-filled and preserved. A mucoperiosteal flap over the cyst is raised and a window is opened in the bone large enough to give adequate access. The

---

Box 7.7 Advantages and limitations of enucleation of cysts

Advantages
- The cavity usually heals without complications
- Little aftercare is necessary
- The complete lining is available for histological examination

Possible disadvantages
- Infection of the clot filling the cavity
- Recurrence due to incomplete removal of the lining
- Serious haemorrhage (primary or secondary)
- Damage to apices of vital teeth projecting into the cyst cavity
- Damage to the inferior dental nerve
- Opening the antrum when enucleating a large maxillary cyst
- Fracture of the jaw if an exceptionally large mandibular cyst is enucleated

---

cyst is then carefully separated from its bony wall. The entire cyst is removed intact and should be sent in fixative for histological examination. The edges of the bone cavity are smoothed off, free bleeding is controlled and the cavity is irrigated to remove debris. The mucoperiosteal flap is replaced and sutured in place. The sutures should be left for at least 10 days.

Any disadvantages are largely theoretical and in competent hands even very large cysts can be enucleated safely. Recurrence is remarkably rare. There are few contraindications: they are relative rather than absolute.

Marsupialisation Marsupialisation is a largely outmoded treatment for radicular cysts. The cyst is opened essentially as for enucleation, but the lining is sutured to the mucous membrane at the margins of the opening. The aim is to produce a self-cleansing cavity which becomes, in effect, an invagination of the oral tissues. However, considerable aftercare is needed to keep the cavity clean. The cavity is initially packed with ribbon gauze and, after the margins have healed, a plug or extension to a denture is made to close the opening. Food debris has to be regularly washed out but, once the cavity has filled up from the base and sides sufficiently to become self-cleansing, the plug can be removed. The cavity usually becomes closed by regrowth of the surrounding tissue and restoration of the normal contour of the part. However, the orifice may close and the cyst re-form. Also, the complete lining is not available for histological examination.

The main application of marsupialisation is for temporary decompression of exceptionally large cysts where fracture of the jaw is a risk. When enough new bone has formed, the remaining cyst can be enucleated. Occasionally, retention of the tooth in a dentigerous cyst is needed and marsupialisation may allow it to erupt.

PARADENTAL CYSTS

Paradental cysts occasionally result from inflammation round partially erupted teeth, particularly mandibular third molars. They affect males predominantly, usually between the ages of 20 and 25 years. The affected tooth is vital but typically shows pericoronitis. Histologically, the cyst resembles a radicular cyst but for a more intense inflammatory infiltrate in the wall.

Enucleation is effective.

DENTIGEROUS CYSTS

A dentigerous cyst surrounds the crown of a tooth and is a dilatation of the follicle (Figs 7.15 and 7.16). The cyst is attached to the neck of the tooth, prevents its eruption and may displace it for a considerable distance.

Clinical features

Dentigerous cysts are more than twice as common in males as females. They are uncommon in children and most often found between the ages of 20 and 50.

Like other cysts, uncomplicated dentigerous cysts cause no symptoms until the swelling becomes noticeable. Alternatively, a dentigerous cyst may be a chance radiographic finding or found when the cause is sought for a missing tooth. Infection of a dentigerous cyst causes the usual symptoms of pain and accelerated swelling.

Fig. 7.15 **Dentigerous cyst.** This cyst has been removed together with its associated tooth. The cyst surrounds the crown and is attached at the cementoenamel junction.

Fig. 7.16 **Dentigerous cyst.** The cyst has developed around the crown of the buried third molar (left), but has extended forward to involve the root of a vital second molar. It should not, however, be confused with a radicular cyst arising from the latter.

Radiography

The cavity is well circumscribed, rounded and unilocular and contains the crown of a tooth displaced from its normal position (Fig. 7.16). Occasionally, there may be pseudoloculation as a result of trabeculation or ridging of the bony wall. The slow growth of dentigerous cysts usually results in a sclerotic bony outline and a well-defined cortex. The affected tooth is often displaced a considerable distance and a third molar, for instance, may be pushed to the lower border of the mandible. Rarely, if the cyst remains unrecognised for a long period, the enclosed tooth may become resorbed (Fig. 7.17).

These features readily distinguish a dentigerous cyst from a radicular cyst. However, an odontogenic keratocyst or ameloblastoma may occasionally envelop the crown of the tooth and either of these may create the radiographic appearance of a dentigerous cyst (Fig. 7.18). The diagnosis ultimately therefore depends on histological examination.

Aetiology and pathogenesis

Dentigerous cysts are considered to be developmental anomalies but no reproducible genetic defect has been identified. Loss of heterozygosity in the region of the PTCH on chromosome 9q has been claimed in sporadic cysts and dentigerous cysts can

Fig. 7.17 **Resorption of tooth associated with a dentigerous cyst.** The crown of this buried canine within the cyst shows resorption. This is unusual and is seen only in long-neglected cysts, as in this otherwise edentulous patient.

also be associated with various syndromes. Some dentigerous cysts appear to be induced by inflammation.

Attachment of the cyst lining at or near the amelocemental junction suggests that dentigerous cysts arise as a result of cystic change in the remains of the enamel organ after enamel formation is complete. Division between the remnants of the internal enamel epithelium covering the enamel and the external enamel epithelium, forming the greater part of the cyst lining, can occasionally be seen at the attachment of the cyst to the neck of tooth (Figs 7.19 and 7.20).

Progressive growth of the cyst leads to dilatation of the dental follicle. Factors triggering these changes are not known. However,

there is a strong association between failure of eruption of teeth and formation of dentigerous cysts which predominantly affect teeth which are particularly prone to failure of eruption, namely, maxillary canines and mandibular third molars in particular.

Fig. 7.20 **Dentigerous cyst.** To the left is the dentine (D). (E) is the enamel space left after decalcification and is separated from the cyst cavity (C) by a thin layer left by the inner enamel epithelium. The cyst itself appears to have formed as a result of accumulation of fluid between the inner and outer enamel epithelium and by continued proliferation of the latter to form the cyst lining, which joins the tooth at the epithelial attachment.

Fig. 7.18 **A cyst arising in the follicle of an unerupted developing tooth.** Radiographically, the cyst might have appeared to be in a true dentigerous relationship with the crown. However, this is not a dentigerous cyst; its lining does not join the tooth at the amelocemental junction (as in Figures 7.19 and 7.20). A higher-power view would reveal that this is an odontogenic keratocyst.

Fig. 7.19 **Dentigerous cyst.** The cyst surrounds the crown of this molar and the wall is attached to its cementoenamel junction. There is a uniform, thin epithelial lining with minimal inflammatory infiltrate. Cholesterol clefts are numerous in the lumen, a result of the formation of cholesterol crystals in the wall.

Fig. 7.21 **Section through the full thickness of the wall of a dentigerous cyst.** There is minimal inflammation and the epithelium is only two or three cells thick. Beyond the fibrous tissue the outermost layer of the wall is formed by woven bone, a feature common to most types of intraosseous cyst.

The lining of dentigerous cysts typically consists of thin, sometimes bilaminar, stratified epithelium (Fig. 7.21), frequently with numerous mucous cells. This epithelium may occasionally keratinise by metaplasia. The fibrous wall is similar to that of radicular cysts, but inflammatory changes are typically absent (Fig. 7.22).

Fig. 7.22 Dentigerous cyst. In this uncomplicated cyst there is no inflammation and the wall comprises a layer of fibrous tissue lined by a thin layer of stratified squamous epithelium two cells thick.

Management principles

If the tooth is in a favourable position and space is available, it may occasionally be possible to marsupialise a dentigerous cyst to allow the tooth to erupt. Alternatively, the tooth can be transplanted to the alveolar ridge or, if appropriate, extracted and the cyst enucleated.

Key features of dentigerous cysts are summarised in Box 7.8.

Box 7.8 Dentigerous cyst: key features

- Arise in bone and contain the crown of an unerupted tooth which is usually displaced
- Are most frequently associated with unerupted third molars and canines
- Clinical and radiographic features usually provide an accurate preoperative diagnosis but confirmation is histological
- May be mistaken radiographically for an odontogenic keratocyst or ameloblastoma
- Respond to enucleation or marsupialisation and do not recur after treatment

---

ERUPTION CYST

An eruption cyst occasionally forms over a tooth about to erupt. Strictly speaking, an eruption cyst is a soft-tissue cyst but probably arises from enamel organ epithelium after enamel formation is complete and is, in effect, a superficial dentigerous cyst.

Clinical features

Eruption cysts affect children and involve teeth having no predecessors (deciduous teeth or permanent molars). The cyst lies superficially in the gingiva overlying the unerupted tooth

and appears as a soft, rounded, bluish swelling (Fig. 7.23). The epithelial lining is separated from the alveolar mucosa by a thin layer of fibrous tissue (Fig. 7.24).

Management

The cyst roof may be removed to allow the tooth to erupt, but most eruption cysts probably burst spontaneously and never come to surgery.

Fig. 7.23 An eruption cyst over an erupting upper molar. There has been bleeding into the cyst cavity as a result of trauma.

Fig. 7.24 Roof of an eruption cyst. At the upper surface is the keratinised epithelium of the alveolar ridge and, below, separated by a thin layer of relatively uninflamed fibrous tissue, the lining of an eruption cyst.

KERATINISING ODONTOGENIC CYSTS → Summaries pp. 135, 136

Keratinising jaw cysts are uncommon but important because of the strong tendency of some of them – unlike most other cysts – to recur after removal. Keratinising cysts are divided into two types, those with a parakeratinised and those with an orthokeratinised epithelial lining. Parakeratinised cysts are called odontogenic keratocysts ('keratocystic odontogenic tumour'), have a tendency to recur and may be either sporadic or associated with multiple abnormalities in the Gorlin syndrome. Orthokeratinised cysts were previously considered a variant of odontogenic keratocyst but have a low risk of recurrence and are now classified separately. The two types are compared in Table 7.1.

Table 7.1 The two types of keratinising odontogenic cysts

Feature	Odontogenic keratocyst ('keratocystic odontogenic tumour')	Orthokeratinised odontogenic cyst
Type of keratinisation	Parakeratin	Orthokeratin
Relative frequency (%)	88	12
Sex %		
Male = 61.5% overall	62	57
Female = 38.5% overall	38	43
Age at presentation (years)	34	40
Association with impacted tooth (%)	48	76
Midline location (%)	6	16
Pain (%)	15	9
Radiographic appearance	Usually multilocular	Frequently monolocular
Recurrence rate (%)	43	4

The presence of bright white keratin is a useful diagnostic feature clinically. It may be appreciated on opening a cyst for biopsy or if the cyst is punctured (Fig. 7.25) and its nature may be confirmed by histology. It should not be mistaken for pus.

Fig. 7.25 Keratinising odontogenic cyst. Perforation of and pressure on the cyst roof has caused keratin, which fills the lumen, to extrude and has helped to confirm the diagnosis.

ODONTOGENIC KERATOCYST → Summaries pp. 135, 136

Clinical features

Most series have recorded a peak incidence between ages 20 to 30 years, but other large series have shown peaks between 50 and 70 years. The mandible is usually affected. At least 50% of odontogenic keratocysts form in the angle of the mandible, extending forwards into the body and upwards into the ramus. Odontogenic keratocysts, like other jaw cysts, are symptomless until the bone is expanded or they become infected.

A very useful diagnostic feature is the insidious pattern of growth. These cysts do not have a high internal pressure like radicular cysts and expand preferentially along the the medullary cavity, the path of least resistance. Thus, a cyst in the mandible may extend through much of the ramus and body without significant expansion of the jaw. Hence, clinical signs often fail to appear until the cyst is well advanced, and relatively extensive cysts are occasionally found by chance in radiographs.

Radiography

Odontogenic keratocysts appear as well-defined radiolucent areas, with a more or less rounded or scalloped margin. Some are unilocular but the majority are multiloculated (Fig. 7.26) and those with many locules may simulate an ameloblastoma (Fig. 7.27). The bony wall appears sharply demarcated and corticated. Occasionally, an odontogenic keratocyst may envelop an unerupted tooth and be indistinguishable radiographically from a dentigerous cyst (see Fig. 7.18). Roots of adjacent teeth may become displaced by large cysts but usually the cyst will extend around roots and the inferior dental canal without displacing them or causing significant expansion (Fig. 7.28).

Key features of odontogenic keratocysts are summarised in Box 7.9.

Pathogenesis and histopathology

Odontogenic keratocysts probably arise from any of the odontogenic epithelia including the dental lamina, the various rests of odontogenic epithelium or, as originally believed, from the enamel organ before tooth formation. However, it is difficult to reconcile such origins with the appearance of odontogenic

Fig. 7.26 Odontogenic keratocyst. Part of a panoramic tomogram showing typical appearances. The cyst is multilocular and has extended a considerable distance along the medullary cavity without appreciable expansion or displacement of the teeth.

keratocysts in middle age and their relatively rapid epithelial turnover. These theories about the source of the keratocyst epithelium are therefore speculative.

Box 7.9 Odontogenic keratocyst: key features

- 5–11% of jaw cysts
- Incidence peaks in 2nd and 3rd decades, mean age 38 years
- Form intraosseously, most frequently in the posterior alveolar ridge or angle of mandible. Mandible 75%, predominantly premolar and molar region
- May grow round a tooth
- Sometimes multilocular radiographically
- Spread extensively along marrow spaces before expanding the jaw
- Frequently recur after enucleation
- Definitive diagnosis only by histopathology, although clinical and radiographic features may allow fairly accurate preoperative diagnosis
- May be confused with ameloblastoma or with dentigerous cysts radiographically
- May be part of the basal cell naevus (Gorlin) syndrome

Fig. 7.27 Odontogenic keratocyst with multiple locules. Note the cortication around each cavity. The appearances resemble ameloblastoma, though the lack of expansion gives a clue to the correct diagnosis. Courtesy Mr EJ Whaites.

Fig. 7.28 Odontogenic keratocyst. Huge lesion extending from coronoid to the opposite molar region with minimal tooth displacement or expansion of bone.

Odontogenic keratocysts are caused by mutation, deletion or other inactivation of the patched (PTCH) gene on chromosome 9q, a tumour suppressor gene. This gene is discussed in more detail in the following section. Loss of PTCH gene activity releases a brake on the cell cycle, mediated through the hedgehog pathway. This results in a relatively high proliferative activity in the epithelial lining of odontogenic keratocysts. This has two effects. First, the cysts appear to enlarge by mural growth rather than osmotic pressure exerted by the cyst's contents. Second, epithelial proliferation is probably a factor determining the frequency with which keratocysts recur.

Growth of keratocysts is by extension of finger-like processes into marrow spaces rather than by expansion. Growth of the wall being greater than expansion of the cyst cavity causes the lining to become much folded (Fig. 7.29). The cyst enlarges slowly but relentlessly along the path of least resistance, expanding to fill the medullary cavity without displacing teeth or expanding the cortex until a late stage. As noted above, this growth pattern is characteristic, quite different from the pushing growth of radicular and dentigerous cysts, and aids radiological diagnosis.

The histological appearances of the lining of odontogenic keratocysts are characteristic (Box 7.10); biopsy is the diagnostic

Box 7.10 Typical histological features of odontogenic keratocyst

- Epithelial lining of uniform thickness
- Flat lower border of epithelium
- Clearly defined basal layer of tall cells in parakeratinised cysts (Fig. 7.30)
- Thin eosinophilic layer of parakeratin
- Cyst lining typically much folded (Fig. 7.29)
- Epithelial lining weakly attached to the fibrous wall
- Thin fibrous wall
- Satellite cysts in the wall (Fig. 7.29)
- Inflammatory cells typically absent or scanty

Fig. 7.29 Odontogenic keratocyst. Typical folded cyst outline with a satellite cyst lying in the wall. The fibrous tissue is uninflamed and thin.

investigation (Fig 7.30). However, if inflammation develops, the epithelial lining undergoes hyperplasia, loses its characteristic features and resembles that of a radicular cyst (Figs 7.31 and 7.32), making histological diagnosis more difficult. As there is often focal inflammation in cysts, as large a sample as possible should be obtained for diagnosis.

The possible neoplastic nature of odontogenic keratocysts

There has always been a tendency to regard these cysts as aggressive on grounds of recurrence and the fact that they may grow to a very large size before detection. This, together with the fact that odontogenic keratocysts are caused by inactivation of a tumour suppressor gene has led to them being reclassified

Fig. 7.30 Odontogenic keratocyst. High power, showing the typical features of the epithelial lining: a flat basement membrane; elongated palisaded basal cells with focal reserve polarity; 10–20 cells in thickness and with a corrugated parakeratotic surface.

Fig. 7.32 Inflamed odontogenic keratocyst. Higher power of a more inflamed cyst with complete loss of diagnostic histological features. The epithelial lining resembles that of a radicular or inflamed dentigerous cyst with only a hint of keratin on the left to give a clue to the correct diagnosis.

(A)

(B)

Fig. 7.31 Inflamed odontogenic keratocyst. Some areas of the lining show typical features (A) but, in (B) inflammation has induced epithelial thickening and loss of the basal palisading and keratin.

as neoplasms and renamed *keratocystic odontogenic tumor*. The term odontogenic keratocyst has a long history and has gained widespread acceptance and so is retained here pending further research.

While the genetic arguments are in some ways convincing, neoplasms are defined on the basis of their relentless growth and not by their molecular genetics. The odontogenic keratocyst responds well to marsupialisation provided all of the locules are opened to the surface. This is not neoplastic behaviour and the status of odontogenic keratocysts continues to be debated.

The features that have been proposed to suggest a neoplastic nature are listed in Box 7.11.

Box 7.11   Evidence that odontogenic keratocyst may be neoplastic

- High proliferative activity of epithelial lining
- Caused by mutation or deletion of PTCH tumour suppressor gene
- May contain defects of p16, p53 and other tumour suppressor genes
- Associated with other neoplasms in the basal cell naevus syndrome
- Infiltrative ('aggressive') growth pattern
- Squamous cell carcinoma may rarely develop within an odontogenic keratocyst
- Recurrence

Management

Diagnosis must be confirmed by biopsy.

Treatment will then depend largely on the extent of the cyst and the degree of multilocularity. Unilocular and small multilocular cysts can be treated conservatively and are usually enucleated and the bony cavity curetted. This must be vigorous to try to ensure that every fragment of cyst lining has been removed, but is difficult as the lining is friable (particularly if inflamed) and the cyst outline is complex. Larger cysts have a higher risk of recurrence as complete removal is more difficult. When the cyst extends around multirooted teeth they may have to be sacrificed to ensure complete removal. Very large cysts may require resection and reconstruction with a bone graft.

A useful additional precaution is the treatment of the cavity with a fixative (Carnoy's solution). This can be applied either before enucleation to kill and toughen the lining for removal or to the bony walls after curettage to destroy residual epithelial cells.

Odontogenic keratocysts that have perforated the cortex grow into the soft tissues and are then even more difficult to eradicate. An even greater danger is that of penetration of the skull base by cysts from the maxilla.

Clearly, it is important to warn patients of the possible need for further operations and that they should have regular radiological examinations at intervals for an indefinite period regardless of the method of treatment. Any recurrences should be treated in a similar manner when they develop. However,

using these methods, the morbidity is low and most teeth in relation to the cyst can be conserved.

Recently, more conservative treatments have been adopted. Marsupialisation followed by enucleation of the residual cyst has been advocated. This causes shrinkage of the cyst, rendering the lining less friable and less adherent. Even large odontogenic keratocysts treated by decompression and insertion of drains can shrink dramatically with remodelling also of adjacent bone. In many such cases, cysts disappear radiographically and macroscopically. Reduction in size is usually associated with ingrowth of oral epithelium into the cavity, replacing the typical keratinised epithelium with non-keratinising stratified squamous epithelium. Teeth displaced by the cyst often regain an upright position.

Complete resolution after marsulialisation takes a long time, up to 20 months, and it requires cooperative patients who will irrigate the cavity and keep it open and clean until it resolves. However, use as a primary treatment is increasing because the morbidity is considerably less than radical surgery.

Recurrence

Recurrence rates after enucleation are affected by various factors (Box 7.12) including those in the preceding section. Even with vigorous treatment, there is no absolute certainty of a complete cure. Rarely, odontogenic keratocysts have recurred in bone grafts after excision.

Box 7.12   Possible reasons for recurrence of keratocysts

- Thin, fragile linings, difficult to enucleate intact
- Finger-like cyst extensions into cancellous bone
- Satellite (daughter) cysts sometimes present in the wall
- More rapid proliferation of keratocyst epithelium
- Formation of additional cysts from other dental lamina remnants (pseudo-recurrence)
- Inferior standard of surgical treatment
- Possibly a neoplasm

A major factor leading to recurrence is the difficulty in removing every trace of the epithelial lining. Its more vigorous proliferative activity than that of other cyst linings may allow a few remaining epithelial cells to readily form another cyst. Formation of another cyst from other dental lamina remnants is not strictly a recurrence, but the fact that recurrences can appear up to 40 years after enucleation suggests this may happen. Otherwise, recurrence is often within the first 5 years after treatment. Vigorous treatment is likely to reduce the risk of recurrence, but there is no absolute certainty of a cure and patients should be followed up with regular radiographic examinations.

The basal cell naevus syndrome (Gorlin–Goltz syndrome) → Summary p. 136

This syndrome, often called the Gorlin syndrome, is heritable as an autosomal dominant trait. It consists essentially of the triad of multiple basal cell naevi, odontogenic keratocysts of the jaws and skeletal anomalies. However, many other defects may be associated.

It is caused by any one of many mutations in, or occasionally deletions in, the patched (PTCH) gene on chromosome 9q. This gene is important in developmental patterning and families with the syndrome have inactivation of one allele causing the skeletal anomalies. The gene is also a tumour suppressor gene and controls the cell cycle via the hedgehog (HH) signalling pathway. Inactivation or mutation of the second copy of the gene is associated with development of multiple basal cell carcinomas and odontogenic keratocysts. Mutations of the same gene may also be found in a variety of other neoplasms such as trichoepitheliomas and medulloblastomas and these are occasionally associated with the syndrome. Mutations within PTCH may also be found in sporadic odontogenic keratocysts.

The main features of the syndrome are listed in Box 7.13, though a great many other abnormalities may be present as the phenotype varies between families. There is no clear correlation between the features seen and the particular gene mutation.

In view of the great variety of abnormalities that may be present, the effects on the patient depend on the predominant

manifestation. Thus, in some cases, there are innumerable basal cell carcinomas. Though termed 'naevoid', these tumours differ from typical basal carcinomas only in their early onset, sometimes in childhood. Other patients have many jaw cysts, necessitating repeated operations. Cleft lip or palate or both is seen in a small proportion of these patients. Otherwise, the importance of this syndrome, from the dental viewpoint,

---

Box 7.13 Key features of Gorlin–Goltz syndrome

- Characteristic facies with frontal and parietal bossing and broad nasal root (Fig. 7.33)
- Multiple keratocysts of the jaws (Figs 7.34 and 7.35)
- Multiple, naevoid (early onset) basal cell carcinomas of the skin
- Skeletal anomalies (usually of a minor nature) such as bifid ribs and abnormalities of the vertebrae
- Intracranial anomalies may include calcification of the falx cerebri and abnormally shaped sella turcica
- Cleft lip and palate in approximately 5%

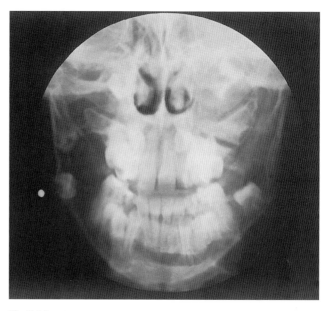

Fig. 7.34   **PA jaws of the same patient with the basal cell naevus (Gorlin's) syndrome shown in Figure 7.33.** Odontogenic keratocysts are present in the ramus and angle of the mandible on both sides, that on the right causing significant expansion.

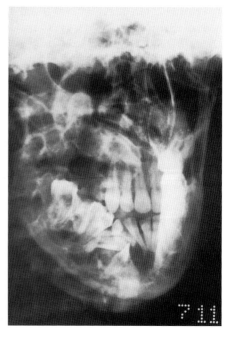

Fig. 7.35   **Oblique lateral radiograph of a patient with the basal cell naevus (Gorlin's) syndrome.** A very large odontogenic keratocyst involves the whole ramus and body, causing considerable expansion, especially at the lower border.

Fig. 7.33   **Basal cell naevus (Gorlin's syndrome).** The typical facies with a broad nasal root and mild frontal bossing.

is treatment of the keratocysts and to warn the patient of the likelihood of development of further cysts which must be dealt with by orthodox means as they arise. If neglected, these cysts can cause complications like other jaw cysts. Histologically, they are indistinguishable from the more common type of odontogenic keratocyst. The great majority are true parakeratinised odontogenic keratocysts and therefore have a strong tendency to recur after enucleation.

ORTHOKERATINISED ODONTOGENIC CYST (ORTHOKERATINISED ODONTOGENIC KERATOCYST)

The second type of keratinising jaw cyst is an orthokeratinised cyst that has been called the orthokeratinised variant of odontogenic keratocyst or the orthokeratinised odontogenic cyst (Fig. 7.36). It is less common than the parakeratinised type.

This cyst differs in a number of respects from the true odontogenic keratocyst, having a lower proliferative activity and no association with basal cell naevus syndrome. Differences are summarised in Table 7.1, and the most important difference is that orthokeratinised cysts are far less likely to recur than parakeratinised cysts. A large proportion arise in a dentigerous relationship, associated with a lower third molar.

There is probably no justification for less thorough conservative treatment than for the parakeratotic type. However, resection is not required.

GINGIVAL CYSTS

Dental lamina cysts of the newborn (Bohn's nodules)

Up to 80% of newborn infants have small nodules or cysts in the gingivae, due to proliferation of the epithelial rests of Serres (Fig. 7.37). Most resolve spontaneously.

Fig. 7.36 Orthokeratinised odontogenic cyst. Uninflamed wall with a thickly orthokeratinised epithelium. Keratin fills the lumen but the characteristic features of odontogenic keratocyst are not present; note the lack of palisaded basal cells.

Cysts (Epstein's pearls) may also arise from non-odontogenic epithelium along the midpalatine raphe. These may enlarge sufficiently to appear as creamy-coloured swellings a few millimetres in diameter, but also resolve spontaneously in a matter of months.

Fig. 7.37 Gingival cyst of the newborn (Bohn's nodules). This section from an embryo shows cyst formation in the rests of Serres superficial to the developing teeth. The cysts are lined by keratinising epithelium.

Gingival cysts of adults

Gingival cysts are exceedingly rare. They usually form after the age of approximately 40. Clinically, they form domeshaped swellings less than 1 cm in diameter and sometimes erode the underlying bone (Fig. 7.38). They are lined by very thin, flat, stratified squamous epithelium and may contain fluid or layers of keratin. They are unlikely to recur after enucleation.

Fig. 7.38 Gingival cyst of adult. Typical presentation as a superficial cyst in the attached gingiva of a premolar tooth.

LATERAL PERIODONTAL CYSTS

These uncommon intraosseous cysts are developmental and form beside a vital tooth. They are usually seen by chance in routine radiographs and resemble other odontogenic cysts radiographically, apart from their position beside a tooth (Fig. 7.39), near the crest of the ridge. They cause no symptoms unless they erode through the bone to extend into the gingiva.

Microscopically, the lining is squamous or cuboidal epithelium, frequently only one or two cells thick, but sometimes with focal thickenings. Some of the cells may have clear cytoplasm and resemble those seen in the dental lamina.

The cyst should be enucleated and the related tooth can be retained if healthy. Features are summarised in Box 7.14.

Botryoid odontogenic cysts

The botryoid odontogenic cyst is probably a variant of, but even more rare than, the lateral periodontal cyst. It typically affects the mandibular premolar to canine region in adults over 50.

Microscopically, it is typically multilocular with fine fibrous septa. The lining consists of flattened non-keratinised epithelium interspersed with clear, glycogen-containing cells and sporadic bud-like proliferations protruding into the cyst. It should be enucleated or conservatively excised as it has a strong tendency to recur.

GLANDULAR ODONTOGENIC CYST (SIALO-ODONTOGENIC CYST)

The glandular odontogenic cyst is another rare entity with some features in common with botryoid odontogenic and lateral periodontal cysts. Its distinguishing feature is small glands in thickenings of the epithelial lining that are lined by mucous cells and secrete mucin. It is frequently also multilocular and has a strong tendency to recur.

Fig. 7.39 Lateral periodontal cyst. Typical radiographic appearance showing a well-demarcated rounded radiolucency between the roots of the lateral incisor and canine, the roots of which have been displaced.

Box 7.14	Key features of lateral periodontal cyst and variants

Lateral periodontal cysts
- Developmental cysts that form beside a vital tooth
- Usually seen by chance in routine radiographs
- Resemble other odontogenic cysts radiographically, apart from position near the crest of the ridge
- Cause no symptoms but can erode through the bone to extend into the gingiva
- Microscopically, the lining is squamous or cuboidal epithelium, frequently only one or two cells thick, sometimes with focal thickenings
- Some cells may have clear cytoplasm
- Respond to enucleation
- The related tooth can be retained if healthy

Botryoid odontogenic cysts
- Probably a variant of lateral periodontal cyst, but more rare
- Typically affect the mandibular premolar to canine region in adults over 50
- Microscopically, typically multilocular* with fine fibrous septa
- Lined by flattened non-keratinised epithelium interspersed with clear, glycogen-containing cells
- Also sporadic bud-like proliferations protrude into the lumen
- Have a strong tendency to recur after enucleation
- Should be conservatively excised

Glandular odontogenic cyst
- Also rare and with many features in common with botryoid odontogenic cysts
- Frequently multilocular*
- Microscopically, pools of mucin and mucous cells present in the epithelium
- Has a strong tendency to recur
- Should be conservatively excised

*Multilocularity not necessarily visible in radiographs

NASOPALATINE DUCT CYSTS

The nasopalatine duct connects the organ of Jacobson in the nasal septum to the palate in many animals. Jacobson's organ is joined centrally to an accessory olfactory bulb. Cats, for instance, may sometimes be noticed to sense an interesting odour by inhaling through the mouth and, in most species, Jacobson's organ is used to assess the state of sexual readiness of potential mates. Disappointingly therefore, Jacobson's organ has disappeared in man and only a few epithelial cells lying along the line of the nasopalatine duct, persist. These cells can give rise to nasopalatine duct cysts.

Nasopalatine cysts, which form in the midline of the anterior maxilla, are uncommon. The nasopalatine, incisive canal, median palatine, palatine papilla and median alveolar cysts are variants of the same lesion, varying slightly in position in relation to the postulated line of the incisive canal.

Clinical features

Nasopalatine duct cysts are slow growing and resemble other cysts of the jaws clinically, apart from their site. Occasionally, they cause intermittent discharge with a salty taste. If allowed to grow sufficiently large, nasopalatine cysts may cause a swelling in the midline of the anterior part of the palate (Fig. 7.40), particularly when superficial (so-called palatine papilla cyst).

Radiography shows a rounded radiolucent area with a well-defined often sclerotic margin in the anterior part of the midline of the maxilla (Fig. 7.41). They occasionally appear heart-shaped because of radiographic superimposition of the nasal spine. They are usually symmetrical but may be slightly larger to one side. The anterior palatine fossa must be distinguished from a small nasopalatine cyst. The maximum size of a normal fossa is up to 6 or 7 mm.

Key features of nasopalatine duct cysts are summarised in Box 7.15.

> **Box 7.15 Nasopalatine duct cyst: key features**
>
> - Often asymptomatic, chance radiographic findings
> - Form in the incisive canal region
> - Arise from vestiges of the nasopalatine duct and may be lined by columnar respiratory epithelium
> - The long sphenopalatine nerve and vessels may be present in the wall
> - Can usually be recognised radiographically
> - Histological examination necessary to exclude other cyst types arising at this site
> - Do not recur after enucleation

Fig. 7.40 Nasopalatine cyst. Typical presentation with a dome-shaped bluish enlargement overlying the incisive canal.

Fig. 7.41 Nasopalatine cyst. The usual appearance is a rounded or pear-shaped area of radiolucency, mainly in the midline.

Pathogenesis and pathology

Nasopalatine cysts arise from the epithelium of the nasopalatine duct in the incisive canal. In man, vestiges of a primitive organ of smell in the incisive canal can be found in the form of incomplete epithelium-lined ducts, cords of epithelial cells, or merely epithelial rests.

The epithelial lining is usually either stratified squamous epithelium or ciliated columnar (respiratory) epithelium or both together (Fig. 7.42). Mucous glands are often and neurovascular bundles are sometimes present in the wall (Fig. 7.43). These are the long sphenopalatine nerve and vessels which pass through the incisive canal and are often removed with the cyst.

Treatment

Nasopalatine duct cysts should be enucleated. Recurrence is unlikely.

Fig. 7.42 Nasopalatine cyst. The lining, in part at least, may consist of respiratory (ciliated columnar) epithelium, as here. Alcian Blue staining reveals blue mucin in goblet cells.

Fig. 7.43 Nasopalatine cyst. Nerves and blood vessels of the incisive canal in the cyst wall.

NASOLABIAL CYSTS

This very uncommon cyst forms outside the bone in the soft tissues, deep to the nasolabial fold. It probably arises from remnants of the nasolabial duct and is occasionally bilateral.

The lining is pseudo-stratified columnar epithelium with or without some stratified columnar epithelium. If allowed to grow sufficiently large, the cyst produces a swelling of the upper lip and distorts the nostril. Treatment is usually by simple excision but, occasionally, may be complicated if the cyst has perforated the nasal mucosa and discharged into the nose.

CYSTIC NEOPLASMS → Summaries pp. 135, 157

Unicystic ameloblastoma

Most ameloblastomas contain microcysts but the unicystic variant has a lining of flattened tumour cells which resemble those of non-neoplastic cysts and a nodule of tumour in the wall or bulging into the lumen. Unicystic ameloblastomas frequently mimic dentigerous cysts radiographically (Ch. 8).

Calcifying odontogenic cyst

This uncommon lesion may be a cystic neoplasm; solid variants are rare (Ch. 8). The cyst lining consists of epithelium, often with palisading of the basal cells which may resemble ameloblasts. The most striking feature is areas of abnormal keratinisation producing swollen cells whose outlines and nuclei become progressively paler (ghost cells).

NEOPLASTIC CHANGE WITHIN CYSTS

Neoplasms, either ameloblastomas or carcinomas, could conceivably arise from the epithelial lining of cysts. There is scant evidence that ameloblastomas arise in this way and the idea almost certainly results from incorrect radiographic interpretation or faulty histological diagnosis.

There are a few well-authenticated cases of carcinomas arising from cyst linings, but they are exceedingly rare. It is essential to exclude other possibilities before such a diagnosis is made. Since cysts of the jaws are common, a neoplasm might develop coincidentally nearby and grow until it involves and fuses with the cyst wall.

SO-CALLED GLOBULOMAXILLARY CYSTS

These exceedingly rare cysts have been traditionally ascribed to proliferation of sequestered epithelium along the line of fusion of embryonic processes. It is now accepted that this view of embryological development is incorrect and there is no evidence that epithelium becomes buried in this fashion. Most so-called globulomaxillary cysts are usually found to be odontogenic cysts of various types.

CYSTS OF THE SOFT TISSUES

Some cysts described earlier form in or extend into the soft tissues overlying the jaws. However, most soft tissue cysts are non-odontogenic. The most common soft tissue cysts are mucoceles (extravasation or retention cysts) and the ranula which originate in minor salivary glands (Ch. 18), but the sublingual dermoid is a developmental anomaly.

Sublingual dermoid

These cysts probably form as a result of some abnormality of development of the branchial arches or pharyngeal pouches.

Clinical features

Dermoid cysts develop between the hyoid and jaw or may form immediately beneath the tongue (Fig. 7.44). They are sometimes filled with desquamated keratin giving them a semi-solid, putty-like consistency. A sublingual dermoid is more deeply placed than a ranula; the latter is obviously superficial, having a thin wall and a bluish appearance. A dermoid causes no symptoms until large enough to interfere with speech or eating. Nevertheless, a large swelling can be accommodated in the floor of the mouth without disability and can be completely concealed by the tongue in its normal resting position.

Pathology

The lining of epidermoid cysts is keratinising stratified squamous epithelium alone. Less often, cysts also have dermal appendages in the wall and are then referred to as dermoid cysts. Still others are lined partly by keratinising stratified squamous epithelium and partly by respiratory (ciliated columnar stratified) epithelium.

These cysts should be dissected out.

Fig. 7.44 Sublingual dermoid cyst. This is an unusually large specimen but appears even larger because the patient is raising and protruding her tongue. This cyst, unlike a ranula, can be seen to have a thick wall because it has arisen in the deeper tissues of the floor of the mouth.

SUGGESTED FURTHER READING

Ackerman GL, Cohen M, Altini M 1987 The paradental cyst: a clinicopathological study of 57 cases. Oral Surg Oral Med Oral Pathol 64:308–312

Altini M, Shear M 1992 The lateral periodontal cyst: an update. J Oral Pathol Med 21:245–250

Blanas N, Freund B, Schwartz M et al 2000 Systematic review of the treatment and prognosis of the odontogenic keratocyst. Oral Surg Oral Med Oral Pathol Radiol Endod 90:553–558

Browne RM (ed) 1991 Investigative pathology of odontogenic cysts. CRC Press, Boca Raton

Cawson RA, Langdon JD, Eveson JW 1996 Surgical pathology of the mouth and jaws. Wright, Oxford

Cawson RA, Binnie WH, Barrett AW, Wright JM 1998 Lucas's pathology of tumors of the oral tissues. Churchill Livingstone, Edinburgh

Cawson RA, Binnie WH, Barrett AW, Wright JM 2001 Oral disease, 3rd edn. Mosby-Wolfe, London

Craig GT 1976 The paradental cyst. A specific inflammatory odontogenic cyst. Br Dent J 141:9–14

Crowley TE, Kaugars GE, Gunsolley JC 1992 Odontogenic keratocysts: a clinical and histologic comparison of the parakeratin and orthokeratin variants. J Oral Maxillofac Surg 50:22–26

Friedrichsen SW 1993 Long-term progression of a traumatic bone cyst. A case report. Oral Surg Oral Med Oral Pathol 76:421–424

Gurol M, Burkes J, Jacoway J 1995 Botryoid odontogenic cyst: analysis of 33 cases. J Periodontol 66:1069–1073

Hernandez GA, Castro A, Castro G, Amador E 1993 Aneurysmal bone cyst versus hemangioma of the mandible. Report of a long-term follow-up of a self-limiting case. Oral Surg Oral Med Oral Pathol 76:790–796

Hussain K, Edmondson HD, Browne RM 1995 Glandular odontogenic cysts. Diagnosis and treatment. Oral Surg Oral Med Oral Pathol 79:593–603

Kuroi M 1980 Simple bone cyst of the jaw: review of the literature and report of a case. J Oral Surg 38:456–459

Li T-J, Browne RM, Matthews JB 1994 Quantification of PCNA+ cells within odontogenic jaw cyst epithelium. J Oral Pathol Med 23:184–189

Meiselman F 1994 Surgical management of the odontogenic keratocyst: conservative approach. J Oral Maxillofac Surg 520:960–963

Philipsen HP, Reichart PA 1998 Unicystic ameloblastoma. A review of 193 cases from the literature. Oral Oncol 34:317–325

Semba I, Kitano M, Mimura T, Sonoda S, Miyawaki A 1994 Glandular odontogenic cyst: analysis of cytokeratin expression and clinicopathological features. J Oral Pathol Med 23:377–382

Shear M, Speight P. 2007 Cysts of the oral and maxillofacial regions, 4th edn. Blackwell Publishing, Oxford

Swanson KS, Kaugars GE, Gunsolley JC 1991 Nasopalatine duct cyst: an analysis of 334 cases. J Oral Maxillofac Surg 49:268–271

Weathers DR, Waldron CA 1973 Unusual multilocular cysts of the jaws (botryoid odontogenic cysts). Oral Surg Oral Med Oral Pathol 36:235–241

William TP, Connor FA 1994 Surgical management of the odontogenic keratocyst: aggressive approach. J Oral Maxillofac Surg 520:964–966

Woolgar JA, Rippin JW, Browne RM 1987 A comparative histological study of odontogenic keratocysts in basal cell naevus syndrome and control patients. J Oral Pathol 16:75–80

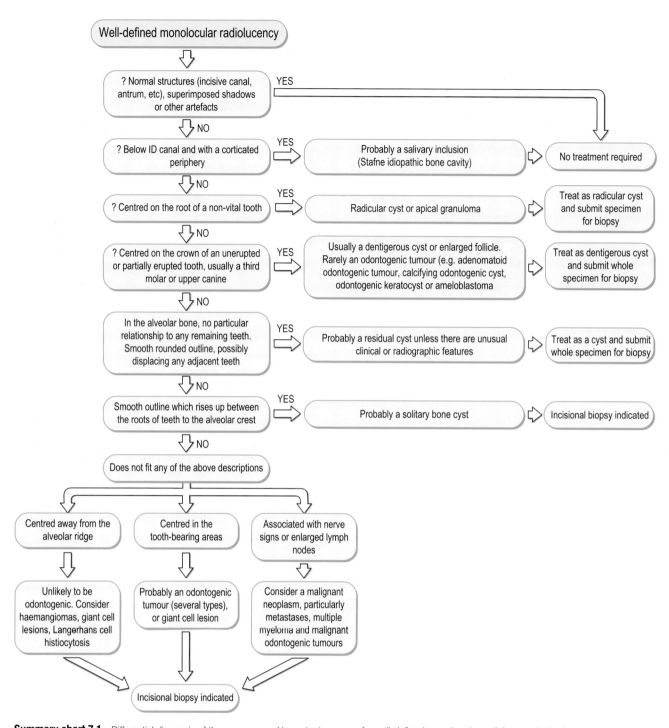

Summary chart 7.1 Differential diagnosis of the common and important causes of a well-defined monolocular radiolucency in the jaws.

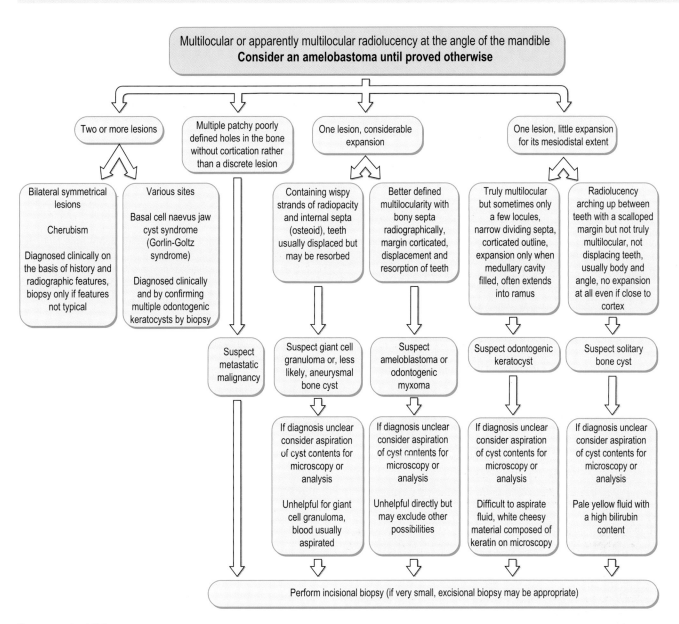

Summary chart 7.2 Differential diagnosis of a multilocular radiolucency at the angle of the mandible.

Odontogenic tumours and tumour-like lesions of the jaws

Tumours or tumour-like swellings of the jaws can be odontogenic, derived from odontogenic tissues, or non-odontogenic (Box 8.1).

Odontogenic tumours are the most common neoplasms of the jaws. There are many types and the majority are rare. Classifications are complex. A simplified version of the current World Health Organization classification is shown in Box 8.2 and the whole classification is given in Appendix 8.1 together with brief details of the rarer lesions. It should be noted that this is a classification of *tumours*, not only of neoplasms, and that it therefore includes lesions of differing types and behaviour.

AMELOBLASTOMAS → Summary p. 136

Several types of ameloblastoma are recognised. This section describes the commonest type, the solid or multicystic type. Unicystic ameloblastomas are dealt with in the next section and the very rare peripheral and desmoplastic ameloblastomas are included in Appendix 8.1

Ameloblastomas are the most common neoplasms of the jaws (Box 8.3). They are usually first recognised between the ages of 30 and 50 and are rare in children and old people. Eighty per cent form in the mandible; of these 70% develop in the

---

Box 8.1   Important causes of tumours (swellings) of the jaws

- Cysts, predominantly odontogenic cysts
- Odontogenic tumours
- Giant cell lesions
- Fibro-osseous lesions
- Primary (non-odontogenic) neoplasms of bone
- Metastatic neoplasms

Box 8.2   Important types of odontogenic tumours

Benign epithelial neoplasms
- Ameloblastoma and its variants
- Squamous odontogenic tumour
- Calcifying epithelial odontogenic tumour
- Adenomatoid odontogenic tumour
- Calcifying cystic odontogenic tumour (calcifying odontogenic cyst)

Benign mixed epithelial and connective tissue neoplasms
- Ameloblastic fibroma

Benign connective tissue neoplasms
- Odontogenic fibroma
- Odontogenic myxoma
- Cementoblastoma

Malignant epithelial neoplasms
- Odontogenic carcinomas
- Clear cell odontogenic carcinoma

Malignant connective tissue neoplasms
- Odontogenic sarcomas

Hamartomas
- Odontomas

Dysplasias
- Cemento-osseous dysplasia

Box 8.3   Ameloblastoma: key features

- Neoplasm of odontogenic epithelium
- The most common odontogenic neoplasm
- Usually presents between ages 30 and 50
- Locally invasive but does not metastasise
- Typically asymptomatic and appears as a multilocular cyst radiographically
- Most commonly forms in posterior mandible
- Treated by excision with a margin of normal tissue
- Maxillary ameloblastomas can invade the cranial base and be lethal

Fig. 8.1   Ameloblastoma. Typical presentation. There is a rounded, bony swelling of the posterior alveolar bone, body and angle of the mandible. There is no ulceration, a feature only seen in very large tumours that have perforated the cortex.

posterior molar region and often involve the ramus. They are symptomless until the swelling becomes obtrusive (Fig. 8.1).

> **Practical point** The possibility that any radiolucency at the angle of the mandible might be an ameloblastoma should not be dismissed until the diagnosis is confirmed by biopsy

Radiographically, ameloblastomas typically form rounded, cyst-like, radiolucent areas with moderately well-defined margins and typically appear multilocular (Fig. 8.2) or with a honeycomb pattern. Lingual expansion may sometimes be seen, but is not pathognomonic of ameloblastoma. However, differentiation from non-neoplastic cysts and other tumours or tumour-like lesions of the jaws is not possible by radiography alone.

Genetic aspects

The causes of ameloblastomas are not known. However, there is evidence that various genes normally expressed during tooth formation are dysregulated in ameloblastoma. Deletion of an ameloblast adhesion molecule and enamel matrix protein called ameloblastin can cause odontogenic tumours similar to ameloblastoma in animals but is not yet linked to human ameloblastoma. Many other genes have been proposed to play a role in pathogenesis including heat shock proteins, inducible nitric oxide synthase and matrix metalloproteinases, but none is the likely primary cause.

Pathology

Conventional ameloblastomas are usually a mixture of solid neoplasm and cysts (Fig. 8.3), though either component may predominate. If only one cavity is present, the lesion is a uni-cystic amelobastoma (below).

Solid and multicystic ameloblastomas may have a variety of histological patterns. All have the common feature of islands or strands of epithelium with a peripheral layer of pre-ameloblast-like cells that, at least focally, have nuclei at the opposite pole

to the basement membrane (reversed polarity). The histological patterns have not been convincingly shown to affect the tumour's behaviour and, apart from sometimes complicating microscopic diagnosis, they are of no significance.

The *follicular* pattern is the most common and most readily recognisable type, with islands and trabeculae of epithelial cells in a connective tissue stroma (Fig. 8.4). The outer layer consists of a well-organised single layer of tall, columnar, ameloblast-like cells with reversed polarity, surrounding a core of loosely arranged polyhedral or angular cells, resembling stellate reticulum (Fig. 8.5). In the *plexiform* pattern the epithelium forms strands and trabeculae of small, darkly staining epithelial cells in a sparsely cellular connective tissue stroma (Fig. 8.6).

Cyst formation is common and there are usually several large cysts up to a few centimeters in diameter. Apparently solid ameloblastomas have numerous microscopic cysts. Cysts may develop either within the epithelial islands or result from cystic degeneration of the connective tissue stroma (Fig. 8.7).

Fig. 8.3 Ameloblastoma of the conventional solid/multicystic type in a resection specimen showing multiple cysts.

Fig. 8.2 Ameloblastoma. The typical radiological appearance of ameloblastoma is a multilocular cyst or multiple cyst cavities of different sizes, as shown here.

Fig. 8.4 Ameloblastoma. Islands of follicular ameloblastoma comprising 'stellate reticulum' and a peripheral layer of elongated ameloblast-like cells.

137

Fig. 8.5 **Ameloblastoma.** At high power in this follicular ameloblastoma the palisaded, elongate peripheral cells with reversed polarity are seen to be very similar in appearance to ameloblasts.

Fig. 8.6 **Ameloblastoma, plexiform type.** There are thin, interlacing strands of epithelium but typical ameloblasts are not seen.

Fig. 8.7 **Ameloblastoma.** Plexiform ameloblastoma composed of interconnecting strands of epithelium surrounding islands of connective tissue. Several of the stromal islands have degenerated to form small cystic cavities.

Other less common histological variants include the *acanthomatous* type with squamous metaplasia of the centre of epithelial islands (Fig. 8.8) producing prickle cells, and sometimes keratin, rather than a stellate reticulum-like tissue. The *basal cell* variant is rare and consists of more darkly staining cells predominantly in a trabecular pattern with little evidence of palisading at the periphery. They have been mistaken for basal cell carcinomas. The *granular cell pattern* is also rare. It resembles the follicular type, but the epithelium, particularly in the central areas of the tumour islands, forms sheets of large eosinophilic granular cells (Fig. 8.9).

Although ameloblastoma is considered benign, a proportion have islands of tumour that extend into the surrounding medullary spaces. This growth pattern is reminiscent of invasion by

Fig. 8.8 **Squamous metaplasia in an ameloblastoma.** Stellate reticulum-like cells have undergone squamous metaplasia to form keratin.

Fig. 8.9 **Ameloblastoma.** Granular cell change in an ameloblastoma. Ameloblastoma and stellate reticulum-like cells have undergone degenerative change to form large pink granular cells. In some tumours this change is extensive and the term 'granular cell ameloblastoma' is applied.

a malignant tumour but extends only a few millimetres beyond the main bony cavity (Fig. 8.10).

Additional types of ameloblastoma are listed in Appendix 8.1.

Management

The diagnosis must be confirmed by biopsy. Treatment is by wide excision, preferably taking 1–2 cm of apparently normal bone around the margin. Complete excision of a large ameloblastoma may therefore require partial resection of the jaw, often with the condyle, and bone grafting. Smaller lesions may be excised leaving the lower border of the jaw intact and extending the resection subperiosteally. Bony repair then causes much of the jaw to re-form.

Excision with a bony margin ensures that any extension into surrounding bone is removed and guarantees a cure. Enucleation is usually followed by recurrence and should be reserved for unicystic ameloblastomas (below).

Regular radiographic follow-up is essential as any recurrence may not appear for several years. Limited re-operation can be performed if necessary. The patient must be warned of the necessity for regular follow-up and, possibly, of a further operation. Spread of ameloblastomas into the soft tissues is difficult to manage (Fig. 8.11).

Maxillary ameloblastomas are particularly dangerous, partly because the bones are considerably thinner than those of the mandible and present weak barriers to spread. Maxillary ameloblastomas tend to form in the posterior segment and to grow upwards to invade the sinonasal passages, pterygomaxillary fossa, orbit and eventually the cranium and brain. They are thus occasionally lethal.

Key features of ameloblastomas are summarised in Box 8.3.

Unicystic ameloblastoma

The unicystic ameloblastoma is defined as an ameloblastoma that presents as a single cyst. The importance of differentiating this type is that enucleation carries a low risk of recurrence.

Unfortunately, making the diagnosis of unicystic ameloblastoma is difficult. An ameloblastoma with only one bony cavity radiographically can be a conventional solid or multicystic ameloblastoma. This will not become apparent until the lesion has been opened or examined histologically.

It is therefore important to bear in mind the various configurations of an ameloblastoma that might account for a unilocular presentation radiologically. These are shown in Figure 8.12.

Fig. 8.10 **Ameloblastoma.** Islands of ameloblastoma penetrating surrounding bone at the periphery of the lesion. Such bony infiltration demands that ameloblastoma is excised with a margin rather than curetted.

Fig. 8.11 **Ameloblastoma.** Soft tissue spread after repeated inadequate excisions.

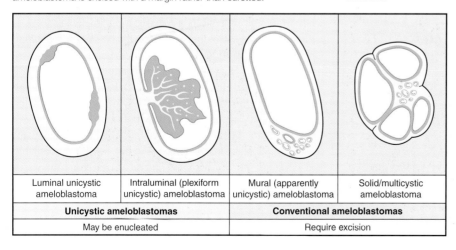

Luminal unicystic ameloblastoma	Intraluminal (plexiform unicystic) ameloblastoma	Mural (apparently unicystic) ameloblastoma	Solid/multicystic ameloblastoma
Unicystic ameloblastomas		**Conventional ameloblastomas**	
May be enucleated		Require excision	

Fig. 8.12 **Explanations for a unicystic presentation of ameloblastoma radiologically.** The two patterns on the left are true unicystic ameloblastomas while that on the right is a conventional ameloblastoma with one very large cyst. See the text for a further explanation of the significance.

An ameloblastoma where the epithelium is limited to a single layer lining the lumen is termed a *luminal type of unicystic ameloblastoma*. If there are papillary projections into the cyst lumen, but no islands within the wall, this is termed an *intraluminal unicystic* or *plexiform unicystic ameloblastoma*. In these types, ameloblastoma epithelium is limited to the lumen or inner cyst wall and the lesion may be enucleated.

The danger of making this diagnosis on radiological grounds alone is shown by the third diagram. Here a conventional ameloblastoma has developed one very large dominant cyst. However, there is a focus of solid/multicystic ameloblastoma in one area of the wall that might penetrate its full thickness or into surrounding bone. This is the *mural type* of (apparently unicystic) ameloblastoma. This is not a true unicystic ameloblastoma. It is a conventional ameloblastoma that could easily be misdiagnosed as one.

Unicystic ameloblastoma is diagnosed predominantly between the ages of 10 and 20, earlier than conventional ameloblastoma, and almost all arise in the posterior mandible. The

single well-defined cavity resembles a dentigerous cyst in over 80% of cases (Fig. 8.13), but may also present as a radicular, residual or other types of cyst.

The histological appearances of all three true unicystic ameloblastomas are similar and are shown in Figure 8.14. The tumour cells forming the cyst wall are flattened and easily mistaken for those of a non-neoplastic cyst.

Unicystic ameloblastomas may be enucleated because the epithelium is enclosed by the fibrous cyst wall. Nevertheless, a 10% recurrence rate after 10 years can be expected. In the mural type of unicystic ameloblastoma, there is a risk that ameloblastoma extends through the cyst wall. This would predispose to recurrence and re-excision of the bony cavity would have to be considered if histological examination showed penetration of the full thickness of the cyst wall.

The diagnosis of unicystic ameloblastoma can only be made confidently after removal because it requires detailed histological examination of the wall. The whole wall needs to be evaluated to define the extent and a single biopsy of a stretched cyst lining is insufficient for diagnosis. The treatment of apparently unilocular ameloblastomas by enucleation therefore has to be peformed before definitive diagnosis and it carries an element of risk. It would be very unfortunate if a conventional ameloblastoma containing one large cyst were enucleated in error as this would risk recurrence, perhaps in soft tissue, and a protracted course. In view of the dangerous sequelae of ameloblastoma in the maxilla, enucleation at that site would always be unwise.

Metastasising ameloblastoma and ameloblastic carcinoma

Both of these exceptionally rare tumours are little more than pathological curiosities – though not to the patient of course.

Metastasising ameloblastoma is a histologically typical ameloblastoma which, though apparently benign, nevertheless gives rise to distant lesions. The metastases are usually in the lung and they have the typical benign microscopic appearances of the primary. Some cases appear to have resulted from aspiration implantation at surgery and others follow surgical disruption at the primary site or repeated incomplete removal. Neither the primary tumour nor its 'metastases' significantly differ histologically from conventional, non-metastasising ameloblastomas. It is therefore not possible to predict on the basis of morphology alone, whether an ameloblastoma will metastasise. The diagnosis of metastasising ameloblastoma can only be made after a metastasis has developed. However, the chances of it so doing are remote. As the 'metastases' are really benign, local excision of the secondary deposit should be curative.

Ameloblastic carcinoma is a tumour which initially resembles an ameloblastoma histologically, but loses differentiation and develops into a carcinoma. It spreads to lymph nodes or beyond. Later, the microscopic appearances become very poorly differentiated or similar to squamous cell carcinoma. Rarely, the progressive loss of differentiation can be seen in successive specimens from the same patient and confirms the diagnosis

Fig. 8.13 Unicystic ameloblastoma. This ameloblastoma forms a monolocular radiolucency enveloping the crown of an unerupted tooth. The radiological appearance mimics a dentigerous cyst, reinforcing the maxim that ameloblastoma should be considered in the differential diagnosis of every radiolucency at the angle of the mandible.

Fig. 8.14 Unicystic ameloblastoma. Part of the lining of a large unicystic ameloblastoma. The epithelium is often stretched and loses its typical features, with only a few ameloblast-like basal cells.

(Fig. 8.15). The treatment is that of an intraosseous carcinoma but the prognosis is poor if metastases are present.

Fig. 8.15 **Ameloblastic carcinoma.** Very rarely a malignant variant of the ameloblastoma is encountered. Histologically, they may be indistinguishable from other carcinomas but, in some cases, as here, a peripheral layer of palisaded ameloblast-like cells remains, indicating the tumour's nature.

ADENOMATOID ODONTOGENIC TUMOUR →
Summary p. 157

Adenomatoid odontogenic tumour is uncommon, completely benign and probably a hamartoma.

Clinically, adenomatoid odontogenic tumours are found either in late adolescence or young adulthood. Females are twice as frequently affected as males. The tumour is most frequently sited in the anterior maxilla and forms a very slow-growing swelling. Alternatively, it may be noticed by chance on a radiograph where it frequently presents as a dentigerous or radicular cyst (Fig. 8.16). Most specimens are only a few centimetres in diameter.

Pathology

A well-defined capsule encloses whorls and strands of epithelium, among which are microcysts, resembling ducts cut in cross-section and lined by columnar cells similar to ameloblasts (Figs 8.17 and 8.18). These microcysts may contain homogeneous eosinophilic material. Microcysts have led to the tumours being called adenomatoid, but they are not ducts and are never seen cut longitudinally. Fragments of amorphous or crystalline calcification may also be seen among the sheets of epithelial cells.

These lesions shell out readily, enucleation is curative and recurrence is almost unknown.

Key features of adenomatoid odontogenic tumour are summarised in Box 8.4.

Box 8.4 **Adenomatoid odontogenic tumour: key features**

- Rare
- Hamartoma of odontogenic epithelium
- Usually presents between ages 15 and 20
- Most common in the anterior maxilla
- Often appears radiographically as a unilocular dentigerous cyst
- Responds to enucleation

Fig. 8.16 Adenomatoid odontogenic tumour, a typical cyst-like presentation in the anterior maxilla.

Fig. 8.17 **Adenomatoid odontogenic tumour.** Low magnification shows duct-like microcysts and convoluted structures. The stroma is scanty.

Fig. 8.18 **Adenomatoid odontogenic tumour.** At higher power the duct-like spaces which give the tumour its name are seen.

141

CALCIFYING EPITHELIAL ODONTOGENIC TUMOUR

→ Summaries pp. 157, 190

This tumour, with bizarre microscopic features, is often termed a Pindborg tumour, after its discoverer. Though rare, it is important, because it has been mistaken for a poorly differentiated carcinoma microscopically.

Clinically, adults are mainly affected at an age of about 40 or more. The typical site is the posterior body of the mandible, which is twice as frequently involved as the maxilla. Symptoms are usually lacking until a swelling appears. Radiographs show a radiolucent area with poorly defined margins. Despite the name, a lesion may be completely radiolucent or develop increasing radiopacity as it matures.

Pathology

Calcifying epithelial odontogenic tumours consist of sheets or strands of epithelial cells in a connective tissue stroma (Fig. 8.19). The epithelial cells are polyhedral and typically have distinct outlines and intercellular bridges. Gross variation in nuclear size, including giant nuclei, is frequently striking (Fig. 8.20). These nuclei are usually hyperchromatic and, though mitoses are rare, produce an alarming resemblance to a poorly differentiated carcinoma. However, unlike most carcinomas, a stromal inflammatory reaction is typically absent. Within the tumour, there are typically homogeneous hyaline areas, with the staining characteristics of amyloid. These may calcify and form concentric rings in and around degenerating epithelial cells and may form large masses. Clear cells may also be present.

Calcifying epithelial odontogenic tumours are not encapsulated, are locally invasive and behave similarly to ameloblastomas. Diagnosis depends on histological examination. It is particularly important to distinguish this pleomorphic tumour from a poorly differentiated carcinoma to avoid overtreatment. Complete excision of the tumour with a border of normal bone should be curative, but recurrence follows incomplete excision.

Fig. 8.19 Calcifying epithelial odontogenic tumour (Pindborg tumour). The tumour is composed of strands and sheets of polyhedral epithelial cells lying in pale pink-staining amyloid-like material. Some of this material has mineralised, stains a darker blue colour and gives rise to radiopacities within the lesion.

Key features of calcifying epithelial odontogenic tumour are summarised in Box 8.5.

Box 8.5 Calcifying epithelial odontogenic tumour: key features

- Rare neoplasm of odontogenic epithelium
- Usually presents between ages 40 and 70
- Many bizarre pleomorphic and hyperchromatic nuclei and formation of amyloid-like material
- Solid tumour, mixed radiolucency
- Most commonly forms in posterior mandible
- Locally invasive but does not metastasise
- Treated by excision with a small margin

Fig. 8.20 Calcifying epithelial odontogenic tumour. At higher power the epithelial cells are seen to have sharply defined cell membranes resembling squamous epithelium and pleomorphic hyperchromatic nuclei. The pale pink material is amyloid-like.

CLEAR CELL ODONTOGENIC CARCINOMA

This very rare neoplasm affects elderly patients (60 to 74 years). Symptoms include mild pain or tenderness, or loosening of teeth of either jaw associated with expansion of the jaw and a ragged area of radiolucency.

Pathology

Clear cell odontogenic carcinoma is poorly circumscribed and consists mainly of clear cells with a central nucleus and a well-defined cell membrane. They form large sheets, separated by thin fibrous septa (Fig. 8.21). Inflammatory cells are scanty but areas of haemorrhage may be seen. Nervous tissue may be enveloped and the tumour invades surrounding tissues.

Important differences from calcifying epithelial odontogenic tumour are the lesser degree of nuclear pleomorphism and the lack of calcifications or amyloid-like material.

Treatment

This tumour is capable of metastasising to regional nodes and distant organs and has occasionally been fatal. Wide excision followed by radiotherapy is required (Fig. 8.22).

CALCIFYING (GHOST CELL) ODONTOGENIC CYST

The calcifying odontogenic cyst is rare and the solid form is even less common. It is a benign neoplasm but has a malignant variant.

Fig. 8.21 **Clear cell odontogenic carcinoma.** This rare epithelial odontogenic tumour is composed of pale-staining clear cells.

Fig. 8.22 **Clear cell odontogenic carcinoma.** This neglected tumour has fungated through the cheek.

Clinically, almost any age and either jaw can be affected. The site is most often anterior to the first molar but, occasionally, it is the gingival mucosa and the underlying bone is merely indented. On radiographs, the appearance is usually cystic but it may be multilocular or contain flecks of calcification. Occasionally, roots of adjacent teeth are eroded.

Pathology

The lining of cystic areas consists of squamous epithelium with cuboidal or ameloblast-like basal cells (Figs 8.23 and 8.24). This epithelium is sometimes thick and can contain areas resembling stellate reticulum. Solid variants of this tumour may therefore resemble an ameloblastoma.

The most conspicuous feature is abnormal keratinisation producing areas of swollen, eosinophilic cells which become progressively paler, leaving only their outlines (ghost cells) or

Fig. 8.23 **Calcifying odontogenic cyst.** The fibrous wall and epithelium run along the left with the lumen filled by ghost cells centrally. Some ghost cells have become incorporated into the fibrous wall on the right and are calcifying.

Fig. 8.24 **Calcifying odontogenic cyst.** There is a thin lining of epithelium with a basal layer of palisaded ameloblast-like columnar cells with stellate reticulum-like suprabasal cells. The lumen (above) is filled by ghost cells shed into the cyst cavity.

hyaline masses (Fig. 8.25). The ghost cells typically calcify in patchy fashion and, where this keratin-like material comes into contact with connective tissue, it excites a foreign body reaction. Approximately 10% of calcifying odontogenic cysts are associated with odontomas or other odontogenic tumours.

The behaviour of a calcifying odontogenic cyst is similar to that of a non-neoplastic cyst, overlying bone is only occasionally eroded and enucleation is usually effective.

Key features are summarised in Box 8.6.

Box 8.6   Calcifying odontogenic cyst: key features

- Rare
- Probably a neoplasm of odontogenic epithelium
- Wide age range
- Radiographically unilocular often undistinguishable from non-neoplastic jaw cysts
- Calcifications in the cyst wall may suggest the diagnosis
- Forms at any site in alveolar ridge, usually posteriorly
- Occasionally forms in soft tissue of the gingiva
- Diagnosis by finding ghost and ameloblast-like cells histologically
- Usually responds to enucleation like a non-neoplastic cyst
- Solid lesions may be more aggressive

SQUAMOUS ODONTOGENIC TUMOUR

This rare tumour mainly affects young adults and involves the alveolar process of either jaw, close to the roots of erupted teeth.

Radiographically, the squamous odontogenic tumour can mimic severe bone loss from periodontitis or produce a cyst-like area.

Pathology

Circumscribed, rounded, or more irregular islands of squamous epithelium with flattened peripheral cells are set in a fibrous stroma (Fig. 8.26). Foci of keratin or parakeratin may form in the epithelium which may also contain laminated calcifications or globular eosinophilic structures.

This tumour is benign, though there may occasionally be invasion of adjacent structures by maxillary lesions. However, curettage and extraction of any teeth involved appears usually to be effective.

AMELOBLASTIC FIBROMA

This tumour, though rare, is important as a relatively common and sometimes destructive odontogenic tumour in the young.

Clinically, ameloblastic fibromas usually affect young persons (average age 15 years). They are slow growing and usually asymptomatic, but eventually expand the jaw. Radiographically, they can appear as a multi- or unilocular cysts in the posterior body of the mandible.

Fig. 8.26   Squamous odontogenic tumour. The lesion is composed of islands of squamous epithelium without peripheral palisaded cells.

Fig. 8.25   Calcifying odontogenic cyst, fibrous wall below, lumen above. The epithelial cells in this area are inconspicuous, the epithelium being almost replaced by numerous ghost cells. Arrows indicate the nuclear remnants and holes that give these cells their name.

Pathology → Summary p. 157

Both the epithelium and connective tissue are neoplastic. The epithelium consists of ameloblast-like or more cuboidal cells surrounding others resembling stellate reticulum or more compact epithelium. The epithelium is sharply circumscribed by a basal membrane and forms islands, strands or mushroom-like proliferations in a loose but cellular, fibromyxoid connective tissue, which resembles the immature dentine papilla (Figs 8.27 and 8.28).

An ameloblastic fibroma may rarely be combined with mixed calcifying dental tissues (ameloblastic fibro-odontoma) and radiographs typically show the densely opaque dental tissues in the otherwise radiolucent area.

Ameloblastic fibroma and fibro-odontoma are benign. They do not infiltrate bone and separate readily from their bony walls. Conservative resection is effective but, if incomplete, recurrence follows. However, there is a potential for malignant change.

Key features are summarised in Box 8.7.

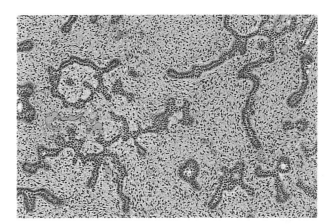

Fig. 8.27 Ameloblastic fibroma. The appearance is somewhat similar to that of ameloblastoma, but the pattern of budding strands is distinctive and the connective tissue resembles the undifferentiated mesenchyme of the dental papilla.

Box 8.7 Ameloblastic fibroma: key features

- Rare
- Neoplasm of both odontogenic epithelium and mesenchyme
- Usually seen in children or young adults
- Solid lesion but appears as unilocular or multilocular radiolucency
- Treated by excision with a small margin
- Can undergo malignant change

Ameloblastic sarcoma (ameloblastic fibrosarcoma)

This is the rare malignant counterpart of ameloblastic fibroma. It is invasive and destructive but has little tendency to metastasise. Reports suggest that approximately 50% arise from ameloblastic fibromas, often after repeated inadequate surgery.

Fig. 8.28 Ameloblastic fibroma. At higher power the resemblance to dental papilla, ameloblasts and stellate reticulum is seen more clearly.

ODONTOGENIC MYXOMA → Summary p. 136

The odontogenic myxoma is peculiar to the jaws and consists of dental mesenchyme.

Clinically, young people are predominantly affected. The tumour gives rise to a fusiform swelling and a radiolucent area with scalloped margins or a soap-bubble or honeycomb appearance (Fig. 8.29).

Pathology

Myxomas consist of scanty spindle-shaped or angular cells with long, fine, anastomosing processes, distributed in loose mucoid material (Figs 8.30 and 8.31). A few collagen fibres may also form and there may be small, scattered epithelial rests. The margins of the tumour are ill-defined and peripheral bone is progressively resorbed.

Myxomas are benign, but can infiltrate widely. Wide excision is required but, in spite of vigorous treatment, some tumours

Fig. 8.29 Odontogenic myxoma of the mandible. An occlusal view showing the finely trabeculated, honeycomb appearance and gross expansion of the mandible. Evidence of residual tumour was still present after 35 years in spite of vigorous treatment, both surgery and radiotherapy, in its earlier stages.

persist and have been seen over 30 years after the original operations. By this time they appear inactive and are symptomless.

Rare variants with a more cellular and pleomorphic microscopic picture may be categorised as myxosarcomas but appear to have little or no potential for metastasis.

Key features are summarised in Box 8.8.

Box 8.8 Odontogenic myxoma: key features

- Rare
- Neoplasm of odontogenic mesenchyme
- Usually seen in young adults
- Benign but prone to recurrence
- Forms a multilocular, sometimes soap-bubble radiolucency
- Most common site is posterior mandible
- Treated by excision

ODONTOGENIC FIBROMA

The odontogenic origin of this rare tumour is suggested by its endosteal site and, sometimes, the presence of epithelial rests.

Clinically, odontogenic fibroma more frequently affects the mandible. It forms a slow-growing asymptomatic mass which may eventually expand the jaw. If found by chance in a radiograph, it appears as a sharply defined, rounded lucent area in a tooth-bearing region.

Pathology

Odontogenic fibromas consist of spindle-shaped fibroblasts and bundles of whorled collagen fibres (Fig. 8.32) and may contain strands of odontogenic epithelium.

Fig. 8.30 Odontogenic myxoma. This cross-section of the mandible through a myxoma shows extensive bony resorption and gross expansion. The pale-staining myxoid lesion gives the tumour an empty appearance.

Odontogenic fibromas are benign and shell out from their surroundings.

TUMOURS AND DYSPLASIAS OF CEMENTUM →
Summaries pp. 157, 172

Cementoblastoma

Cementoblastoma is a neoplasm of cementum. Lesions formerly categorised as cementomas or cemental dysplasias are now categorised as fibro-osseous lesions as discussed below, as is cemento-ossifying fibroma.

Cementoblastoma is a benign neoplasm and forms a mass of cementum-like tissue as an irregular or rounded mass attached to the root of a tooth, usually a mandibular first molar.

Clinically, cementoblastomas mainly affect young adults, particularly males, typically below the age of 25. They are slow-growing and the jaw is not usually expanded. A cementoblastoma only rarely causes gross bony swelling and pain.

Fig. 8.31 Odontogenic myxoma. High-power view showing the typical appearance of sparse fibroblasts lying in a myxoid of ground substance-rich matrix.

Fig. 8.32 Odontogenic fibroma. This rare mesenchymal odontogenic tumour consists of fibrous tissue containing rests and strands of odontogenic epithelium resembling those found in the periodontal ligament.

Radiographically, there is typically a radiopaque mass, with a thin radiolucent margin, attached to the roots of a tooth (Fig. 8.33). The mass may be rounded or irregular in shape and mottled in texture. Resorption of related roots is common, but the tooth remains vital.

Pathology

The mass consists of cementum which often contains many reversal lines, resembling Paget's disease. Cells are enclosed within the cementum and in the irregular spaces are many osteoclasts and osteoblast-like cells (Figs 8.34 and 8.35). The cellular appearance may sometimes appear so active as to be mistaken for an osteosarcoma.

Peripherally, there is a broad zone of unmineralised tissue and a connective tissue capsule. These appearances are essentially the same as those of an osteoblastoma, a rare bone tumour. They are only distinguishable by the cementoblastoma's relationship to a tooth (Fig. 8.36).

Cementoblastomas are benign and, if completely excised and the tooth extracted, there should be no recurrence. Incomplete removal leads to continued growth.

Key features are summarised in Box 8.9.

> **Box 8.9** Cementoblastoma: key features
>
> • Neoplasm of cementoblasts (odontogenic mesenchyme)
> • Usually seen in young adults
> • Benign
> • Radiopaque with a narrow lucent rim
> • Most commonly at the apex of a vital lower first molar
> • Treated by enucleation

Cemento-ossifying fibroma → Summaries pp. 157, 172

Cemento-ossifying fibromas are benign neoplasms of bone (or the specialised odontogenic bone cementum). Historically, classifications included two separate lesions, cementifying fibroma and ossifying fibroma, but these were merged because it was realised that the two lesions were almost indistinguishable. In the current WHO classification, the entity is called ossifying fibroma. However, the term cemento-ossifying fibroma is retained here because it remains in widespread use and because it avoids confusion with the ossifying fibroma of long bones, a very different lesion. Cemento-ossifying fibroma arises exclusively in the jaws, facial bones and skull.

Cemento-ossifying fibroma is uncommon and typically causes a painless swelling in the mandibular premolar or molar region. Patients are usually between 20 and 40 years, but the

Fig. 8.33 Periapical radiograph showing the typical appearances of a cementoblastoma. A radiopaque mass with a radiolucent rim is attached to the root apex. By kind permission of Mr E Whaites.

Fig. 8.34 Cementoblastoma. A dense mass of interconnected trabeculae of osteoid is fused to the resorbed roots of the first permanent molar.

Fig. 8.35 Cementoblastoma. At high power at the periphery of the lesion there are seams of osteoid radiating from the centre of the lesion (to the right) with a thick layer of atypical cementoblasts on their surface. The capsule of the lesion is to the left.

age range is wide. Females are affected several times more frequently than males.

Cemento-ossifying fibroma is a fibro-osseous lesion (Ch. 10). Histologically, it has similarities to fibrous dysplasia and cemento-osseous dysplasias and it cannot always be differentiated from them on the basis of its microscopic appearances alone.

Like other fibro-osseous lesions, the cemento-ossifying fibroma starts as a small radiolucency and expands slowly. Calcification develops centrally as the lesion enlarges. Most become densely calcified given time and appear largely radiopaque. At all stages, the lesion has a sharply defined margin, often with a thin radiolucent rim surrounded by a narrow zone of cortication. This circumscription is a key diagnostic feature and can be detected both radiographically (Figs 8.37 and 8.38)

and histologically (Figs 8.39 and 8.40). Roots of related teeth can be displaced.

Microscopy

Cemento-ossifying fibromas are well demarcated from the surrounding bone. The appearances are widely variable and range from predominantly fibrous tumours with variable degress of cellularity and scanty calcifications to densely calcified nodules with little stroma.

Fig. 8.38 **Cemento-ossifying fibroma.** This example is more densely mineralised and the peripheral radiolucent rim is readily apparent.

Fig. 8.36 Resorbed root at the centre of a cementoblastoma showing continuity of cementum with the mineralised tissue of the lesion.

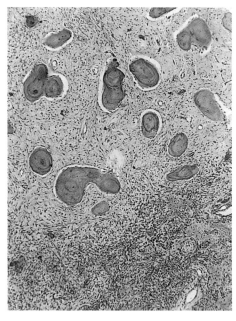

Fig. 8.39 **Cemento-ossifying fibroma.** This example contains densely mineralised and darkly staining islands of cementum-like tissue lying in cellular fibrous tissue. Towards the actively growing periphery of the lesion (lower part) the fibrous tissue is more cellular and is forming woven bone.

Fig. 8.37 **Cemento-ossifying fibroma.** The tumour forms a characteristic rounded well-circumscribed lesion radiographically. This example is cloudily radiolucent and slow-growing, as can be seen by the displacement of the teeth.

The types of calcifications include trabeculae of woven bone with osteoblastic rimming, which frequently form a reticular pattern. Other patterns are dystrophic calcifications or predominantly acellular, rounded calcifications resembling cementicles (Fig. 8.39). These calcifications gradually grow, fuse and, ultimately, form a dense mass (Fig. 8.40). Most so-called cementifying fibromas show mixed spherical calcifications and bone trabeculae.

Histologically, cemento-ossifying fibroma may be indistinguishable from limited areas of fibrous dysplasia or cemento-osseous dysplasias. However, the clinical and radiographic finding of a well-defined margin should allow the distinctions to be made.

Management

The patterns of calcifications have no effect on the tumour's behaviour. Cemento-ossifying fibromas can usually be readily enucleated, separating from bone in the plane of their capsule. Occasionally, large tumours that have distorted the jaw require local resection and bone grafting, but recurrence is rare.

Densely mineralized lesions are relatively avascular and can become a focus for chronic osteomyelitis following extraction of an associated tooth or biopsy. If this happens, removal of some surrounding bone may be required if the infection cannot be controlled.

Psammomatoid ossifying fibroma

This variant of cemento-ossifying fibroma has also been called juvenile (active) ossifying fibroma. It used to be thought to be primarily a disease of those aged 20 or less and developed a reputation for recurrence following treatment. However, it is now known that these lesions can develop at all ages. They affect the maxilla, facial bones and base of skull more frequently than the mandible.

Lesions tend to be asymptomatic but expansion appears greater than in the conventional cemento-ossifying fibroma.

Histologically, the lesion consists of a highly cellular fibroblastic stroma containing compact, rounded calcifications, larger than, but reminiscent of, the so-called psammoma bodies in thyroid carcinomas, hence the name (Fig. 8.41). These small mineralised balls do not fuse together as the lesion matures.

This variant should be treated by enucleation and curettage exactly as conventional cemento-ossifying fibroma. There is a risk of recurrence, perhaps because these lesions often arise in thin facial bones that make treatment difficult. However, any recurrence is usually eradicated by a second or third curettage so that conservative surgery is all that is required.

Juvenile ossifying fibroma

This histological pattern is commoner in children. The loose, fibroblastic stroma contains very fine, lace-like trabeculae of immature osteoid entrapping plump osteoblasts. Mitoses may be seen and focal collections of giant cells are common. The histological appearances are similar to osteoblastoma or even osteosarcoma, but this misdiagnosis can be avoided by noting the radiological circumscription.

This type may be treated in the same way as the conventional cemento-ossifying fibroma.

NON-NEOPLASTIC ODONTOGENIC LESIONS

Fig. 8.40 Cemento-ossifying fibroma. In this mature lesion, there are large coalescing islands of dense bone and little fibrous tissue. Note the well-demarcated periphery of fibrous tissue which has shelled away from the adjacent bone during removal.

Fig. 8.41 Cemento-ossifying fibroma, psammomatoid type comprising small darkly stained mineralised nodules of bone in a cellular fibrous tissue.

CEMENTO-OSSEOUS DYSPLASIAS

These are non-neoplastic proliferations. They are of periodontal ligament origin and all the variants involve the same pathological processes and differ mainly in their extent and radiographic appearances.

Periapical cemental dysplasia → Summary p. 190

Periapical cemental dysplasia affects women (particularly the middle-aged) more than 10 times as frequently as men and is also more common in black patients. It typically involves the mandibular incisor region, but can affect several sites or be generalised.

The condition is asymptomatic and can be seen early in radiographs as rounded radiolucent areas related to the apices of the teeth. These simulate periapical granulomas but related teeth are vital. Later, increasing calcification, starting centrally, causes the masses to become densely radiopaque (Fig. 8.42), but all stages of development may be seen in multiple lesions.

Pathology

The lesions resemble cemento-ossifying fibromas histologically and consist, in their early stages, of cellular fibrous tissue containing foci of cementum-like tissue. Progressive calcification leads to the formation of a solid, bone-like mass. Early lesions need to be distinguished from periapical granulomas by dental investigation. Further treatment is unnecessary, as the disorder is self-limiting.

Florid cemento-osseous dysplasia → Summary p. 190

This is probably a florid form of periapical cemental dysplasia and affects a similar group of persons. The sclerotic masses are frequently symmetrical and may involve all four quadrants. They are asymptomatic unless they become infected, but can expand the jaw and occasionally develop solitary bone cysts in their interior.

Radiographically, florid cemento-osseous dysplasia appears as radiopaque, somewhat irregular masses without a radiolucent border and in the past has been mistaken for chronic osteomyelitis (Fig. 8.43).

Microscopically, the appearances are generally similar to periapical cemental dysplasia.

Focal cemento-osseous dysplasia → Summary p. 190

This term is given to changes similar to florid osseous dysplasia but forming a single lesion.

Management of cemento-osseous dysplasias

Infection of these lesions by unwise extractions or other means must be avoided. Osteomyelitis resulting from such causes is difficult to treat because of the widespread sclerosis in the late stages. Wide excision may then be required to allow resolution. Treatment is otherwise not indicated except, rarely, for cosmetic reasons or if solitary bone cysts cause expansion.

Fig. 8.43 Florid cemento-osseous dysplasia. Section of a panoramic tomogram showing the typical appearances of multiple irregular radiopaque masses centred on the roots of the teeth. The periphery of each is radiolucent and the surrounding bone shows some sclerosis. Similar lesions were present in the contralateral molar region and on some maxillary teeth.

Fig. 8.42 Periapical cemento-osseous dysplasia. Three films taken over a period of years showing, (A) the early radiolucent stage resembling periapical granulomas, (B) intermediate stage with patchy mineralisation and (C) the late stage with well-defined masses of cementum in the centre of lesions. By kind permission of Mr EJ Whaites.

Gigantiform cementoma

This extremely rare condition may be a variant of cemento-osseous dysplasia. It is inherited and produces extremely large and disfiguring lesions, usually in more than one quadrant.

ODONTOMAS (ODONTOMES) → Summary p. 172

Odontomas are developmental malformations (hamartomas) of dental tissues, not neoplasms. Like teeth, once fully calcified they do not develop further. Even when the morphology is grossly distorted (as in complex odontomas), the pulp, dentine, enamel and cementum are in normal anatomical relationships with one another and, also like teeth, odontomas may erupt.

Odontomas affect the maxilla slightly more frequently than the mandible and are often recognised in early adolescence by the dense opacity of the enamel component in routine radiographs. When odontomas have erupted, infection can develop in one of the many stagnation areas and abscess formation commonly follows. In other cases, odontomas displace teeth or block their eruption or become involved in cyst formation.

Compound odontomas

These consist of many separate, small, tooth-like structures (denticles), probably produced by localised, multiple budding-off from the dental lamina and formation of many tooth germs (Fig. 8.44).

Clinically, a compound odontoma usually forms in the anterior part of the jaws and gives rise to a painless swelling. The denticles may be seen radiographically as separate densely-calcified bodies (Fig. 8.45).

Histologically, the denticles are embedded in fibrous connective tissue and have a fibrous capsule (Figs 8.46 and 8.47).

The mass should be enucleated as a potential obstruction to tooth eruption or cyst formation.

Fig. 8.45 **Compound odontoma.** The denticles overlap each other in the radiograph but are, nevertheless, just visible as individual tooth-like structures.

Fig. 8.46 **Compound odontoma.** A denticle of dentine surrounded by enamel matrix is lying within more irregular calcified tissues.

Fig. 8.47 **Compound odontoma.** Sections from various areas of the odontoma, seen in the radiograph shown in Figure 8.45, show denticles of dentine and enamel cut in various planes, and more irregular calcified tissues, within a connective tissue capsule.

Fig. 8.44 Compound odontoma, a cluster of small deformed teeth or denticles.

Complex odontoma

Complex odontomas consist of an irregular mass of hard and soft dental tissues, having no morphological resemblance to a tooth and frequently forming a cauliflower-like mass.

Clinically, complex odontomas are usually seen in young persons, but may escape diagnosis until late in life. Typically, a hard painless swelling is present, but the mass may start to erupt and infection follows. The mass may also undergo cystic change or resorption. Radiographically, when calcification is complete, an irregular radiopaque mass is seen containing areas of densely radiopaque enamel (Fig. 8.48).

Histologically, the mass consists of all the dental tissues in a disordered arrangement, but frequently with a radial pattern. The pulp is usually finely branched so that the mass is perforated, like a sponge, by small branches of pulp (Fig. 8.49).

Key features are summarised in Box 8.10.

The mass should be removed by conservative surgery.

Box 8.10 Odontoma: key features

- Hamartomas of odontogenic epithelium and mesenchyme
- Usually found between ages 10 and 20 years
- Benign
- Develop like surrounding teeth with initial (crypt-like) radiolucent phase, intermediate stage of mixed radiolucency, finally densely radiopaque
- May be compound (many small teeth) or complex (disordered mass of dental hard tissue)
- Most common sites are anterior maxilla and posterior mandible
- Respond to enucleation

Other types of odontomas

In the past, complex classifications have been devised to include such developmental anomalies as *dilated*, *invaginated* and *geminated* odontomas. These abnormalities are, in part, obviously tooth-like. Dilated and gestant odontomas arise by invagination of cells of the enamel organ or of the epithelial sheath of Hertwig, which actively proliferate until they expand the developing tooth. Gestant odontomas range in severity from a cingular pit in an otherwise normal upper lateral incisor to the so-called *dens in dente*. Minor morphological anomalies such as these have been discussed in Chapter 2.

'Dentinoma'. Calcified masses called 'dentinomas' have rarely been described. However, dentine forms only under the

Fig. 8.48 Complex odontoma. In this radiograph, the odontoma overlies the crown of a buried molar and shows the typical dense amorphous area of radiopacity. Note the radiolucent rim of follicle and lamina dura of a 'crypt' extending around the lesion.

Fig. 8.49 Complex odontoma. A disorganised mass of dentine, enamel and cementum penetrated by fine divisions of pulp.

inductive effect of ameloblasts and the existence of dentinomas is no longer accepted.

Mixed odontogenic tumours. Very occasionally odontomas and odontogenic tumours are combined.

SUGGESTED FURTHER READING

Ackermann GL, Altini M, Shear M 1988 The unicystic ameloblastoma: a clinicopathological study of 57 cases. J Oral Pathol Med 17: 541–546

Baden E, Doyle J, Mesa M, Fabie M, Lederman D, Eichen M 1993 Squamous odontogenic tumour. Report of three cases including the first extraosseous case. Oral Surg Oral Med Oral Pathol 75:733–738

Bang G, Koppang HS, Hansen LS et al 1989 Clear cell odontogenic carcinoma: report of three cases with pulmonary and lymph node metastases. J Oral Pathol Med 18:113–118

Bredenkamp JK, Zimmerman MC, Mickel RA 1989 Maxillary ameloblastoma. A potentially lethal neoplasm. Arch Otolaryngol Head Neck Surg 115:99–104

Bruce RA, Jackson IT 1991 Ameloblastic carcinoma. Report of an aggressive case and review of the literature. J Cranio Max Fac Surg 19:267–271

Buchner A 1991 The central (intraosseous) calcifying odontogenic cyst: an analysis of 215 cases. J Oral Maxillofac Surg 49:330–339

Buchner A, Merrell PW, Hansen LS, Leider AS 1991 Peripheral (extraosseous) calcifying odontogenic cyst. A review of forty-five cases. Oral Surg Oral Med Oral Pathol 72:65–70

Cawson RA 1972 Myxoma of the mandible with a 35 year follow-up. Br Oral Surg 10:59–63

Cawson RA, Binnie WH, Barrett AW, Speight P, Wright JM 1998 Lucas's pathology of tumors of the oral tissues. Churchill Livingstone, Edinburgh

Cawson RA, Binnie WH, Barrett AW, Wright JM 2001 Oral disease, 3rd edn. Mosby-Wolfe, London

Daley TD, Wysocki GP 1994 Peripheral odontogenic fibroma. Oral Surg Oral Med Oral Pathol 78:329–336

Franklin CD, Pindborg JJ 1976 The calcifying epithelial odontogenic tumor. A review and analysis of 113 cases. Oral Surg 42:753–765

Gardner DG, Corio RL 1984 Plexiform unicystic ameloblastoma. A variant of ameloblastoma with low-recurrence rate after enucleation. Cancer 53:1730–1735

Gerol M, Burkes EJ 1995 Peripheral ameloblastoma. J Periodontol 66:1065–1068

Gorlin RJ, Pindborg JJ, Redman RS, Williamson JJ, Hansen LS 1964 The calcifying odontogenic cyst – A new entity and possible analogue of the cutaneous epithelioma of Malherbe. Cancer 17:723–729

Handlers JP, Abrams AM, Melrose RJ, Danforth R 1991 Central odontogenic fibroma: clinicopathologic features of 19 cases and review of the literature. J Oral Maxillofac Surg 49:46–54

Holmlund A, Anneroth G, Lundquist G, Nordenram A 1991 Ameloblastomas originating from odontogenic cysts. J Oral Pathol Med 20:318–321

Hong SP, Ellis GL, Hartman KS 1991 Calcifying odontogenic cyst: a review of ninety-two cases with reevaluation of their nature as neoplasms, the nature of ghost cells, and subclassification. Oral Surg Oral Med Oral Pathol 72:56–64

Kaugars GE, Miller ME, Abbey LM 1989 Odontomas. Oral Surg Oral Med Oral Pathol 67:172–176

Keszler A, Dominguez FV, Giannunzio G 1995 Myxoma in childhood: an analysis of 10 cases. J Oral Maxillofac Surg 53:518–521

McCoy BP, Carroll MKO, Hall JM 1992 Carcinoma arising in a dentinogenic ghost cell tumor. Oral Surg Oral Med Oral Pathol 74:371–378

Muller S, Parker DC, Kapadia SB, Budnick SD, Barnes EL 1995 Ameloblastic fibrosarcoma of the jaw. A clinicopathologic and DNA analysis of five cases and review of the literature. Oral Surg Oral Med Oral Pathol 79:469–477

Peltola J, Magnusson B, Hopponen R-P, Borrman H 1994 Odontogenic myxoma – a radiographic study of 21 tumours. Br J Oral Maxillofac Surg 32:298–301

Philipsen HP, Reichart PA 1998 Unicystic ameloblastoma. A review of 193 cases from the literature. Oral Oncol 34:317–325

Philipsen HP, Reichert PA, Zhang KJ, Nikai H, Yu QX 1991 Adenomatoid odontogenic tumor: biologic profile base on 499 cases. J Oral Pathol Med 20:149–158

Pindborg JJ, Kramer IRH, Shear M 1992 Histological typing of odontogenic tumours, 2nd edn. World Health Organization. Springer Verlag, Berlin

Reichart PA, Philipsen HP, Sonner S 1995 Ameloblastoma: biological profile of 3677 cases. Oral Oncol Eur J Cancer 31B:86–99

Ulmansky M, Hjorting-Hansen E, Praetorius F, Haque MF 1994 Benign cementoblastoma. A review and five new cases. Oral Surg Oral Med Oral Pathol 77:48–55

Williams HK, Mangham C, Speight PM 1999 Juvenile ossifying fibroma. An analysis of eight cases and a comparison with other fibro-osseous lesions. J Oral Pathol Med 29:13–18

Williams TP 1993 Management of ameloblastoma: a changing perspective. J Oral Maxillofac Surg 51:1064–1070

**APPENDIX
8.1**

WHO classification of odontogenic tumours 2005

Malignant tumours	
Odontogenic carcinomas	
Metastasising (malignant) ameloblastoma	See text of Chapter 8
Ameloblastic carcinoma – primary	See text of Chapter 8
Ameloblastic carcinoma – secondary, dedifferentiated, intraosseous and peripheral	See text of Chapter 8
Primary intraosseous carcinoma • Primary intraosseous carcinoma derived from keratocystic odontogenic tumour • Primary intraosseous carcinoma derived from odontogenic cysts	A squamous carcinoma that originates in odontogenic epithelium, in a cyst or other odontogenic tumour. Of the cysts, odontogenic keratocyst (keratocystic odontogenic tumour) is that most likely to undergo malignant change
Clear cell odontogenic carcinoma	See text of Chapter 8
Ghost cell odontogenic carcinoma	A malignant variant of dentinogenic ghost cell tumour or calcifying odontogenic cyst, recognised by histological similarity or presence of pre-existing lesion
Odontogenic sarcomas	
Ameloblastic fibrosarcoma Ameloblastic fibrodentino- and fibro-odontosarcoma	Both extremely rare malignant variants of the fibroma and fibrodentinoma respectively, the latter containing some dentine-like material histologically. These are low grade, recur but rarely metastasise. They often develop when the benign counterpart is repeatedly but incompletely removed
Benign tumours	
Composed of odontogenic epithelium but without odontogenic ectomesenchyme	
Ameloblastoma, solid/multicystic	See text of Chapter 8
Ameloblastoma, extraosseous/peripheral	Rare soft tissue variant, usually in gingiva. Readily excised, recurrence is unusual
Ameloblastoma, desmoplastic	Extremely rare. Unusual ameloblastoma variant containing a dense fibrous stroma, as common in the maxilla as the mandible, mottled radiolucency that is difficult to define and without the typical histological features of ameloblastoma
Ameloblastoma, unicystic	See text of Chapter 8
Squamous odontogenic tumour	See text of Chapter 8
Calcifying epithelial odontogenic tumour	See text of Chapter 8
Adenomatoid odontogenic tumour	See text of Chapter 8
Keratocystic odontogenic tumour	New name for odontogenic keratocyst, parakeratinised type. See text of Chapter 7
Composed of odontogenic epithelium with odontogenic ectomesenchyme with or without hard tissue formation	
Ameloblastic fibroma	See text of Chapter 8
Ameloblastic fibro-dentinoma	Rare variant of ameloblastc fibroma containing dentine-like material. The same histological appearance may also be found as a hamartoma overlying the crowns of unerupted molar teeth
Ameloblastic fibro-odontoma	See text of Chapter 8
Odontoma, complex and compound	See text of Chapter 8
Odontoameloblastoma	Extremely rare, an otherwise typical ameloblastoma but with formation of dental hard tissues

Calcifying cystic odontogenic tumour	New name for calcifying odontogenic cyst, now reclassified as a neoplasm. See text of Chapter 8
Dentinogenic ghost cell tumour	A solid neoplasm with histological similarities to the calcifying cystic odontogenic tumour. Infiltrative margin, recurs
Composed of odontogenic mesenchyme and/or ectomesenchyme with or without epithelium	
Odontogenic fibroma	See text of Chapter 8
Odontogenic myxoma and myxofibroma	See text of Chapter 8
Cementoblastoma	See text of Chapter 8
Bone related lesions	
Ossifying fibroma	New name for cemento-ossifying fibroma. See text of Chapter 8
Fibrous dysplasia	See text of Chapter 10
Osseous dysplasias	See text of Chapter 8
Central giant cell granuloma	See text of Chapter 9. Arises most frequently in the jaws but also in other bones, not definitely odontogenic
Cherubism	See text of Chapter 10
Aneurysmal bone cyst	See text of Chapter 10
Simple bone cyst	WHO preferred name for solitary bone cyst. See text of Chapter 10
Other tumours	
Melanotic neuroectodermal tumour of infancy	See text of Chapter 9

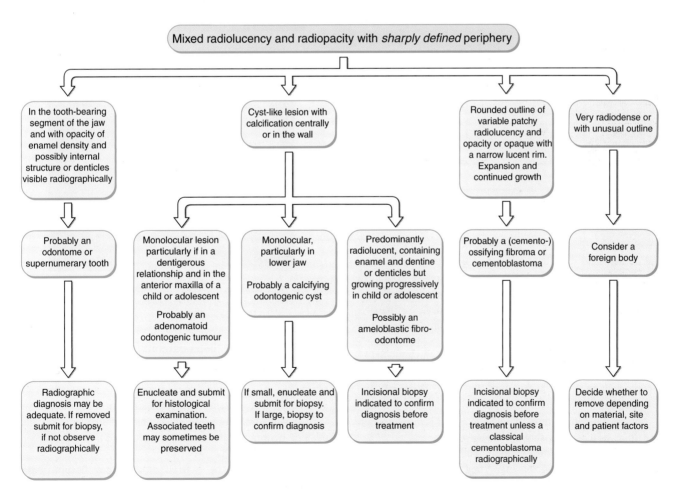

Summary chart 8.1 Differential diagnosis and management of sharply defined mixed radiolucencies in the jaws.

Non-odontogenic tumours of the jaws

Almost any type of tumour can arise in the jaws, but most of them are considerably more common in other parts of the skeleton. Only the more important examples (Box 9.1) are considered here.

Box 9.1 Non-odontogenic tumours of bone

Primary – benign
- Osteoma
- Osteochondroma
- Cemento-ossifying fibroma
- Central giant cell granuloma
- Haemangioma
- Melanotic neuroectodermal tumour

Primary – malignant
- Osteosarcoma
- Chondrosarcoma
- Ewing's sarcoma
- Multifocal or potentially multifocal:
    Myeloma
    Langerhans cell histiocytosis

Metastatic
- Carcinoma

OSTEOMA AND OTHER BONY OVERGROWTHS →
Summary p. 172

True tumours consisting of bone (either compact or cancellous) are occasionally seen, but localised overgrowths of bone (exostoses) are more common. They consist of lamellae of compact bone, but large specimens may have a core of cancellous bone. Small exostoses may form irregularly on the surface of the alveolar processes (Fig. 9.1) and specific variants are *torus palatinus* and *torus mandibularis*. They differ from other exostoses only in that they develop in characteristic sites and are symmetrical.

Torus palatinus commonly forms towards the posterior of the midline of the hard palate (Fig. 9.2). The swelling is rounded and symmetrical, sometimes with a midline groove. It is not usually noticed until middle age and, if it interferes with the fitting of a denture, should be removed.

Tori mandibularis form on the lingual aspect of the mandible opposite the mental foramen. They are typically bilateral, forming hard, rounded swellings (Fig. 9.3). The management is the same as that of torus palatinus.

Fig. 9.1 Exostoses. Bony exostoses, aside from tori, are found most frequently buccally on the alveolar bone and are often symmetrically arranged.

Fig. 9.2 Torus palatinus. Palatal tori range from small smooth elevations to lobular swellings such as this. The bone is covered by only a thin mucosa which is prone to trauma.

Compact and cancellous osteoma

Compact osteomas consist of lamellae of bone, sometimes in layers like an onion but not in Haversian systems (Fig. 9.4). This dense bone contains occasional vascular spaces and grows very slowly. Cancellous osteomas consist of slender trabeculae of bone, with interstitial marrow spaces and a lamellated cortex (Fig. 9.5).

Osteomas should be excised only if they become large enough to cause symptoms or interfere with the fitting of a denture.

Fig. 9.3 Mandibular tori. The typical appearance of bilateral tori lingual to the lower premolars.

Fig. 9.5 Cancellous osteoma of the mandible. The tumour has arisen from a relatively narrow base lingually to the molars but has been moulded forward during growth by pressure of the tongue. The trabecular pattern of cancellous bone can be seen. A torus mandibularis arises further forward on the jaw, arises from a broad base and is usually bilateral.

OSTEOCHONDROMA (CARTILAGE-CAPPED OSTEOMA)

These bony overgrowths grow by ossification beneath a cartilaginous cap. Most arise from the region of the coronoid or condylar process and form a hard bony protuberance which can interfere with joint function. The cartilaginous cap may not be visible in radiographs. Almost any age can be affected.

Pathology

The lesion is subperiosteal and has a cap of hyaline cartilage where the cartilage cells are sometimes regularly aligned or irregular and contain minute foci of ossification (Fig. 9.6). As age advances, the mass progressively ossifies.

These tumours are benign and usually cease to grow after skeletal maturation. Removal is therefore curative.

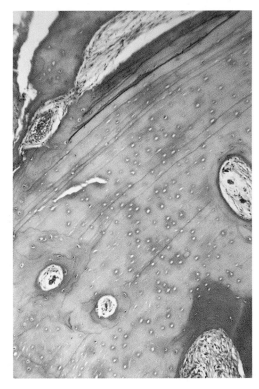

Fig 9.4 Compact osteoma. Dense bone is laid down in lamellae with occasional vascular spaces, but there is no attempt to form Haversian systems.

CEMENTO-OSSIFYING FIBROMA → Summary p. 157

Cemento-ossifying fibroma has been discussed in Chapter 8, as its presence in the jaw and cemental content suggest an odontogenic origin.

GIANT CELL GRANULOMA → Summary p. 136

The giant cell granuloma is a localised tumour of fibrous tissue containing numerous osteoclasts. It is not related to the giant cell tumour (osteoclastoma), which by contrast is an aggressive neoplasm of long bones.

Pathogenesis

The earlier name 'giant cell reparative granuloma' derives from the unconvincing idea (also applied to solitary bone cysts)

Gardner's syndrome

Gardner's syndrome comprises multiple osteomas of the jaw, polyposis coli with a high malignant potential and often other abnormalities such as dental defects and epidermal cysts or fibromas. It is inherited as an autosomal dominant trait but penetrance is weak.

Early recognition of these oral features should prompt bowel radiography or endoscopy and possibly prophylactic colectomy.

Fig. 9.6 Osteochondroma. There is a superficial cap of hyaline cartilage which undergoes endochondral ossification to form normal trabeculae of lamellar bone. The marrow spaces contain normal marrow continuous with those in the underlying bone.

Fig. 9.7 Giant cell granuloma. This maxillary lesion has perforated the cortex and formed an ulcerated bluish soft-tissue mass on the alveolar ridge. The underlying alveolar bone is considerably expanded.

Fig. 9.8 Giant cell granuloma. Characteristic radiographic appearance of an expansile radiolucency with scalloped margins containing numerous thin internal septa of wispy bone and osteoid.

Fig. 9.9 Giant cell granuloma. This tissue is vascular and contains much extravasated blood, around which giant cells are clustered.

that it was a reaction to trauma which caused intramedullary haemorrhage. The cause is unknown though they are generally considered hyperplastic or reactive rather than neoplastic. Identical lesions occur in Noonan syndrome, the genetic cause of which is known to be mutation of the PTPN11 gene and a chromosomal translocation t(X;4) has been identified in a long bone lesion.

Giant cell granuloma is usually seen in young people under 20 and in females twice as frequently as males. The mandible, anterior to the first molars, where the teeth have had deciduous predecessors, is the usual site. There is frequently only a painless swelling, but growth is sometimes rapid and the mass can, rarely, erode through the bone, particularly of the alveolar ridge, to produce a purplish soft-tissue swelling (Fig. 9.7).

Radiographs show a rounded cyst-like radiolucent area, often faintly loculated or with a soap-bubble appearance (Fig. 9.8). Roots of teeth can be displaced or occasionally resorbed.

Pathology and management

Giant cell granuloma forms a lobulated mass of proliferating vascular connective tissue packed with giant cells (osteoclasts) (Figs 9.9 and 9.10). Signs of bleeding into the mass and deposits of haemosiderin are frequently seen. Fibroblastic proliferation or prominent osteoid and bone formation are common. There are no changes in blood chemistry.

Curettage of giant cell granulomas is usually adequate and wide excision unnecessary; small fragments that may be left behind may cause little trouble, rarely require further treatment and may resolve spontaneously. Recurrence follows incomplete removal and a further limited operation may become necessary.

Key features are summarised in Box 9.2.

Other giant cell lesions of the jaws

Several other jaw lesions (Box 9.3) can resemble a giant cell granuloma microscopically and must be considered in the differential diagnosis.

HAEMANGIOMA OF BONE → Summary p. 135

Haemangiomas are rare tumours of bone, but a relatively high proportion are in the mandible, particularly in women.

Clinically, haemangiomas cause progressive painless swellings which, when the overlying bone is resorbed, may become pulsatile. Teeth may be loosened and there may be bleeding, particularly from the gingival margins involved by the tumour.

Radiographically, the features of haemangioma are extremely varied. They range from a sharply defined cyst-like appearance to poorly defined pseudoloculated radiolucencies or a soap-bubble appearance. A serpiginous outline is particularly suggestive.

Pathology

Haemangiomas of bone are essentially similar to those in soft tissues. They are usually cavernous (Fig. 9.11), but there is also an arteriovenous type (fast-flow angioma) which has large feeder arteries, tends to expand rapidly and is likely to bleed severely if opened.

Management

A haemangioma may not be suspected if its vascularity is not obvious. Opening it or extracting a related tooth may therefore release torrents of blood, occasionally with fatal results. However, once the diagnosis has been made, wide en bloc resection is the only practical treatment. If there are identifiable feeder vessels selective arterial embolisation makes surgery considerably safer and may be all that is required.

Fig. 9.10 Giant cell granuloma. High power showing the osteoclast-like giant cells with numerous, evenly dispersed nuclei.

Fig. 9.11 Haemangioma of bone. The marrow spaces contain very large blood-filled sinuses with thin walls; the lesion is poorly localised and permeates between the bony trabeculae.

Fig. 9.12 **Melanotic neuroectodermal tumour of infancy.** The anterior maxilla of this neonate contains an expansile radiolucency which has displaced tooth germs and eroded the alveolar bone.

Fig. 9.13 **Melanotic neuroectodermal tumour of infancy.** Pale pink-staining epithelial cells, some of which are pigmented (centrally), arranged in clusters and surrounded by small, round, darkly staining tumour cells.

MELANOTIC NEUROECTODERMAL TUMOUR OF INFANCY (PROGONOMA) → Summary p. 337

This rare tumour, which arises from the neural crest, may appear in the anterior maxilla in the first few months of life. It is usually painless and slowly expansive, but occasionally grows rapidly.

Radiographically, there is an area of bone destruction, frequently with ragged margins, and displacement of the developing teeth (Fig. 9.12).

Genetics

A molecular genetic study has shown chromosomal deletions at 1p together with translocations t(11;22) in a small number of cases. What genes are affected by these chromosomal anomalies is unknown. However, these changes are distinct from other neuroectodermal tumours, such as neuroblastoma or Ewing's sarcoma, demonstrating that this lesion is a distinct entity.

Microscopy

Melanotic neuroectodermal tumour consists of slit-like or larger spaces lined by cuboidal, melanin-containing cells in a fibrous stroma. Small round cells, which are non-pigmented, form clusters in the stroma or lie in the alveolar spaces (Figs 9.13 and 9.14). Some degree of atypia and infrequent mitotic figures are often seen. The round cells resemble neuroblasts and may be associated with neurofibrillary material indicating neural differentiation.

Ultrastructurally, pigmented cells show both epithelial and melanocytic features. Cells with melanosomes in various stages of maturation, and cells with neuroblastic features, including neurosecretory granules and cytoplasmic processes may be seen.

Frequent mitotic figures and loss of differentiation of the melanocyte-like cells suggest more aggressive behaviour. In a tumour that recurred and later disseminated widely after treatment, only the melanocyte-like cells remained at autopsy.

Fig. 9.14 **Melanotic neuroectodermal tumour of infancy.** Higher power showing the melanin pigment granules within a strand of epithelium.

Management

Radiography, CT scans and MRI are not diagnostic in themselves, but the appearance of a destructive maxillary tumour in the maxilla in an infant, together with submucosal pigmentation and high levels of urinary vanillylmandelic acid are distinctive. Serum levels of epinephrine, norepinephrine, vanillylmandelic acid and neuron-specific enolase may be high but typically return to normal after treatment. The clinical and radiographic features of melanotic neuroectodermal tumour of infancy are so distinctive that preliminary biopsy which may provoke the tumour into greater activity should not be necessary.

These tumours are frequently described as benign, but up to 15% may recur and a very few have metastasised and disseminated widely. Histology is an unreliable guide to behaviour, as even those tumours which show histologically malignant features may do well. Nevertheless, a high mitotic index, and possibly CD99 expression, may indicate more aggressive behaviour.

Surgery is the treatment of choice, but the extent of the resection is controversial and can range from local excision and curettage to total maxillectomy. The tumour is non-encapsulated but usually separates easily from the bone at operation. Conservative

Fig. 9.15 Osteosarcoma. The picture shows the progress of the tumour over a period of 3 months. The patient died with metastases in the lungs, about a month after the second picture was taken. (Taken before the advent of colour photography.)

treatment is usually curative but, even when excision is incomplete, recurrence is rare. Regional lymph node dissection may be necessary only for rare cases where there has been lymphatic invasion. Radiotherapy and chemotherapy (undesirable in an infant) have been shown to be ineffective in controlling this tumour.

Key features are summarised in Box 9.4.

Box 9.4   **Melanotic neuroectodermal tumour of infancy: key features**

- Very rare
- Congenital or appears in first few months
- Presents as expansion of anterior maxilla, typically bluish in colour
- Benign but destroys bone
- Usually responds to conservative excision or curettage

MALIGNANT NEOPLASMS OF BONE

Osteosarcoma → Summary p. 190

Osteosarcoma is highly malignant and the most common primary (non-odontogenic) neoplasm of bone, but overall is rare, especially in the jaws.

Osteosarcomas rarely have identifiable causes but a few develop late in life after irradiation or Paget's disease of bone, but the latter type rarely affects jaws.

Osteosarcoma of the jaws is typically seen between the ages of 30 and 40. Males are slightly more frequently affected and the body of the mandible is a common site. There is typically a firm swelling which grows noticeably in a few months and becomes painful (Fig. 9.15). Teeth may be loosened and there may be paraesthesia or loss of sensation in the mental nerve area. Metastases to the lungs may develop early.

Fig. 9.16 Osteosarcoma. Radiograph of the jaw removed from the patient seen in Figure 9.15 shows the irregular bone destruction and pattern of new bone formation which replaces the normal structure.

Radiographically, appearances are variable but irregular bone destruction usually predominates over bone formation. Bone formation in a soft-tissue mass is highly characteristic (Fig. 9.16). A sun-ray appearance or Codman's triangles at the margins, due to lifting of the periosteum and new bone formation, are rarely seen and not specific to osteosarcoma. Radiographs of the chest should also be taken, as secondary deposits may be present.

Genetics

The most frequent known causative mutations in osteosarcoma are in the retinoblastoma gene RB1. Osteosarcoma arising in Paget's disease is associated with different causative mutations. There are also genetic syndromes that predispose to osteosarcoma so that mutation or loss of several genes may be able to induce this malignancy.

Fig. 9.17   Osteosarcoma. Trabeculae of abnormal woven bone surrounded by atypical cells in which mitoses are frequent and pleomorphism is conspicuous.

Fig. 9.18   Osteosarcoma. A post-mortem specimen of lung from the same patient shown in Figure 9.15. Malignant cells infiltrate the alveoli and are forming woven bone (left).

Pathology

The neoplastic osteoblasts vary in size and shape, they may be small and angular or large and hyperchromatic (Fig. 9.17). Mitoses may be seen, particularly in the more highly cellular areas. Giant cells may be conspicuous, but many cells are non-descript. Bone formation does not necessarily predominate and osteoid formation is the main diagnostic criterion and is seen in metastases (Fig. 9.18). Cartilage and fibrous tissue are usually

also present and sometimes predominate but usually only in part of the tumour. A small biopsy may, therefore, show only a single tissue, such as cartilage, and be mistaken for a chondrosarcoma.

Key features are summarised in Box 9.5.

Box 9.5   Osteosarcoma of the jaws: key features
• Rare
• Patients' mean age is about 35
• Occasionally follows irradiation
• Usually affects the mandible
• Radiographically, bone formation is seen in a soft tissue mass
• Treated by radical surgery, sometimes with additional chemotherapy
• Slightly better prognosis than osteosarcoma of the long bones

Management

Osteosarcoma is rapidly invasive and can metastasise early. Treatment is by early mandibulectomy or maxillectomy together with wide excision of any soft-tissue extensions of the tumour. This may be combined with radiotherapy and/or chemotherapy. The prognosis depends mainly on the extent of the tumour at operation and deteriorates with spread to the soft tissues, to lymph nodes (in about 10% of cases), or to the base of the skull. In approximately 50%, there is local recurrence within a year of treatment and a sharp deterioration in prognosis. The 5-year survival rate may range from 40% for tumours less than 5 cm in diameter to zero for tumours over 15 cm.

CHONDROMA AND CHONDROSARCOMA →
Summary p. 190

Chondroma of the jaws is rare and chondrosarcoma should always be suspected because the histological features of low-grade chondrosarcomas are bland and they may easily be mis-diagnosed as chondromas. Most head and neck chondromas arise in the maxillary bones or base of skull.

Histologically, chondromas consist of hyaline cartilage, but the cells are irregular in size and distribution. Calcification or ossification may develop.

Management

Excision should include a wide margin of normal tissue, because of the difficulty in distinguishing benign from malignant tumours.

Chondrosarcoma

Chondrosarcomas of the jaws affect adults at an average age of about 45. The anterior maxilla is the site in 60% of cases.

Pain, swelling or loosening of teeth associated with a radiolucent area are typical. The radiolucency can be well or poorly circumscribed, or may appear multilocular. Calcifications are frequently present and may be widespread and dense.

Fig. 9.19 **Chondrosarcoma.** Lobules of abnormal hyaline cartilage are formed in a disorganised fashion by sheets of malignant cells.

Fig. 9.20 **Chondrosarcoma.** Higher power of cartilage with a chondrosarcoma showing the abnormal chondrocytes and disorganised mineralisation.

Pathology

The cartilage in jaw tumours is usually comparatively well formed or, less often, poorly differentiated or myxoid (Fig. 9.19). The chondrocytes are pleomorphic, often binucleate and may show mitotic activity (Fig. 9.20).

Maxillofacial chondrosarcomas are aggressive and local recurrence or persistent tumour is the main cause of death. Lungs or other bones are the usual sites of distant spread, but fewer than 10% of these tumours metastasise.

Chondrosarcomas must be widely excised as early as possible, but this can be difficult in the maxillofacial region. Inadequate excision usually leads to recurrences beyond the original site and deterioration of the prognosis. The response to radiotherapy is usually poor.

Mesenchymal chondrosarcoma is an uncommon but highly malignant variant. It is a highly cellular tumour in which there are only small foci of tissue recognisable as poorly-formed cartilage. It is sometimes very vascular.

EWING'S SARCOMA

Ewing's sarcoma is a member of the peripheral primitive neuroectodermal tumour group. It is rare but, when it affects the head and neck region, has a predilection for the body of the mandible.

Clinically, patients are usually children or young adults. Typical symptoms are bone swelling and often pain, progressing over a period of months. Teeth may loosen and the overlying mucosa ulcerate. Fever, leukocytosis, a raised ESR and anaemia may be associated and indicate a poor prognosis.

Genetics

The genetics of Ewing's sarcoma are complex. Though the disease does not have a familial pattern, a predisposition is inherited on chromosome 22. Cells in almost all tumours have one of several similar characteristic reciprocal translocations, usually t(11;22)(q24;q12), and detecting this is a useful diagnostic test. The translocation fuses two genes (Ewing's sarcoma gene EWS and Fli1) that then produce an abnormal transcription factor responsible for transforming the cells.

Pathology

Ewing's sarcoma cells resemble lymphocytes but are about twice their size and are of neuroectodermal origin. They have a darkly staining nucleus and a rim of cytoplasm, which is typically vacuolated and stains for glycogen. The cells form diffuse sheets or loose lobules, separated by septa. Distant spread is usually to the lungs and other bones. Lymph nodes are occasionally involved.

The initial treatment is chemotherapy followed by wide excision and radiotherapy. Chemotherapy improves the survival but, unfortunately, increases the risk of lymphoid tumours in later life. If the disease is localised, 70% of patients will survive 5 years, but the survival in those with disseminated disease is less than 20%.

MYELOMA

Multiple myeloma is a neoplasm of plasma cells which produce a monoclonal immunoglobulin. It causes multiple foci of bone destruction, bone pain and tenderness. Rarely, a jaw lesion can cause the initial symptoms. Proliferation of myeloma cells in the marrow frequently causes anaemia and sometimes thrombocytopenia. Infections may result from depressed production of normal immunoglobulins. Occasionally, myeloma is detected before symptoms appear, by the chance finding, in a routine examination, of a greatly raised ESR as a result of overproduction of immunoglobulin – usually IgG.

Genetics

Myeloma arises by one of several mechanisms involving chromosomal translocations. These bring together one of a variety of oncogenes, often the cell cycle regulator cyclin D1, with genes for immunoglobulins, both transforming the cell and inducing the excessive immunoglobulin synthesis. Multiple myeloma occasionally affects two or more members of a family.

Pathology

Myeloma appears as sheets of neoplastic plasma cells that may be well or poorly differentiated (Fig. 9.21). Because the cells are monoclonal they secrete only one type of immunoglobulin light chain, either kappa or lambda and this is helpful in diagnosis (Fig. 9.22). Diagnosis depends on marrow biopsy and confirmation by serum electrophoresis showing a monoclonal band (Fig. 9.23). Light chain overproduction is common and leads to Bence-Jones proteinuria and often amyloidosis.

Fig. 9.21 **Multiple myeloma.** The lesion is composed of a uniform and dense infiltrate of neoplastic plasma cells with darker than normal staining nuclei.

Fig. 9.22 **Multiple myeloma.** Immunocytochemistry for λ light chain results in a brown positive stain in all cells, indicating a monoclonal and therefore neoplastic proliferation of plasma cells.

Dental aspects

A myelomatous deposit in the jaws or amyloid deposition (see below) in the oral soft tissues can be the first manifestation of the disease. A deposit in the jaw appears as a painful, punched-out area of radiolucency and rarely can cause a pathological fracture. A solitary plasmacytoma can also form a mass in jaws (see below). Bleeding or purpura due to thrombocytopenia, anaemia or infections may also complicate treatment. Bisphosphonate jaw necrosis is increasingly seen as a complication of treatment.

Treatment

Occasionally, the effects of hypergammaglobulinaemia are noticed by chance in a routine blood examination; treatment at this stage is more likely to be successful but, in any case, bone lesions may not appear until years later.

Initially, all patients will be treated with melphalan or combination chemotherapy including steroids and there is frequently a good initial response. Remission is maintained and prolonged with drugs such as interferon, thalidomide or lanilidomide. However, thalidomide frequently causes deep vein thromboses, rashes, bradycardia or neuropathy. During remission, the patient's own bone marrow may be harvested. Relapse can then be treated by high-dose chemotherapy or radiotherapy followed by bone marrow transplant, using autologous marrow or peripheral blood stem cells. There is no cure but patients fit enough for aggressive treatment may live many years during which there may be relapses and remissions.

Spread to bone marrow is common and localised lesions may be treated with radiotherapy or occasionally surgery. When bone metastases are widespread or symptomatic they may be treated

Fig. 9.23 Immunoelectrophoresis comparing patient's (P) and control (C) serum for their content of κ and λ (L) lightchains. The patient has a raised level of κ light chain.

with bisphosphonates to reduce bone resorption, reduce bone pain and hypercalcaemia and prevent fractures and collapse of vertebrae. High-potency bisphosphonates given intravenously include pamidronate and zoledronic acid and this treatment carries a risk of bisphosphonate-induced jaw necrosis (see Ch. 6).

SOLITARY (EXTRAMEDULLARY) PLASMACYTOMA

Approximately 80% of these rare tumours form in the soft tissues of the head and neck region. Multiple myeloma develops in up to 50% of patients within 2 years.

Solitary plasmacytoma of bone occasionally affects the jaw. Bone pain, tenderness, or a swelling and a sharply defined area of radiolucency are typical. Treatment is by radiotherapy. The prognosis is significantly better than for soft-tissue plasmacytoma. Over 65% of patients survive for 10 or more years, but the majority eventually develop multiple myeloma.

Histologically, the appearances of solitary and multiple myeloma are the same.

Key features are summarised in Box 9.6.

Box 9.6   Multiple myeloma: key features

- Myeloma is a malignant bone-seeking neoplasm of plasma cells
- Radiographically, punched-out lesions appear particularly in the skull
- Similar lesions may appear in the jaws
- Malignant plasma cells show varying degrees of dedifferentiation
- Monoclonal immunoglobulin (usually IgG) produced
- Anaemia, purpura or immunodeficiency may be associated
- Light chain production can lead to amyloidosis causing macroglossia in 20%
- Short-term benefit only from combination chemotherapy
- Solitary (soft tissue or intraosseous) myelomas rare but may affect maxillofacial region. They progress to multiple myeloma

---

Amyloidosis

Amyloidosis is a typical product of myeloma and is the deposition in the tissues of an abnormal protein with characteristic staining properties. In over 20% of cases of overproduction of immunoglobulin light chains, amyloid is deposited in the mouth, particularly the tongue, to cause macroglossia or localised swellings or both (Figs 9.24 and 9.25) (see Ch. 14).

LANGERHANS CELL HISTIOCYTOSIS (HISTIOCYTOSIS X) → Summary p. 135

Langerhans cells are dendritic antigen-presenting cells within epithelia that derive from the bone marrow. In this group of conditions they proliferate and localise in bone, organs and skin. Three main forms are recognised and their features are shown in Table 9.1 but, in practice, this is a continuous spectrum of disease severity.

Fig. 9.24   Amyloidosis. These slightly yellow nodules on the lateral border of an enlarged tongue are characteristic of amyloidosis.

Fig. 9.25   Amyloid deposited in tongue mucosa. (A) The H&E-stained section shows a broad band of amorphous tissue between the epithelium and underlying muscle (1). This stains bright red with eosin where it is densest (2). (B) Congo Red stain also stains the densest deposits red. (C) When the Congo Red section is viewed under polarized light, the amyloid shows green birefringence.

Table 9.1 Presentations of Langerhans cell histiocytosis

Classification	Presentation	Features
Chronic unifocal form	Solitary eosinophilic granuloma	Adults, usually bones (80%+), lymph nodes or lungs affected
Chronic multifocal form	Multifocal eosinophilic granuloma (including Hand–Schuller–Christian disease)	Young adults and adolescents. Single system involvement but multiple lesions, usually in skull, skin, nodes, brain, liver
Acute disseminated form	Letterer–Siwe disease	Young children and infants. Multiple organ systems and bone

Key features of oral lesions are summarised in Box 9.7.

Box 9.7 Langerhans cell histiocytosis: oral lesions

- Isolated or multifocal tumours of Langerhans cells
- Eosinophilic granulomas form sharply demarcated radiolucencies
- Alveolar bone around teeth may be destroyed (teeth floating in air appearance)
- May also mimic juvenile periodontitis radiographically
- Diagnosis is by biopsy
- Solitary lesions respond to curettage or resection

The cause is unknown though viral infection has long been suspected. It is possible that the trigger may affect other cells such as lymphocytes and that the Langerhans cell proliferation reflects an abnormal immune regulation. Although it is not considered neoplastic, the condition is clonal; all lesional cells are derived from a single precursor.

In all these tumours, diagnosis may be confirmed by immunocytochemistry for the CD1a surface marker on Langerhans cells or by demonstrating the characteristic cytoplasmic Birbeck granules by electron microscopy.

Oral involvement is present in approximately 10% in both children and adults and the mandible is affected in nearly 75%, either alone or in polyostotic disease. Other perioral sites of involvement are the cervical lymph nodes which can become enlarged either in isolation, in association with restricted bone lesions or more frequently with multisystem disease. Cervical lymphadenopathy can sometimes be massive. Langerhans cell histiocytosis restricted to the oral mucosa is extremely rare.

Overall, the behaviour of Langerhans cell histiocytosis is unpredictable, but the younger the patient and the greater the number of organ systems affected, the worse the prognosis.

Solitary eosinophilic granuloma

Solitary eosinophilic granuloma of the jaw causes localised bone destruction with swelling and often pain (Fig. 9.26).

Fig. 9.26 **Langerhans cell histiocytosis.** This localised lesion (eosinophilic granuloma) has produced an ulcerated mass on the maxillary alveolar ridge. The clinical appearances are non-specific.

Fig. 9.27 **Langerhans cell histiocytosis.** This localised lesion (eosinophilic granuloma) shows the characteristic appearance of a well-defined radiolucency scooped out of the alveolar bone. The margin is corticated in places, but less well-defined elsewhere.

Occasionally, gross periodontal destruction exposes the roots of the teeth. A rounded area of radiolucency with indistinct margins (Fig. 9.27) and an appearance of teeth 'floating in air' are typical. Adults are mainly affected and the lesion is most frequently in the mandible.

Pathology

There are varying proportions of histiocyte-like Langerhans cells and eosinophils, sometimes with other types of granulocytes (Fig. 9.28). The Langerhans cells have pale, vesiculated and often lobulated nuclei and weakly eosinophilic cytoplasm (Fig. 9.29). For diagnosis, positive staining of Langerhans cells for S-100 protein and CD1a antigen and Birbeck granules seen by electron microscopy are confirmatory. Biopsy is required for diagnosis.

The response to curettage is usually good and spontaneous regression is also possible.

Fig. 9.28   Langerhans cell histiocytosis. Clusters of eosinophils in a background of paler-staining Langerhans cells.

Fig. 9.29   Langerhans cell histiocytosis. Higher power showing the pale-staining Langerhans cells with their characteristic folded, bilobed (coffee bean) nuclei.

Multifocal eosinophilic granuloma

Usually the skull, axial skeleton and femora, and also sometimes the viscera (hepatosplenomegaly) or the skin may be involved. When the skull is affected, there are multiple lesions in the jaws and base of skull and a minority of patients present with the Hand–Schuller–Christian triad of exophthalmos, diabetes insipidus and lytic skull lesions. The histological features are the same as eosinophilic granuloma.

Letterer–Siwe syndrome

This aggressive form of histiocytosis affects infants or young children and behaves like a lymphoma of Langerhans cells. Progression to widespread disease, with involvement of skin, viscera and bones, can be rapidly fatal, despite treatment by irradiation and/or chemotherapy.

Management

The natural history ranges from isolated lesions with spontaneous regression, to widespread disease and a rapidly fatal outcome despite treatment, particularly in the very young.

Spontaneous regression is most likely in single-system disease in jaws and other sites. Under the circumstances, surgical excision of uncomplicated eosinophilic granuloma of the jaws should probably be avoided provided that the diagnosis has been confirmed by biopsy. However, follow-up should be prolonged.

In those over 2 years, the mortality is probably about 15%, but in younger infants the mortality may be 50%. Monocytosis or thrombocytopenia are also associated with a high mortality.

In addition to biopsy of oral lesions, physical examination, skeletal survey and blood picture are needed to show any dissemination and its degree.

Isolated jaw lesions tend to regress spontaneously over a period of months to years, but usually a more rapid solution is required or intervention is necessary because of pain, pathological fracture or loss of teeth. Curettage usually suffices or biopsy alone may initiate healing. Intralesional injection of corticosteroids may be given as adjunctive treatment and may be safe and effective for monostotic disease. Irradiation may be given if other measures fail. Prolonged follow-up is desirable because of the risk of recurrences.

For multisystem disease, a combination of cytotoxic agents (often vinca alkaloids), corticosteroids and irradiation of active bone lesions is required. Nevertheless, some cases, particularly in young children, are refractory to currently available treatments so that such treatments as marrow transplantation, gene transfer therapy and monoclonal antibodies against the CD1a antigen are under trial. Haematopoietic stem cell transplantation is currently being used.

Thalidomide has also been used and has been effective in some cases of disseminated disease.

LYMPHOMAS

As discussed later, lymphomas of the oral soft tissues are uncommon except in association with HIV infection. They are also a serious complication of Sjögren's syndrome (Ch. 18). Primary lymphomas of bone are rare (see Ch. 22).

METASTATIC TUMOURS → Summaries pp. 136, 190

Blood-borne metastasis from carcinoma of various organs (Box 9.8) is common particularly in late disease.

Rarely, a malignant deposit in the jaw causes the first symptoms and can lead to diagnosis of the primary. More often, the

---

Box 9.8   The commonest primary sites for malignant neoplasms that metastasise to the jaws

- Breast
- Bronchus
- Prostate
- Thyroid
- Kidney

Fig. 9.30 **Metastatic carcinoma of the mandible.** Swelling developed in the ramus quite suddenly in this apparently fit patient. Investigations showed a deposit of poorly differentiated carcinoma in the jaw and signs of a bronchial carcinoma.

Fig. 9.31 **Metastatic bronchogenic carcinoma.** This small metastasis in the alveolar bone has produced a poorly demarcated, patchy radiolucency and destroyed the lamina dura around a root apex. Such small lesions have been mistaken for periapical granulomas radiographically.

Fig. 9.32 **Metastatic carcinoma in the mandible.** A large and poorly defined radiolucent metastasis has destroyed most of the posterior body of the mandible, resulting in a pathological fracture.

Fig. 9.33 **Metastatic carcinoma in the jaw.** Section across a mandible shows a deposit of carcinoma which has destroyed the cortex of the bone.

neoplasm has been treated earlier. In either case, a metastasis in the jaw indicates life-threatening disease. Patients are usually middle-aged or elderly.

Common symptoms are pain or swelling of the jaw (Fig. 9.30) and there may be paraesthesia or anaesthesia of the lip. There is typically an area of radiolucency with a hazy outline (Figs 9.31 and 9.32). It sometimes simulates an infected cyst or may be quite irregular and simulate osteomyelitis.

Sometimes the entire mandible may have a moth-eaten appearance. Bone sclerosis is a typical result of prostatic carcinoma.

Pathology

Secondary deposits are usually adenocarcinomas but depend on the nature of the primary growth. Osteoclastic bone destruction at the periphery of the deposit is the most common effect (Fig. 9.33). After histological confirmation of the diagnosis, a careful history, especially of previous operations, may be required.

General and blood examinations and a skeletal survey will show the extent of the disease. The primary growth should be treated if still feasible. In most cases, bony metastases imply that palliative treatment is the best that can be achieved though, in the case of hormone-dependent cancers such as prostate or breast, further hormonal treatment may be effective in inducing relatively long remission. Irradiation may sometimes make the lesion in the jaw regress for a time and lessen pain.

SUGGESTED FURTHER READING

Auclair PL, Cuenin P, Kratochvil FJ, Slater LJ, Ellis GL 1988 A clinical and histomorphologic comparison of the central giant cell granuloma and the giant cell tumor. Oral Surg Oral Med Oral Pathol 66:197–208

Barrera-Franco JL,Flores-Flores G, Mosquedo-Taylor A 1993 Mandibular metastasis as the first manifestation of hepatocellular carcinoma: report of a case and review of the literature. J Oral Maxillofac Surg 51:318–321

Bennett J, Thomas G, Evans AW et al 2000 Osteosarcoma of the jaws: a 30-year retrospective review. Oral Surg Oral Med Oral Pathol Oral Radiol Endod 90:323–333

Bunel K, Sindet-Pedersen S 1993 Central hemangioma of the mandible. Oral Surg Oral Med Oral Pathol 75:565–570

Cawson RA, Langdon JD, Eveson JW 1996 Surgical pathology of the mouth and jaws. Wright, Oxford

Cawson RA, Binnie WH, Barrett AW, Wright JM 1998 Lucas's pathology of tumors of the oral tissues. Churchill Livingstone, Edinburgh

Cawson RA, Binnie WH, Barrett AW, Wright JM 2001 Oral disease, 3rd edn. Mosby-Wolfe, London

Dagenais M, Pharoah MJ, Sikorski PA 1992 The radiographic characteristics of histiocytosis X. A study of 29 cases that involve the jaws. Oral Surg Oral Med Oral Pathol 74:230–236

Emile J-F, Wechsler J, Brousse N et al 1995 Langerhans cell histiocytosis. Definitive diagnosis with the use of monoclonal antibody O10 on routinely paraffin-embedded samples. Am J Surg Pathol 19:636–641

Epstein JB, Voss NJS, Stevenson-Moore P 1984 Maxillofacial manifestations of multiple myeloma. An unusual case and review of the literature. Oral Surg Oral Med Oral Pathol 57:267–271

Fartarsch M, Vigneswaran N, Diepgen TL, Hornstein OP 1990 Immunohistochemical and ultrastructural study of histiocytosis X and non-X histiocytoses. J Am Acad Dermatol 23:885–892

Favara BE, Jaffe R 1994 The histopathology of Langerhans' cell histiocytosis. Br J Cancer 70(Suppl. XXIII):S17–S23

Fechner RE, Mills SE 1992 Tumors of the bones and joints. Atlas of tumor pathology. Third series. Fascicle 8. Armed Forces Institute of Pathology, Washington DC

Flick WG, Lawrence FR 1980 Oral amyloidosis as initial symptom of multiple myeloma. Oral Surg Oral Med Oral Pathol 49:18–20

Furutani M, Ohnishi M, Tanaka Y 1994 Mandibular involvement in patients with multiple myeloma. J Oral Maxillofac Surg 52:23–25

Garrington GE, Collett WK 1988 Chondrosarcoma. I. A selected literature review. J Oral Pathol 17:1–11

Garrington GE, Collett WK 1988 Chondrosarcoma. II. Chondrosarcoma of the jaws: analysis of 37 cases. J Oral Pathol 17:12–20

Garrington GE, Scofield HH, Cornyn J, Hooker SP 1967 Osteosarcoma of the jaws. Analysis of 56 cases. Cancer 20:377–391

Hackney FL, Aragon SB, Aufdemorte TB, Holt RG, Sickels JEV 1991 Chondrosarcoma of the jaws: clinical findings, histopathology and treatment. Oral Surg Oral Med Oral Pathol 71:139–143

Harris M 1993 Central giant cell granulomas regress with calcitonin therapy. Br J Oral Maxillofac Surg 31:89–94

Hartman KS 1980 Histiocytosis X. A review of 114 cases with oral involvement. Oral Surg Oral Med Oral Pathol 49:38–54

Hawkins PN 1994 Amyloidosis. Medicine Int 22:76–82

Henry CH, Granite EL, Rafetto LK 1992 Osteochondroma of the mandibular condyle: report of a case and review of the literature. J Oral Maxillofac Surg 50:1102–1108

Hirshberg A, Leibovich P, Buchner A 1994 Metastatic tumors to the jaw bones: analysis of 390 cases. J Oral Pathol Med 23:337–341

Kanazawa H, Shoji A, Yokoe H, Midorikawa S, Takamiya Y 1993 Solitary plasmacytoma of the mandible. Case report and review of the literature. J Cranio Max Fac Surg 21:202–206

Kilpatrick SE, Wenger DE, Gilchrist GS, Shives TC, Woolan PC 1995 Langerhans' cell histiocytosis (Histiocytosis X) of bone. A clinicopathologic analysis of 263 pediatric and adult cases. Cancer 76:2471–2484

Kyle RA 2000 The role of bisphosphonates in multiple myeloma. Ann Intern Med 132:734–736

Lambertenghi-Delilliers G, Bruno E, Cortelezzi A, Fumagalli L, Morosini A 1988 Incidence of jaw lesions in 193 patients with multiple myeloma. Oral Surg Oral Med Oral Pathol 65:533–537

Li X, Tanaka K, Nakatani F et al 2005 Transactivation of cyclin E gene by EWS-Fl1 and antitumor effects of cyclin dependent kinase inhibitor on Ewing's family tumor cells. Int J Cancer 116:385-394

Lieberman PH, Jones CR, Steinman RM et al 1996 Langerhans' cell (eosinophilic) granulomatosis. A clinicopathologic study encompassing 50 years. Am J Surg Pathol 20:519–552

Lucas DR, Unni KK, McLeod RA, O'Connor MI, Sim FH 1994 Osteoblastoma: a clinicopathologic study of 306 cases. Hum Pathol 25:117–134

Millar BG, Browne RM, Flood TR 1990 Juxtacortical osteosarcoma of the jaws. Br J Oral Maxillofac Surg 28:73–79

Mintz GA, Abrams AM, Carlsen GD, Melrose RJ, Fister HW 1981 Primary malignant giant cell tumor of the mandible. Report of a case. Oral Surg Oral Med Oral Pathol 51:164–171

Mosby EL, Lowe MW, Cobb CM, Ennis RL 1992 Melanotic neuroectodermal tumor of infancy: review of the literature and report of a case. J Oral Maxillofac Surg 50:886–894

Ormiston IW, Piette E, Tideman H, Wu PC 1994 Chondrosarcoma of the mandible presenting as periodontal lesions: report of 2 cases. J Cranio Max Fac Surg 22:231–235

Regezi JA, Zarbo RJ, McClatchey KD, Courtney RM, Crissman JD 1987 Osteosarcomas and chondrosarcomas of the jaws: immunohistochemical correlations. Oral Surg Oral Med Oral Pathol 64:302–307

Reinish EI, Raviv M, Srolovitz H, Gornitsky M 1994 Tongue, primary amyloidosis and multiple myeloma. Oral Surg Oral Med Oral Pathol 77:121–125

Tai YT, Li XF, Catley L et al 2005 Immunomodulatory drug lenalidomide (CC-5013, IMiD3) augments anti-CD40 SBN-40-induced cytotoxicity in human multiple myeloma: clinical implications. Cancer Res 65:11712-11720

Thongngarm T, Lynch C, McMurray RW 2000 Primary non-Hodgkin's lymphoma of bone. J Rheumatol 27:2923–2924

Whitaker SB,Waldron CA 1993 Central giant cell lesions of the jaws. A clinical, radiologic and histopathologic study. Oral Surg Oral Med Oral Pathol 75:199–208

Willman CL, Busque L, Griffith BB, Favara BE, McClain KL, Duncan MH et al 1994 Langerhans cell histiocytosis (histiocytosis X) – a clonal proliferative disease. N Engl J Med 331:154–160

Wood RE, Nortje CJ, Hesseling P, Grotepass F 1990 Ewing's tumor of the jaw. Oral Surg Oral Med Oral Pathol 69:120–127

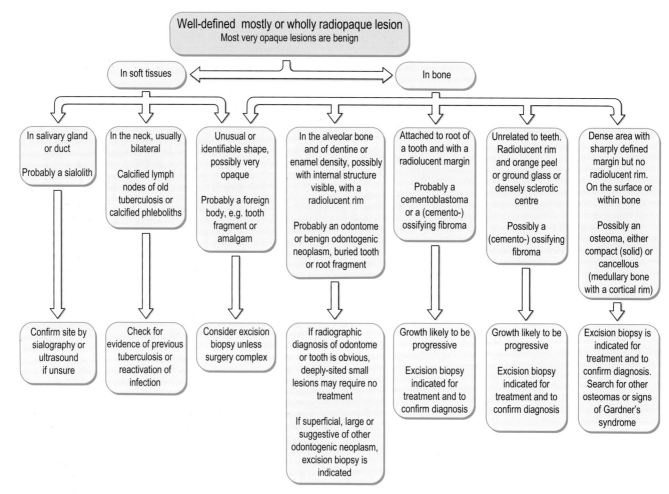

Summary chart 9.1   Differential diagnosis of a well-defined radiopaque lesion in the jaws and soft tissues.

Summary chart 9.2 Differential diagnosis of an ill-defined or diffuse radiographic lesion in the jaws.

Genetic, metabolic and other non-neoplastic bone diseases

GENETIC DISEASES OF BONE

Osteogenesis imperfecta (brittle bone syndrome)

The term brittle bone *syndrome* should not be confused with the considerably more common disease of osteoporosis which is frequently termed brittle bone *disease*. In osteogenesis imperfecta, which is usually transmitted as an autosomal dominant trait, the bones are excessively fragile.

Genetics

The usual causal genes are COL1A1 and COL1A2. The procollagen alpha helix is defective and fails to polymerise into normal type 1 collagen and mineralise. Osteoblasts do not form bone in adequate amounts, leading to fractures. However, there is molecular and clinical diversity and types V, VI and VII disease are caused by other gene defects. Abnormal dentine (dentinogenesis imperfecta) is present, particularly in type III disease, which is associated with the COL1A2 mutation.

The bones are thin and lack the usual cortex of compact bone (Fig. 10.1), but development of epiphyseal cartilages is unimpaired so that bones can grow to their normal length. Nevertheless, they may become grossly distorted by multiple fractures and result in dwarfism. The most severe cases (type II) usually die at birth or soon after: mild cases (type V) may have little disability. In the more common form (type I), the many fractures can cause severe deformity (Figs 10.2 and 10.3). The sclera of the eyes may also appear blue because their thinness

Fig. 10.1   Osteogenesis imperfecta. A section from the vault of the skull of a stillborn infant with type II disease; the most severe form of osteogenesis imperfecta shows that the bone is small in amount, primitive (woven) in character and shows no attempt at differentiation into cortical plates and medullary space.

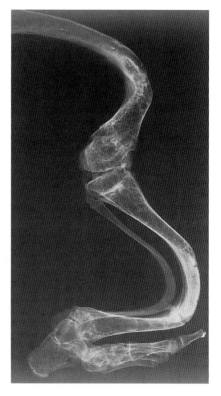

Fig. 10.2   Osteogenesis imperfecta. Leg of an infant with a severe type of osteogenesis imperfecta showing severe bending as a result of multiple fractures under body weight.

allows the pigment layer to show through (Fig. 10.4). Deafness also develops.

Adults with mild osteogenesis imperfecta account for about 25% of fractures in this disease. They also tend to suffer from back and joint pain usually due to osteoarthritis; about 60% have joint hypermobility but otherwise, the majority have good health.

Fig. 10.3 Clinical appearance of a severely affected child with osteogenesis imperfecta type III in which there is progressive deformity.

Fig. 10.4 Blue sclera in osteogenesis imperfecta.

Dental aspects

Obvious dentinogenesis imperfecta is sometimes associated, but all patients have some degree of abnormality of the dentine microscopically (see Ch. 2). In types III and IV, the craniofacial form is abnormal as a result of differential growth deficiency and bending of cranial structures. An abnormally ventral position of the sella region is due to bending of the cranial base and a closing mandibular growth rotation. Vertical underdevelopment of dentoalveolar structures and the condylar process are the main reasons for the relative mandibular prognathism.

Management

Success has been claimed for gene therapy using normal stromal marrow cells which can differentiate into a multiplicity of cell types including bone cells. Treatment with a bisphosphonate may be given to improve bone formation (see Ch. 6). No other treatment is effective, in which case all that can be done is to protect the child from even minor injuries and to minimise deformity by attending to fractures. Care must be taken during dental extractions, but fractures of the jaws are uncommon in this disease.

Key features are summarised in Box 10.1.

Box 10.1 Osteogenesis imperfecta: key features

- Thin fragile bones due to inadequate type I collagen formation
- Usually an autosomal dominant trait
- Autosomal recessive types (II, III, IV) – severe fragility
- Multiple fractures typically lead to gross deformities
- Dentinogenesis imperfecta associated especially in type IV
- Jaw fractures are uncommon

Osteopetrosis – marble bone disease

Osteopetrosis is a rare genetic disease in which the bones become solidified and dense (Fig. 10.5), but brittle. There is inactivity of osteoclasts and absence of normal modelling resorption. Medullary spaces are minute (Fig. 10.6) and the epiphyseal ends of the bones are club-shaped. Because of the deficiency of marrow space, the liver and spleen take on blood-cell formation, but anaemia is common and defective white cells can lead to abnormal susceptibility to infection.

Dental aspects

There may be compression of cranial nerve canals so that trigeminal or facial nerve neuropathies can result. Despite its density, bone can be brittle so that the jaw may fracture during extractions. Osteomyelitis is a recognised complication and prevention of dental infections is important. There is no effective treatment apart from marrow transplantation.

Key features are summarised in Box 10.2.

CHAPTER 10

> **Box 10.2   Osteopetrosis: key features**
>
> - Rare genetic defect of osteoclastic activity
> - Bones lack medullary cavities but are fragile
> - Extramedullary haemopoiesis in liver and spleen but anemia common
> - Osteomyelitis a recognised complication
> - Bone marrow transplantation offers the main hope

Achondroplasia

Achondroplasia is the most common type of genetic skeletal disorder and manifests itself as short-limbed individuals who historically became circus dwarfs. The essential defect is inability to form bone from cartilage at the epiphyses and base of the skull. This is due to a homozygous G1138A mutation at the 380 position in the fibroblast growth factor receptor 3 gene. This mutation, also termed G380R, is detectable prenatally to enable the diagnosis of the homozygous mutant type which is lethal in the newborn.

Dental aspects

While the limbs are excessively short in relation to the trunk, the head, which is normal in size, appears disproportionately large. Defective growth at the base of the skull causes the middle third of the face to be retrusive and the profile to be concave. The mandible is often protrusive and, as a result of the disparity of growth of the jaws, there is usually severe malocclusion and sometimes posterior open bite. Associated macroglossia and migratory glossitis have also been described.

There is no effective treatment, but the occlusion may be improved by orthodontic treatment.

Key features are summarised in Box 10.3.

Cleidocranial dysplasia

In this rare familial disorder, there is defective formation of the clavicles, delayed closure of fontanelles and sometimes

Fig. 10.6   Osteopetrosis. Almost solid bone with only small lacunae has replaced the medullary space.

Fig. 10.5   Osteopetrosis. In contrast to osteogenesis imperfecta the bone is excessively thick and dense as a result of defective resorption.

Box 10.3 Achondroplasia: key features

- A common type of genetic dwarfism
- Failure of proliferation of cartilage in epiphyses and base of skull
- Short limbs but normal-sized skull
- Middle third of face retrusive due to deficient growth of skull base
- Malocclusion may need correction

---

retrusion of the maxilla. Partial or complete absence of clavicles allows the patient to bring the shoulders together in front of the chest (Fig. 10.7).

Fig. 10.7 Cleidocranial dysplasia. Defective development of the clavicles allows this abnormal mobility of the shoulders. Other members of the family were also affected.

Dental aspects

Cleidocranial dysplasia is one of the few identifiable causes of delayed eruption of the permanent dentition. Many permanent teeth may remain embedded in the jaw (Fig. 10.8) and frequently become enveloped in dentigerous cysts (see Ch. 7). Bulging frontal, parietal and occipital bones and hypoplastic middle third of the face can produce a bird-face appearance.

Key features are summarised in Box 10.4.

Box 10.4 Cleidocranial dysplasia: key features

- Rare genetic disorder causing defective formation of clavicles, delayed closure of fontanelles and other defects
- Many or most permanent teeth typically remain embedded in the jaw
- Many additional unerupted teeth also present
- Sometimes many dentigerous cysts

Cherubism → Summaries pp. 136, 173

Cherubism causes multiple multilocular bone lesions in the mandible and maxilla that start in childhood, enlarge and then regress.

Cherubism is caused by one of several mutations in the SH3BP2 gene on chromosome 4p and is inherited as an autosomal dominant trait. The gene product is thought to be a signalling molecule but its exact function is unclear.

Though a dominant condition, there may be no family history because of variable expressivity and penetrance. As a result of weaker penetrance of the trait in females, the disease is approximately twice as common in males. Non-familial cases may also be new mutations. Usually, only isolated cases are encountered, but a family with no fewer than 20 affected members has been reported. The disorder may be seen almost worldwide, but appears to be rare in Japan.

Fig. 10.8 Cleidocranial dysplasia. There are many additional teeth but widespread failure of eruption and possibly development of dentigerous cysts.

Fig. 10.9 **Cherubism.** The typical 'cherubic' bulging of the cheeks can be seen.

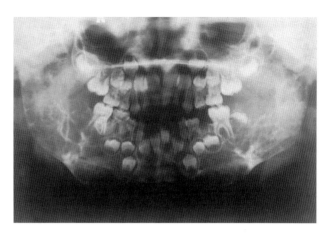

Fig. 10.10 **Cherubism.** Both rami, much of the body of the mandible and the posterior maxillae are expanded by multilocular radiolucent lesions which have displaced and destroyed developing teeth.

The onset is typically between the ages of 6 months to 7 years, but rarely is delayed until late teenage or after puberty. Typically, symmetrical swellings are noticed at the age of 2 to 4 years in the region of the angles of the mandibles and, in severe cases, in the maxillae. The symmetrical mandibular swellings give the face an excessively chubby appearance (Fig. 10.9). The alveolar ridges are expanded and the mandibular swellings may sometimes be so gross lingually as to interfere with speech, swallowing or even breathing, but the rapidity of progress is variable. Teeth are frequently displaced and may be loosened.

Maxillary involvement is usually associated with widespread mandibular disease and is uncommon. Extensive maxillary lesions cause the eyes to appear to be turned heavenward; this together with the plumpness of the face, is the reason for these patients being likened to cherubs. The appearance of the eyes is due to such factors as the maxillary masses pushing the floors of the orbits and eyes upwards and also exposing the sclera below the pupils. Expansion of the maxillae may also cause stretching of the skin and some retraction of the lower lids. Rarely, destruction of the infra-orbital ridges weakens support for the lower lid. Maxillary involvement can also cause the palate to assume an inverted 'V' shape.

Despite lack of inflammation, there is frequently cervical lymphadenopathy, due to reactive hyperplasia and fibrosis. This is typically seen in the early stages and may completely subside by puberty.

Radiographic changes may be seen considerably earlier than clinical signs and are usually more extensive than the clinical swelling. The angles of the mandible are particularly involved, but the process extends towards the coronoid notch and sometimes also forwards along the body (Fig. 10.10). The lesions simulate multilocular cysts as a result of fine bony septa extending between the soft tissue masses. Panoramic radiographs help to determine the extent of the disease, but it is more clearly visualised by CT scanning.

Maxillary involvement is shown by diffuse rarefaction of the bone, but spread of lesions can cause opacity of the sinuses. A distinctive radiographic sign is exposure of the posterior part of the hard palate in lateral skull films, as a result of forward displacement of the teeth. Even after complete clinical resolution of the facial swelling, bone defects may persist radiographically. Growth is rapid for a few years, then slows down until puberty is reached. There is then slow regression until, by adulthood, normal facial contour is typically completely restored. However, radiolucent areas may persist longer. Severe cases may suffer permanent deformity, particularly if bony support for the eye has been destroyed.

Pathology

The lesions consist of multinucleate giant cells (Fig. 10.11) and resemble giant cell granulomas or hyperparathyroidism. With the passage of time, giant cells become fewer and there is bony repair of the defect (Fig. 10.12).

Management

Because of natural regression of the disease, treatment can usually be avoided. If disfigurement is severe the lesions respond to curettage or to paring down of excessive tissue but, in the early stages particularly, will recur.

Key features are summarised in Box 10.5.

Fig. 10.11 **Cherubism.** An early lesion showing multinucleate giant cells lying in haemorrhagic oedematous fibrous tissue. The appearances are indistinguishable histologically from giant cell granuloma.

Fig. 10.12 **Cherubism.** In a late lesion, there is formation of woven bone by the fibrous tissue and giant cells are less numerous. Eventually bone remodelling will restore the contour and quality of the bone.

Box 10.5 **Cherubism: key features**

- Inherited as autosomal dominant trait
- Jaw swellings appear in infancy
- Angle regions of mandible affected symmetrically giving typical chubby face
- Symmetrical involvement of maxillae also in more severe cases
- Radiographically, lesions appear as multilocular cyst-like areas
- Histologically, lesions consist of giant cells in vascular connective tissue
- Lesions regress with skeletal maturation and normal facial contour restored

---

Hypophosphatasia

Hypophosphatasia is an uncommon recessive genetic disorder. The early-onset type causes rickets-like skeletal disease with defective mineralisation. Defective cementogenesis results in premature loss of teeth and this is sometimes the only sign of the disease (see Fig. 2.30). Plasma alkaline phosphatase levels are low, but urinary phosphoethanolamine excretion is raised. Late-onset hypophosphatasia is sometimes a dominant trait and its main manifestation is fragility of the bones.

Sickle cell anaemia and thalassaemia major

Bone changes are uncommon but, when severe, these diseases (see Ch. 25), particularly thalassaemia, can cause bony malformations of the maxillofacial region. In particular, expanded erythropoiesis causes thickening but osteoporosis of the bones of the skull. In sickle cell anaemia, infarcts in the jaws are painful. Symptomatically and radiographically, they can mimic osteomyelitis. Bone infarcts may appear relatively radiolucent at first, but become sclerotic and opaque areas in the skull or jaws are left by earlier infarcts.

In thalassaemia, the diploic spaces of the skull are enlarged due to marrow expansion and have a hair-on-end appearance radiographically and a thin cortex. The maxillae may also be expanded causing severe malocclusion. The zygomatic bones are pushed outwards and the nasal bridge depressed in severe cases.

Hyperparathyroidism–jaw tumour syndrome

This syndrome is an extremely rare autosomal dominant disease. Unlike sporadic hyperparathyroidism (see above), giant cell lesions do not develop.

Instead, cemento-osseous lesions form in the jaws. In addition to the jaw lesions, parathyroid adenomas or carcinomas, renal cysts, renal tumours and uterine tumours may be associated (see Ch. 31).

Management

The main problem is that of the parathyroid and other tumours. Parathyroid adenomas usually respond to surgery, but management of parathyroid carcinoma is more difficult. The prognosis is also affected by the behaviour of associated tumours of the kidneys or uterus.

The jaw lesions usually shell out quite readily, but some have recurred, probably as a result of incomplete excision. Otherwise, they may sometimes regress spontaneously after removal of the parathyroid tumour, though this may take months or even years.

Gigantism and acromegaly

Overproduction of pituitary growth hormone, usually by an adenoma, before the epiphyses fuse, gives rise to gigantism with overgrowth of the whole skeleton. After fusion of the epiphyses, overproduction of growth hormone gives rise to acromegaly. The main features are continued growth at the mandibular condyle, causing gross prognathism, macroglossia, thickening of the facial soft tissues and overgrowth of the hands and feet (see Ch. 31).

Fluorosis

Excessive amounts of fluorides in the drinking water, as in certain parts of Northern India, cause severe mottling of the teeth and also sclerosis of the skeleton. The intervertebral ligaments and muscle insertions calcify, causing stiffness (particularly of the back) and pain. Histologically, the bone changes are somewhat similar to those of Paget's disease.

METABOLIC BONE DISEASE

Rickets

Vitamin D is essential for the absorption and metabolism of calcium and phosphorus. Deficiency during the period of bone development causes rickets with defective calcification and development of the skeleton, but rarely of the teeth (Ch. 30).

Defective calcium and phosphorus metabolism may also result from chronic renal disease (either hereditary or inflammatory) causing abnormal excretion of these minerals. Defective development of bone (renal rickets) can result.

The onset of rickets is usually in infancy. The main defects are broadening of the growing ends of bones and prominent costochondral junctions due to the epiphyseal defects (Fig. 10.13). The weakened bones bend readily. Typical changes in the skulls are wide fontanelles, bossing of the frontal and parietal eminences and thinning of the back of the skull. Radiographs show the wide, thick epiphyses and deformities (Fig. 10.13). There are usually normal serum calcium but low phosphorus levels, or either may be depressed. The alkaline phosphatase level is raised.

Pathology

Throughout the bone, but especially at the ends of the shafts, trabeculae become surrounded by newly formed, uncalcified osteoid matrix. In the zone of provisional calcification, mineralisation of cartilage fails and the cartilage cells continue to proliferate until the epiphyseal plate becomes greatly thickened, wide and highly cellular (Fig. 10.14). Blood vessels invade and branch irregularly among the proliferating cartilage cells. They are accompanied by connective tissue which further disorganises the epiphysis.

Dental aspects

Teeth have priority over the skeleton for minerals and dental defects rarely result from rickets. Hypocalcification of dentine, with a wide band of predentine and excessive interglobular spaces, may be seen in unusually severe rickets. Eruption of teeth may also be delayed in such cases. Rachitic children are not abnormally susceptible to dental caries and 'shortage of calcium' as a cause of dental caries is a myth.

Treatment

Vitamin D, the equivalent of 2000 to 3000 i.u. daily, should be given. The diet should also be adequate in other components. Orthopaedic treatment may be needed to correct deformities.

Vitamin D-resistant rickets

This term is given to familial hypophosphataemia. The skull sutures may be wide but the dental changes are more striking.

Fig. 10.13   Rickets. Overgrowth of cartilage (as shown in the section in Figure 10.14) causes the epiphyseal plate to be broad, thick and irregular, and the ends of the bone become splayed. The growing end of the bone is ill-defined and calcification defective.

Fig. 10.14   Rickets. Microscopically, the epiphyseal plate has become disorganised with loss of the well-drilled lines of chondrocytes. There is also fibrous proliferation, but no calcification.

The pulp chambers are abnormally large and calcification of dentine is defective. Pulpitis, often due to minimal caries, and apparently spontaneous dental abscesses are typical complications. Preventive dental care using fissure sealants and other means is therefore essential.

Scurvy

Scurvy, caused by vitamin C deficiency, leads to defective formation of collagen and osteoid matrix; such matrix as forms is well calcified. Infantile scurvy, with skeletal defects, is largely of historical interest in Britain but has been described, for instance, in an infant whose mother had eccentric ideas about diet. A case with gingival bleeding was described in 2000.

The amount of osteoid matrix formed is small but highly calcified so that the ends of the long bones are sharply defined radiologically. Weakness of the connective tissue and the haemorrhagic tendency (purpura) cause detachment of the periosteum by bleeding and bone pain. The haematoma becomes calcified as shown in the radiograph (Fig. 10.15).

Severe scurvy also causes swollen, bleeding gingivae (see Ch. 5) and early tooth loss (see Ch. 30).

Hyperparathyroidism → Summary p. 173

Primary hyperparathyroidism is usually caused by hyperplasia or adenoma of the parathyroids, but is uncommon. Overproduction of parathormone (PTH) mobilises calcium and raises the plasma calcium level.

Post-menopausal women are mainly affected. The major symptoms result from renal damage which leads to hypertension or other cardiovascular disease. Peptic ulcer symptoms or mere malaise are also common. Bone disease is rarely seen now, because of earlier treatment, but small lesions may be detectable radiographically. Among dental patients a cyst-like swelling of the jaw with the histological features of a giant-cell lesion is the classical way by which hyperparathyroidism has been detected, but is rare. It is essential not to miss this diagnosis, because of the risk of irreversible renal damage in the absence of treatment. The possibility of secondary hyperparathyroidism (see below) should also be excluded.

Radiographically, the main effects are thinning of bone trabeculae, subperiosteal resorption of the bone of the fingers and resorption of the terminal phalangeal tufts. In severe disease, radiolucent cyst-like areas (osteitis fibrosa cystica) often with a multiloculated appearance are a typical but rare finding (Figs 10.16 and 10.17). Alveolar bone may also be resorbed but re-forms with treatment (Figs 10.18 and 10.19).

Pathology

Histologically, the cyst-like areas are foci of osteoclasts in a highly vascular stroma (Fig. 10.20). Extensive haemosiderin deposits cause the lesion to appear as a brown tumour.

These foci are indistinguishable from giant cell granulomas of the jaws. Unlike the latter, there are characteristic changes in blood chemistry (Box 10.6) and sometimes multifocal involvement of other bones. Occasionally, bone lesions cause pathological fractures. The increased excretion of calcium leads ultimately to renal calcinosis or stone formation and renal damage. Other clinical features also result from the hypercalcaemia. Blood chemistry examination is essential in patients found to have giant-cell lesions of the jaws, especially adults of middle age or over.

Fig. 10.15 Scurvy. In contrast to rickets, calcification is unimpeded and there is a thick layer of calcified cartilage at the end of the bone. Osteoid formation, on the other hand, is poor, so that little bone can be formed. The attachment of the periosteum to the bone is weak, so that it is easily separated; haemorrhage beneath it (as here) is due to scorbutic purpura and this becomes calcified.

Fig. 10.16 Hyperparathyroidism. A patient of 51 with hyperparathyroidism as a result of a parathyroid adenoma. There is an area of bone destruction simulating a multilocular cyst.

Fig. 10.17   Hyperparathyroidism. Osteitis fibrosa cystica in the humerus of the same patient with a parathyroid adenoma. Note also the loss of trabecular pattern and cortex.

Fig. 10.18   Hyperparathyroidism. A periapical view reveals the relative radiolucency of the bone. There is loss of lamina dura around the roots, loss of trabeculae centrally and coarsening of the trabecular pattern elsewhere.

Box 10.6   Biochemical findings in primary hyperparathyroidism

- Raised plasma calcium (2.8 mmol/l or more)
- Low plasma phosphorus (less than 0.8 mmol/l)
- Raised plasma parathyroid hormone levels
- Raised plasma alkaline phosphatase (over 100 IU/l)

Secondary hyperparathyroidism results from prolonged stimulation of the parathyroids by a persistently depressed plasma

Fig. 10.19   Hyperparathyroidism. The same patient after treatment shows improved bone density and reformation of the lamina dura and cortex.

Fig. 10.20   Hyperparathyroidism. Multinucleate osteoclast-like giant cells are lying in a haemorrhagic fibrous tissue. The appearances are indistinguishable from giant cell granuloma histologically.

calcium. The most common cause is chronic renal failure.

Secondary hyperparathyroidism is now a more frequent cause of osteolytic bone lesions than primary, but shows the same histological picture of osteoclastic proliferation. Such lesions may also be a sign of rejection of a renal transplant (Fig. 10.21).

Hyperparathyroidism is also present in 95% of patients with type 1 multiple endocrine adenoma (MEN 1) syndrome as discussed in Chapter 31.

Management

In primary hyperparathyroidism, surgical removal of the parathyroids is curative. For secondary hyperparathyroidism, the renal failure should be treated if possible. Bone lesions may respond to oral administration of vitamin D, whose metabolism is abnormal as a result of the renal disease. If hypercalcaemia is very longstanding, parathyroid hyperplasia may be

Fig. 10.21 **Hyperparathyroidism.** In this patient with hyperparathyroidism as a result of rejection of a kidney graft, there is a well-defined area of bone loss.

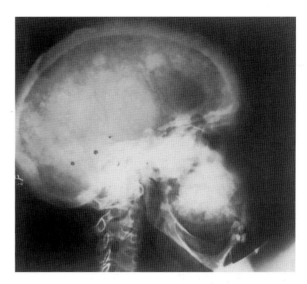

Fig. 10.22 **Paget's disease of the skull and maxilla.** The thickening of the bone and the irregular areas of sclerosis and resorption, which give it a fluffy appearance, are in striking contrast to the unaffected mandible.

irreversible (so-called tertiary hyperparathyroidism) and need to be treated by parathyroidectomy.

Key features are summarised in Box 10.7.

> **Box 10.7** **Hyperparathyroidism: key features**
>
> - Overproduction of parathyroid hormone due to hyperplasia or adenoma of parathyroid glands leads to mobilisation of bone calcium
> - Significant bone disease now uncommon
> - Common effects are malaise, hypertension or peptic ulcer
> - Jaw lesions are rare, but appear radiographically as multilocular cyst-like areas sometimes with multifocal involvement of other bones
> - Histologically, bone lesions consist of vascular foci of giant cells, indistinguishable from giant cell granulomas
> - Diagnosis confirmed by raised serum calcium, parathyroid hormone and alkaline phosphatase but low serum phosphorus

---

OTHER BONE DISEASES

Paget's disease of bone (osteitis deformans) →
Summaries pp. 173, 190

Paget's disease causes bone distortion and weakening, particularly in the elderly. Patients past middle age are affected most severely. In Britain, up to 3% of people over 40 may have radiographic signs of Paget's disease, but clinical disease is less common.

Intranuclear inclusions compatible with a paramyxo- or other virus have been demonstrated in both osteoblasts and osteoclasts and a viral cause appears possible. However, there may be multiple causes. Mutations in the TNFRSF11A gene

on chromosome 18q and the SQSTM1 gene on chromosome 5q can both cause Paget's disease. The former encodes the RANK protein, which is required for osteoclast formation, and the latter interferes with another component of the same pathway. There are also familial and juvenile forms and several other genes are implicated.

Clinically, bones most frequently affected are sacrum, spine, skull, femora and pelvis. The disease may be widespread and is usually symmetrical, but sometimes a single bone is affected. In the uncommon severe form, the main features are an enlarged head, thickening of long bones, which bend under stress, and tenderness or aching pain which can be severe and almost intractable.

Pathology

Bone resorption and replacement becomes rapid, irregular, exaggerated and purposeless. The changes progress erratically, but the ultimate result is thickening of affected bones without localised swellings. In the early stages, there is typically resorption which is later followed by sclerosis, but since closely adjacent parts of the bone may show different stages of the disease, a common result is patchy areas of osteoporosis and of sclerosis (Figs 10.22 and 10.23).

Destruction and new bone formation may alternate rapidly and the change in bony activity is marked histologically by blue-staining reversal lines. Their irregular pattern characteristically produces a jigsaw puzzle ('mosaic') appearance in the bone (Figs 10.24 and 10.25).

The main histological changes are the irregular pattern of reversal lines, many osteoblasts and osteoclasts, the latter are abnormally large and with more nuclei than normal. There is also fibrosis of the marrow spaces and increased vascularity.

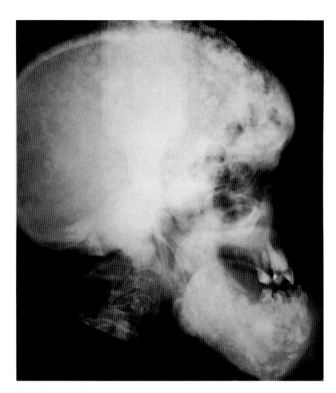

Fig. 10.23   Paget's disease. A very severely affected individual with extensive sclerosis and enlargement of all skull bones and jaws including, unusually, the mandible.

Fig. 10.24   Paget's disease of bone. There is a well-marked irregular ('mosaic') pattern of reversal lines due to repeated alternation of resorption and apposition. The marrow has been replaced by fibrous tissue; many osteoblasts and osteoclasts line the surface of the bone.

Fig. 10.25   Paget's disease affecting the jaw results in destruction of the lamina dura surrounding the teeth and, at a later stage, causes hypercementosis and sometimes ankylosis.

In the late stages, affected bones are thick, the cortex and medulla are obliterated and the whole bone is spongy in texture.

Serum calcium and phosphorus levels are usually normal, but the alkaline phosphatase level is particularly high and may reach 700 iu/l. The development of osteosarcoma is a recognised but rare complication of Paget's disease and rarely affects the jaws. Many patients live to an advanced age in spite of their disabilities.

Dental aspects

The vault of the skull is more frequently affected than the facial skeleton and the maxilla considerably more frequently than the mandible (see Fig. 10.22). Narrowing of foramina can occasionally cause cranial nerve deficits.

When the jaws are affected, the alveolar process becomes symmetrically and grossly enlarged (Figs 10.26 and 10.27). There may also be gross and irregular hypercementosis of teeth, which may become fused to sclerotic areas of the bone. Attempts to extract affected teeth may succeed only by tearing away a large mass of bone. Severe bleeding or osteomyelitis of ischaemic bone may follow.

The main radiographic features are lower density of the bone in the early stages and sclerosis in the later stages. Changes are patchily distributed and loss of normal trabeculation causes the bone to have a characteristic cotton-wool appearance. In affected skulls, pagetic bone lacunae are separated from normal bone by a lucent rim detectable in both conventional radiographs and CT scans.

Treatment is with calcitonin or bisphosphonates, or both. Calcitonins, such as salcatonin, have to be given by injection

Fig. 10.26   Paget's disease of bone. Characteristic features of the involved maxilla are the broadening and deepening of the alveolar process, generalised enlargement and spacing of the teeth.

Fig. 10.27   Paget's disease. A rare example of severe mandibular involvement.

and are more effective for reducing bone pain and osteolysis, but can cause nausea and an unpleasant taste. Calcitonin is also given preoperatively to reduce bleeding from the highly vascular bone and may help to relieve cranial nerve deficits. Bisphosphonates (such as sodium etidronate) can be given orally and depress bone turnover by slowing both the dissolution and growth of hydroxyapatite crystals. Osteonecrosis sometimes results from use of oral bisphosphonates, though occasional cases have been reported (see Ch. 6).

Risedronate is used particularly for Paget's disease in postmenopausal women. Associated adverse effects include facial oedema or, less frequently, Stevens–Johnson syndroma, swollen tongue, palpitations and episcleritis.

An uncommon complication is development of osteosarcoma which has a poor prognosis so that in a large series the survival rate was only 14% after 2.5 years. Osteosarcomatous change in the jaws is rare in comparison with other bones but does develop occasionally.

Key features are summarised in Box 10.8.

Box 10.8   Paget's disease: key features

- Persons past middle age affected
- Common radiographic finding. Less common as clinical disease
- Enlargement of skull, thickening but weakness of long bones and bone pain are typical of severe disease
- Maxilla occasionally, but mandible rarely affected
- Teeth may show gross irregular hypercementosis
- Radiographically, patchy sclerosis and resorption give a cotton-wool appearance
- Histologically, irregular resorption and apposition leaves jigsaw puzzle ('mosaic') pattern of reversal lines
- Serum alkaline phosphatase up to 700 u/l

FIBRO-OSSEOUS LESIONS

A fibro-osseous lesion is one in which bone is replaced by cellular fibrous tissue, which gradually matures with the formation of woven bone, lamellar bone or very dense amorphous mineralisation.

The group includes disorders ranging from fibrous dysplasia to the circumscribed lesions of cemento-ossifying fibroma and the cemental dysplasias (Box 10.9). Cherubism is sometimes included but has been described earlier. Behaviour varies but growth in early life with spontaneous arrest and increasing ossification, roughly coinciding with skeletal maturation, is typical of non-neoplastic fibro-osseous lesions. Neoplastic lesions show progressive growth. Because of their histological similarities, the diagnosis depends greatly on the clinical and radiographic findings.

Box 10.9   Fibro-osseous lesions

Fibrous dysplasia
- Monostotic
- Polyostotic

Cemento-osseous dysplasias (Ch. 8)
- Periapical cemental dysplasia
- Focal cemento-osseous dysplasia
- Florid cemento-osseous dysplasia

Fibro-osseous neoplasms
- Cemento-ossifying fibroma (Ch. 8)

Fibrous dysplasia → Summary p. 173

Fibrous dysplasia is caused by mutation in the GNAS1 gene, which encodes a G protein signalling molecule. The mutation activates the affected cell. Mutation is not inherited but somatic and occurs early in development so that patients are mosaics for the mutation, with both normal and affected cells. If the gene is mutated very early, many affected daughter cells are present in different organs and Albright's syndrome results. Later mutation generates fewer abnormal daughter cells, mostly osteoblasts, and polyostotic disease develops. A later mutation affects osteoblasts in only a single bone.

Monostotic fibrous dysplasia → Summary p. 173

Monostotic fibrous dysplasia is the commonest form, six times commoner than the polyostotic form. It gives rise to a bony swelling caused by a poorly circumscribed area of fibro-osseous proliferation. This typically starts in childhood but usually undergoes arrest in early adulthood. The jaws are the most frequent sites in the head and neck region and a common site overall. Males and females are almost equally frequently affected.

When the jaws are involved, a painless, smoothly rounded swelling, usually of the maxilla, is typical (Fig. 10.28). Initially, the teeth are aligned but, if the mass becomes large, it will

disturb function and cause malocclusion by displacing teeth. Lesions affecting the maxilla may spread to involve contiguous skull bones causing deformity of the orbit, base of skull and cranial nerve lesions (craniofacial fibrous dysplasia).

Radiographically, the features depend on the stage. Early lesions are patchy radiolucencies but develop into weak radiopacities, with a ground glass or fine orange-peel texture as the lesion mineralises. The degree of radiopacity increases and late lesions are sclerotic and lack the trabecular pattern of normal bone. Sometimes a fingerprint pattern of coarse trabeculae may be seen. The cortex and lamina dura are affected by the process and their definition is lost radiographically. The cortex is expanded but thin and barely discernable during growth (Fig. 10.29). The key features are that the margins merge imperceptibly with the surrounding normal bone and that there is always expansion (Fig. 10.30).

Pathology

The lesions consist of loose cellular fibrous tissue containing slender trabeculae of woven bone of variable shape which

Fig. 10.28 **Fibrous dysplasia.** Typical presentation with a poorly-defined, rounded expansion of the maxilla with no displacement of teeth and intact overlying mucosa.

Fig. 10.29 **Fibrous dysplasia.** This well-established lesion with a rounded swelling merges imperceptibly with normal bone surrounding the canine. There is loss of lamina dura and cortex in the affected area and the fine trabecular pattern produces an orange-peel or thumb-print appearance.

Fig. 10.30 **Fibrous dysplasia affecting the left mandible with a patchy radiolucency.** No lesion border can be identified.

merge imperceptibly into surrounding normal bone (Figs 10.31 and 10.32).

Osteoblasts are scattered throughout the substance of the trabeculae rather than surrounding them. The bone remains woven in type for many years and lamellar bone is seen only in old inactive lesions. Some calcified spherules and occasional loose foci of giant cells can also be seen.

Biopsy is required to confirm a fibro-osseous lesion, but cannot distinguish fibrous dysplasia from other fibro-osseous lesions with certainty. Identification of the GNAS1 mutation by DNA sequencing of cells from the lesion is diagnostic.

Fig. 10.31 **Fibrous dysplasia.** Slender trabeculae of woven bone, said to resemble Chinese characters in shape, lying in a very cellular fibrous tissue. With maturation there is progressively more bone formation.

Fig. 10.32 **Fibrous dysplasia.** There is loss of lamina dura around the teeth and its replacement by lesional bone. These numerous small trabeculae give rise to the ground-glass and orange-peel appearances radiographically.

Treatment

The disease is self-limiting, but lesions become quiescent rather than resolve and can reactivate in later life. The lesion is not demarcated and cannot be excised. Disfiguring lesions may be pared down to a normal contour, but this should be delayed until the process has become inactive, usually around the end of the second decade. Surgery to active or recently active lesions risks reactivation and rapid growth. There is a small risk of sarcomatous change.

Key features are summarised in Box 10.10.

> **Box 10.10** **Monostotic fibrous dysplasia: key features**
>
> - Persons under 20 years mainly affected
> - Localised swelling usually of maxilla
> - Radiographically, normal bone trabeculation replaced by ground glass or orange-peel pattern
> - Lesions merge imperceptibly with normal bone at the margins
> - Histologically, normal bone replaced by fibrous connective tissue containing slender trabeculae of bone
> - Usually becomes inactive with skeletal maturation

Polyostotic fibrous dysplasia → Summary p. 173

Polyostotic fibrous dysplasia is rare and, unlike the monostotic form, females are affected three times more frequently than males.

Polyostotic fibrous dysplasia involves the head and neck region in up to 50% of cases. A jaw lesion may then be the most conspicuous feature and polyostotic disease may not be suspected initially. In a young girl in particular, investigation for other skeletal lesions and pigmentation is indicated.

Histologically and radiographically, the individual lesions are indistinguishable from the monostotic form.

Albright's syndrome

Albright's syndrome comprises polyostotic fibrous dysplasia, skin pigmentation and endocrine abnormalities. Endocrine dysfunction is usually manifest as precocious puberty, but other thyroid, pituitary and adrenal anomalies may develop, including malignant neoplasms.

Skin pigmentation consists of brownish macules with irregular outlines that frequently overlie affected bones and appear especially on the back of the neck, trunk, buttocks, or thighs, but hardly ever on the oral mucosa.

Histologically and radiographically, the individual bone lesions are indistinguishable from the monostotic form.

Cemento-osseous dysplasias → Summary p. 190

These are of periodontal ligament origin and are discussed in Chapter 8. The histological appearances are similar but they differ mainly in their extent and radiographic appearances.

Solitary bone 'cyst' (solitary bone cavity) →

Summaries pp. 135, 136

Solitary bone cysts are mostly seen in teenagers and uncommon after the age of 25. They form painless swellings or are chance radiographic findings. The lesion is found more commonly in long bones but, when the jaws are affected, they are found almost exclusively in the mandible.

Radiographically, these cavities form rounded, radiolucent areas which generally tend to be less sharply defined than odontogenic cysts and have two unusual features. First, the area of radiolucency is typically much larger than the size of the swelling suggests. Second, the cavity arches up between the roots of the teeth and may as a consequence be first seen on a bite-wing radiograph (Figs 10.33 and 34).

Fig. 10.33   Solitary bone cyst. Typical appearance showing a moderately well-defined but non-corticated radiolucency extending up between the roots of the teeth.

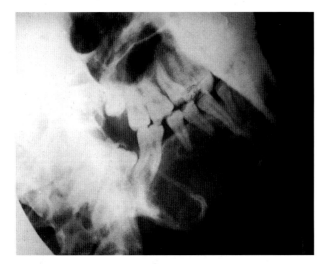

Fig. 10.34   Solitary bone cyst. Oblique lateral view showing a large rounded expansile radiolucent lesion extending from the first premolar to the angle. This cyst is more expansile than usual and shows the variability of presentation of a solitary bone cyst.

Pathology

Solitary bone cysts used to be known as 'haemorrhagic' or 'traumatic' bone cysts and postulated to result from injury to, and haemorrhage within, the bone of the jaw. This was then supposed to be followed by failure of organisation of the clot and of repair of the bone. However, there is little evidence to support this theory. Blood-filled bone cavities form in the jaws as a consequence of enucleation of true cysts, but solitary bone cysts do not arise as a result. Further, a common form of treatment is to open solitary bone cysts to allow bleeding into the cavity. Normal healing then follows. It seems hardly likely that intra-bony haemorrhage can both cause and cure these lesions. Futile speculation about these lesions should not obscure the fact that their cause remains unknown. The cavity has a rough bony wall. There may be a thin connective tissue lining or only a few red cells, blood pigment or giant cells adhering to the bone surface (Fig. 10.35). There are often no cyst contents but there may sometimes be a little fluid. The 'cyst' has no epithelial lining

Key features of solitary bone cysts are summarised in Box 10.11.

Box 10.11   Solitary bone cyst: key features

- Often chance radiographic findings. Rarely expand the jaw
- Are of unknown aetiology
- Have no epithelial lining. Appear empty at operation or contain pale fluid
- Diagnosis suggested by radiographic features (especially extension between tooth roots) and findings at operation
- Histology confirms the lack of epithelial lining
- Resolve after surgical opening and closure, or occasionally spontaneously

---

Management

Solitary bone cysts are not seen in elderly patients and in those that have refused surgery, so that it is apparent that these lesions

Fig. 10.35   Solitary bone cyst. The scanty cyst lining comprises bone and a thin layer of fibrous tissue. Epithelium is not present and in some cases even the fibrous lining is lacking.

resolve spontaneously. It may be necessary, however, to open the cavity, if only to confirm the diagnosis. The characteristic lack of cyst fluid and the unlined bony wall are usually enough to provide a diagnosis, but it is preferable, if possible, to remove any connective tissue lining for histological examination. Opening of the cavity is followed by healing, probably as a result of bleeding. Natural regression, if permitted, seems probable and reparative changes have been seen in excised specimens.

Cysts similar to solitary bone cysts may develop in florid cemento-osseous dysplasia and cause more expansion than typical solitary bone cysts.

Osteoporotic bone marrow defect

This is an anatomical variant rather than a lesion and is included here because it may be misdiagnosed radiographically for solitary bone cyst (Fig. 10.36).

The defect is simply a very large marrow space filled with haemopoetic or fatty marrow. No treatment is required but large and radiographically well-defined examples are often submitted to biopsy for diagnosis.

Aneurysmal bone 'cyst' (cavity) → Summary p. 136

Aneurysmal bone cysts are exceedingly rare in the jaws. Little is known of their pathogenesis and the most likely possibility is that they are vascular malformations.

Clinical features

Most patients are between 10 and 20 years of age and there appears to be no strong predilection for either sex. The mandible

is usually affected. The main manifestation is usually a painless swelling and a radiolucent area, which may be balloon-like or occasionally show a suggestion of trabeculation or loculation.

Key features of aneurysmal bone cysts are summarised in Box 10.12.

Box 10.12   Aneurysmal bone cyst: key features

- Rare in the jaws
- Jaw lesions are usually in the mandibular ramus and angle
- Affect patients usually between 10 and 20 years
- Are of unknown aetiology
- Form very expansile soap-bubble radiolucencies which may be mistaken clinically and radiographically for ameloblastoma or odontogenic keratocyst
- Histologically, consist of a mass of blood-filled spaces with scattered giant cells
- Are treated by curettage but sometimes recur

There is a moderate degree of consensus that aneurysmal bone cyst is a non-neoplastic, fibro-dysplastic lesion. However, clonal chromosomal aberrations and rearrangements have been found and it has recently been suggested that at least some lesions are neoplastic. Fortunately, these considerations do not affect the fact that these are rare lesions which typically respond to simple curettage with only a small risk of recurrence.

Pathology

The aneurysmal bone cyst is in no sense a cyst except in its radiographic appearance. No epithelial lining is present. Histologically, there is a highly cellular mass of blood-filled spaces which has been likened to a blood-filled sponge (Fig. 10.37). The extreme cellularity, mitotic activity and frequent presence of many giant cells may lead to confusion with a sarcoma. It is essential that this mistake should not be made and the patient subjected, as a consequence, to unnecessarily radical and possibly hazardous treatment. Treatment consists of thorough curettage which may need to be repeated, as the lesion occasionally recurs.

Fig. 10.36   Osteoporotic bone marrow defect affecting a typical site. Large lesions with well-defined borders such as this are often subjected to unnecessary biopsy.

Fig. 10.37   Aneurysmal bone cyst. Cyst wall composed of loose fibrous tissue containing occasional giant cells and large blood-filled spaces.

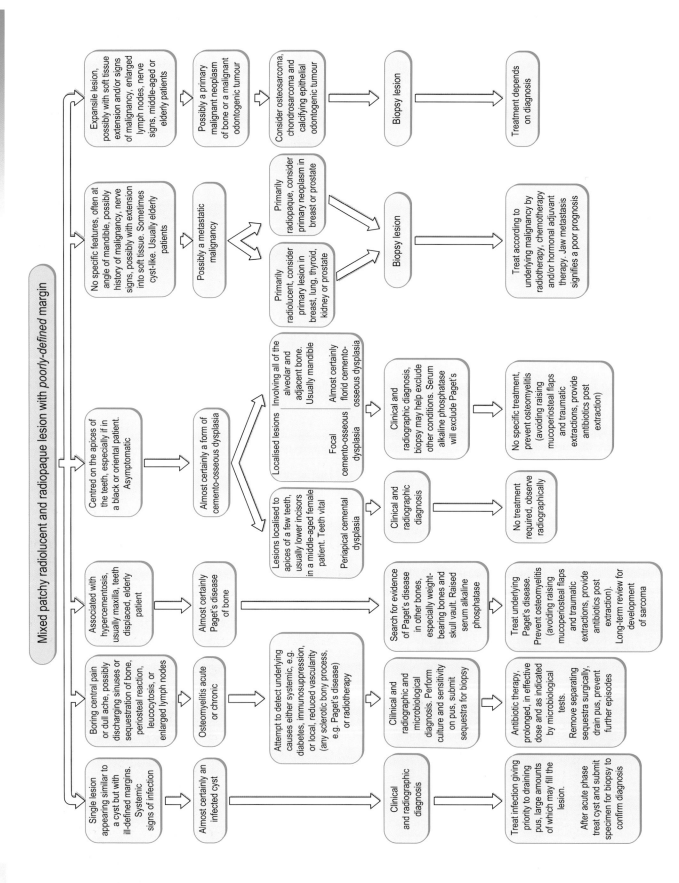

Summary chart 10.1 Mixed patchy radiolucent and radiopaque lesion with poorly defined margin.

Aspects of bone diseases of dental significance are summarised in Box 10.13.

PATHOLOGY OF OSSEOINTEGRATION

Osseointegrated implants have revolutionised dentistry and are also inserted to retain facial prostheses, obturators and bone-conduction hearing aids.

Osseointegration is defined as a direct structural and functional connection between viable bone and the surface of a load-bearing implant. This is possible only using implants made from a limited number of metals, principally titanium, niobium and some of their alloys. The correct implant shape is also necessary to provide maximum surface area and transmit load effectively to the bone.

Successful osseointegration is achieved by bone growing almost to contact the implant. No periodontal membrane is present and the implant is held tightly by friction and a thin layer of collagen and proteoglycan bone matrix about 100 nm thick (Fig. 10.38). The implant surface does not itself induce

Fig. 10.38 Successful osseointegration, bone (unstained right) in contact with implant thread (left). The tiny gap between the two is not appreciated with light microscopy.

bone formation but, in medullary bone, both trabeculae of bone and marrow spaces may contact the implant.

Because there is no periodontal ligament there are no proprioceptive or pain fibres. There is no possibility of implant movement to cushion acute impact or to allow movements to adapt to functional forces. Thus, implants placed in growing jaws submerge like ankylosed teeth or move unpredictably and orthodontic movement is not possible. However, bone trabeculae do remodel around an implant in response to stress transmitted directly to the bone.

Implants penetrate the mucosa without allowing bacteria into the tissues because they develop a periodontal cuff that bears some similarity to the normal gingiva. Again, there are no collagen fibres joining the soft tissue to the implant. Instead, a dense cuff of collagen fibres runs circumferentially around the implant or its abutment. A non-keratininsed junctional epithelium forms against the titanium surface and a gingival sulcus of variable depth may be present. This epithelium is derived from the surrounding mucosa and adheres to the implant through hemidesmosomes in the same way as normal junctional epithelium adheres to tooth.

There are said to be no absolute contraindications to implant placement, but the factors listed in Box 10.14 should be considered potential problems because they are associated with a higher rate of implant failure. The infective endocarditis risk is unknown. Implant placement is a sterile procedure of lower risk than manipulating teeth and, provided the implants are well maintained, the risk of infection is very low.

Failure of implants is defined by progressive bone loss and increasing mobility and usually manifests shortly after placement or initial loading. Increased probing depths are often also present. Failure of integration during the healing period may be caused by movement, such as from that from early loading.

Failure in the longer term is principally from bone loss as a result of excessive loading or peri-implantitis.

Excessive loading may result from bruxism, non-axial forces from poorly designed superstructures or having too few implants to resist normal occlusal forces. Excessive loading tends to cause deep angular bone loss around the implant. The mechanisms are unclear, but may involve microfractures of the superficial bone around the implant. Fracture of the implant itself is rare though components of the superstructure may fail mechanically.

Plaque-induced inflammation and bone loss around implants is called peri-implantitis and the microbial flora and host responses are similar to those in gingivitis and periodontitis. Infrabony pockets do not develop because there are no contact points or interdental papillae to form a local plaque trap. Bone loss is horizontal or forms a broad saucer-shaped defect that affects the entire implant circumference (Fig. 10.39). Peri-implant disease is surprisingly rare.

Fig. 10.39 Peri-implant disease. There is pocketing with a bead of pus exuding onto the gingival margin between the implants and a broad ring of bone loss evident radiographically. These older cylindrical coated implants were prone to peri-implantitis. Courtesy of Prof R Palmer.

Box 10.15   Complications of implant placement

- Incorrect placement
    Perforation of cortex, haematoma, emphysema
    Antral or nasal perforation, sinusitis
    Damage to inferior dental neurovascular bundle
- Infection, acute and chronic
    Consequent alveolar bone loss
- Complications of associated surgery
    Oroantral communication following sinus lift procedures

Other causes of failure are listed in Box 10.15. In addition, implants are more likely to fail in the maxilla than the mandible, if there is movement during healing or if the bone is overheated by the drill during placement.

Occasionally, patients are seen with non-osseointegrated implants such as blade implants or pins of various metals. These older types of implant usually failed rapidly as a result of infection (Fig. 10.40).

Fig. 10.40   Gross infection around old types of implant. There is a subperiosteal implant in contact with almost all the maxillary alveolus. Note the extensive bone loss below it, visible most clearly at the left tuberosity. There are two blade implants in the mandible, both with bone loss extending down the stem to involve the blade. The patient is at risk from severe infection and continued bone destruction until the implants are removed. Courtesy of Prof R Palmer.

SUGGESTED FURTHER READING

Cawson RA, Langdon JD, Eveson JW 1996 Surgical pathology of the mouth and jaws. Wright, Oxford

Cawson RA, Binnie WH, Barrett AW, Wright JM 2001 Oral disease, 3rd edn. Mosby-Wolfe, London

Chindia ML, Ocholla TJ, Imalingat B 1991 Osteopetrosis presenting with paroxysmal trigeminal neuralgia. A case report. Int J Oral Maxillofac Surg 20:199–200

Cornelius EA, McClendon JL 1969 Cherubism – hereditary fibrous dysplasia of the jaw. Roentgenographic features. Am J Roentgenol 106:136–143

Droz-Desprez D, Azou C, Bordigoni P, Bonnaure-Mallet M 1992 Infantile osteopetrosis: a case report on dental findings. J Oral Pathol Med 21:422–425

Ebata K, Usami T, Tohnai I, Kaneda T 1992 Chondrosarcoma and osteosarcoma arising in polyostotic fibrous dysplasia. J Oral Maxillofac Surg 50:761–764

Freemont AJ 1996 The pathology of osteogenesis imperfecta. J Clin Pathol 49:618–619

Frohberg U, Tiner BD 1995 Surgical correction of facial deformities in a patient with cleidocranial dysplasia. J Craniofac Surg 6:49–53

Hitomi G, Nishide N, Mitsui K 1996 Cherubism: diagnostic imaging and review of the literature in Japan. Oral Surg Oral Med Oral Pathol Oral Radiol Endod 81:623–628

Koury ME, Regezi JA, Perrott DH, Kaban LB 1995 'Atypical' fibro-osseous lesions: diagnostic challenges and treatment concepts. Int J Oral Maxillofac Surg 24:162–169

Lala R, Matarazzo P, Bertelloni S et al 2000 Pamidronate treatment of bone fibrous dysplasia in nine children with McCune-Albright syndrome. Acta Paediatr 89:188–193

Mangion J, Rahman N, Edkins S et al 1999 The gene for cherubism maps to chromosome 4p16.3. Am J Hum Genet 65:151–157

Melrose RJ, Abrams AM, Mills BG 1976 Florid osseous dysplasia. A clinicopathologic study of thirty-four cases. Oral Surg Oral Med Oral Pathol 41:62–68

Peters WJN 1979 Cherubism: a study of twenty cases in one family. Oral Surg Oral Med Oral Pathol 47:307–311

Ruggieri P, Sim FH, Bond JR, Unni KK 1994 Malignancies in fibrous dysplasia. Cancer 73:1411–1424

Schneider LC, Mesa ML 1990 Differences between florid osseous dysplasia and chronic diffuse sclerosing osteomyelitis. Oral Surg Oral Med Oral Pathol 70:308–312

Shapiro F 1993 Osteopetrosis. Current clinical considerations. Clin Orthop Rel Res 294:34–44

Summerlin D-J, Tomich OE 1994 Focal cemento-osseous dysplasia: a clinicopathological study of 221 cases. Oral Surg Oral Med Oral Pathol 78:611–620

Talley DB 1952 Familial fibrous dysplasia of the jaws. Oral Surg 5:1012–1019

Tamura Y, Welch DC, Zic JA et al 2000 Scurvy presenting as painful gait with bruising in a young boy. Arch Pediatr Adolesc Med 154:732–735

von Wovern N 2000 Cherubism: a 36 year follow-up of 2 generations in different families and review of the literature. Oral Surg Oral Med Oral Pathol Oral Radiol Endod 90:765–772

Waldron CA 1993 Fibro-osseous lesions of the jaws. J Oral Maxillofac Surg 51:828–835

Williams HK, Mangham C, Speight PM 1999 Juvenile ossifying fibroma. An analysis of eight cases and a comparison with other fibro-osseous lesions. J Oral Pathol Med 29:13–18

Younai F, Eisenbud L, Sciubba JJ 1988 Osteopetrosis: a case report including gross and microscopic findings in the mandible at autopsy. Oral Surg Oral Med Oral Pathol 65:214–221

Disorders of the temporomandibular joints and periarticular tissues

Temporomandibular joint (TMJ) disorders can cause various combinations of limitation of movement of the jaw, pain, locking or clicking sounds. Pain, in particular, is a frequent cause of limitation of movement. These complaints are rarely due to organic disease of the joint and many are due to trauma. However, these functional disorders must be considered in the differential diagnosis. Important causes of limitation of mandibular movement are summarised in Boxes 11.1 and 11.2.

Box 11.1   Causes of limitation of mandibular movement

Intracapsular causes*
- Infective arthritis
- Juvenile arthritis
- Traumatic arthritis and disk damage
- Intracapsular condylar fracture

Pericapsular causes*
- Irradiation and other causes of fibrosis
- Dislocation
- Condylar neck fracture
- Infection and inflammation in adjacent tissues

Muscular
- TMJ dysfunction syndrome
- Myalgia caused by bruxism
- Haematoma from ID block
- Tetanus

Other
- Oral submucous fibrosis
- Systemic sclerosis
- Zygomatic and maxillary fractures
- Drugs
- Craniofacial anomalies involving the joint

*Apart from irradiation, intracapsular and periarticular causes may be acute and reversible or, alternatively, lead to fibrous ankylosis of the joint. Infection and trauma are the most common causes.

Box 11.2   Important causes of intracapsular ankylosis ('true ankylosis')

Trauma
- Intracapsular comminuted fracture of the condyle disorganises the joint. Bleeding may be followed by organisation and bone formation. Early mobilisation of such injuries should prevent bony ankylosis
- Penetrating wounds
- Forceps delivery at birth

Infection
- Otitis media/mastoiditis
- Osteomyelitis of the jaws
- Haematogenous – pyogenic arthritis

Arthritides
- Systemic juvenile arthritis
- Psoriatic arthropathy
- Osteoarthritis (rarely)
- Rheumatoid arthritis (rarely)

Neoplasms
- Chondroma
- Osteochondroma
- Osteoma

Miscellaneous
- Synovial chondromatosis

---

to mean ankylosis. Inability to open the mouth fully is usually temporary and causes are summarised below.

TEMPORARY LIMITATION OF MOVEMENT (TRISMUS)

Infection and inflammation in or near the joint

The main cause is acute pericoronitis with associated muscle spasm. Mumps can also cause transient and unnoticed limitation of movement. Rare causes include suppurative arthritis, osteomyelitis, cellulitis and suppurative parotitis. Submasseteric abscess results in profound trismus and infection in the pterygoid, lateral pharyngeal or submandibular spaces may also cause varying degrees of trismus.

Mandibular block injections may cause inflammation of the muscles around the joint and oedema, either because of

Trismus may be defined as inability to open the mouth due to muscle spasm, but the term is usually used for limited movement of the jaw from any cause and usually refers to temporary limitation of movement. The term *ankylosis* usually refers to persistent limitation of movement and can be either bony or fibrous. However, the term *trismus* is sometimes loosely used irritation by the local anaesthetic or by introduction of infection, but rarely do so.

Injuries

Unilateral condylar neck fracture usually produces only mild limitation of opening with deviation of the jaw to the affected side, but closing into intercuspal occlusion may be difficult. Bilateral displaced condylar fractures cause an anterior open bite with limited movement. Rarely, a fall on the chin can result in unilateral or bilateral dislocation of the condylar head into the middle cranial fossa and severe restriction of all movements. Less severe injuries frequently result in an effusion into the temporomandibular joint; both wide opening and complete closure are then obstructed.

Any unstable mandibular fracture causes protective muscle spasm and limitation of movement. Patients suffering from displaced Le Fort II or III fractures often complain of limited opening whereas, in reality, they are fully open with the jaws wedged apart by the displaced middle third. Reduction of the fracture allows closure.

Tetanus and tetany

These are rare causes of masticatory muscle spasm. Trismus (lockjaw) is a classical early sign of tetanus which, though rare, must be excluded because of its high mortality. This possibility should be considered whenever a patient develops acute severe limitation of movement of the jaw without local cause, but has had a penetrating wound, even if small, elsewhere.

Tetany is most likely to be seen as a result of anxiety and hyperventilation syndrome.

Temporomandibular pain dysfunction syndrome

Pain dysfunction syndrome is one of the most common causes of temporary limitation of movement of the temporomandibular joint, as discussed later.

Hysterical trismus

Inability to open the mouth is occasionally the main symptom in disturbed patients.

Drugs

Phenothiazine neuroleptics can cause tardive dyskinesia with uncontrollable, involuntary grimacing or chewing movements. Tardive dyskinesia is typically a result of long-term treatment: unlike drug-related Parkinsonism, there is little response to treatment. Metoclopramide, which has phenothiazine-like properties, can cause limitation of movement of the jaw.

Management

In all these conditions the essential measure is to relieve the underlying cause.

DISLOCATION

The temporomandibular joint may become fixed in the open position by anterior dislocation; this is due to forcible opening of the mouth by a blow on the jaw, or during dental extractions under general anaesthesia. In the latter case, the condition should be noticed immediately. It must be corrected before the patient recovers consciousness, by pressing downwards and backwards on the lower posterior teeth. Occasionally, a patient will dislocate spontaneously while yawning. Epileptic patients sometimes also dislocate during fits.

Occasionally, the dislocation remains unnoticed and, surprisingly, a patient may tolerate the disability and discomfort for weeks or even months (Figs 11.1–11.3). In these cases, effusion into the joint, following injury, becomes organised to form fibrous adhesions. When this happens, manual reduction may be impossible and open reduction, with division of adhesions, must be carried out.

Recurrent dislocation

Recurrent dislocation of the temporomandibular joint is more common and is typically seen in adolescent girls and young adults. It is a typical feature of floppy joint syndromes, notably Ehlers–Danlos and Marfan's syndromes, or there may be no underlying systemic disorder.

Augmentation of the eminence by bone graft or down-fracture of the eminence are overall the most successful procedures.

Fig. 11.1 **Dislocation of the jaw.** Radiography of a temporomandibular joint of the same patient showed complete dislocation of the condyle in front of the eminentia articularis. (Figures 11.1–11.3 by courtesy of the late Professor I Curson).

Fig. 11.2 Longstanding dislocation of the jaw: the teeth had been extracted about a month previously; in spite of the patient's inability to close her mouth and the distorted appearance, the dislocation remained unrecognised.

Fig. 11.3 Reduction of the dislocation (performed by open operation because of development of fibrous adhesions) restores the patient's normal appearance and movements of the jaw.

Ehlers–Danlos syndrome

Ehlers–Danlos syndrome (see Ch. 2) is a heritable disease of collagen formation causing, among other features, hyperextensibility of the skin, easy bruising and loose jointedness. Ten subtypes are recognised. Mitral valve prolapse is associated in types I and II in particular.

A very small minority of patients with pain dysfunction syndrome appear to have Ehlers–Danlos syndrome. In addition to the risk of TMJ dislocation, other features as discussed earlier are summarised in Box 11.3.

Box 11.3   Ehlers–Danlos syndrome: important features

- Hypermobility of joints (in types I, VI and VII especially)
- Risk of TMJ subluxation
- Bleeding tendencies and purpura especially in type IV
- Mitral valve prolapse and risk of infective endocarditis in types I and II
- Severe early-onset periodontitis in type VII
- Often, teeth with short or distorted roots and pulp stones

PERSISTENT LIMITATION OF MOVEMENT

Management of ankylosis depends on its aetiology and can be classified for surgical purposes as shown in Box 11.4.

Irradiation

The penetrating power of modern sources, such as cobalt 60 or linear accelerators, is such that high doses can damage

---

Box 11.4   Management of ankylosis

Mechanical interference with opening ('pseudoankylosis'). Causes include:
- Trauma: depressed fracture of the zygomatic bone or arch
- Hyperplasia: developmental overgrowth of the coronoid process
- Neoplasms: osteochondroma, osteoma, osteosarcoma of the coronoid process
- Miscellaneous: myositis ossificans, congenital anomalies

Extracapsular ankylosis ('false ankylosis'). Causes include:
- Trauma: periarticular fibrosis (wounds/burns). Posterior or superior dislocation. Longstanding anterior dislocation
- Infection: chronic periarticular suppuration
- Neoplasia: fibrosarcoma of the capsule. Chondroma or chondrosarcoma
- Periarticular fibrosis
  Irradiation
  Oral submucous fibrosis
  Progressive systemic sclerosis

---

deep tissues without a superficial burn. Radiation involving the region of the masticatory muscles, for the treatment of a maxillary tumour for instance, often leads to fibrosis of muscle and adhesions to the surrounding fascial layers, causing fibrous ankylosis.

Treatment is difficult and may involve division of muscle attachments from the jaw or section of the angle or body of the mandible to produce a false joint. Bone surgery is complicated by the risk of osteoradionecrosis and infection (see Ch. 6).

Oral submucous fibrosis

Oral submucous fibrosis is an important condition that causes not only limitation of opening, but is also premalignant. Symmetrical fibrosis of such sites as the buccal mucosa, soft palate and the pillars of the fauces renders the mucosa immobile and prevents opening. Fibrosis extends deeply into muscles of mastication and is progressive. Ultimately, opening the mouth may become so limited that eating and dental treatment become increasingly difficult and tube feeding may become necessary. There is no effective treatment. This condition is considered in detail in Chapter 16.

Progressive systemic sclerosis (scleroderma)

Systemic sclerosis is an uncommon connective tissue disease characterised by widespread subcutaneous and submucous fibrosis. Though the most obvious feature is the progressive stiffening of the skin, the gastrointestinal tract, lungs, heart and kidneys can also be affected.

Systemic sclerosis is a connective tissue (collagen vascular) disease associated with a variety of autoantibodies (see Ch. 25).

Clinically, women between the ages of 30 and 50 are predominantly affected. Raynaud's phenomenon is the most common early manifestation, often associated with arthralgia. A hallmark of the disease is involvement of the hands causing such changes as atrophy of or ischaemic damage to the tips of the fingers and contractures preventing straightening of the fingers (see Fig. 1.3).

The skin becomes thinned, stiff, tethered, pigmented and marked by telangiectases. The head and neck region is involved in over 75% and, in a minority, symptoms start there. Narrowing of the eyes and taut, mask-like limitation of movement (Mona Lisa face) can give rise to a characteristic appearance. The lips may be constricted (fish mouth) or become pursed with radiating furrows. Occasionally, involvement of the periarticular tissues of the temporomandibular joint together with the microstomia may greatly limit opening of the mouth, but this is typically much less frequent and severe than in the case of oral submucous fibrosis. Involvement of the oral submucosa may cause the tongue to become stiff and narrowed (chicken tongue), but the clinical effects on the oral tissues are typically relatively minor compared with those seen in oral submucous fibrosis. Widening of the periodontal ligament space is another abnormality characteristic of systemic sclerosis but seen in fewer than 10% of cases. The mandibular angle may be resorbed or rarely there is gross extensive resorption of the jaw. Sjögren's syndrome also develops in a significant minority.

Histologically, there is great thickening of the subepithelial connective tissue, degeneration of muscle fibres and atrophy of minor glands. The collagen fibres are swollen and eosinophilic. There are scattered infiltrates of chronic inflammatory cells which are frequently perivascular and arterioles typically show fibrointimal thickening of their walls.

Complications and prognosis

The main disabilities caused by systemic sclerosis are dysphagia and pulmonary, cardiac or renal involvement. Visceral disease, particularly dysphagia and reflux oesophagitis, are common and are sometimes the initial symptoms. Pulmonary involvement leads to impaired respiratory exchange and, eventually, dyspnoea and pulmonary hypertension. Cardiac disease can result from the latter or myocardial fibrosis. Renal disease secondary to vascular disease is typically a late effect; it leads to hypertension and is an important cause of death. The overall 5-year survival rate is 70%.

No specific treatment is available. Immunosuppressive drugs are ineffective. Penicillamine may be given to depress fibrous proliferation but can cause loss of taste, oral ulceration, lichenoid reactions and other complications. Symptomatic measures such as those described for oral submucous fibrosis can be used to prevent undue limitation of jaw movement. Complications such as renal failure are managed by conventional means.

Management

Once ankylosis has become established, the objectives of surgery are to establish joint movement and function, to prevent relapse, to restore appearance and occlusion in the adult and to achieve normal growth and occlusion in the child by interceptive surgery and orthodontics.

In osteoarthrectomy, a block of bone is removed and relapse is prevented by interposition of a temporalis muscle flap, silicone rubber, or metal. In the growing patient, joint reconstruction using a free costo-chondral bone graft gives better results as, in many cases, the graft will grow with the patient, preventing subsequent facial deformity.

ARTHRITIS AND OTHER CAUSES OF PAIN IN OR AROUND THE JOINT

The main causes are:

Injury. Dislocation, joint effusion or fractures of the neck of the condyle can cause pain of varying severity, but surprisingly often, fractures in this region pass unnoticed.

Infection and inflammation. Acute pyogenic arthritis is exceedingly rare but exceedingly painful.

Rheumatoid and other arthritides. The temporomandibular joints tend to be much less severely affected than other small joints. If specifically asked, many patients with rheumatoid arthritis admit to temporomandibular joint symptoms but, overall, pain is not conspicuous. Pain associated with osteoarthritis of this joint is even more uncommon (see below).

Vascular disease. Cranial arteritis is an important cause of ischaemia and pain in the masticatory muscles while chewing.

Muscle spasm. The most common cause of pain in the region of the temporomandibular joint is so-called pain dysfunction syndrome as discussed later.

Salivary gland disease. Painful conditions of the parotids (inflammatory or neoplastic) can cause pain in this region.

Ear disease. Otitis externa, otitis media and mastoiditis are potent causes of pain referred to the temporomandibular joint.

Rheumatoid arthritis

The main feature of this common multisystem disease is chronic inflammation of many joints, pain, progressive limitation of movement, varying degrees of constitutional upset and immunological abnormalities.

Rheumatoid arthritis is the only important inflammatory disease of the temporomandibular joints, but is, nevertheless, an infrequent cause of significant symptoms there.

Clinical features

Women are affected, particularly in the third and fourth decades. Loss of weight, malaise and depression are common. The smaller joints are mainly affected (particularly those of the hands) and the distribution tends to be symmetrical.

The main symptoms of temporomandibular joint involvement are crepitus and limitation of movement, but severe pain is surprisingly uncommon. The temporomandibular joints are never involved alone and the other affected joints usually dominate the picture. One large survey found 71% of patients with rheumatoid arthritis to have clinical abnormalities of the temporomandibular joints, while 79% showed radiographic abnormalities. Despite the fact that these were middle-aged patients with longstanding disease, pain was not significantly more common than in control patients. The main clinical abnormalities were limitation of opening or crepitus, both of which were considerably more common than in other patients.

Radiography shows flattening of the condyles with loss of contour and irregularity of the articular surface as typical findings. The joint space may be widened by exudate in the acute phases but later narrowed. The underlying bone may be

osteoporotic and the margins of the condyles may be irregular. There may be limitation of condylar movement.

Histologically, there is proliferation and hypertrophy of the synovial lining cells and infiltration of the synovium by dense collections of lymphocytes and plasma cells (Fig. 11.4). The inflammatory cells are often arranged as focal aggregates with germinal centres. There is effusion into the synovial fluid which contains neutrophils and fibrinous exudate from the hyperaemic vessels onto the surface of the synovial membrane. A vascular, inflamed mass of granulation tissue (pannus) spreads over the surfaces of the articular cartilages from their margins and is followed by death of chondrocytes and loss of intercellular matrix. Fibrous adhesions form between the joint surfaces and the meniscus. The meniscus may eventually be destroyed and inflammatory changes in the ligaments and tendons can rarely lead to fibrous ankylosis and loss of stability of the joint.

Management

Diagnosis is based on the clinical, radiographic and autoantibody findings. Serum IgG is usually raised and a variety of autoantibodies, particularly rheumatoid factor and antinuclear antibodies, may be detected.

Dental aspects

Generally speaking, though rheumatoid arthritis is a common disease, specific treatment of TMJ symptoms is unlikely to be necessary. The mainstay of treatment is the use of non-steroidal anti-inflammatory drugs, but any gross abnormalities of occlusion, such as overclosure, should be corrected to reduce stress on the temporomandibular joints. Sjögren's syndrome is associated in approximately 15%. Important features of rheumatoid arthritis are summarised in Box 11.5.

Box 11.5 Rheumatoid arthritis: important features

- Onset in middle age. Sometimes acute
- Morning stiffness
- Symmetrical involvement of several joints
- Involvement of hand joints with ulnar deviation
- Joint inflammation and rheumatoid nodules
- Rheumatoid factor frequently positive
- Muscle wasting and osteoporosis
- Frequently malaise, fatigue, fever and anaemia
- Pain and disability usually severe, but not in the TMJ
- Sjögren's syndrome in about 15%

Osteoarthritis

Osteoarthritis is predominantly a disorder of cartilaginous repair, particularly of the elderly, in which there is a defect of cartilage repair exacerbated by trauma. Heavy stress, particularly on weight-bearing joints, is the main cause of pain, but frequently joints with radiographic signs of osteoarthritis are painless (Fig. 11.5). A characteristic feature is the presence of Heberden's nodes (bony swellings) of the terminal interphalangeal joints.

Fig. 11.4 Rheumatoid arthritis. Inflamed villi of pannus growing across the surface of a temporomandibular joint severely affected by rheumatoid arthritis. The condylar surface is destroyed.

Fig. 11.5 **Osteoarthritis.** The fibrocartilage layer is split and the underlying bone shows resorption and repair centrally.

> **Box 11.6** **Important features of osteoarthritis**
>
> - Onset mainly over 60 years
> - Insidious development over months or years
> - Pain mainly on movement of weight-bearing joints
> - Usually one or a few joints involved
> - Heberden's nodes
> - Palpable coarse crepitus of affected joints
> - Bony swelling and deformity
> - Muscle weakness and wasting
> - Little or no inflammation or systemic symptoms

Dental aspects

Osteoarthritis of the temporomandibular joint is mainly a post-mortem finding in elderly patients, is occasionally seen by chance in radiographs, but is not a cause of significant symptoms. Nevertheless, the conviction that osteoarthritis is a significant cause of temporomandibular joint pain, even in young persons, is widely held in the USA in particular, and surgical intervention was common. However, the tide of litigation that followed has led to more conservative measures and an International Conference on Temporomandibular Joint Surgery commented disarmingly that 'it was noted that facts are commonly not allowed to interfere in discussions of TMJ problems'. Although some degree of consensus was reached at this conference, it was apparent that neither the pathogenesis nor the effectiveness of surgical treatment of this condition were firmly established. More frequently now, other interventions such as intra-articular steroid injections are used.

In the rare event that a patient has pain associated with osteoarthritis of the temporomandibular joint, any factor contributing to stress on the joint should be relieved. Anti-inflammatory analgesics are the main line of treatment.

The concept of TMJ 'internal derangement' is also open to a variety of interpretations. Some regard it as an underlying cause of pain. However, internal derangements seen radiographically are frequently painless. It therefore remains too controversial a subject to discuss here.

Important features of osteoarthritis are summarised in Box 11.6.

Other types of arthritis

Many other types of arthritis can affect the temporomandibular joints but rarely do so. They include psoriatic arthritis, the juvenile arthritides, gout, ankylosing spondylitis, Lyme disease and Reiter's disease. Psoriatic arthropathy can cause ankylosis of the temporomandibular joint. Some of the variants of juvenile arthritis, such as Still's disease, are severe and disabling. Destruction of the condylar head, severely limited opening and secondary micrognathia have been reported. Management is essentially that of the underlying disease.

Cranial (giant cell) arteritis

Cranial arteritis sometimes causes ischaemic pain in the masticatory muscles in elderly patients and should be considered in patients over middle age who complain of headache and pain on mastication.

Clinically, women, usually after the age of 55, are predominantly affected. The disease may start with malaise, weakness, low-grade fever and loss of weight. Severe throbbing headache is the most common symptom. The temporal artery frequently becomes red, tender, firm, swollen, and tortuous. In 20% of patients, there is ischaemic pain in the masticatory muscles, comparable to and often misnamed 'jaw claudication' (claudication is literally, limping). More important is involvement of the ophthalmic artery causing disturbances of vision or sudden blindness. Polymyalgia rheumatica may be associated. There is then weakness and pain of the shoulder or pelvic girdles associated with the febrile symptoms. The ESR is usually greatly raised.

Histologically, inflammation involves the arterial media and intima. The infiltration by mononuclear cells is typically associated with multinucleate cells. Intimal damage leads to formation of thrombi, which usually become organised and there may be severe damage to the internal elastic lamina, sometimes going on to complete destruction (Figs 11.6–11.8). Healing is by fibrosis, particularly of the media, thickening of the intima and partial recanalisation of the thrombus. Lesions skip short lengths of an artery and a biopsy should be at least 3 cm long.

Management

The possibility of complications, particularly blindness, which develops in up to 50% of untreated patients, makes it essential to start treatment early. Systemic corticosteroids (starting with 60 mg/day) should be given on the basis of inflamed scalp vessels and a high (>70 mm/hour) ESR. Corticosteroids are usually quickly effective and should be continued until the ESR falls to normal.

Fig. 11.6 **Giant cell (temporal) arteritis.** The structure of the artery is disrupted by inflammatory cells and the lumen is much reduced in size.

GC

EL

Fig. 11.7 **Giant cell (temporal) arteritis.** At higher power the internal elastic lamina of the artery may be seen together with giant cells, lymphocytes and neutrophils in the media. GC, giant cell; EL, elastic lamina.

Fig. 11.8 **Giant cell (temporal) arteritis.** At high power multinucleate giant cells, lymphocytes and neutrophils may be seen among the remnants of the artery's internal elastic lamina (arrowed).

Pain dysfunction syndrome

Pain dysfunction syndrome predominantly affects young or youngish women and is characterised by pain, clicking sounds from the joint, or limitation of movement (Box 11.7). It is overall the most common cause of complaints related to the temporomandibular joint.

Box 11.7 **Typical features of pain dysfunction syndrome**

- Female to male preponderance of nearly 4 to 1
- Most patients are between 20 and 40 years
- Onset is usually gradual
- Onset occasionally ascribed to violent yawning, laughing or a similar incident
- Pain usually one-sided, rarely severe
- Typically, a dull ache is made worse by mastication
- Pain typically felt in front of the ear
- Frequently also limitation of opening, or 'locking' of the jaw
- Ultimately self-limiting

The area may be tender to pressure and a clicking sound, when the mouth is opened or closed, is common. Sometimes pain is felt lower down over the ramus, occasionally at the angle of the jaw and more rarely still, other sites nearby. Defects of occlusion can often be found as in any other patients.

Aetiology

Abnormalities of occlusion, such as lack of posterior occlusal support from loss of molar teeth, are often blamed, but there is no evidence that they are a cause. In spite of the problems created by dentures, for instance, edentulous patients seem rarely, if ever, to be affected. Trauma, particularly minor injuries such as may be caused by violent yawning, laughing, or dental treatment, is occasionally a possible factor, but the evidence does not seem strong. Illustrative of some of the difficulties in identifying this complaint and its causes is that its prevalence reported in different surveys ranges from 12% to 86% of adults.

All the evidence suggests that pain dysfunction syndrome is of dubious aetiology that typically affects only a restricted group of the population. It is self-limiting and does not progress to permanent damage or degenerative arthritis later in life. Elderly patients are remarkably free from temporomandibular joint symptoms. Defective neuromuscular coordination, causing areas of spasm of the masticatory muscles, appears to be the main cause.

Investigation

In view of the absence of objective signs, diagnosis is largely by exclusion. Organic causes (as enumerated above) of pain or limitation of movement of the joint should be ruled out by investigation. As in all cases of pain in the region of the jaws, referred pain from the teeth should be carefully excluded.

The temporomandibular joint should be palpated for tenderness or swelling which, if present, suggest organic disease. Crepitus may be felt but is not specific and is not necessarily a sign of significant joint disease. Radiographs of the joints may be taken to make sure that movements are not excessive in either direction and are equal on both sides. However, the main value of radiographs is to exclude such changes as fluid accumulation (widening of the joint space) or damage or deformity of the joint surfaces, indicating organic disease. Trigeminal neuralgia can be occasionally triggered by movement of the jaw and should be suspected in older patients, particularly when the pain is severe and paroxysmal. Response to treatment with carbamazepine or gabapentin is virtually diagnostic.

Management

In the USA, this complaint has been investigated and treated (often by surgery) so excessively vigorously that the resulting litigation has forced a search for a consensus on management. It is now accepted that the indications for active intervention, particularly surgery or 'occlusal therapy', are of questionable value. Moreover, there is a strong placebo effect in any form of treatment. The main principles of management of pain dysfunction syndrome are summarised in Box 11.8.

Box 11.8   Principles of management of pain dysfunction syndrome

- Reassurance
- Habit management and physical therapy
- Occlusal appliances
- Analgesics

Any abnormal biting habits should be identified and controlled. Faulty neuromuscular control should be dealt with by exercises to correct faulty patterns of activity as shown by such abnormalities as deviations on closure.

In practice, fitting an acrylic overlay appliance is simple and usually effective. It also tends to relieve abnormal grinding habits. It should cover the occlusal surfaces of the teeth and allow free occlusion without cuspal interference. Short-term use of simple analgesics may also be helpful.

'Costen's syndrome'

This antiquated term applies to headache, ear symptoms (tinnitus or deafness) and burning pain in the tongue and throat and was ascribed to over-closure causing excessive backward movement of the head of the condyle. This syndrome does not exist, but the term 'Costen's syndrome' persists in medicine and is often thought to be synonymous with pain dysfunction syndrome.

Condylar hyperplasia

Condylar hyperlasia is a rare, usually unilateral, overgrowth of the mandibular condyle. It causes facial asymmetry, deviation of the jaw to the unaffected side on opening and a crossbite. The condition usually manifests itself after puberty and is slowly progressive. Pain in the affected joint is variable. If the condition is still active at the time of diagnosis, an intracapsular condylectomy should be performed to destroy the active growth centre. If the disease has stabilised – usually at the end of puberty or shortly afterwards – corrective osteotomies should restore the occlusion and facial symmetry (Fig. 11.9).

Neoplasms

Tumours of the temporomandibular joint are rare, but may arise from the condyle – either the bone or articular cartilage – or from the joint capsule. Metastatic tumours such as those from the breast, prostate and thyroid occasionally metastasise to the condylar head (see Ch. 6).

Though otherwise rare in the facial skeleton, osteochondroma (Fig. 11.10) is probably the most common tumour of the condyle or coronoid process. Osteoma and chondroma and their malignant counterparts may develop, but apart from their interference with joint function and disturbance of occlusion, their behaviour and management are the same as when they arise elsewhere in the jaws. Condylectomy may be required for a neoplasm such as an osteochondroma and an external approach is used.

Loose bodies in the temporomandibular joints

Loose bodies are rare in the temporomandibular joints compared with other joints. Many types of loose bodies are recognised, but the main causes are osteochondritis dissecans and synovial chondromatosis.

Fig. 11.9   Condylar hyperplasia. The condyle retains an immature structure with a thick cartilage layer, calcification and new bone formation, reflecting the continued growth.

Fig. 11.10 Osteochondroma of the condyle. Two cartilage-capped exostoses arising near the condyle have grown progressively sideways to form a distorted condylar head several centimetres across.

Osteochondritis dissecans

This is the main cause of loose bodies in joints, most commonly in the knee. It is believed to result from trauma causing an area of subchondral bone to undergo avascular necrosis with subsequent degenerative changes in the overlying articular cartilage. This area subsequently separates to produce one or several loose bodies. In the temporomandibular joint, the patient has discomfort and episodes of locking. The loose body may be seen on tomography, arthrography or arthroscopy. Surgical removal of the loose body, which is always in the lower joint compartment, relieves the symptoms.

Synovial chondromatosis

In this disease, foci of cartilage develop in the synovial membrane; it is thought to be a benign neoplasm. Synovial chondromatosis rarely affects the temporomandibular joint, but can cause swelling and limitation of movement, with deviation to the affected side on opening. Conventional radiographs may show radiopaque masses in the region of the joint capsule, but if no abnormality may be seen, MRI should reveal multiple cartilaginous nodules and distension of the capsule. Both upper and lower joint compartments are involved and, exceptionally rarely, the process may extend into the cranial cavity.

Histologically, there is proliferation and atypia of chondrocytes in the subsynovial connective tissue with formation of microscopic or larger nodules of cartilage. These nodules enlarge, may calcify and escape into the joint cavity. The appearance of the chondrocytes is such that it is possible to mistake the lesion for a chondrosarcoma if the pathologist is not made aware of the clinical history and operative findings. It has been shown immunohistochemically that most of the nuclei of the chondrocytes are inactive and that malignancy can be excluded.

Removal of the loose bodies and the whole of the affected synovium are curative. Incomplete excision can be followed by recurrence.

SUGGESTED FURTHER READING

Bjornland T, Refsum SB 1944 Histopathologic changes in the temporomandibular joint disk in patients with chronic arthritic disease. A comparison with internal derangement. Oral Surg Oral Med Oral Pathol 77:572–578

Borle RM, Borle SR 1991 Management of oral submucous fibrosis: a conservative approach. J Oral Maxillofac Surg 49:788–791

Buckingham RB, Braun T, Harinstein D et al 1991 Temporomandibular joint dysfunction: a close association with systemic joint laxity (the hypermobile joint syndrome). Oral Surg Oral Med Oral Pathol 72:514–519

Cawson RA, Langdon JD, Eveson JW 1996 Surgical pathology of the mouth and jaws. Wright, Oxford

Cawson RA, Binnie WH, Barrett AW, Wright JM 2001 Oral disease, 3rd edn. Mosby-Wolfe, London

Chalmers IM, Blair GS 1973 Rheumatoid arthritis of the temporomandibular joint. A clinical and radiological study using circular tomography. Quart J Med XLII:369–386

Denucci DJ, Dionne RA, Dubner R 1996 Identifying a neurobiologic basis for drug therapy in TMDs. JADA 127:581–593

Forssell H, Happonen R-P, Forssell K, Virolainen E 1985 Osteochondroma of the mandibular condyle, report of a case and review of the literature. Br J Maxillofac Surg 23:183–189

Goldstein BH 1999 Temporomandibular disorders. A review of current understanding. Oral Surg Oral Med Oral Pathol Oral Radiol Endod 88:379–385

Goss AN 1993 Toward an international consensus on temporomandibular joint surgery. Report of the Second International Consensus Meeting, April 1992, Buenos Aires, Argentina. Int J Oral Maxillofac Surg 22:78–81

Harris M, Feinmann C, Wise M, Treasure F 1993 Temporomandibular joint and orofacial pain: clinical and medicolegal management problems. Br Dent J 174:129–136

Harris RJ 1988 Lyme disease involving the temporomandibular joint. J Oral Maxillofac Surg 46:78–79

Holmlund A, Reinholt F, Bergstedt H 1992 Synovial chondromatosis of the temporomandibular joint. Report of a case. Oral Surg Oral Med Oral Pathol 73:266–268

Kaban LB, Belfer ML 1981 Temporomandibular joint dysfunction: an occasional manifestation of serious psychopathology. J Oral Surg 39:742–746

Kerscher A, Piette E, Tideman H, Wu PC 1993 Osteochondroma of the coronoid process of the mandible. Oral Surg Oral Med Oral Pathol 75:559–564

Könönen M 1992 Signs and symptoms of craniomandibular disorders in men with Reiter's disease. J Craniomandib Disord Facial Oral Pain 6:247–253

Koorbusch GF, Zeitler DL, Fotos PG, Doss JB 1991 Psoriatic arthritis of the temporomandibular joints with ankylosis. Oral Surg Oral Med Oral Pathol 71:267–274

Larheim TA, Haanaes HR 1981 Micrognathia, temporomandibular joint changes and dental occlusion in juvenile rheumatoid arthritis of adolescents and adults. Scand J Dent Res 89:328–329

Leighty SM, Spach DH, Myall RWT, Burns JL 1993 Septic arthritis of the temporomandibular joint: review of the literature and report of two cases in children. Int J Oral Maxillofac Surg 22:292–297

Lustmann J, Zeltser R 1989 Synovial chondromatosis of the temporomandibular joint. Review of the literature and case report. J Oral Maxillofac Surg 18:90–94

Maher R, Lee AJ, Warnakulasuriya KAAS et al 1994 Role of areca nut in the causation of oral submucous fibrosis: a case-control study in Pakistan. J Oral Pathol Med 23:65–69

Miles DA, Kaugars GA 1991 Psoriatic involvement of the temporomandibular joint. Literature review and report of two cases. Oral Surg Oral Med Oral Pathol 71:770–774

Pillai R, Balaram P, Reddiar KS 1992 Pathogenesis of oral submucous fibrosis. Relationship to risk factors associated with oral cancer. Cancer 69:2011–2020

Rosati LA, Stevens C 1990 Synovial chondromatosis of the temporomandibular joint presenting as an intracranial mass. Arch Otolaryngol Head Neck Surg 116:1334–1337

Sun S, Helmi E, Bays R 1990 Synovial chondromatosis with intracranial extension. Oral Surg Oral Med Oral Pathol 70:5–9

White RD, Makar J, Steckler RM 1992 Synovial sarcoma of the temporomandibular joint. J Oral Maxillofac Surg 50:1127–1230

Self-assessment questions and learning guides

These self-assessment questions and learning guides are based on the material in the previous section, but may also link to material covered elsewhere. They are not intended to be comprehensive, but give an indication of the understanding and problem solving abilities expected at an undergraduate level. You will not find all the information you require to answer these questions in the relevant chapters and tables. Use these questions to guide your additional reading and learning.

CHAPTER 1

- How might poor history taking inhibit a patient from providing the information you seek?
- Which features in a pain history might suggest pain of odontogenic, neurological or vascular origin?
- What is the difference between a medical history and a medical history questionnaire?
- What features of the extraoral head and neck examination might suggest systemic disease?
- What are the advantages and disadvantages of the various methods for testing the vitality of teeth? How is it possible to be certain about the vitality of a specific tooth?
- What features in the examination of the hands suggest systemic disease?
- Could you undertake a mucosal biopsy and submit the specimen for diagnosis correctly?
- What features in the history and examination would prompt you to send a biopsy for immunofluorescence testing?
- Which blood investigations might be useful to investigate a patient with oral ulceration?
- How should a sample of pus for culture and antibiotic sensitivity be collected?
- When constructing a differential diagnosis, how would you decide the appropriate order for the various possible diagnoses?
- Which oral conditions may be diagnosed on the basis of the history alone?
- Which normal oral structures may be mistaken for lesions?

CHAPTER 2

- What are the causes of failure of eruption and early loss of deciduous teeth?
- How will you differentiate developmental defects of the teeth from those with other causes?
- Do you know how to plot a family tree for a genetic condition?
- Why are only females affected by vertical ridging of the teeth in amelogenesis imperfecta?
- The challenges of restoring dentitions affected by amelogenesis imperfecta and dentinogenesis imperfecta are different. Explain why in terms of the tooth structure.
- How might radiographic features of the jaws predict colon carcinoma?
- How would you distinguish tetracycline staining and fluorosis?
- Why might a cleft palate indicate a cardiac defect? What are the underlying mechanisms that link these conditions?

CHAPTER 3

- How may caries be prevented by reference to the four major aetiological factors?
- Can caries activity be predicted by investigating the oral or plaque flora?
- Can you explain how different sugars and differing bacterial flora affect the Stephan curve?
- Why is frequency of carbohydrate intake so important in dental caries?
- What are the effects of dietary fluoride on dental caries?
- How does an intact layer of plaque over a carious lesion affect its structure?
- What is the importance of cavitation to the treatment of dental caries?
- How does enamel etching for restorative procedures differ from dental caries?
- Why do patients with erosion caused by dietary acid intake not usually have problems with excessive dental caries?

- How does the viability of the dentine and pulp protect against the sequelae of dental caries?
- How can the activity of an individual carious lesion be estimated clinically?
- How does knowledge of enamel caries influence treatment decisions?
- How does knowledge of dentine caries influence treatment decisions?

CHAPTER 4

- How is pulpitis diagnosed and how may it be differentiated from periapical periodontitis?
- What conditions may mimic the symptoms of pulpitis?
- What operative procedures foster resolution of reversible pulpitis?
- Can you trace the possible pathways from pulpitis to life-threatening infection?
- Why, even when dental caries is untreated, are these life-threatening complications so rare?
- How does differentiating internal from external resorption aid treatment?
- What is the aetiology of tooth-wear and how may it be associated with general health?

CHAPTER 5

- How do the plaque flora and host immunological responses to plaque mature through life?
- What is the significance of the histological stages of gingivitis and periodontitis?
- What is the current state of the controversy between the specific plaque and non-specific plaque hypotheses?
- What is the rate of progression of chronic adult periodontitis?
- What conditions predispose to periodontitis in children and in adults?
- What are the pathological differences between acute necrotising ulcerative gingivitis and chronic adult periodontitis?
- How does HIV infection predispose to periodontal destruction?
- What clinical features of gingivitis or periodontitis might suggest underlying HIV infection?
- Which systemic medical conditions may present with gingival signs and symptoms?
- A middle-aged adult presents with advancing periodontal destruction in a previously healthy mouth. How would you investigate this patient?
- What diseases have similar presentations to plaque-induced gingivitis and periodontitis?

CHAPTER 6

- Osteomyelitis of the jaws often has local or systemic predisposing causes. How would you identify these?
- How do the radiographic changes in osteomyelitis develop with time?
- What are the differences between chronic osteomyelitis and florid cemento-osseous dysplasia?
- Why is dry socket not considered a form of osteomyelitis?
- Which microbial species are associated with facial infections of odontogenic origin?
- Which of the various odontogenic soft tissue infections of the face may be life-threatening and why?
- What investigations are required when a patient presents with a soft tissue infection of suspected odontogenic origin?

CHAPTER 7

- What is cortication radiologically and what does it mean if a lesion is corticated?
- What features of the history and examination would lead you to suspect a cyst rather than any other localised radiolucency in the jaws?
- How may hyaline or Rushton bodies aid cyst diagnosis?
- When should you undertake an incisional biopsy of a cyst?
- Which cysts have diagnostic histological features?
- How does the growth pattern of a cyst aid diagnosis?
- What are the arguments for and against considering the odontogenic keratocyst an odontogenic tumour?
- How does the orthokeratinising odontogenic cyst differ from the odontogenic keratocyst?
- A young adult presents with bilateral odontogenic keratocysts. How would you investigate and manage this patient?
- Which types of cyst may recur following treatment?
- How would you differentiate a sublingual dermoid cyst from a ranula?
- How may ranulas be treated conservatively?

CHAPTER 8

- When presented with a lesion in the jaws, what features would suggest an odontogenic tumour rather than a cyst, primary bone tumour or other cause?
- How is a unicystic ameloblastoma defined and how may one be diagnosed?
- There is a recent tendency to treat ameloblastoma conservatively. How is this achieved and what are the advantages and disadvantages of this approach?
- Which odontogenic tumours would be expected to recur following removal by enucleation and curettage?
- Which odontogenic tumour might present as localised periodontitis?

- The odontogenic myxoma is benign but requires excision with a margin for effective treatment. Why?
- Which odontogenic tumours contain radiopacities?
- You notice a radiopaque lesion attached to the root of a tooth; how would you investigate and manage this patient?
- How would you investigate and treat a patient with a radiolucency near the angle of the mandible?

CHAPTER 9

- A lesion in a child is found to be a giant cell lesion on biopsy. How does the site affect treatment?
- How would you further investigate a patient whose intra-osseous lesion proved to be a giant cell lesion on biopsy?
- What radiological features might suggest an intra-osseous haemangioma?
- How does the clinical course of osteosarcoma of the jaws differ from that of osteosarcoma of the long bones?
- How does the position of a radiolucency either above or below the inferior dental canal aid differential diagnosis?
- It is often said that a sharply demarcated radiopaque lesion in bone is almost certainly benign. Is this correct?

CHAPTER 10

- How is osteogenesis imperfecta linked to dentinogenesis imperfecta and why are the teeth not affected in some types of osteogenesis imperfecta?

- What are the causes of failure of eruption of teeth?
- What abnormalities are seen in the bones and teeth in the different forms of rickets?
- What investigations would aid the differentiation of a central giant cell granuloma from a brown tumour of hyperparathyroidism?
- What conditions may be confused with Paget's disease radiographically and how may they be differentiated?
- What is the cause of fibrous dysplasia and how may it be differentiated from cemento-ossifying fibroma?

CHAPTER 11

- How would you investigate a patient complaining of trismus?
- How would you investigate a patient complaining of limited jaw opening?
- What radiographs and other imaging techniques are appropriate for assessment of the temporomandibular joints?
- Does a normal temporomandibular joint radiograph exclude joint disease?
- How would you investigate and treat a case of temporomandibular pain dysfunction syndrome with particular emphasis on excluding organic disease?

SOFT TISSUE DISEASE

Diseases of the oral mucosa: introduction and mucosal infections

A few mucosal diseases, such as lupus erythematosus, are important indicators of severe underlying systemic disease and rare conditions, such as acanthosis nigricans, can be markers of internal malignancy. Pemphigus vulgaris is potentially lethal, as is HIV infection – which can give rise to a variety of mucosal lesions. Biopsy is mandatory, particularly in the bullous diseases as, in such cases, the diagnosis can only be confirmed by microscopy. In other cases, microscopic findings can be less definite, but often (as in the case of major aphthae for example) serve to exclude more dangerous diseases. Mucosal ulceration – a break in epithelial continuity – is a frequent feature of stomatitis. Important causes are summarised in Table 12.1. However, ulceration is not a feature of all mucosal diseases as discussed below.

PRIMARY HERPETIC STOMATITIS → Summary p. 221

Primary infection is caused by Herpes simplex virus, usually type 1, which, in the non-immune, can cause an acute vesiculating stomatitis. However, most primary infections are subclinical. Thereafter, recurrent (reactivation) infections usually take the form of herpes labialis (cold sores or fever blisters).

Transmission of herpes is by close contact and up to 90% of inhabitants of large, poor, urban communities, develop antibodies to herpes virus during early childhood. In many British and US cities, by contrast, approximately 70% of 20-year-olds may be non-immune, because of lack of exposure to the virus. In such countries, the incidence of herpetic stomatitis has declined and it is seen in adolescents or adults, rather than children. It is more common in the immunocompromised, such as HIV infection, when it can be persistent or recurrent.

Clinical features

The early lesions are vesicles which can affect any part of the oral mucosa, but the hard palate and dorsum of the tongue are favoured sites (Figs 12.1 and 12.2). The vesicles are dome-shaped and usually 2–3 mm in diameter. Rupture of vesicles leaves circular, sharply defined, shallow ulcers with yellowish or greyish floors and red margins. The ulcers are painful and may interfere with eating.

The gingival margins are frequently swollen and red, particularly in children, and the regional lymph nodes are enlarged and tender. There is often fever and systemic upset, sometimes severe, particularly in adults.

Table 12.1 Important causes of oral mucosal ulcers		
	Vesiculo-bullous diseases	**Ulceration without preceding vesiculation**
Infective	Primary herpetic stomatitis Herpes labialis Herpes zoster and chickenpox Hand-foot-and-mouth disease	Cytomegalovirus-associated ulceration Some acute specific fevers Tuberculosis Syphilis
Non-infective	Pemphigus vulgaris Mucous membrane pemphigoid Linear IgA disease Dermatitis herpetiformis Bullous erythema multiforme	Traumatic Aphthous stomatitis Behçet's disease HIV-associated mucosal ulcers Lichen planus Lupus erythematosus Chronic ulcerative stomatitis Eosinophilic ulceration Wegener's granulomatosis Some mucosal drug reactions Carcinoma (Ch. 17)

Fig. 12.1 **Herpetic stomatitis.** Pale vesicles and ulcers are visible on the palate and gingivae, especially anteriorly, and the gingivae are erythematous and swollen.

Fig. 12.2 **Herpetic stomatitis.** A group of recently ruptured vesicles on the hard palate, a characteristic site. The individual lesions are of remarkably uniform size but several have coalesced to form larger irregular ulcers.

Fig. 12.3 **Herpetic vesicle.** The vesicle is formed by accumulation of fluid within the prickle cell layer. The virus-infected cells, identifiable by their enlarged nuclei, can be seen in the floor of the vesicle and a few are floating freely in the vesicle fluid.

Fig. 12.4 **A smear from a herpetic vesicle.** The distended degenerating nuclei of the epithelial cells cluster together to give the typical mulberry appearance.

Oral lesions usually resolve within a week to ten days, but malaise can persist so long that an adult may not recover fully for several weeks.

Pathology

Vesicles are sharply defined and form in the upper epithelium (Fig. 12.3). Virus-damaged epithelial cells with swollen nuclei and marginated chromatin (ballooning degeneration) are seen in the floor of the vesicle and in direct smears from early lesions (Fig. 12.4). Incomplete division leads to formation of multinucleated cells. Later, the full thickness of the epithelium is destroyed to produce a sharply defined ulcer (Fig. 12.5).

Diagnosis

The clinical picture is usually distinctive (Box 12.1). A smear showing virus-damaged cells is additional diagnostic evidence. A rising titre of antibodies reaching a peak after 2–3 weeks provides absolute but retrospective confirmation of the diagnosis.

Treatment

Aciclovir is a potent antiherpetic drug and is life-saving for potentially lethal herpetic encephalitis or disseminated infection. Aciclovir suspension used as a rinse and then swallowed should accelerate healing of severe herpetic stomatitis if used sufficiently early. Bed rest, fluids and a soft diet may sometimes be required.

Fig. 12.5 **Herpetic ulcer.** The vesicle has ruptured to form an ulcer (right) and the epithelium at the margin contains enlarged, darkly staining virus-infected cells liberating free virus into the saliva.

Fig. 12.6 **Herpes labialis.** (A) Typical vesicles. (B) Crusted ulcers affecting the vermilion borders of the lips.

> **Box 12.1** **Herpetic stomatitis: key features**
>
> - Usually caused by H. simplex virus type 1
> - Transmitted by close contact
> - Vesicles, followed by ulcers, affect any part of the oral mucosa
> - Gingivitis sometimes associated
> - Lymphadenopathy and fever of variable severity
> - Smears from vesicles show ballooning degeneration of viral-damaged cells
> - Rising titre of antibodies to HSV confirms the diagnosis
> - Aciclovir is the treatment of choice

In mild cases, topical tetracycline suspension, rinsed round the mouth several times a day, relieves soreness and may hasten healing by controlling secondary infection.

Unusually prolonged or severe infections or failure to respond to aciclovir (200–400 mg/day by mouth for 7 days) suggest immunodeficiency and herpetic ulceration persisting for more than a month is an AIDS-defining illness.

HERPES LABIALIS → Summary p. 221

After the primary infection, the latent virus can be reactivated in 20–30% of patients to cause cold sores (fever blisters). Triggering factors include the common cold and other febrile infections, exposure to strong sunshine, menstruation or, occasionally, emotional upsets or local irritation, such as dental treatment. Neutralising antibodies produced in response to the primary infection are not protective.

Clinically, changes follow a consistent course with prodromal paraesthesia or burning sensations, then erythema at the site of the attack. Vesicles form after an hour or two, usually in clusters along the mucocutaneous junction of the lips, but can extend onto the adjacent skin (Fig. 12.6).

The vesicles enlarge, coalesce and weep exudate. After 2 or 3 days they rupture and crust over but new vesicles frequently appear for a day or two only to scab over and finally heal,

usually without scarring. The whole cycle may take up to 10 days. Secondary bacterial infection may induce an impetiginous lesion which sometimes leaves scars.

Treatment

In view of the rapidity of the viral damage to the tissues, treatment must start as soon as the premonitory sensations are felt. Aciclovir cream is available without prescription and may be effective if applied at this time. This is possible because the course of the disease is consistent and patients can recognise the prodromal symptoms before tissue damage has started. However, penciclovir applied 2-hourly is more effective.

Herpetic cross-infections

Both primary and secondary herpetic infections are contagious. *Herpetic whitlow* (Fig. 12.7) is a recognised though surprisingly uncommon hazard to dental surgeons and their assistants. Herpetic whitlows, in turn, can infect patients and have led to outbreaks of infection in hospitals and among patients in dental practices. Now that gloves are universally worn when giving

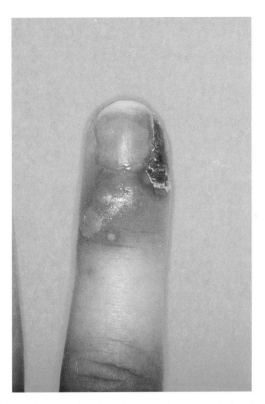

Fig. 12.7 **Herpetic whitlow.** This is a characteristic non-oral site for primary infection as a result of contact with infected vesicle fluid or saliva. The vesiculation and crusting are identical to those seen in herpes labialis.

Fig. 12.8 **Herpes zoster.** A severe attack in an older person shows confluent ulceration on the hard and soft palate on one side.

Fig. 12.9 **Herpes zoster of the trigeminal nerve.** There are vesicles and ulcers on one side of the tongue and facial skin supplied by the first and second divisions. The patient complained only of toothache.

dental treatment, such cross-infections should no longer happen. In immunodeficient patients, such infections can be dangerous, but aciclovir has dramatically improved the prognosis in such cases and may be given on suspicion.

Mothers applying antiherpetic drugs to children's lesions should wear gloves.

HERPES ZOSTER OF THE TRIGEMINAL AREA →
Summary p. 221

Zoster (shingles) is characterised by pain, a vesicular rash and stomatitis in the related dermatome. The varicella-zoster virus (VZV) causes chickenpox in the non-immune (mainly children), while reactivation of the latent virus causes zoster, mainly in the elderly.

Unlike herpes labialis, repeated recurrences of zoster are very rare. Occasionally, there is an underlying immunodeficiency. Herpes zoster is a hazard in organ transplant patients and can be an early complication of some tumours, particularly Hodgkin's disease, or, increasingly, of AIDS, where it is five times more common than in HIV-negative persons and potentially lethal.

Clinical features

Herpes zoster usually affects adults of middle age or over but, occasionally, attacks even children. The first signs are pain and

irritation or tenderness in the dermatome corresponding to the affected ganglion.

Vesicles, often confluent, form on one side of the face and in the mouth up to the midline (Figs 12.8 and 12.9). The regional lymph nodes are enlarged and tender. The acute phase usually lasts about a week. Pain continues until the lesions crust over and start to heal, but secondary infection may cause suppuration and scarring of the skin. Malaise and fever are usually associated.

Patients are sometimes unable to distinguish the pain of trigeminal zoster from severe toothache, as in the patient shown in Figure 12.9. This has sometimes led to a demand for a dental extraction. Afterwards, the rash follows as a normal course of events and this has given rise to the myth that dental extractions can precipitate facial zoster.

Pathology

The varicella-zoster virus produces similar epithelial lesions to those of herpes simplex, but also inflammation of the related posterior root ganglion.

Management

Herpes zoster is an uncommon cause of stomatitis, but readily recognisable (Box 12.2).

Box 12.2 Herpes zoster of the trigeminal area: key features

- Recurrence of VZV infection typically in the elderly
- Pain precedes the rash
- Facial rash accompanies the stomatitis
- Lesions localised to one side, within the distribution of any of the divisions of the trigeminal nerve
- Malaise can be severe
- Can be life-threatening in HIV disease
- Treat with systemic aciclovir, intravenously, if necessary
- Sometimes followed by post-herpetic neuralgia, particularly in the elderly

---

According to the severity of the attack, oral aciclovir (800 mg five times daily, usually for 7 days) should be given at the earliest possible moment, together with analgesics. The addition of prednisolone may accelerate relief of pain and healing. In immunodeficient patients, intravenous aciclovir is required and may also be justified for the elderly in whom this infection is debilitating.

Complications

Post-herpetic neuralgia mainly affects the elderly and is difficult to relieve (Ch. 34).

CYTOMEGALOVIRUS-ASSOCIATED ULCERATION

Cytomegalovirus (CMV) is a member of the herpes virus group. Up to 80% of adults show serological evidence of CMV infection without clinical effects, but it is a common complication of immunodeficiency, particularly AIDS. In the latter it can be life-threatening.

Oral ulcers in which CMV has been identified are sometimes clinically indistinguishable from recurrent aphthae, others have raised, minimally rolled borders. Generally, the ulcers are large, shallow and single, and affect either the masticatory or non-masticatory mucosa. Sometimes, oral ulcers are associated with disseminated CMV infection.

Microscopically, CMV-associated ulcers are non-specific, but cells with typical owl-eye intranuclear inclusions can be seen in the inflammatory infiltrate in the ulcer floor. They are usually recognisable by light microscopy but their nature can be confirmed by immunocytochemistry (see Fig. 1.8), in-situ hybridisation or electron microscopy.

The virus present in oral lesions may merely be a passenger, but their causative role is suggested by reports of response to ganciclovir.

HAND-FOOT-AND-MOUTH DISEASE → Summary p. 221

This common, mild viral infection, which often causes minor epidemics among school children, is characterised by ulceration of the mouth and a vesicular rash on the extremities.

Hand-foot-and-mouth disease is usually caused by strains of Coxsackie A virus. It is highly infectious, frequently spreads through a classroom in schools and may also infect a teacher or parent. The incubation period is probably between 3 and 10 days. Foot-and-mouth disease of cattle is a quite different rhinovirus infection which rarely affects humans but can also cause a mild illness with vesiculating stomatitis.

Clinical features

The small scattered oral ulcers usually cause little pain. Intact vesicles are rarely seen and gingivitis is not a feature. Regional lymph nodes are not usually enlarged and systemic upset is typically mild or absent.

The rash consists of vesicles, sometimes deep-seated, or occasionally bullae, mainly seen around the base of fingers or toes, but any part of the limbs may be affected (Fig. 12.10). The rash is often the main feature and such patients are unlikely to be seen by dentists. In some outbreaks, either the mouth or the extremities alone may be affected.

Serological confirmation of the diagnosis is possible but rarely necessary as the history, especially of other cases, and clinical features are usually adequate. The disease typically resolves within a week. No specific treatment is available or needed but myocarditis or encephalitis are rare complications.

Key features are summarised in Box 12.3.

THE ACUTE SPECIFIC FEVERS

Fevers which cause oral lesions are rarely seen in dentistry. Those which cause vesicular rashes (smallpox and chickenpox) produce the same lesions in the mouth.

Fig. 12.10 **Hand-foot-and-mouth disease.** The rash consists of vesicles or bullae on the extremities; in this patient they are relatively inconspicuous.

> **Box 12.3** **Hand-foot-and-mouth disease: key features**
>
> - Caused mainly by Coxsackie A viruses
> - Highly infectious
> - School children predominantly affected
> - Occasionally spreads to teacher or parent
> - Typically mild vesiculating stomatitis and/or vesiculating rash on extremities
> - Rarely severe enough for dental opinion to be sought
> - Confirmation of diagnosis (if required) by serology
> - No specific treatment available or needed

In the prodromal stage of measles, Koplik's spots form on the buccal mucosa and soft palate and are pathognomonic. Palatal petechiae or ulceration, involving the fauces especially, are seen in glandular fever and are accompanied by the characteristic, usually widespread lymphadenopathy.

KAWASAKI'S DISEASE (MUCOCUTANEOUS LYMPH NODE SYNDROME)

Kawasaki's disease is endemic in Japan but uncommon in Britain. It is frequently unrecognised and has caused significant mortality. Though its epidemiology suggests that it is an infection, this has not been established.

Clinical features

Children are affected and have persistent fever, oral mucositis, ocular and cutaneous lesions and cervical lymphadenopathy (Ch. 26). Oral lesions consist of widespread mucosal erythema with swelling of the lingual papillae (strawberry tongue), but are insignificant compared with the serious cardiac effects (Ch. 27).

TUBERCULOSIS

The recrudescence of tuberculosis in the West is partly a consequence of the AIDS epidemic. Moreover, multiply-resistant mycobacteria are becoming widespread. Oral tuberculosis is rare and a complication of pulmonary disease with infected sputum. Those with HIV infection are an important group of victims, but oral tuberculosis is occasionally seen in immunocompetent persons who are usually elderly men with pulmonary infection and a chronic cough that has progressed unrecognised or who have neglected treatment.

The typical lesion is an ulcer on the mid-dorsum of the tongue; the lip or other parts of the mouth are infrequently affected. The ulcer is typically angular or stellate, with overhanging edges and a pale floor, but can be ragged and irregular (Fig. 12.11). It is painless in its early stages and regional

lymph nodes are usually unaffected. Widespread ulcers in multiple oral sites have been reported in a patient with AIDS.

The diagnosis is rarely suspected until after biopsy.

Pathology

Typical tuberculous granulomas are seen in the floor of the ulcers (Fig. 12.12). Mycobacteria are rarely identifiable in the oral lesion but can be demonstrated in the sputum. Chest radiographs show advanced infection.

Fig. 12.11 **A tuberculous ulcer of the tongue.** The rather angular shape and overhanging edges of the ulcer are typical. The patient was a man of 56 with advanced but unrecognised pulmonary tuberculosis.

Fig. 12.12 **Tuberculous ulcer.** At the margin, numerous granulomas are present in the ulcer bed. The darkly stained multinucleate Langhans giant cells are visible even at this low power.

Tuberculosis or non-tuberculous mycobacterial infection must be considered in patients with AIDS who develop oral ulceration with histological granuloma formation.

Management

Diagnosis is confirmed by biopsy, chest radiography and a specimen of sputum. Mycobacterial infection is confirmed by culture or PCR.

Oral lesions clear up rapidly if vigorous multidrug chemotherapy is given for the pulmonary infection. No local treatment is needed.

Tuberculous cervical lymphadenopathy

See Chapter 26

SYPHILIS

As a result of contact tracing and early treatment, fewer than 150 cases a year of primary or secondary syphilis were seen in England and Wales in the 1980s. However, since the mid-1990s, the prevalence has steadily risen. This is a worldwide trend and the disease has, for example, become widespread in Eastern Europe.

Oral lesions in each stage of syphilis are clinically quite different from each other. Oral lesions have recently been reported in Britain but some may pass unrecognised.

Primary syphilis

An oral chancre appears 3–4 weeks after infection and may form on the lip, tip of the tongue or, rarely, other oral sites. It consists initially of a firm nodule about a centimetre across (Fig. 12.13). The surface breaks down after a few days, leaving a rounded ulcer with raised indurated edges. This may resemble a carcinoma, particularly if on the lip. However, the appearances

vary. A chancre is typically painless but regional lymph nodes are enlarged, rubbery and discrete. A biopsy may only show non-specific inflammation but sometimes there is conspicuous perivascular infiltration.

Serological reactions are negative at first. Diagnosis therefore depends on finding *Treponema pallidum* by dark-ground illumination of a smear from the chancre, but they must be distinguished from other oral spirochaetes. Clinical recognition of oral chancres is difficult but important. They are highly infective, and treatment is most effective at this stage.

After 8 or 9 weeks the chancre heals, often without scarring.

Secondary syphilis

The secondary stage develops 1–4 months after infection. It typically causes mild fever with malaise, headache, sore throat and generalised lymphadenopathy, soon followed by a rash and stomatitis.

The rash is variable, but typically consists of asymptomatic pinkish (coppery) macules, symmetrically distributed and starting on the trunk. It may last for a few hours or weeks and its presence or history is a useful aid to diagnosis. Oral lesions, which rarely appear without the rash, mainly affect the tonsils, lateral borders of the tongue and lips. They are usually flat ulcers covered by greyish membrane and may be irregularly linear (snail's track ulcers) or coalesce to form well-defined rounded areas (mucous patches).

Discharge from the ulcers contains many spirochaetes and saliva is highly infective. Serological reactions (see below) are positive and diagnostic at this stage, but biopsy is unlikely to be informative.

Tertiary syphilis

Late-stage syphilis develops in many patients about 3 or more years after infection. The onset is insidious, and during

Fig. 12.13　Primary chancre. The lower lip is a typical site for extragenital chancres but they are rarely seen.

Fig. 12.14　Tertiary syphilis; gummas of the palate. Necrosis in the centre of the palate has caused perforation of the bone and two typical round punched-out holes.

Table 12.2 Interpretation of serological tests for syphilis

VDRL	FTA-ABS	Usual interpretation
+	−	False-positive
+	+	Active syphilis
−	+	Treated syphilis

the latent period the patient may appear well. A characteristic lesion is the gumma.

Clinically, a gumma, which may affect the palate, tongue or tonsils, can vary from a few to several centimetres in diameter. It begins as a swelling, sometimes with a yellowish centre which undergoes necrosis, leaving a painless indolent deep ulcer. The ulcer is rounded, with soft, punched-out edges. The floor is depressed and pale (wash-leather) in appearance. It eventually heals with severe scarring which may distort the soft palate or tongue, or perforate the hard palate (Fig. 12.14) or destroy the uvula.

Microscopically, there may be no more than a predominance of plasma cells in the inflammatory infiltrate (a common finding in oral lesions) but associated with peri- or endarteritis. Granuloma formation is rare. Also rarely, there may be diffuse chronic inflammatory infiltration of the lingual muscles or coagulative necrosis mimicking caseation. However, the appearances can be completely non-specific. Diagnosis therefore depends on the serological findings.

Leukoplakia of the tongue may also develop during this late stage (Ch. 16) and other effects of syphilis such as aortitis, tabes or general paralysis of the insane may be associated.

Management

Serological confirmation of the infection is essential (Table 12.2). Tests are either specific (such as the FTA-ABS) or non-specific as in the VDRL. The VDRL becomes positive 4–6 weeks after infection and becomes negative only after effective treatment, but false positives can result from several other causes. The FTA-ABS acts as a check against false positive or negative results, but remains positive despite effective treatment for the life of the individual.

The Rapid Plasma Reagin (RPR) titre may also be high in active syphilis, but it is also a non-specific (lipoidal antigen) test. Specific tests include the *Treponema pallidum* haemagglutination assay (THPA), the fluorescent treponemal antibody absorption test (FTA-abs test) and the treponemal enzyme-linked immunosorbent assay (ELISA). Specific and non-specific tests are used in combination to distinguish active syphilis from false positives.

Antibiotics, particularly penicillin, are the mainstay of treatment, but tetracycline and erythromycin are also effective. Treatment should be by a specialist and must be continued until non-specific serological reactions (VDRL) are persistently negative.

CAT-SCRATCH DISEASE

See Chapter 26.

CANDIDOSIS[1]

Candidal infection can cause a spectrum of lesions (Box 12.4) particularly thrush, chronic white plaques (chronic hyperplastic candidosis, 'candidal leukoplakia') or erythematous areas such as denture stomatitis.

Box 12.4 Spectrum of oral candidosis

Acute candidosis
- Thrush
- Acute antibiotic stomatitis

Chronic candidosis
- Denture-induced stomatitis
- Chronic hyperplastic candidosis (Ch. 16)
- Chronic mucocutaneous candidosis (Ch. 15)
- Erythematous candidosis

Angular stomatitis (common to all types of oral candidosis)

Thrush[2] → Summaries pp. 220, 277

Thrush, a disease recognised in infants by Hippocrates, can also affect adults. In the 19th century, Trousseau called thrush a 'disease of the diseased'; this has been dramatically confirmed by its frequency in HIV disease.

Factors predisposing to candidal infection are shown in Box 12.5.

Box 12.5 Oral candidosis: important predisposing factors

- Immunodeficiency (diabetes mellitus or AIDS particularly) or immunosuppression (including steroid inhalers)
- Anaemia
- Suppression of the normal oral flora by antibacterial drugs
- Xerostomia
- Denture wearing
- Smoking

Neonatal thrush results from immaturity of the immune response and infection is probably acquired during passage through the birth canal. Any adult male who develops thrush without apparent cause should be suspected of having HIV infection. However, any form of candidosis can be secondary to HIV infection.

Clinical features

Thrush forms soft, friable and creamy coloured plaques on the mucosa (Fig. 12.15). The distinctive feature is that they can

[1]Candid*osis* not 'candid*iasis*' because it is a my*cosis*. The '-iases' are in general parasitic infections such as trypanosomiasis.
[2]Thrush is not a mere nickname or household term but is of respectable antiquity though its origin is uncertain.

be easily wiped off to expose an erythematous mucosa. Their extent varies from isolated small flecks to widespread confluent plaques. Angular stomatitis is frequently associated, as it is with any form of intraoral candidosis.

Pathology

A Gram-stained smear shows large masses of tangled hyphae, detached epithelial cells and leucocytes (Fig. 12.16). Biopsy shows hyperplastic epithelium infiltrated by inflammatory oedema and cells, predominantly neutrophils. Staining with PAS shows many candidal hyphae growing down through the epithelial cells to the junction of the plaque with the spinous cell layer (Fig. 12.17). At this level there is a concentration of inflammatory exudate and inflammatory cells. More deeply, the epithelium is hyperplastic but attenuated, with long slender processes extending down into the corium, surrounded by a light infiltrate predominantly lymphoplasmacytic.

The microscopic appearances explain both the friable nature of the plaques of thrush and their ready detachment.

Key features are summarised in Box 12.6.

Fig. 12.15 Thrush. The lesions consist of soft, creamy patches or flecks lying superficially on an erythematous mucosa. This soft palate distribution is particularly frequent in those using steroid inhalers.

Fig. 12.16 Direct smear from thrush. The tangled mass of Gram-positive hyphae of *Candida albicans* is diagnostic. A few yeast cells may be present as well, but it is the large number of hyphae that is diagnostic.

> **Box 12.6 Thrush: key features**
>
> * Acute candidosis
> * Secondary to various predisposing factors (Box 12.5)
> * Common in HIV infection and indicates low immunity
> * Creamy soft patches, readily wiped off the mucosa
> * Smear shows many Gram-positive hyphae
> * Histology shows hyphae invading superficial epithelium with proliferative and inflammatory response
> * Responds to topical antifungals or itraconazole

Management

Control of any local cause such as topical antibiotic treatment may alone cause thrush to resolve. If not, a course of nystatin or amphotericin lozenges should allow the oral microflora to return to normal. Failure of resonse to topical antifungals such as nystatin suggests immune deficiency. HIV infection should always be suspected when thrush is seen in an adult male in whom there is no other detectable cause. In such patients, candidosis may respond to fluconazole or itraconazole, but is typically associated with a low CD4 count and indicates a poor prognosis.

Rarely, persistent thrush is an early sign of chronic mucocutaneous candidosis such as candida-endocrinopathy syndrome (Ch. 15).

Fig. 12.17 Thrush. At high power the components of a plaque may be clearly seen. The surface layers of the epithelium are separated by inflammatory oedema and are colonised by fungal hyphae (A) and infiltrated by neutrophils (B).

Angular stomatitis → Summary p. 220

Angular stomatitis is typically caused by leakage of candida-infected saliva at the angles of the mouth. It can be seen in infantile thrush, in denture wearers or in association with chronic hyperplastic candidosis. It is a characteristic sign of candidal infection.

Clinically, there is mild inflammation at the angles of the mouth. In elderly patients with denture-induced stomatitis, inflammation frequently extends along folds of the facial skin extending from the angles of the mouth (Fig. 12.18). These folds have frequently, but unjustifiably, been ascribed to 'closed bite' but, in fact, are due to sagging of the facial tissues with age. Furrows at the angles of the mouth are made deeper by loss of vertical dimension and by loss of support to the upper lip by resorption of the underlying bone. Though establishment of correct vertical dimension and increasing the thickness of the labial flange of the upper denture can slightly lessen these furrows, they can rarely be eliminated in this way. Plastic surgery is required when patients are anxious to have these signs of age removed.

Treatment of intraoral candidal infection alone causes angular stomatitis to resolve. If there is co-infection with *S. aureus*, local application of fusidic acid cream may be required.

Denture-induced stomatitis → Summaries pp. 220, 279

A well-fitting upper denture cuts off the underlying mucosa from the protective action of saliva. In susceptible patients, particularly smokers, this can promote candidosis, seen as a symptomless area of erythema. The erythema is sharply limited to the area of mucosa occluded by a well-fitting upper denture or even an orthodontic plate (Fig. 12.19). Similar inflammation is not seen under the more mobile lower denture which allows a relatively free flow of saliva beneath it. Angular stomatitis is frequently associated and may form the chief complaint.

Smoking also appears to increase susceptibility to this infection.

In the past, denture-induced stomatitis was ascribed to 'allergy' to denture base material, but there is no foundation for this fancy. Methylmethacrylate monomer is mildly sensitising, but even the rare individuals sensitised to it can wear the polymerised material without any reaction.

Pathology

Gram-stained smears show candidal hyphae and some yeast forms which have proliferated in the interface between denture base and mucosa. Histologically, there is typically mild acanthosis with prominent blood vessels superficially and a mild chronic inflammatory infiltrate. The inflammation is probably a response to enzymes such as phospholipases produced by this fungus.

Management

The clinical picture is distinctive, but the diagnosis can be confirmed by finding candidal hyphae in a Gram-stained smear taken from the inflamed mucosa or the fitting surface of the denture. Quantification of candida in saliva is of little value as candidal carriage is common and counts are higher in denture wearers. The infection responds to antifungal drugs, but topical agents such as nystatin or amphotericin can only gain access to the palate if the patient leaves out the denture while the tablets are allowed to dissolve in the mouth.

Porosity in methylmethacrylate denture base also harbours *C. albicans* and dentures may therefore form a reservoir which can reinfect the mucosa. Elimination of *C. albicans* from the denture base is important and can be achieved by soaking the denture in 0.1% hypochlorite or dilute chlorhexidine overnight.

A simpler alternative is to coat the fitting surface of the denture with miconazole gel or varnish while it is being worn. The denture should be removed and scrubbed clean at intervals and miconazole re-applied three times a day. This treatment should be continued until the inflammation has cleared and *C. albicans* has been eliminated. This is likely to take 1–2 weeks, but patients should be warned not to continue this treatment indefinitely.

Fig. 12.18 Angular stomatitis. Cracking and erythema at the commissure is due to leakage of saliva containing *C. albicans*, constantly reinfecting the lesion.

Fig. 12.19 Typical denture stomatitis. Clear demarcation between the erythema of the mucosa covered, in this instance, by an orthodontic appliance. The pallor of the palate behind the posterior margin is clearly seen.

It should be noted that resistance to miconazole is growing. Also the oral gel is absorbed and, like other imidazole antifungal drugs, enhances the anticoagulant effect of warfarin.

Lack of response may be due to poor patient compliance or to an underlying disorder, particularly iron deficiency. If candidal infection is unusually florid or associated with patches of thrush, a blood picture should be requested. Itraconazole or fluconazole orally have a systemic effect and can be used for resistant cases, but topical treatment is safer, less expensive and usually satisfactory.

Key features are summarised in Box 12.7.

Box 12.7   Denture-induced stomatitis: key features

- Candidal infection promoted by well-fitting upper denture
- Enclosed mucosa is cut off from protective action of saliva
- Mucosal erythema sharply restricted to area covered by the denture
- Angular stomatitis frequently associated
- Hyphae proliferate in denture–mucosa interface
- Smear shows Gram-positive hyphae
- Resolves after elimination of *C. albicans* by antifungal treatment

---

Acute antibiotic stomatitis → Summary p. 220

This can follow overuse or topical oral use of antibiotics, especially tetracycline, suppressing normal, competing oral flora. It is infrequently seen now. Clinically, the whole mucosa is red and sore. Flecks of thrush may be present. Resolution may follow withdrawal of the antibiotic but is accelerated by topical antifungal treatment.

Generalised candidal erythema, which is clinically similar, can also be a consequence of xerostomia which promotes candidal infection. It is a typical complication of Sjögren's syndrome. Nystatin suspension or miconazole gel held in the mouth is usually effective.

Erythematous candidosis → Summaries pp. 220, 279

This term applies to patchy red mucosal macules due to *C. albicans* infection in HIV-positive patients (see Fig. 24.3). Favoured sites, in order of frequency, are the hard palate, dorsum of the tongue and soft palate.

Treatment with itraconazole is usually effective.

SUGGESTED FURTHER READING

Alam F, Argiriadou AS, Hodgson TA et al 2000 Primary syphilis remains a cause of oral ulceration. Br Dent J 189:352–354

Alrabiah FA, Sacks SL 1996 New antiherpesvirus agents. Their targets and therapeutic potential. Drugs 52:17–32

Cawson RA, Binnie WH, Barrett AW, Wright J 2001 Oral disease, 3rd edn. Mosby-Wolfe, London

Drew WL 2000 Ganciclovir resistance: a matter of time and titre. Lancet 355:609–610

Epstein JB, Sherlock CH, Wolber RA 1993 Oral manifestations of cytomegalovirus infection. Oral Surg Oral Med Oral Pathol 75:443–451

Glesby MJ, Moore RD, Chaisson RE 1995 Clinical spectrum of herpes zoster in adults infected with human immunodeficiency virus. Clin Infect Dis 21:370–375

Jones AC, Freedman PD, Phelan JA, Baughman RA, Kerpel SM 1993 Cytomegalovirus infections of the oral cavity. Oral Surg Oral Med Oral Pathol 75:76–85

Nachbar FN, Classen V, Nachbar T et al 1996 Orificial tuberculosis detection by polymerase chain reaction. Br J Dermatol 135:106–109

Regezi JA, Eversole R, Barker BF et al 1996 Herpes simplex and cytomegalovirus coinfected ulcers in HIV-positive patients. Oral Surg Oral Med Oral Pathol Oral Radiol Endod 81:55–62

Whitley RJ, Weiss H, Gnann JW 1996 Acyclovir with and without prednisone for the treatment of herpes zoster. A randomized, placebo-controlled trial. Ann Intern Med 125:376–383

**APPENDIX
12.1**

Treatment of candidosis

Confirm diagnosis with smear (most types) or biopsy (chronic hyperplastic candidosis) unless presentation is typical	
Check history for predisposing causes which may require treatment	
If candidosis is recurrent or not responsive to treatment, test for anaemia, folate and vitamin B_{12} deficiency and perform a urine test for diabetes	

If a denture is worn:

- Stop night-time wear
- Check denture hygiene and advise
- Soak denture overnight in antifungal (dilute hypochlorite, chlorhexidine mouthwash) or, less effective, apply miconazole gel to denture fit surface while worn

If a steroid inhaler is used, check it is being used correctly, preferably with a spacer. Advise to rinse mouth out after use

Drug treatments

Presentation	Generalised acute or chronic	Chronic hyperplastic form	Angular stomatitis	Immunosuppression or otherwise resistant to treatment*
Drug of choice and regime	Nystatin 100 000 units QDS for 7–10 days as suspension or pastilles *or* amphotericin 10 mg QDS as lozenges or suspension 10–14 days	Miconazole gel 24 mg/ml. Apply QDS	Apply miconazole gel 24 mg/ml QDS to the angles of the mouth 10 days or fusidic acid cream	Consider fluconazole 50 mg/day for 7–14 days (longer in immunosuppression) or itraconazole
Notes	Amphotericin is generally preferred over nystatin which has an unpleasant taste	Only effective if lesion accessible for application. For recurrent infection in white patches fluconazole may be required simultaneously	Must treat intraoral infection simultaneously. This is always present even if not evident	Itraconazole (100 mg/day for 14 days) has a higher risk of adverse effects
Cautions	Neither has any significant unwanted effects	Significant doses may be absorbed if applied to denture fit surface. Avoid in pregnancy. Potentiates warfarin anticoagulation, numerous other but less frequent effects	No adverse effects if only small amounts are applied as described above	Avoid in pregnancy and renal disease. Numerous drug interactions possible

If there is conspicuous papillary hyperplasia of the palate, consider treatment (cryosurgery or excision) after treatment when inflammation has subsided. The irregular surface predisposes to recurrence of candidosis.

*Candidal resistance to azole drugs is possible but failure of treatment is more likely to result from non-compliance with local measures such as denture wear and cleaning or an untreated underlying condition

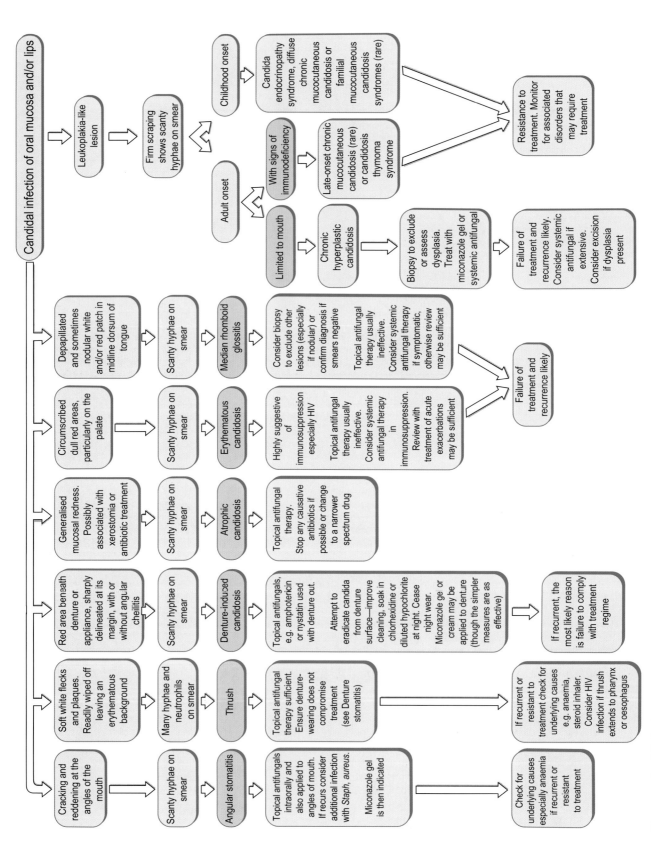

Summary chart 12.1 Summary of the types of oral candidal infection and their management.

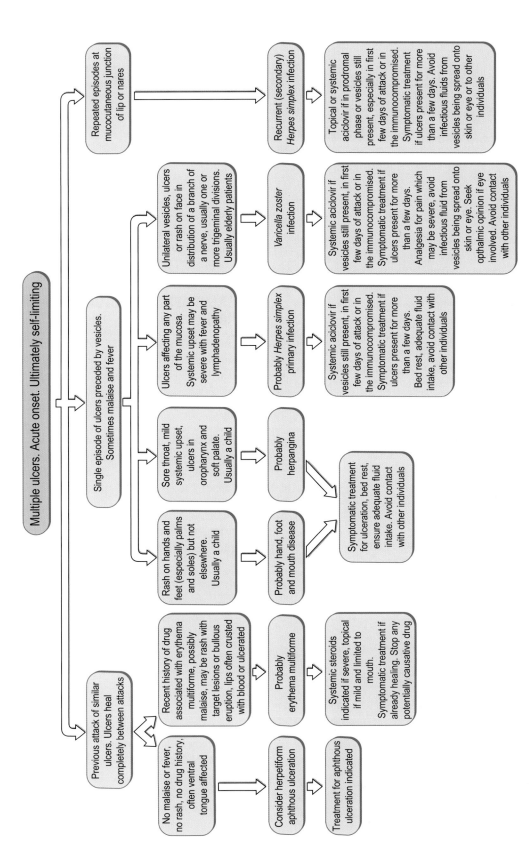

Summary chart 12.2 Differential diagnosis and management of the common and important causes of multiple oral ulcers with acute onset.

Diseases of the oral mucosa: non-infective stomatitis

TRAUMATIC ULCERS → Summaries pp. 246, 247

Traumatic ulcers are usually caused by biting, denture trauma or chemical trauma and arise at trauma-prone sites such as lip, buccal mucosa or adjacent to a denture flange. They are tender, have a yellowish-grey floor of fibrin slough and red margins (Figs. 13.1 and 13.35). Inflammation, swelling and erythema are variable, depending on the cause and time since trauma. There is no induration unless the site is scarred from repeated episodes of trauma. If caused by the sharp edge of a broken-down tooth, they are usually on the tongue or buccal mucosa. Occasionally, a large ulcer is caused by biting after a dental local anaesthetic (see Fig. 33.1).

Traumatic ulcers heal a few days after elimination of the cause. If they persist for more than 7–10 days, or there is any other cause for suspicion as to the cause, biopsy should be carried out.

LINGUAL PAPILLITIS

This condition, also known as transient lingual papillitis or fungiform papillitis, is common but patients rarely seek treatment. One or a cluster of fungiform papillae become slightly swollen, white and intensely painful to touch. The condition

Fig. 13.1   A large traumatic ulcer on the lower lip. Note the colour of the fibrin slough, distinct from the keratin of a white patch, and the well-defined epithelial margin with minimal inflammation.

resolves spontaneously after a few days, sometimes after only one. The cause is unknown but trauma and certain foods are usually blamed. Biopsy does not aid diagnosis.

RECURRENT APHTHOUS STOMATITIS (RECURRENT APHTHAE) → Summaries pp. 221, 246

Recurrent aphthae constitute the most common oral mucosal disease and affect 10–25% of the population, but many cases are mild and no attention is sought for their relief.

Aetiology

The main factors thought to contribute are shown in Box 13.1.

Genetic factors   There is some evidence for a genetic predisposition. The family history is sometimes positive and the disease appears to affect identical twins more frequently than

---

Box 13.1   Possible aetiological factors for recurrent aphthae

- Genetic predisposition
- Exaggerated response to trauma
- Infections
- Immunological abnormalities
- Gastrointestinal disorders
- Haematological deficiencies
- Hormonal disturbances
- Stress

---

non-identical. However, this probably applies to a minority. A variety of HLA associations have been reported, but no one haplotype seems to be consistently associated. In the possibly related Behçet's disease (see below), the evidence for a genetic predisposition is much stronger.

Trauma   Some patients think that the ulcers result from trauma because the early symptoms simulate pricking of the mucosa by (for instance) a toothbrush bristle. Trauma may dictate the site of ulcers in patients who already have the disorder, but most aphthae are in relatively protected sites and the masticatory mucosa is generally spared.

Infections There is no evidence that aphthae are directly due to any microbes and there is scanty evidence that cross-reacting antigens from streptococci or L-forms play any significant role. The hypothesis that there may be defective immunoregulation caused by herpes or other viruses is unproven.

Immunological abnormalities Since the aetiology of recurrent aphthae is unknown, there has been a facile tendency to label them as 'autoimmune'. A great variety of immunological abnormalities have been reported, but there have been almost as many contrary findings and no convincing theory of immunopathogenesis takes into account the clinical features. It is also possible that the immunological abnormalities are as much a consequence of the ulcers as the cause. Evidence of an association with atopic (IgE-mediated) disease is unconfirmed. Circulating antibodies to crude extracts of fetal oral mucosa have been reported, but their titre is unrelated to the severity of the disease and, in many patients, there are no significant changes in immunoglobulin levels. Antibody-dependent cytotoxic mechanisms have been postulated, but not convincingly demonstrated. The histological features of aphthae (see below) have also been invoked to support hypotheses that the disease is either an immune complex-mediated (type III) or a cell-mediated (type IV) reaction according to taste. However, others have failed to confirm the presence of circulating immune complexes and, in any case, the significance of such complexes, which are sometimes detectable in the absence of disease, is notoriously difficult to interpret. Depressed circulating helper/suppressor T-lymphocyte ratios have been reported, but others have found no difference between active and remittant phases of the disorder. Recurrent aphthae also lack virtually all features of and any association with typical autoimmune diseases (Ch. 23). They also fail to respond reliably to immunosuppressive drugs and become more severe in the immune deficiency state induced by HIV infection.

Gastrointestinal disease Aphthae were previously known as 'dyspeptic ulcers', but are only rarely associated with gastrointestinal disease. Any association is usually because of a deficiency, particularly of vitamin B_{12} or folate secondary to malabsorption. An association with coeliac disease (sometimes asymptomatic) has been found in approximately 5% of patients with aphthae, but a secondary haematinic deficiency, particularly folate deficiency, is probably the cause.

Haematological deficiencies Deficiencies of vitamin B_{12}, folate, or iron have been reported in up to 20% of patients with aphthae. Such deficiencies are probably more frequent in patients whose aphthae start or worsen in middle age or later. In many such patients, the deficiency is latent, the haemoglobin is within normal limits and the main sign is micro- or macrocytosis of the red cells. In patients who thus prove to be vitamin B_{12} or folate deficient, remedying the deficiency may bring rapid resolution of the ulcers.

Hormonal factors In a few women, aphthae are associated with the stressful luteal phase of the menstrual cycle, but there is no strong evidence that hormone treatment is reliably effective.

'Stress' Some patients relate exacerbations of ulceration to times of stress and some studies have reported a correlation. However, stress is notoriously difficult to quantify and some studies have found no correlation.

HIV infection Aphthous stomatitis is a recognised feature of HIV infection. Its frequency and severity are related to the degree of immune deficiency, as discussed later.

Non-smoking It has long been established that recurrent aphthae are a disease, almost exclusively, of non-smokers. And this is one of the few consistent findings. Recurrent aphthae may also start when smoking is abandoned. The reasons are unclear but it is believed that smoking has a systemic protective action against this disease.

In brief, therefore, the aetiology of recurrent aphthae is unclear. There is no evidence that they are a form of autoimmune disease in any accepted sense and it is uncertain whether many of the reported immunological abnormalities are cause or effect. However, in a minority of patients there is a clear association with haematological deficiencies. The latter, in turn, may be secondary to small-intestine disease or other cause of malabsorption.

That speculation about the cause of recurrent aphthae has continued for at least half a century, the variety of current theories and the contradictory findings indicate how little is known.

Clinical features

Typical features of recurrent aphthae are summarised in Box 13.2.

Females are not significantly more frequently affected than males. The frequency of ulceration typically reaches a peak in early adult life or a little later, then gradually wanes.

Box 13.2 Typical features of recurrent aphthae

- Onset frequently in childhood but peak in adolescence or early adult life
- Attacks at variable but sometimes relatively regular intervals
- Most patients are otherwise healthy
- A few have haematological defects
- Most patients are non-smokers
- Usually self-limiting eventually

Recurrent aphthae are rare in the elderly, particularly the edentulous. However, older persons may be affected if a haematological deficiency develops. The great majority of patients are clerical, semi-professional, or professional workers and are total non-smokers. Occasionally, aphthae start when smoking is given up.

The usual history is of painful ulcers recurring at intervals of approximately 3 to 4 weeks. Occasionally, they are continuously present. Unpredictable remissions of several months may be noted. Individual minor aphthae persist for 7–10 days then heal without scarring. Aphthae typically affect only the non-keratinised mucosa such as the buccal mucosa, sulcuses, or lateral borders of the tongue, but major aphthae can affect the masticatory mucosa. Ulcers are of three clinically distinguishable types (Box 13.3).

Box 13.3   Types of recurrent aphthae

Minor aphthae (Fig. 13.2)
- The most common type
- Non-keratinised mucosa affected
- Ulcers are shallow, rounded, 5–7 mm across, with an erythematous margin and yellowish floor
- One or several ulcers may be present

Major aphthae (Fig. 13.3)
- Uncommon
- Ulcers frequently several centimetres across
- Sometimes mimic a malignant ulcer
- Ulcers persist for several months
- Masticatory mucosa such as the dorsum of the tongue or occasionally the gingivae may be involved
- Scarring may follow healing (Fig. 13.4)

Herpetiform aphthae (Fig. 13.5)
- Uncommon
- Non-keratinised mucosa affected
- Ulcers are 1–2 mm across
- Dozens or hundreds may be present
- May coalesce to form irregular ulcers
- Widespread bright erythema round the ulcers

The pain of major aphthae can interfere with eating. Moreover, major aphthae are sometimes a feature of HIV disease and add to such patients' burdens.

Pathology

There is alleged to be initial lymphocytic infiltration followed by destruction of the epithelium and infiltration of the tissues by neutrophils. Mononuclear cells may also surround blood vessels (perivascular cuffing). These changes are said to be

Fig. 13.3   Aphthous stomatitis, major type. This large, deep ulcer with considerable surrounding erythema has been present for several weeks.

Fig. 13.4   Recurrent aphthous stomatitis, major type. The same ulcer shown in Figure 13.3, but healing. The ulcer is much smaller but there is scarring and puckering of the surrounding mucosa.

Fig. 13.5   Recurrent aphthous stomatitis, herpetiform type. There are numerous small, rounded and pinpoint ulcers, some of which are coalescing. The surrounding mucosa is lightly erythematous and the overall picture is highly suggestive of viral infection, but the attacks are recurrent and no virus can be isolated.

Fig. 13.2   Aphthous stomatitis, minor form. A single, relatively large shallow ulcer in a typical site. There is a narrow band of periulcer erythema. These features are non-specific and the diagnosis must be made primarily on the basis of the history.

consistent with either type III or IV reactions, but true vasculitis is not seen. Overall, the appearances are non-specific (Fig. 13.6).

Biopsy is of no value in the diagnosis except to exclude carcinoma in the case of major aphthae. Aphthae are not preceded by vesiculation and smears readily distinguish herpetiform aphthae from herpetic ulceration.

Diagnosis and management

The most important diagnostic feature is the history of recurrences of self-healing ulcers at fairly regular intervals (Table 13.1). The only other condition with this history is Behçet's disease. Usually, increasing frequency of ulcers brings the patient to seek treatment. Otherwise, most patients appear well, but haematological investigation is particularly important in older patients. Routine blood indices are informative and usually the most important finding is an abnormal mean corpuscular volume (MCV). If macro- or microcytosis is present, further investigation is necessary to find and remedy the cause. Treatment of vitamin B_{12} deficiency or folate deficiency is sometimes sufficient to control or abolish aphthae.

Apart from the minority with underlying systemic disease, treatment is empirical and palliative only. Despite numerous clinical trials, no medication gives completely reliable relief. Patients should therefore be made to understand that the trouble may not be curable, but can usually be alleviated and usually resolves eventually of its own accord.

Corticosteroids Some patients get relief from Corlan (hydrocortisone hemisuccinate 2.5 mg) pellets allowed to dissolve in the mouth three times a day. Corticosteroids are unlikely to hasten healing of existing ulcers, but probably reduce the painful inflammation. The most rational form of treatment is for patients to take these pellets continuously (whether or not ulcers are present) to enable the corticosteroid to act in the very early, asymptomatic stages. This regimen is only applicable

Table 13.1 Check-list for diagnosis of recurrent aphthae

	Check for	Comments
History	• Recurrences • Pattern? Minor, major or herpetiform type? • Onset as child or teenager • Family history • Distribution only on non-keratinised mucosa • Signs or symptoms of Behçet's disease (ocular, genital, skin, joint lesions (Box 13.4)	The history is all-important
Examination	• Discrete well-defined ulcers • Scarring or soft palate involvement suggesting major aphthae	Exclude other diseases with specific, appearances, e.g. lichen planus or vesiculobullous disease
Special investigations	• Anaemia, iron, red cell folate and vitamin B_{12} status • History of diarrhoea, constipation or blood in stools suggesting gastrointestinal disease, e.g. coeliac disease or malabsorption	Used to exclude underlying conditions, especially in patients with onset in later life

to those who have frequent ulcers (at 2- or 3-week intervals or more frequently). This should be tried for 2 months then stopped for a month to assess any improvement and whether there is any deterioration without treatment.

Triamcinolone dental paste This is a corticosteroid in a vehicle which sticks to the moist mucosa. When correctly applied the vehicle absorbs moisture and forms an adhesive gel which can remain in place for one or several hours, but it is difficult to apply a fragment of this paste to the ulcer and to get it to adhere firmly. It is only useful for patients with infrequent ulcers, for ulcers near the front of the mouth and for patients dextrous enough to be able to follow the instructions. This gel should form a protective layer over the ulcer to help make it comfortable. The corticosteroid is slowly released and has an anti-inflammatory action. Another alternative is the use of a corticosteroid asthma spray to deposit a potent corticosteroid over the ulcer. Topical corticosteroids used as described have no systemic effect.

Tetracycline mouth rinses Trials in both Britain and the USA showed that tetracycline rinses significantly reduced both the frequency and severity of aphthae. For herpetiform aphthae particularly, the contents of a tetracycline capsule (250 mg) can be stirred in a little water and held in the mouth for 2–3 minutes, three times daily. Some patients like to use this mouth rinse

Fig. 13.6 Recurrent aphtha. Section of an early ulcer showing the break in the epithelium, the inflammatory cells in the floor and the inflammatory changes more deeply where numerous dilated vessels can be seen.

regularly for 3 days each week if they have frequent ulcers. An antifungal drug may also need to be given to patients who are susceptible to superinfection by *Candida albicans*.

Chlorhexidine A 0.2% solution has also been used as a mouth rinse for aphthae. Used three times daily after meals and held in the mouth for at least 1 minute, it has been claimed to reduce the duration and discomfort of aphthous stomatitis. Zinc sulphate or zinc chloride solutions may also have a slight beneficial effect.

Topical salicylate preparations Salicylates have an anti-inflammatory action and also have local effects. Preparations of choline salicylate in a gel can be applied to aphthae. These preparations, which are available over the counter, sometimes appear to be helpful.

Possible treatments for recurrent aphthae are summarised in Appendix 13.1.

Treatment of major aphthae Major aphthae, whether or not there is underlying disease such as HIV infection, may sometimes be so painful, persistent and resistant to conventional treatment as to be disabling. Reportedly effective treatments include azathioprine, cyclosporin, colchicine and dapsone, but thalidomide is probably most reliably effective. Their use may be justified for major aphthae even in otherwise healthy persons if they are disabled by the pain and difficulty of eating. However, thalidomide can cause severe adverse effects and is strongly teratogenic and, like the other drugs mentioned, can only be given under specialist supervision.

BEHÇET'S DISEASE → Summary p. 246

Behçet's syndrome was originally defined as a triad of oral aphthae, genital ulceration and uveitis. However, it is a multisystem disorder with varied manifestations and now termed Behçet's disease. It is rare in the UK and USA, but is particularly common in Turkey (Behçet was a Turk) and very common in Japan. It is said that a high prevalance of Behçet's disease exists in races along the Silk Road[1] but this is only a vague generalisation.

The aetiology is unknown but it has features, such as circulating immune complexes, suggesting immune complex disease, but any antigen remains unidentified, though there is some evidence for involvement of a virus, possibly herpes simplex. The immunological changes are similar to those found in aphthous stomatitis.

Patients are usually young adult males between 20 and 40 years old. Patients suffer one of four patterns of disease, namely:

1. Mucocutaneous (oral and genital ulceration)
2. Arthritic (joint involvement with or without mucocutaneous involvement)

3. Neurological (with or without other features) or
4. Ocular (with or without other features).

The racial distribution suggests a strong genetic component and this is confirmed by the fact that each of these presentations is linked to a different HLA tissue type. HLA-B12 and/or DR2 types, for example, are linked to mucocutaneous and arthritic disease. Unfortunately, these HLA associations are of no value in diagnosis, but HLA-B51 is useful as a predictor of ocular lesions, which can lead to blindness. There is also an association with HLA-B5 and HLA-B51(B5101). Diagnostic criteria are listed in Box 13.4.

Oral aphthae are the most consistent feature and are not distinguishable from common aphthae. They are frequently the first manifestation. Behçet's disease should therefore be considered in the differential diagnosis of aphthous stomatitis, particularly in patients in an at-risk racial group, and the

---

Box 13.4   Diagnostic criteria for Behçet's disease

Major criteria
- Recurrent oral aphthae
- Genital ulceration
- Eye lesions (recurrent hypopyon, iritis or iridocyclitis; chorioretinitis)
- Skin lesions (erythema nodosum, subcutaneous thrombophlebitis, hyperirritability)

Minor criteria
- Arthralgia or arthritis
- Gastrointestinal lesions
- Vascular lesions (mainly thrombotic) (Fig. 13.7)
- Central nervous system involvement

Fig. 13.7   Thrombophlebitis in Behçet's disease. Inflammation and pigmentation highlight the sites of veins (arrow) and their valves. This is only one of several possible skin manifestations.

---

[1]The Silk Road was a caravan route, 4000 miles long mostly through desperately inhospitable country, from China to the Lebanon and thence to Western Europe. As well as silk, gold, silver and jewels were brought to Europe. Ideas also travelled and Buddhism for example was brought to China from India.

medical history should be checked for the features shown in Box 13.4. The frequency of other manifestations is highly variable. As a result there are no absolute criteria or reliable tests for the diagnosis, but aphthous stomatitis in combination with any two of the other major features can be regarded as adequate.

Special tests are not helpful in diagnosis, apart from the pathergy test. The test is positive if there is an exaggerated response to a sterile needle puncture of the skin. However, the test must be interpreted by an experienced clinician and tends to be positive only in Mediterranean patients. Moreover, a positive pathergy test does not correlate with the presence of oral lesions or with the overall severity of the disease and is rarely positive in UK patients. It is also not entirely specific for Behçet's disease.

The importance of making the diagnosis is indicated by the life-threatening nature of thrombosis and the risk of blindness or brain damage.

The main pathological finding is vasculitis and anti-endothelial cell (aEC) antibodies are reportedly found in 50% of those with active disease, but their role remains uncertain. The aetiology is largely speculative, but lesions may result from immune-complex mediated vasculitis of small vessels which is said to be present in mucocutaneous and all types of lesion. However, microscopic evidence of vasculitis in the oral ulcers is open to question.

Management

Treatment is difficult and requires a multidisciplinary approach. The oral ulceration may be treated in the same way as the common form. When major aphthae are particularly severe or if there is frequent recurrence, colchicine may be helpful but thalidomide may be most effective particularly for HIV-associated aphthae.

NICORANDIL-INDUCED ORAL ULCERATION

The potassium channel activator Nicorandil, used for angina, causes ulcers very similar to major aphthae but without the recurrent pattern.

Ulcers appear within a year of starting the drug, often a few weeks, and are usually solitary on the lateral tongue, buccal mucosa, gingivae or fauces. They persist for several months unless the drug is withdrawn, when they heal within a few weeks depending on their size. Biopsy shows only non-specific inflammatory features and does not aid diagnosis other than to exclude other causes.

HIV-ASSOCIATED ORAL ULCERATION

Patients with HIV infection (Ch. 24) are susceptible to severe recurrent aphthae which are not otherwise distinguishable from common aphthae. With declining immune function, the ulcers become more frequent and severe and, by interfering with

eating, may contribute to the patient's deterioration. Biopsies should be taken to exclude opportunistic infections, otherwise the aetiology is unknown. Treatment with thalidomide is most frequently effective but, in some cases, cytomegalovirus can be seen in biopsies, and treatment with ganciclovir may be more appropriate.

Necrotising gingival ulceration may also be seen.

LICHEN PLANUS → Summaries pp. 232, 246, 247, 277, 278, 279

Lichen planus is a common chronic inflammatory disease of skin and mucous membranes. It mainly affects patients of middle age or over. Oral lesions have characteristic appearances and distribution.

Aetiology

In spite of histological changes which can be diagnostic, the aetiology of lichen planus remains problematical. The predominantly T-lymphocyte infiltrate suggests cell-mediated immunological damage to the epithelium and a plethora of immunological abnormalities has been reported. Though it has not been possible to demonstrate humoral or lymphocytotoxic mechanisms, the inflammatory infiltrate consists mainly of T-lymphocytes. Both CD4 and CD8 cells are present, but numbers of CD8 cells may rise with disease progression and they are more numerous in relation to the epithelium. Precise trigger mechanisms remain unclear, but lichen planus undoubtedly appears to be a T-lymphocyte mediated disorder.

Disease indistinguishable from lichen planus, induced by drugs (notably gold and anti-malarial agents), also suggests involvement of immunological mechanisms. Oral lichen planus is also a virtually invariable feature and an early sign of graft-versus-host disease (Ch. 23), but this does not clarify any immunological mechanisms.

In some countries, hepatitis C infection is thought to be contributory.

Clinical features

Typical features of lichen planus are summarised in Box 13.5.

The lesions' characteristic appearance and distribution should be taken into account in making the diagnosis.

Striae are most common and typically form sharply-defined snowy-white, lacy, starry, or annular patterns (Fig. 13.8). They may occasionally be interspersed with minute, white papules. Striae may not be palpable or may be firmer than the surrounding mucosa.

Atrophic areas are red areas of mucosal thinning (Fig. 13.9) and often combined with striae.

Erosions are shallow irregular areas of epithelial destruction. These also can be very persistent and may be covered by

Box 13.5   Oral lichen planus: typical features

- Females account for at least 65% of patients
- Patients usually over 40 years
- Untreated disease can persist for 10 or more years
- Lesions in combination or isolation, comprise:
  - Striae
  - Atrophic areas
  - Erosion
  - Plaques
- Common sites are:
  - Buccal mucosae
  - Dorsum of tongue
  - Gingivae (infrequently)
- Lesions usually bilateral and often symmetrical
- Cutaneous lesions only occasionally associated
- Usually, good response to corticosteroids

Fig. 13.9   Lichen planus, atrophic type. There are shallow irregular zones of erythema surrounded by poorly defined striae.

a smooth, slightly raised yellowish layer of fibrin (Fig. 13.10). The margins may be slightly depressed due to fibrosis and gradual healing at the periphery. Striae may radiate from the margins of these erosions.

Plaques are occasionally seen in the early stages particularly on the dorsum of the tongue. Otherwise they may result from persistent disease and mainly affect the buccal mucosa.

Distribution   The buccal mucous membranes, particularly posteriorly, are by far the most frequently affected, but lesions may spread forward almost to the commissures. The next most common site is the tongue, either the edges or the lateral margins of the dorsum, or less frequently the centre of the dorsum. The lips and gingivae may also occasionally be affected, but the floor of the mouth and palate usually escape. Lesions are very often symmetrical, sometimes strikingly so (Fig. 13.11).

Symptoms   Striae alone may be asymptomatic and unnoticed by the patient, or cause roughness or slight stiffness of the mucosa. Atrophic lesions are sore and erosions usually cause more severe symptoms still and may make eating difficult.

Fig. 13.10   Severe erosive lichen planus. Thick plaques of fibrin cover extensive ulcers on the dorsum of the tongue in this case.

Fig. 13.8   Lichen planus, striate pattern. This is the most common site and type of lesion, a lacy network of white striae on the buccal mucosa. The lesions are usually symmetrically distributed.

Fig. 13.11   Erosive lichen planus of the tongue. Two extensive areas of shallow ulceration have formed symmetrically on the tongue. Lingual involvement is seen usually in severe cases where the buccal mucosa and other sites are affected.

Gingival lichen planus → Summary p. 279

The gingivae are occasionally the only site of lichen planus which needs to be distinguished from other forms of gingivitis. Lesions are usually atrophic so that the gingivae appear shiny, inflamed and smooth ('desquamative gingivitis') (Fig. 13.12). Striae are uncommon on the gingivae but sometimes present in other parts of the mouth. Only limited segments of the gingivae may be affected.

Soreness caused by atrophic lesions makes toothbrushing difficult. Plaque accumulation and associated inflammatory changes appear to aggravate lichen planus. The contribution of local irritation to lichen planus is suggested by disappearance of the lesions when the teeth are extracted. Lichen planus of the denture-bearing area is virtually unknown.

Skin lesions

Lichen planus is a common skin disease, but skin lesions are uncommon in those who complain of oral symptoms. Skin lesions typically form purplish papules, 2–3 mm across with a glistening surface marked by minute fine striae and are usually itchy. Typical sites are the flexor surface of the forearms and especially the wrists (Fig. 13.13). Skin lesions help, but are not essential, to confirm the diagnosis of oral lichen planus.

Pathology

Corresponding with their clinical features, lesions fall into three distinct histological types (Box 13.6).

Typical histological features of atrophic lesions are summarised in Box 13.7 and shown in Figures 13.14–13.17.

Erosions merely show destruction of the epithelium, leaving only the fibrin-covered, granulating connective tissue floor of the lesion. Diagnosis depends on seeing atropic lesions or striae nearby.

Diagnosis

The diagnosis of lichen planus can usually be made on the history, the appearance of the lesions and their distribution.

Fig. 13.12 Desquamative gingivitis caused by lichen planus. A well-defined band of patchy erythema extends across the full width of the attached gingiva around several teeth. This change may be localised or widespread. Within the red areas faint white flecks and striae are sometimes visible.

Fig. 13.13 Dermal lichen planus. This, the flexor surface of the wrists, is a characteristic site. The lesions consist of confluent papules with a pattern of minute white striae on their surface.

Box 13.6 Lichen planus: typical histological features of white lesions (striae) (Figs 13.14–13.16)

- Hyperkeratosis or parakeratosis
- Saw-tooth profile of the rete ridges sometimes
- Liquefaction degeneration of the basal cell layer
- Compact, band-like lymphoplasmacytic (predominantly T-cell) infiltrate cells hugging the epithelio-mesenchymal junction
- CD8 lymphocytes predominate in relation to the epithelium

Fig. 13.14 Lichen planus. The rete ridges have the characteristic pointed (saw-tooth) outline which is frequent in the skin but uncommon in mucosal lichen planus.

227

However, dysplastic leukoplakias occasionally have a streaky whitish appearance. A biopsy should be taken, particularly when striae are ill-defined, plaques are present or the lesions are in any other ways unusual.

Fig. 13.15 **Lichen planus.** The basement membrane is thickened and lymphocytes from the dense infiltrate below emigrate into the basal cells of the epithelium where they are associated with focal basal cell degeneration.

Fig. 13.16 **Lichen planus.** Lymphocytes infiltrating the basal cells are associated with basal cell apoptosis, loss of a prominent basal cell layer and prickle cells abutting the basement membrane. A cluster of apoptotic bodies is visible (arrows), each consisting of a shrunken bright pink cell with a condensed and fragmented nucleus.

Box 13.7 Lichen planus: typical histological features of atrophic lesions (Fig. 13.17)

- Severe thinning and flattening of the epithelium
- Destruction of basal cells
- Compact band-like, subepithelial inflammatory infiltrate hugging the epithelio-mesenchymal junction

---

Management

Patients are sometimes concerned that lichen planus is infectious and should be reassured that this is not so.

Topical application of potent anti-inflammatory corticosteroids is usually effective but monitoring is required and these preparations are suitable only for hospital use. Possible alternatives are to use similar corticosteroids (such as beclomethasone) from aerosol inhalers used for asthma. Approximately six puffs each day from an inhaler can be used to deliver enough of the corticosteroid to an ulcer.

Potent corticosteroids used topically may occasionally promote thrush as a side-effect. Triamcinolone dental paste applied to the lesions is an alternative but less effective form of treatment. Gingival lichen planus is the most difficult to treat. The first essential is to maintain rigorous oral hygiene. Corticosteroids should also be used, as already described and, in this situation, triamcinolone dental paste may be useful as it can readily be applied to the affected gingivae. In cases unresponsive to corticosteroids, tacrolimus mouthrinses are likely to be effective. In exceptionally severe cases, if topical treatment fails, treatment with systemic corticosteroids is effective.

A checklist for the management of lichen planus is given in Box 13.8.

Lichenoid reactions → Summaries pp. 232, 247, 277, 278

This term is given to lichen planus-like lesions caused by either systemic drug treatment or those where the histological picture is not completely diagnostic.

A very wide range of drugs can cause lichenoid reactions of the skin, mucous membranes or both (Box 13.9). The clinical features are often indistinguishable from 'true' lichen planus and usually consist only of white striae. When there is severe atrophy or ulceration, detecting a possible causative drug may aid management and a complete drug history is mandatory in all patients thought to suffer from lichen planus. Some

Fig. 13.17 **Lichen planus.** The epithelium is atrophic and greatly thinned. A well-demarcated, dense, broad band of lymphocytes extends along the superficial corium immediately below the epithelium.

features which suggest a drug reaction are shown in Box 13.10.

In practice, it can be difficult or impossible to differentiate lichenoid reactions from lichen planus. Many patients are taking potentially causative drugs, sometimes more than one.

Box 13.8   Checklist for management of lichen planus

- Always check for drugs which might cause a lichenoid reaction. This is indistinguishable clinically but may respond to a change of medication
- When inflammation worsens or symptoms become more severe, consider the possibility of superinfection with *Candida*
- Biopsy lesions which appear unusual, form homogeneous plaques or are in unusual sites
- Check for skin lesions which may aid diagnosis
- Reassure patients that the condition is not usually of great consequence despite the fact that it can cause constant irritating soreness. Tell patients that the severity waxes and wanes unpredictably and the condition may persist for many years
- Be aware that squamous carcinoma may develop in lesions, although very rarely. Follow up lesions associated with reddening, and any unusual in site, appearance or severity

---

Box 13.9   Some drugs capable of causing lichenoid reactions

These are only the more common causes:
- Colloidal gold
- Beta-blockers
- Oral hypoglycaemics
- Allopurinol
- Non-steroidal anti-inflammatory drugs
- Antimalarials
- Methyldopa
- Penicillamine
- Some tricyclic antidepressants
- Thiazide diuretics
- Captopril

Box 13.10   Features suggesting a lichenoid reaction

- Onset associated with starting a drug
- Unilateral lesions or unusual distributions
- Unusual severity
- Widespread skin lesions
- Localised lesion in contact with a restoration

However, these may not be responsible as lichen planus is so common a disease that its presence may be coincidental. Also, the drugs often cannot be stopped because of possible medical adverse effects. Changing to another drug may not be helpful as the alternative may also cause a reaction.

Proof of causation requires withdrawal and rechallenge after healing, but the risk is hardly ever justified. Also, reactions

may persist months or years after administration (especially after colloidal gold injection). Often a causative drug is not even suspected because it has been taken without prescription.

Biopsy can sometimes distinguish lichenoid reactions, but the features are relatively subtle and not completely specific. While biopsy is of value to exclude other conditions, it cannot usually distinguish lichen planus from a lichenoid reaction.

Lichenoid reactions are treated in exactly the same way as lichen planus with withdrawal of drug(s) if possible. Thus, the absolute distinction between lichen planus and a lichenoid reaction is not always necessary for treatment.

Topical lichenoid reactions are most frequently responses to restorative materials, either amalgam or polymeric. The clinical appearances are similar or identical to lichen planus or lupus erythematosus, but lesions are localised to mucosa in contact, not just close to, restorations.

The more sharply defined a lesion is, the more atrophic or ulcerated, and the more closely related to a restoration, the more likely it is that removal of the restoration will be effective.

Corroded amalgam restorations are more likely to trigger reactions, but which components of restorative materials are responsible remains unclear. Several metals in amalgams are haptens and patients with amalgam reactions are more likely to show hypersensitivity to metals on skin testing. Another possible cause is the tiny particles of amalgam in the mucosa, thought to be the result of removal of amalgams by air turbine. However, amalgam particles buried beneath the mucosa frequently do not produce any reaction. Microscopic particles are thrown from the bur with sufficient energy to penetrate the tissues but the significance is unknown.

Lichenoid reactions to restorations are confirmed when healing follows removal of the restoration. Patch testing for metal hypersensitivity and biopsy are not useful for diagnosis as the skin can react to a substance which causes no reaction in the mouth (Ch. 27). The decision whether to remove a restoration or not can therefore be a matter of trial and error.

Malignant change in lichen planus

The risk of and possible frequency of malignant change in lichen planus has long been controversial. Reportedly 1–4% of patients suffer this complication after 10 years, but there is growing controversy about such figures. Doubts about the validity of the diagnosis of lichen planus, in reports of malignant change, have been expressed – dysplastic lesions, for example, may have a streaky appearance that has been mistaken for striae. Also, because lichen planus is so common a disease, the quoted rates for malignant change would greatly exceed the actual incidence of oral cancer.

Specific risk factors have also not been identified with certainty.

The differential diagnosis of oral lichen planus is summarised in Summary chart 13.1.

Summary chart 13.1 Differential diagnosis of oral lichen planus and conditions which mimic it clinically.

LUPUS ERYTHEMATOSUS → Summaries pp. 232, 247

Lupus erythematosus is a connective tissue disease which has two main forms, namely systemic and cutaneous ('discoid'). Either can give rise to oral lesions which may appear similar to those of oral lichen planus.

Systemic lupus erythematosus has varied effects (Ch. 25). Arthralgias and rashes are most common, but virtually any organ system can be affected. A great variety of autoantibodies, particularly antinuclear, is produced.

Discoid lupus is essentially a skin disease with mucocutaneous lesions indistinguishable clinically from those of systemic lupus. These may be associated with arthralgias but rarely significant autoantibody production.

Clinically, oral lesions appear in about 20% of cases of systemic lupus and can, rarely, be the presenting sign (Fig. 13.18). Typical lesions are white, often striate, areas with irregular atrophic areas or shallow erosions, but the patterns, particularly those of the striae, are typically far less sharply defined than in lichen planus. They are often patchy and unilateral and may be in the vault of the palate which lichen planus typically spares.

Lesions can form variable patterns of white and red areas. There may also be small slit-like ulcers just short of the gingival margins. In about 30%, Sjögren's syndrome develops and, rarely, cervical lymphadenopathy (Ch. 26) is the first sign.

Fig. 13.18 Lupus erythematosus. The clinical presentation is often very similar to lichen planus, with ulceration, atrophy and striae. Lesions on the soft palate or with radiating striae, as here, should be investigated for lupus erythematosus.

Fig. 13.20   Lupus erythematosus. The histological picture is similar to that seen in lichen planus, with a subepithelial band of lymphocytes, basal cell degeneration and epithelial atrophy. The dense perivascular infiltrates of lymphocytes in the deeper tissues are characterstic of lupus erythematosus.

Fig. 13.19   Lupus erythematosus stained with PAS to show the thickened basement membrane.

Pathology

Lesions show irregular patterns of epithelial atrophy and acanthosis. Liquefaction degeneration of the basal cell layer is typical and there is PAS-positive thickening of the basement membrane zone and around blood vessels due to deposition of antigen/antibody complexes (Fig. 13.19). In the corium, there is oedema and often a hyaline appearance. The inflammatory infiltrate is highly variable in density, typically extends deeply into the connective tissue and may have a perivascular distribution (Fig. 13.20).

Lupus erythematosus shows more irregular patterns of acanthosis and lacks the band-like distribution of lymphocytes in the papillary corium of lichen planus.

In frozen sections, a band of immunoglobulins and complement (C3) with a granular texture deposited along the basement membrane may be shown by immunofluorescence. This deposit also underlies normal epithelium in systemic lupus. In paraffin sections, immunoglobulin deposits may be detectable using immunoperoxidase staining. Obvious vasculitis may be seen in systemic, but not in discoid lupus erythematosus.

Diagnosis of systemic lupus erythematosus should be confirmed by the pattern of antinuclear autoantibodies. The most specific is that to double-stranded (native) DNA. Haematological findings in active SLE include a raised ESR, anaemia and, often, leukopenia or thrombocytopenia.

Oral lesions of discoid lupus erythematosus may respond in some degree to topical corticosteroids. However, oral lesions in acute systemic lupus erythematosus may not respond to doses of corticosteroids adequate to control systemic effects of the disease. Under such circumstances, palliative treatment is needed until disease activity abates.

CHRONIC ULCERATIVE STOMATITIS

This uncommon mucosal disease is associated with IgG antibodies to squamous epithelium nuclear protein. The target antigen is also known as CUSP and is related by gene sequence to the p73 cell cycle control protein.

Clinically, females over 40 years are mainly affected. Lesions are usually erosions, but sometimes lichen planus-like. Some examples have, in fact, been mistaken for lichen planus clinically, so that it seems possible that antinuclear antibody chronic ulcerative stomatitis may be more common than is appreciated. Skin involvement is uncommon.

Histologically, the appearances may be similar to erosive lichen planus. However, immunofluorescence shows speckled antinuclear antibodies in the perilesional mucosa and shaggy deposits of fibrinogen in the basement membrane zone. Serum shows antinuclear antibody in high titre that reacts with guinea pig oesophagus substrate but the titre does not correspond with clinical severity.

The most effective treatment appears to be with chloroquine or hydroxychloroquine, supplemented if necessary with prednisolone. However, complete clearance is not always achieved or resolution may be followed by relapses. Immunological changes also persist after clearance of the lesions. Doses of chloroquine phosphate or hydroxychloroquine sulphate should be kept below 4 mg/kg or 6.5 mg/kg respectively to minimise the risk of ocular damage.

Key features of chronic ulcerative stomatitis are summarised in Box 13.11.

Box 13.11   Chronic ulcerative stomatitis: key features

- Females over 40 years mainly affected
- Lesions resemble striae or erosions of lichen planus
- Direct immunofluorescence shows speckled IgG antibodies to squamous epithelial nuclear protein
- Circulating epithelial nuclear antibodies in high titre
- Chloroquine or hydroxychloroquine moderately effective

PEMPHIGUS VULGARIS → Summaries pp. 246, 247

Pemphigus is an uncommon autoimmune disease causing vesicles or bullae on skin and mucous membranes. It is usually fatal if untreated. Females usually aged 40–60 years are predominantly affected. Lesions often first appear in the mouth but spread widely on the skin. Vesicles are fragile and infrequently seen intact in the mouth. Residual erosions often have ragged edges and are superficial, painful and tender (Fig. 13.21). Gently stroking the mucosa can cause a vesicle or bulla to appear (Nikolsky's sign).

Progress of the disease is very variable. It may sometimes be fulminating with rapid development of widespread oral ulceration, spread to other sites such as the eyes within a few days, and very soon afterwards to the skin.

Skin lesions consist of vesicles or bullae varying from a few millimetres to a centimetre or so across (Fig. 13.22). The bullae at first contain clear fluid which may then become purulent or haemorrhagic. Rupture of vesicles leaves painful ragged erosions. Protein, fluid and electrolytes are lost from the raw areas and they readily become secondarily infected. Without treatment, death usually follows, but immunosuppressive treatment is usually life-saving.

Pathology

An immunopathogenesis can be more convincingly demonstrated in pemphigus vulgaris than in any other oral disease and the histological findings are summarised in Box 13.12 and shown in Figure 13.23.

The epithelial cells that lose their attachments become rounded in shape and the cytoplasm contracts around the nucleus. Small

Fig. 13.22   Pemphigus vulgaris. The characteristic bullae often appear in the mouth but soon spread over the skin, forming widespread moist or crusted lesions when they rupture. (Taken before the advent of colour photography.)

Fig. 13.21   Pemphigus vulgaris. Typical oral presentation with erythema, erosions and persistent ulcers. The surrounding epithelium is friable and disintegrates on gentle stroking.

Fig. 13.23   Pemphigus. The edge of a bulla formed by separation of the epithelium just above the basal cells. There is acantholysis centrally and a layer of basal cells remains covering the dermal papillae.

> **Box 13.12** Pemphigus vulgaris: pathology
>
> - Loss of intercellular adherence of suprabasal spinous cells (acantholysis)
> - Formation of clefts immediately superficial to the basal cells
> - Extension of clefts to form intraepithelial vesicles (Fig. 13.23)
> - Rupture of vesicles to form ulcers
> - High titre of circulating antibodies to epithelial 'intercellular cement substance' (desmoglein 3)
> - Binding of antibodies to intercellular substance detectable by fluorescence microscopy

groups of these rounded-up acantholytic (Tzanck) cells can often be seen histologically in the contents of a vesicle or in a smear from a recently ruptured vesicle.

Pemphigus antibodies are tissue-specific and react only to the epithelial cell surface antigen, an intercellular adhesion molecule (ICAM), desmoglein 3 and can be detected by immunofluorescence (Fig. 13.24). The mechanism of breakdown of intercellular attachments appears to result from synthesis of proteases by the epithelial cells.

Management

The diagnosis must be confirmed as early as possible. Biopsy is essential and the changes are sufficiently characteristic to make a diagnosis. Immunofluorescence microscopy should be used to exclude similar but less common diseases. Once the diagnosis has been confirmed, immunosuppressive treatment is required. There is little consensus about dosage but a typical

regimen is 80–100 mg/day of predisolone plus azathioprine (1–1.5 mg/kg daily). Azathioprine is given to allow doses of the corticosteroid to be lowered and reduce their side-effects. Treatment can only be stopped if relapse fails to follow withdrawal; immunosuppressive treatment itself causes a significant mortality. With combined immunosuppressive treatment, the average mortality is approximately 6%. More recently, mycophenolate mofetil has been used with benefit and has significantly fewer adverse effects.

The main features of the several variants of pemphigus are summarised in Appendix 13.2.

Key clinical features are summarised in Box 13.13.

> **Box 13.13** Pemphigus vulgaris: key clinical features
>
> - Females predominantly affected, usually aged 40–60 years
> - Lesions often first in the mouth but spread widely on the skin
> - Lesions consist of fragile vesicles and bullae
> - Ruptured vesicles form irregular erosions on the mucosa
> - Nikolsky's sign may be positive
> - Widespread skin involvement is fatal if untreated
> - Good response to prolonged immunosuppressive treatment

MUCOUS MEMBRANE PEMPHIGOID → Summaries pp. 246, 247

Mucous membrane pemphigoid is an uncommon chronic disease causing bullae and painful erosions (Box 13.14). The term *cicatricial pemphigoid* is an older and less apt name for mucous membrane pemphigoid because scarring is not a prominent

> **Box 13.14** Mucous membrane pemphigoid: typical features
>
> - Females mainly affected and usually elderly
> - Oral mucosa often the first site
> - Involvement of the eyes, may cause scarring and blindness
> - Skin involvement absent or minimal
> - Indolent, non-fatal disease
> - Oral bullae are subepithelial and frequently seen intact

Fig. 13.24 **Pemphigus vulgaris.** Frozen tissue stained with fluorescent antibody to IgG shows green fluorescence along the lines of the interpithelial attachments of the keratinocytes typical of pemphigus. See Figure 1.6.

feature in the mouth. Conversely, in the eye, scarring may be extensive and impair sight. Skin involvement is uncommon and much more likely to indicate the condition *bullous pemphigoid*, in which the mouth is rarely affected.

Lesions (Fig. 13.25) are rarely widespread and progress is slow. 'Desquamative gingivitis' can be a manifestation (Fig. 13.26). Intact bullae are not often seen (Fig 13.27). Nikolsky's sign is typically positive and a striking clinical finding is sometimes that the epithelium slides away from the underlying tissue when pressed by a sharp scalpel during biopsy. In the mouth, bleeding into bullae can cause them to appear as blood blisters. Rupture of erosions leaves raw ulcers with well-defined margins, often with small tags of torn epithelium at their margins. Individual erosions persist for some weeks then slowly heal.

Fig. 13.25 Mucous membrane pemphigoid. Typical oral presentation with persistent erythema and ulceration of the palate. On close examination tags of epithelium are sometimes seen at the ulcer margins.

Fig. 13.26 Desquamative gingivitis as a result of mucous membrane pemphigoid. There is patchy reddening involving the attached gingivae around several teeth and in places the erythema extends to the alveolar mucosa. Unlike desquamative gingivitis caused by lichen planus, there are no flecks or striae and occasionally tags of separating epithelium may be found.

Fig. 13.27 Mucous membrane pemphigoid, an intact bulla at the junction of the attached gingiva and alveolar mucosa. The bulla fluid is lightly blood stained and visible through the intact pale yellow epithelial roof.

Further erosions may develop nearby and this process may persist for a year or more. Lesions may remain localised to the mouth for very long periods and may never involve other sites.

The main features of the subtypes of pemphigoid are summarised in Appendix 13.3.

Pathology

Histologically, there is loss of attachment and separation of the full thickness of the epithelium from the connective tissue at basement membrane level. Epithelium, though separated, remains for a time intact and forms the roof of a bulla (Fig. 13.28). The floor of the bulla is formed by connective tissue alone, infiltrated with inflammatory cells. The disease is immunologically mediated and binding of autoantibody or, more frequently, of complement components along the basement membrane zone can be demonstrated (Fig. 13.29). Circulating autoantibodies are detectable in some patients by indirect immunofluorescence, but their low levels usually require sensitive techniques.

Management

The diagnosis is confirmed by biopsy and immunofluorescence microscopy, but it is preferable to obtain an intact vesicle or bulla. Because of the possible risk to sight, ocular examination is necessary if early changes in the eyes are suspected.

Mucous membrane pemphigoid limited to the oral mucosa of mild or moderate severity should be treated with dapsone as a first-line treatment in preference to systemic steroids. However, side-effects may limit treatment. Mild disease or disease in remission can often be effectively controlled with topical corticosteroids. Doses are small and without systemic effects. Minor eye involvement also responds to dapsone, but severe eye disease requires potent immunosuppression with

Fig. 13.28 Mucous membrane pemphigoid. Biopsy from clinically normal mucosa. The full thickness of the epithelium has separated cleanly from the underlying connective tissue to form a microscopic fluid-filled bulla. The weakened attachment of epithelium to connective tissue has separated with the slight trauma involved in biopsy.

Fig. 13.29 Mucous membrane pemphigoid. Frozen tissue stained with fluorescent anti-C3 shows a line of fluorescence along the basement membrane indicating complement activation there. Intact mucosa is required for immunofluoresence and biopsy is best performed in apparently normal mucosa, not in a lesion. See Figure 1.6.

steroids and azathioprine, cyclophosphamide or mycophenylate mofetil to induce remission.

'DESQUAMATIVE GINGIVITIS' → Summary p. 279

The term *'desquamative gingivitis'* is a clinical description, not a diagnosis. It is used for conditions in which the gingivae appear red or raw. Usually the whole width of the attached gingiva around varying numbers of teeth is affected (see Figs 13.12 and 13.26).

Lichen planus is the most common cause. The gingivae then appear smooth, red and translucent due to the thinness of the atrophic epithelium. In older patients, mucous membrane pemphigoid may cause gingival erosions. Pemphigus vulgaris is another possible cause. In all cases, the appearances are strikingly different from simple marginal gingivitis and the correct diagnosis should be confirmed by biopsy.

OTHER CAUSES OF EPITHELIAL SHEDDING

Rare causes of vesiculo-bullous disease include epidemolysis bullosa (see Table 13.2).

Superficial epithelial desquamation can be mistaken for blistering by patients. It may be caused by detergents in toothpastes, particularly sodium lauryl suphate and patients may elect to change brand. However, the sloughing is often unnoticed or blamed on astringent or sharp foods and appears to be of no significance.

ERYTHEMA MULTIFORME → Summaries pp. 221, 246

This is a mucocutaneous disease but, among dental patients, oral lesions are the most prominent or the only ones present (Box 13.15).

Target lesions are red macules a centimetre or more in diameter with a bluish cyanotic centre. In severe cases, skin lesions are bullous. The attack usually lasts for 3 or 4 weeks with new

---

Box 13.15   Erythema multiforme: typical clinical features

- Occasionally triggered by herpetic infection or drugs
- Adolescents or young adults, particularly males, mainly affected
- Mild fever and systemic upset may be associated
- Lips frequently grossly swollen, split, crusted and bleeding (Fig. 13.30)
- Widespread irregular fibrin-covered erosions and erythema in the mouth (Fig. 13.31)
- Conjunctivitis may be associated
- Cutaneous lesions may consist of widespread erythema alone (Fig. 13.32) or characteristic target lesions
- Attacks may recur at intervals of several months
- Remittent but usually ultimately self-limiting

Fig. 13.30 Erythema multiforme. Ulceration of the vermilion border of the lip with bleeding, swelling and crusting is characteristic.

Fig. 13.31 Erythema multiforme. There is ulceration, erythema, sloughing of epithelium and a small vesicle centrally. The anterior part of the mouth and the lips are typically affected.

crops of lesions developing over a period of about 10 days. Recurrences, usually at intervals of several months, for a year or two are characteristic and are sometimes increasingly severe.

In the most severe cases, ocular damage may impair sight and occasionally cause blindness. With widespread skin blistering, this condition is known as toxic epidermal necrolysis. Very rarely, renal damage can be fatal.

Aetiology and pathology

The aetiology is not clear and though the disease may be reaction to a variety of causes, no convincing mechanism has been proposed. Infections, particularly herpetic, can be triggering factors. Drugs, particularly sulphonamides and barbiturates, have also been implicated, but a positive drug history is also rare. Even when drugs have been taken, coincidence cannot always be excluded and, in most patients, no precipitating cause can be found.

The histological appearances are variable. Widespread necrosis of keratinocytes with eosinophilic colloid change in the superficial epithelium may be conspicuous. This may progress to intraepithelial vesicle or bulla formation (Fig. 13.33). However, subepithelial vesiculation is more frequent (Fig. 13.34). Degenerative changes in the epithelium are associated with infiltration by inflammatory cells which also involve the corium and may have a perivascular distribution. Leakage of immunoglobulins from blood vessels has been reported, but vasculitis is not seen histologically.

Management

Patients should be warned of the possibility of recurrences but that the disease usually runs a limited course.

There is no specific treatment. Systemic corticosteroids may give symptomatic relief. Antibiotics are usually also given in severe cases with the idea of preventing secondary infection. Levamisole has also been reported to be effective. In some cases aciclovir is effective.

'ALLERGIC' STOMATITIS

Many otherwise harmless substances coming into contact with the skin cause hypersensitisation in susceptible subjects. When this has happened further contact causes an inflammatory reaction. Examples are eczema or contact dermatitis caused by a wide variety of household and industrial materials. Some mucous membranes such as the eyes can also become sensitised in this way, but the different parts of the body differ widely in their response. Sulphonamide ointments, for example, are highly sensitising to the skin but cause little trouble in the eyes. The oral mucous membrane appears to show yet other differences and appears to be unable to mount reactions comparable with contact dermatitis and there is no such condition as oral eczema. Most so-called allergic reactions of the mouth are due to direct irritation by the substance.

Even patients who are sensitised to a material such as nickel can tolerate it in the mouth; it may then cause a characteristic rash but not oral lesions. Amalgam restorations cause no trouble in patients sensitised to mercury, though the material should not be allowed to come into contact with the skin (Ch. 25). Similar considerations apply to methylmethacrylate. Those few people who are sensitised to the monomer can wear acrylic den-

Fig. 13.33 **Erythema multiforme.** At higher power there is necrosis of prickle cells producing intraepithelial vescicles.

Fig. 13.34 **Erythema multiforme.** There is a dense inflammatory infiltrate immediatley below the epithelium and around blood vessels in the deeper corium. The epithelium is separating from the connective tissue, here along the basement membrane, and there is ulceration centrally.

Fig. 13.32 **Erythema multiforme.** As the name suggests, the rash is variable and ranges from patchy erythema, as here, to the more characteristic target lesions and bullae.

tures with impunity. Inflammation under acrylic dentures, often in the past described as 'acrylic allergy', is usually candidal infection or a direct irritant effect of unpolymerised monomer. Authenticated cases of contact hypersensitisation of the oral mucous membrane are so few as to make it questionable whether the oral mucosa can mount this type of reaction. If it does so it must be phenomenally rare.

REITER'S DISEASE (SERONEGATIVE ARTHROPATHY)

The 'classical' triad comprises arthritis, urethritis and conjunctivitis. It was first noticed after an attack of gastrointestinal infection in a Prussian officer in the trenches in World War I. Sexually transmitted *Chlamydia* infection or gut infections such as with *Salmonella* usually precede arthritis by about 1 to 3 weeks. Patients are typically males between the ages of 20 and 40 years; 80% of them are HLA-B27 positive. Pain and swelling typically affect the knees, ankles and feet; back pain is associated in approximately 50%.

Antibiotics are given to eliminate gut or other triggering infections; non-steroidal anti-inflammatories are frequently effective for controlling joint pain but corticosteroids may be required.

Dental aspects

The temporomandibular joints are probably not involved. Oral manifestations are uncommon and consist of scalloped or circinate white lines somewhat resembling one type of migratory glossitis but involving any part of the mouth. In other cases there may be shallow erosions. Lesions are typically painless and frequently unnoticed.

MUCOCUTANEOUS LYMPH NODE SYNDROME (KAWASAKI'S DISEASE)

Kawasaki's disease is endemic in Japan and appears to be relatively common in other countries in the Far East such as Taiwan; there have also been outbreaks in Hawaii and the USA, where it has surpassed rheumatic fever as the leading cause of childhood-acquired heart disease. In Britain, it may cause approximately 100 deaths per annum.

The distribution of cases suggests an infectious cause, but no agent has been identified with certainty. Recently (2006), significant titres of antigens to *Staphylococcus aureus* and *Streptococcus pyogenes* have been found in 65 Japanese children so that multiple superantigens may be involved in the pathogenesis.

Typical clinical features are summarised in Box 13.16.

The overall mortality may be 1–3%, from heart failure secondary to coronary artery disease or dysrhythmias secondary to myocardial ischaemia, and coronary artery aneurysms which develop in over 50%. However, mortality is closely related to

Box 13.16 **Typical features of Kawasaki's disease**

- Children under 5 years old affected
- Fever persisting for more than 5 days
- Generalised, often morbilliform rash
- Red, swollen and indurated palms and soles
- Erythematous stomatitis
- Swelling and cracking of the lips and pharynx
- Unilateral mass of swollen cervical lymph nodes
- Abdominal symptoms frequently
- Deterioration of mood ('extreme misery')
- Heart involvement in approximately 20%

failure to recognise the disease in its early stages; with greater awareness of the disease the mortality may be improving. Nevertheless, in a recent series of 20 patients in Europe, two children died despite treatment.

Management

The diagnosis usually depends on the clinical and, particularly, electrocardiographic findings.

There is no specific treatment, but aspirin, despite the possible risk of Reye's syndrome, is frequently given to lessen vascular damage and thromboses. However, a single large dose of intravenous gammaglobulin, given with aspirin and sometimes corticosteroids, in the early acute stages appears to be the most effective means of reducing the risk of coronary artery damage. Coronary artery aneurysms respond well to thrombolytic therapy.

MISCELLANEOUS MUCOSAL ULCERS

Eosinophilic ulcer (atypical or traumatic eosinophilic granuloma)

Tumour-like ulcerated lesions with a microscopic picture resembling a traumatic ulcer but with a prominent eosinophil inflammatory reaction and large, sometimes apparently atypical endothelial cells or histiocytes may occur. These arise particularly on the tongue, but also in the gingivae and, occasionally, other sites. Sometimes there is a history of trauma and, experimentally, crush injury to muscle can induce a proliferative response with tissue eosinophilia.

Clinically, the ulcerated mass may be mistaken for a carcinoma, but is typically soft: almost any age can be affected. Eosinophilic ulcers heal slowly.

Pathology

There is typically a dense aggregation of eosinophils and cells which resemble histiocytes beneath the ulcerated surface. The histiocytes lack the ultrastructural features and surface markers of Langerhans cells but are occasionally pleomorphic.

The differential diagnosis is from Langerhans cell histiocytosis, which can be excluded by the absence of Langerhans cells markers (Ch. 9), and lymphoma. In practice, lesions usually heal spontaneously within 3 to 10 weeks and management of an isolated soft tissue mass having these histological characteristics should be expectant.

Fig. 13.35 Chemical burn. The gingivae are white and necrotic following injudicious use of a caustic agent. On the patient's right side full-thickness ulceration is present.

Ruptured blood blisters (localised oral purpura)

Rupture of blood blisters leaves painful ulcers. Bullae of mucous membrane pemphigoid sometimes fill with blood but must be distinguished from localised oral purpura or systemic purpura (Ch. 23).

Wegener's granulomatosis

Mucosal ulceration is occasionally a feature of this disease but mainly in its established stage (Ch. 28). Clinically, ulceration may be widespread but is otherwise non-specific.

Oral reactions to drugs

A great variety of drugs (see Box 13.9) can cause mucosal reactions, either as local effects (Fig. 13.35) or through systemic mechanisms which are often obscure. Systemically mediated reactions include ulceration, lichenoid reactions and erythema multiforme. These reactions are discussed in more detail in Chapter 35.

Some uncommon mucocutaneous diseases

In many of these conditions, the oral lesions are rare or insignificant in comparison with the skin disease (Table 13.2). See also pemphigus and pemphigoid variants in Appendices 13.2 and 13.3.

Factitious ulceration (self-inflicted oral lesions)

Factitious ulcers in the mouth are traumatic but considerably less common than the usual type. They are typically a consequence of a disturbed mental state ('a call for attention'). Rarely, factitious oral ulceration has been a prelude to suicide.

The most common type of self-inflicted oral injuries has been so-called self-extraction of teeth. The diagnosis of self-inflicted injuries may be difficult but suspicious features are shown below.

Features suggestive of factitious oral lesions

- Lack of correspondence with any recognisable disease
- Bizarre configuration with sharp outlines
- Usually in an otherwise healthy mouth
- Clinical features inconsistent with the history
- In areas accessible to the patient

Investigation may be needed to exclude organic disease. Underlying emotional disturbance is typically well-concealed. Frequently the diagnosis can be confirmed only by discreet observation after admission to hospital. The patient's family doctor should be told of the need for specialist psychiatric accessment.

Table 13.2	Some uncommon mucosal diseases			
Disease	**Cause**	**Oral features**	**Treatment**	
Epidermolysis bullosa	Autosomal recessive – gravis type due to type VII collagen defect (junctional type usually lethal at birth)	Subepithelial bullae leading to severe intraoral scarring after minimal trauma especially in recessive types	None wholly effective. Protect against any mucosal abrasion	
Pyostomatitis vegetans	Complication of inflammatory bowel disease particularly ulcerative colitis	Yellowish miliary pustules in thickened, erythematous mucosa release pus, leaving shallow ulcers. Suprabasal clefting and intraepithelial vesiculation or abscesses containing eosinophils. Sometimes intercellular Ig. Peripheral eosinophilia up to 20% of WBC	Control of inflammatory bowel disease or systemic prednisolone	
Gonorrhoea	*N. gonorrhoeae* sexually transmitted	Oropharyngeal erythema or ulcers rarely seen	Amoxycillin, spectinomycin or a 4-quinoline	
Reiter's disease	Urethritis, conjunctivitis, arthritis. Post-infective reaction	Painless circinate white lesions, histologically psoriasis-like	Oral lesions self-limiting	
Leprosy	*Mycobacterium leprae*	Oral ulcers or nodules. Seen mainly in Asia	Dapsone	

Keratosis follicularis (Darier's disease; warty dyskeratoma)	Genetic. Autosomal dominant	Intraepithelial bullae containing granulocytes and acantholytic cells. Pebbly lesions mainly of palate due to hyperkeratosis, acantholysis with 'corps ronds' and 'grains' (dyskeratosis)	Oral lesions not troublesome but respond to retinoids

SUGGESTED FURTHER READING

Allen CM 1998 Is lichen planus really premalignant? Oral Surg Oral Med Oral Pathol Oral Radiol Endod 85:347

Amagai M 2000 Towards a better understanding of pemphigus autoimmunity. Brit J Dermatol 143:237–243

Calabrese L, Fleischer AB 2000 Thalidomide: current and potential clinical applications. Am J Med 108:487–495

Carson PJ, Hameed A, Ahmed AR 1996 Influence of treatment on the clinical course of pemphigus vulgaris. J Am Acad Dermatol 34:645–652

Cawson RA, Binnie WH, Barrett AW, Wright J 2001 Oral disease, 3rd edn. Mosby-Wolfe, London

Cervera R, Navarro M, López-Soto A et al 1994 Antibodies to endothelial cells in Behçet's disease: cell binding activity heterogeneity and association with clinical activity. Ann Rheum Dis 53:265–267

Chan LS, Yancey KB, Hammerberg C et al 1993 Immune-mediated subepithelial blistering diseases of mucous membranes. Arch Dermatol 129:448–455

Chorzelski TP, Olszewska M, Jarzabek-Chorzelski M, Jablonsa S 1998 Is chronic ulcerative stomatitis an entity? Clinical and immunological findings in 18 cases. Eur J Dermatol 8:261–265

Church LF, Schosser RH 1992 Chronic ulcerative stomatitis associated with stratified epithelial specific antinuclear antibodies. A case report of a newly described entity. Oral Surg Oral Med Oral Pathol 73:579–582

Cribier B, Garnier C, Lausriat D, Heid E 1994 Lichen planus and hepatitis C virus infection: an epidemiologic study. J Am Acad Dermatol 31:1070–1072

Eisen D, Ellis CN, Duell EA, Griffiths CEM, Voorhees JJ 1990 Effect of topical cyclosporine rinses on oral lichen planus. A double blind analysis. N Engl J Med 323:290–294

Enk AH, Knop J 1999 Mycophenolate is effective in the treatment of pemphigus vulgaris. Arch Dermatol 135:54–56

Hietanen J, Pihlman K, Linder E, Reunala T 1987 No evidence of hypersensitivity to dental restorative materials in oral lichen planus. Scand J Dent Res 95:320–327

Ho VC, Gupta AK, Ellis CN, Nickoloff BJ, Vorrhees JJ 1990 Treatment of severe lichen planus with cyclosporine. J Am Acad Dermatol 22:64–68

Horie N, Shimoyama T, Kato T et al 2000 Eosinophilic ulcer of the tongue: a case report with immunohistochemical study. Oral Med Pathol 4:25–29

Huilgol SC, Bhogal BS, Black MM 1995 Immunofluorescence of the immunobullous disorders. Eur J Dermatol 5:186–195

Karjalainen TK, Tomich CE 1989 A histopathologic study of oral mucosal lupus erythematosus. Oral Surg Oral Med Oral Pathol 67:547–554

Laine J, Kalimo K, Forssell H, Happonen R-P 1992 Resolution of oral lichenoid lesions in patients allergic to mercury compounds. Br J Dermatol 126:10–15

Lee K-H, Bang D, Choi E-S et al 1999 Presence of circulating antibodies to a disease-specific antigen on cultured human dermal microvascular endothelial cells in patients with Behçet's disease. Arch Dermatol Res 291:374–381

Lee LA, Walsh P, Prater CA et al 1999 Characterisation of an autoantigen associated with chronic ulcerative stomatitis: the CUSP autoantigen is a member of the p53 family. J Invest Dermatol 133:146–151

Lozada-Nur F 2000 Oral lichen planus and oral cancer: is there enough evidence? Oral Surg Oral Med Oral Pathol Oral Radiol Endod 89:265–266

Lozada-Nur F, Gorsky M, Silverman S 1989 Oral erythema multiforme: clinical observations and treatment of 95 patients. Oral Surg Oral Med Oral Pathol 67:36–40

MacPhail LA, Greenspan D, Feigal DW, Lennette ET, Greenspan J 1991 Recurrent aphthous ulcers in association with HIV infection. Description of ulcer types and analysis of T-lymphocyte subsets. Oral Surg Oral Med Oral Pathol 71:678–683

Porter SR, Scully C, Flint S 1988 Hematologic status in recurrent aphthous stomatitis compared with other oral disease. Oral Surg Oral Med Oral Pathol 66:41–44

Porter SR, Bain SE, Scully CM 1992 Linear IgA disease manifesting as recalcitrant desquamative gingivitis. Oral Surg Oral Med Oral Pathol 74:179–182

Porter SR, Kirby A, Olsen I et al 1997 Immunologic aspects of dermal and oral lichen planus. A review. Oral Surg Oral Med Oral Pathol Oral Radiol Endod 83:358–366

Porter SR, Scully C, Pedersen A 1998 Recurrent aphthous stomatitis. Crit Rev Oral Biol Med 9:306–321

Rehberger A, Püspök A, Stallmeister T et al 1998 Crohn's disease masquerading as aphthous ulcers. Eur J Dermatol 8:274–276

Sakane T, Takeno M, Suzuki N et al 1999 Behçet's disease. N Engl J Med 341:1284–1291

Scully C, Porter SR 1989 Recurrent aphthous stomatitis: current concepts of etiology, pathogenesis and treatment. J Oral Pathol Med 18:21–27

Scully C, Carrozzo M, Gandolfo S et al 1999 Update on mucous membrane pemphigoid. A heterogeneous immune-mediated subepithelial blistering entity. Oral Surg Oral Med Oral Pathol Oral Radiol Endod 88:56–68

Scully C, de Almeida OP, Porter SR et al 1999 Pemphigus vulgaris: the manifestations and long-term management of 55 patients with oral lesions. Br J Dermatol 140:84–90

Van der Meij EH, Reibel J, Slootweg PJ et al 1999 Interobserver and intraobserver variability in the histologic assessment of oral lichen planus. J Oral Pathol Med 28:274–277

Van der Meij EH, Schepman KP, Smeele LE et al 1999 A review of the recent literature regarding malignant transformation of oral lichen planus. Oral Surg Oral Med Oral Pathol Oral Radiol Endod 88:307–310

Van Gestel A, Koopman R, Wijnands M, van de Putte L, van Riel P 1994 Mucocutaneous reactions to gold: a prospective study of 74 patients with rheumatoid arthritis. J Rheumatol 21: 1814–1819

Vente C, Reich K, Ruuprecht R et al 1999 Erosive lichen planus: response to topical treatment with tacrolimus. Br J Dermatol 14:338–342

Vincent SD, Lilly GE, Baker KA 1993 Clinical, historic, and therapeutic features of cicatricial pemphigoid. A literature review and open therapeutic trials with corticosteroids. Oral Surg Oral Med Oral Pathol 76:453–459

Williams JV, Marks JG, Billingsley EM 2000 Use of mycophenolate mofetil in the treatment of paraneoplastic pemphigus. Br J Dermatol 142:506–509

APPENDIX
13.1

Treatment for aphthous stomatitis

- Exclude underlying causes, e.g. iron, vitamin B_{12} and folate deficiency. Treat these first
- Exclude possibility of Behçet's disease; if likely, refer to specialist centre
- Select treatments appropriate to severity and patients' expectations of treatment. Patients may need to try several before they find one that works well for them
- Before drug treatment, reassure patients that RAS is common, not serious but troublesome with no significance for general health. Advise to avoid spicy, sharp and salty food and acid and carbonated drinks (or use a straw) when ulcers are present. Such reassurance and advice may be sufficient for those with only occasional ulcers
- Select a treatment from those below. Those in the darker shaded boxes are not suitable for treatment in general dental practice because of the need to monitor for adverse effects but could be prescribed in conjunction with the patient's medical practitioner
- Preparations marked * are available without prescription in the UK. Triamcinolone in Orabase can only be supplied over the counter in a 5 g tube for 5 days use
- Note that children less than 6 years old cannot rinse and expectorate effectively

Treatment	Instructions	Indication/problems
Covering agents, e.g. carboxymethylcellulose paste (Orabase)*, carmellose sodium*	Apply QDS to dried areas around ulcer with moist finger. Allow film to hydrate before contact with adjacent mucosa. Use as required	Infrequent ulcers anteriorly in sulci, ideally single ulcers. Handling is difficult, patient must be dextrous. Unpleasant texture and taste. Symptomatic treatment only by protecting ulcer
Topical gels, e.g. Carbenoxolone (Bioral)*, choline salicylate (Bonjela)*, aminacrine and lignocaine (various)*	Use according to manufacturer's instructions	Ulcers must be accessible. Carbenoxolone is claimed to speed healing but the others are symptomatic treatments only. Choline salicylate is not associated with Reye's syndrome and may be used in children. Large amounts can cause salicylate poisoning in small children
Mouthwashes, e.g. obtundents (benzydamine)* or antiseptics (chlorhexidine)*	Use according to manufacturer's instructions. Hold in mouth for 1–2 minutes for maximum effect	Infrequent ulcers or crops of ulcers (recurring >6-weekly), useful when ulcers are widely separated around the mouth or inaccessible to pastes and gels. Benzydamine is a symptomatic treatment only. Antiseptics may shorten healing time, presumably by reducing bacterial colonisation of the ulcer surface. Benzydamine may sting and chlorhexidine has unpleasant taste and causes staining
Low-potency steroid, e.g. hydrocortisone sodium succinate (Corlan) pellets 2.5 mg	Hold pellet on ulcer and allow to dissolve in contact, QDS	Single ulcers or crops of clustered ulcers. Ulcer must be accessible, usually in sulcus. No significant adverse effects, safe in children. If used regularly have slight therapeutic effect and may reduce recurrence. Very slow to dissolve
Low-potency steroid paste, e.g. triamcinolone 0.1% in Orabase*	As covering agents	See covering agents. If used regularly has slight therapeutic effect and may reduce recurrence rate. Much of the symptomatic effect derives from the Orabase vehicle
Tetracycline mouthwash	Dissolve soluble tetracycline capsule contents (very few preparations available) 250 mg in 5–10 ml water and rinse for 2–3 minutes QDS 5 days	Particularly useful for herpetiform ulceration. Not for those aged less than 12 years. Long courses predispose to candidosis
Steroid aerosols, e.g. beclomethasone diproprionate (100 micrograms/puff)	1 puff per ulcer QDS max, maximum 8 puffs per day	Useful to deliver potent steroids to inaccessible areas, e.g. oropharynx. Spreads dose fairly widely and so more useful in widespread ulceration from lichen planus than in RAS. Risk of steroid adverse effects with prolonged use
Steroid mouthwash, e.g. betamethasone	Dissolve 0.5 mg in 5 ml water and rinse for 2–3 minutes QDS	Useful for widespread ulcers and when severity merits potent therapeutic treatment, e.g. crops of ulcers 6-weekly or more frequently,

APPENDIX 13.1

Treatment for aphthous stomatitis

sodium phosphate	from onset of prodrome and while ulcer or symptoms present. For severe ulceration may be used six times daily	RAS major or severe pain. Significant risk of steroid adverse effects with prolonged use – important to spit out after use. In severe cases, dose may be swallowed for a short period for additional systemic effect
Systemic drugs, e.g. steroids, azathioprine, colchicine, thalidomide, intralesional steroid injection (major RAS only)	Various regimes	Reserved for the most severe minor RAS, major RAS and ulcers refractory to other treatments. Colchicine and thalidomide are particularly effective in Behçet's disease and RAS major Significant risk of adverse effects – reserved for treatment in specialist centres

APPENDIX
13.2

Pemphigus variants

These may resemble pemphigus vulgaris clinically, but differ in their histological features, target antigens and response to treatment.

Paraneoplastic pemphigus

Associated particularly with lymphomas, leukaemias and Castleman's disease. Severe mucosal involvement. Varied skin lesions. Suprabasal intraepithelial acantholysis. IgG deposits on cell surfaces throughout the epithelium. IgG deposits along BMZ. Circulating IgG autoantibodies. Several target antigens including desmogleins 1 and 3. Usually resolves with removal of the tumour, but stomatitis sometimes intractable.

IgA pemphigus

Rare mucosal involvement. Skin vesicles or pustules. Neutrophil infiltration and acantholysis of epithelium. Circulating IgA autoantibodies in 50%. Usually responds to dapsone.

Pemphigus herpetiformis

Occasional mucosal involvement. Pruritic skin lesions. Eosinophilic spongiosis and intraepithelial pustules, with or without acantholysis. Target antigens, desmoglein 1 and sometimes desmoglein 3. Responds to dapsone, sometimes with immunosuppressive treatment.

Pemphigus foliaceus

No mucosal involvement. Target antigen desmoglein 1.

APPENDIX
13.3

Subtypes of pemphigoid

Linear IgA disease

Predominantly cutaneous but mucosal involvement frequent; ocular disease rare. Subepithelial blistering with mixed inflammatory infiltrate including eosinophils. Linear band of IgA along BMZ. Circulating IgA autoantibodies in low titre.

Bullous pemphigoid

Skin bullae with rare oral involvement. Not histologically distinguishable from mucous membrane pemphigoid.

Anti-epiligrin pemphigoid

Mucocutaneous blistering, but rare ocular or laryngeal involvement. Intense linear IgG deposition along BMZ. Circulating IgG antibodies. Target antigen, laminin 5 and its subunits. Immunosuppressive treatment may be required.

Anti-p105 pemphigoid

Severe mucosal and skin blistering may have sudden onset. Subepithelial blistering with papillary neutrophil infiltration. Linear deposits of IgG and C3 along BMZ. Circulating IgG antibodies against a 105-kDa component of BMZ.

Note: The last two entities have been only recently recognised, so that they have not yet been fully characterised.

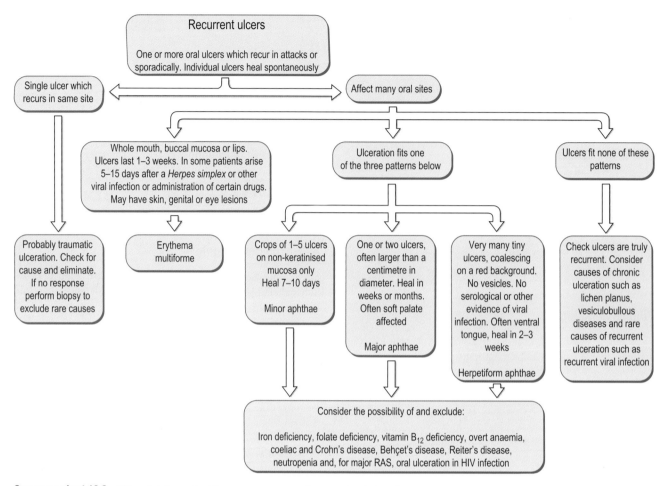

Summary chart 13.2   *Differential diagnosis of the common causes of recurrent oral ulceration.*

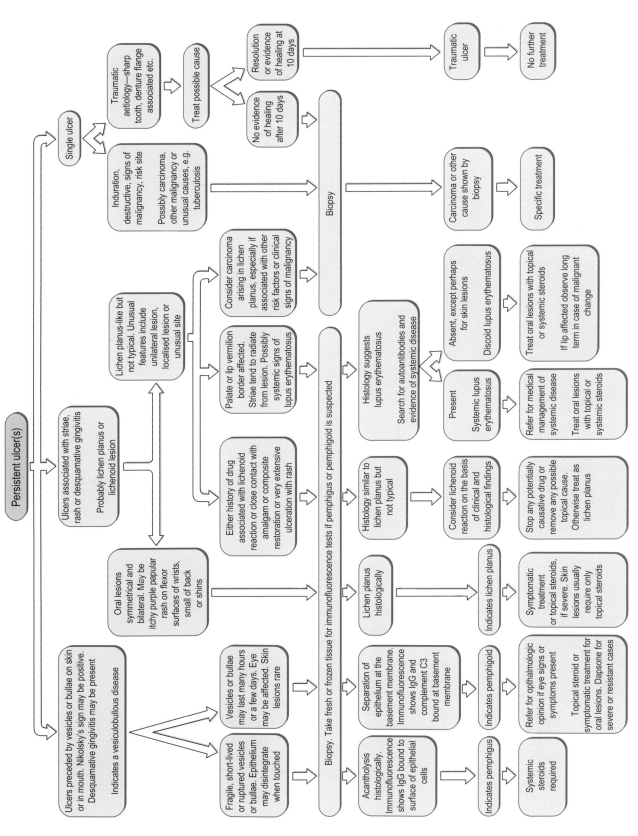

Summary chart 13.3 Differential diagnosis and management of persistent oral ulceration.

Tongue disorders

The tongue can be involved in generalised stomatitis, as in herpetic stomatitis for example, and show lesions similar to those in other parts of the mouth. The tongue is also the site of lesions or the source of symptoms peculiar to itself. For unknown reasons, it can manifest the earliest symptoms of anaemia or latent defects of haemopoiesis.

Patients are also aware that doctors traditionally look at the tongue. As a result, they look at their own and as a consequence sometimes worry about insignificant changes or think normal features, such as the foliate papilla, are a cause for concern.

THE SORE TONGUE

There are several clinical types of sore tongue (Box 14.1).

Box 14.1   **Clinical types of sore tongue**

- Ulcers (of any type) involving the tongue
- Glossitis (red and sore tongue)
- The sore, physically normal tongue
- Geographical tongue (erythema migrans)

Ulceration of the tongue

The tongue may be involved in, or even the predominantly affected site of, various types of stomatitis such as herpes simplex or, more frequently, lichen planus (see Figs 13.10 and 13.11). The tongue may also be the site of solitary ulcers, particularly carcinoma which, when far back, may be difficult to see. The lateral borders are affected and carcinoma of the dorsum of the tongue is exceptionally rare.

When there are definable lesions of these kinds, diagnosis is usually straightforward and depends on clinical examination and sometimes biopsy.

Glossitis

Glossitis is the term used for the red, smooth and sore tongue particularly characteristic of anaemia. These features are a combination of signs (redness and smoothness) and a symptom

(soreness) which are not always associated. Tongues can be sore in the absence of visible changes or smooth but asymptomatic from a variety of causes (Box 14.2).

Box 14.2   **Important causes of glossitis**

- Anaemia
- Vitamin B group (especially B_{12}) deficiencies
- Candidosis

Iron deficiency and pernicious anaemia are the main causes (Fig. 14.1). Women are more frequently affected. Detailed haematological examination is essential. These investigations are important, as a fall in haemoglobin level may lag behind other changes. Thus, there may be glossitis, haematological signs of a deficiency state, but a haemoglobin level within normal

Fig. 14.1   Glossitis in iron-deficiency anaemia. The tongue is smooth, due to atrophy of the papillae, and is red and sore. Anaemia is the commonest diagnosable cause of glossitis and must always be looked for by haematological examination.

limits. Abnormalities of the red cells may be seen in a stained film, but the red cell MCV (mean corpuscular volume) is frequently a useful guide. Serum levels of iron and ferritin, B$_{12}$ or folate (as the case may be) are depressed. When abnormalities such as these are found, specific treatment quickly relieves the symptoms.

Glossitis with angular stomatitis is characteristic of riboflavin deficiency and sometimes of nicotinic acid deficiency, but these are rare. The diagnosis of vitamin deficiency should not be made on oral signs alone in an otherwise healthy patient. These B group vitamins are frequently given in an attempt to relieve sore tongue but are virtually invariably ineffective. Their ineffectiveness makes it clear that deficiency of these vitamins is not the cause.

Candidosis can cause the tongue to be red, sore and oedematous. This is typical of acute antibiotic stomatitis (Fig. 14.2) and often then associated with angular stomatitis and other features of candidosis. This condition is rarely seen now that antibiotics are used less indiscriminately than in the past and topical oral antibiotics have now been discredited for oral infections. In Sjögren's syndrome, the tongue becomes red and acquires a cobblestone texture (see Fig. 18.12).

Lichen planus can produce a smooth tongue due to atrophy of the papillae (particularly late in longstanding disease), but there is then no soreness and typically no erythema. There is often a bluish-white sheen to the surface of the tongue and other signs of lichen planus may be seen in other parts of the mouth (Fig. 14.3).

The sore, physically normal tongue

This type creates the most difficult problems. The symptoms are frequently psychogenic, but it is essential to exclude organic disease, particularly a haematological deficiency.

Haematological deficiencies. Soreness can precede visible, physical changes (Fig. 14.4). The haemoglobin is frequently within normal limits, but there are other abnormalities as described earlier. Treatment of the deficiency quickly relieves the symptoms.

Psychogenic disorders. Soreness of the tongue frequently appears to be psychogenic and is sometimes termed 'burning mouth syndrome'. Some regard it as a variant of atypical facial pain and it is discussed in Chapter 34.

Geographical tongue (erythema migrans linguae) →
Summaries pp. 277, 279

In this condition, there is the recurrent appearance and disappearance of red areas on the tongue. The cause is unknown but, sometimes, there is a clear family history of its presence in

Fig. 14.3 Smooth tongue due to lichen planus. This is a late change due to longstanding disease. The tongue is smooth due to atrophy of the papillae, but has a faint silvery sheen. There are usually no symptoms at this stage.

Fig. 14.2 Glossitis in antibiotic stomatitis. The tongue is red, smooth and sore as in anaemic glossitis, but the appearance is partly due to inflammatory oedema. Similar changes affect the rest of the mucosa and other features of candidosis, such as thrush, are often present.

Fig. 14.4 A normal-looking but persistently sore tongue in a doctor's wife who had had repeated but inadequate haematological investigations which failed to detect early pernicious anaemia.

several generations. The abnormality can sometimes therefore be seen in infancy, but is probably not often noticed then. Most cases are seen in middle-aged patients. It seems improbable (but not impossible) that the condition has remained unnoticed for so long. In many patients, geographical tongue seems to be a developmental anomaly, but there also appears to be an association with psoriasis.

Clinically, an irregular, smooth, red area appears, usually with a sharply-defined edge, where the filiform papillae stop short (Fig. 14.5). It extends for a few days, then heals, only to appear again in another area (Fig. 14.6). Sometimes the lesion is annular with a slightly raised pale margin and several of these areas may coalesce to form a scalloped pattern. Most patients have no symptoms, but some adults complain of soreness. One possible reason is that the patient has become anxious that cancer is the cause and needs to be reassured. In others, soreness may be due to an underlying haematological deficiency state and the lesion is coincidental.

However, even children with geographical tongue sometimes complain that it is sufficiently hypersensitive to prevent them eating certain foods. The areas of epithelial thinning and inflammatory changes may therefore cause symptoms in some.

Fig. 14.5 Erythema migrans. Typical appearance with irregular depapillated patches centred on the lateral border of the tongue. Each patch has a narrow red and white rim.

Fig. 14.6 Erythema migrans. The change of pattern can be seen, on a later occasion, in the same patient as in Figure 14.5.

Soreness in association with geographical tongue may also be psychogenic and may then respond to appropriate treatment. Some evidence suggests a significant association between geographical tongue and emotional disturbance. However, there remains a group where no cause for the soreness can be found and no treatment seems to be effective.

Histologically, there is thinning of the epithelium in the centre of the lesion with mild hyperplasia and hyperkeratosis at the periphery (Fig. 14.7); there are chronic inflammatory cells in the underlying connective tissue. Sometimes the changes are the same as those of psoriasis.

Fig. 14.7 Erythema migrans. The edge of a lesion showing normal mucosa to the right and, to the left, the epithelium densely infiltrated by neutrophils. This epithelium at the advancing edge will be shed, leaving the depapillated red patch.

THE FOLIATE PAPILLAE

The foliate papillae are bilateral, pinkish soft nodules on the lateral borders of the tongue at the junction of the anterior two-thirds and the posterior third (Ch. 1). They enclose lymphoid follicles which sometimes become hyperplastic or inflamed and sore (see Figs 1.1 and 1.2). The appearance sometimes alarms patients who need to be reassured that they are normal structures.

LINGUAL VARICOSITIES

Dilated tortuous veins may be seen along the ventral surface of the tongue and tend to become more prominent with age (Fig. 14.8). They may be noticed by patients who need to be reassured that they are not abnormal.

HAIRY TONGUE

The filiform papillae can become elongated and hair-like, forming a thick fur on the dorsum of the tongue. The filaments may be up to half a centimetre long and pale brown to black in colour (Fig. 14.9). Adults are affected but the cause is unknown. Heavy smoking, excessive use of antiseptic mouth-washes and defective diet have been blamed, but their effect is questionable. The discoloration is probably caused by pigment-producing bacteria and fungi but not *Candida albicans*.

Treatment is difficult. The measure most likely to succeed is to persuade the patient to scrape off the hyperplastic papillae and vigorously cleanse the dorsum of the tongue with a firm toothbrush. This removes large numbers of microorganisms mechanically and also, by removing the overgrown papillae, makes conditions less favourable for their proliferation.

Black tongue

The dorsum of the tongue may sometimes become black without overgrowth of the papillae. This may be staining due to drugs, such as iron compounds used for the treatment of anaemia, but is then transient. Occasionally, the sucking of antiseptic lozenges causes the tongue to become black and this may be due to pigment-producing organisms, particularly aspergillus strains.

Furred tongue

The tongue can become coated with desquamating cells and debris, in those who smoke heavily, in many systemic upsets, especially of the gastrointestinal tract, and infections in which the mouth becomes dry and little food is taken. A furred tongue is often seen in the childhood fevers, especially scarlet fever.

Fig. 14.8   Lingual varices. The formation of varicosities in the vessels of the undersurface of tongue and floor of mouth is a common finding with age. Occasionally such varices may be the site of thrombosis.

MEDIAN RHOMBOID GLOSSITIS → Summaries pp. 220, 279

Median rhomboid glossitis is an abnormality in the midline of the dorsum of the tongue at the junction of the anterior two-thirds with the posterior third. The site suggests that it is developmental, but it is not seen in children and no longer accepted that it results from persistence of the tuberculum impar. Median rhomboid glossitis is typically pink in colour. Sometimes candidal infection is superimposed to cause the lesion to be white.

Clinically, median rhomboid glossitis is seen in adults and is typically symptomless. It appears as a nodular red or pink area of depapillation (Fig. 14.10). Alternatively, it may be white (Fig. 14.11). The lesions is usually flat or appears slightly depressed. In some cases there is nodular fibrous and epithelial hyperplasia.

Its chief importance is that the histological features have sometimes been mistaken for a carcinoma, particularly when nodular, and treated accordingly. Quite apart from the need for proper histological assessment, carcinoma virtually never develops in this site.

Fig. 14.9   Hairy tongue. In this patient there are numerous elongated papillae but a brown rather than black pigmentation.

Fig. 14.10   Median rhomboid glossitis. The typical lozenge-shaped area of depapillation in the midline of the tongue.

Fig. 14.11 **Median rhomboid glossitis.** There is a whitish patch of depapillation with sharply demarcated borders in the midline of the tongue.

Fig. 14.12 Median rhomboid glossitis with epithelial hyperplasia, light inflammation below and a band of scar tissue (A).

Fig. 14.13 **Median rhomboid glossitis.** There is hyperplasia with elongate rete processes, hyperparakeratosis and an inflammatory infiltrate of lymphocytes and plasma cells in the connective tissue. There are no signs of candidal infection.

Histologically, the appearances are variable. There is usually epithelial atrophy and often broad parallel-sided rete process hyperplasia with an inflammatory infiltrate and a broad band of dense scarred fibrous tissue below (Fig. 14.12). Fungal hyphae should be sought but are often not found (Fig 14.13). Other lesions show epithelial atrophy with loss of filiform papillae and less inflammation.

Management

Reassurance is usually the main requirement. Candidosis can be recognised by finding hyphae in a Gram-stained smear and can be treated with an antifungal drug. However, a pink or lobulated abnormality will remain. Observation is required to detect any enlargement of the area, but a need for biopsy is unlikely.

MACROGLOSSIA

Important causes are summarised in Box 14.3.

Amyloidosis

Amyloidosis is an important cause of macroglossia since it is usually associated with life-threatening disease, particularly multiple myeloma (Ch. 9). Amyloidosis is the deposition in the tissues of an abnormal protein with characteristic staining

Fig. 14.14 Macroglossia due to a congenital haemangioma.

properties. It can result from overproduction of immunoglobulin light chains, usually by multiple myeloma. In over 20% of such cases, amyloid is deposited in the mouth, particularly the tongue, to cause macroglossia or localised swellings or both

---

Box 14.3 **Important causes of macroglossia**

- Congenital haemangioma or lymphangioma (Fig. 14.14 and Ch. 20)
- Down's syndrome (Ch. 33)
- Cretinism (Ch. 31)
- Acromegaly (Ch. 31)
- Amyloidosis (Ch. 9)
- Lingual thyroid (Ch. 31)

(see Figs 9.24 and 9.25). Macroglossia due to amyloid can be so gross as to protrude from the mouth. Purpura and anaemia may be associated.

Pathology

Amyloid appears as weakly eosinophilic, hyaline homogeneous material. It is typically perivascular and stains with Congo red, which also shows a characteristic apple-green birefringence under polarised light (see Fig. 9.25). There is also fluorescence with thioflavine T and a characteristic fibrillary structure by electron microscopy.

Widespread amyloidosis can cause fatal renal failure, but progress of the disease may be delayed by chemotherapy. Alternatively, the patient may die from myeloma when it is the cause of amyloidosis.

SUGGESTED FURTHER READING

Dawson TAJ, Pielou WD 1967 Geographic tongue in three generations. Br J Dermatol 79:678–681

Field EA, Speechley JA, Rugman FR 1995 Oral signs and symptoms in patients with undiagnosed vitamin B_{12} deficiency. J Oral Pathol Med 24:468–470

Kleinhauz IEM, Baht R, Littner M 1994 Antecedents of burning mouth syndrome (glossodynia) – recent life events vs psychopathologic events. J Dent Res 73:567–572

Morris LF, Phillips CM, Binnie WH et al 1992 Oral lesions in patients with psoriasis. Cutis 49:339–344

O'Connor N, Bunch C 1995 Laboratory diagnosis in haematology. Medicine Int 23:489–494

Pippard MJ, Heppleston AD 1996 Microcytic and macrocytic anaemias. Medicine Int 24:4–10

Rojo L, Silvestre FJ, Bagan JV, De Vincente T 1994 Prevalence and psychopathology in burning mouth syndrome. Oral Surg Oral Med Oral Pathol 78:312–316

Benign chronic white mucosal lesions

The appearance of most mucosal white lesions is due to hyperkeratosis; any excess keratin, becoming sodden with saliva, appears white. Apart from the lingual filiform papillae, visible keratinisation of any significant degree is abnormal in the mouth.

Chronic mucosal white plaques have sometimes been termed *leukoplakias*. This term literally means no more than a white plaque but, in the past, was widely but mistakenly regarded as implying premalignancy. However, only a small minority of white patches are premalignant (Ch. 16). The majority, without malignant potential, are discussed here (Table 15.1).

LEUKOEDEMA → Summary p. 278

Leukoedema is a bilateral, diffuse, translucent greyish thickening, particularly of the buccal mucosa. It is a variation of normal, present in 90% of blacks and variable numbers of whites.

Histologically, there is thickening of the epithelium with intracellular oedema of the spinous layer.

Treatment is unnecessary but reassurance may be required.

Table 15.1 Important causes of benign mucosal white lesions

Prevalence	Lesion	Cause
Common	Leukoedema	Normal variation
	Frictional keratosis	Friction
	Cheek biting	Cheek biting
	Fordyce's granules	Developmental
	Stomatitis nicotina	Pipe smoking
	Thrush	Candidal infection
Uncommon	Chemical	Caustic chemicals
	Hairy leukoplakia	Epstein–Barr virus
	White sponge naevus	Genetic
	Chronic mucocutaneous candidosis	Candidal infection/ immunodeficiency
	Psoriasis	Uncertain
	Oral keratosis of renal failure	Uncertain
	Verruciform xanthoma	Uncertain
	Skin grafts	Iatrogenic

FRICTIONAL KERATOSIS AND CHEEK BITING →
Summaries pp. 277, 278

White patches can be caused by prolonged mild abrasion of the mucous membrane by such irritants as a sharp tooth, cheek biting or dentures.

Clinical features

At first, the patches are pale and translucent (Fig. 15.1), but later become dense and white, sometimes with a rough surface. Habitual cheek biting causes an area of buccal mucosa to appear patchily red and white with a rough surface (Fig. 15.2).

Pathology

The epithelium is moderately hyperplastic with a prominent granular cell layer and thick hyperkeratosis but no dysplasia (Fig. 15.3). There are often scattered chronic inflammatory cells in the corium.

Management

Removal of the irritant causes the patch quickly to disappear. Biopsy is necessary only if the patch persists. Frictional keratosis

Fig. 15.1 Frictional keratosis. A poorly–defined patch of keratosis on the buccal mucosa is due to friction from the sharp buccal cusp of a grossly carious upper molar.

Fig. 15.2   Cheek–biting. There is whitening of the buccal mucosa and a shredded surface.

Fig. 15.4   Fordyce's spots. Clusters of creamy, slightly elevated papules on the buccal mucosa.

Fig. 15.3   Frictional keratosis. There is a slight hyperplasia of the basal cells and a thick layer of orthokeratin at the surface.

Fig. 15.5   Fordyce's spots. Each spot is a histologically normal superficial sebaceous gland without a hair follicle.

is completely benign and there is no evidence that continued minor trauma alone has any carcinogenic potential.

FORDYCE'S GRANULES → Summary p. 278

Sebaceous glands are present in the oral mucosa in at least 80% of adults, particularly the elderly. They grow in size with age and appear in the oral mucosa as soft, symmetrically distributed, creamy spots a few millimetres in diameter, particularly in older persons (Fig. 15.4). The buccal mucosa is the main site, but sometimes the lips and, rarely, even the tongue are involved.

These glands are sometimes mistaken for disease, but patients can be reassured that they are of no significance. If a biopsy is carried out, it shows a normal sebaceous gland with two or three lobules (Fig. 15.5).

PIPE SMOKER'S KERATOSIS ('STOMATITIS NICOTINA') → Summary p. 277

Smoker's keratosis is seen among heavy, long-term pipe smokers and some cigar smokers.

Clinical features

The appearances are distinctive in that the palate is affected, but any part protected by a denture is spared. Changes are then seen only on the soft palate.

CHAPTER
15

Fig. 15.6 Stomatitis nicotina (smoker's palate). There is a generalised whitening with sparing of the gingival margin. The inflamed openings of the minor salivary glands form red spots on the white background.

Fig. 15.7 Stomatitis nicotina (smoker's palate). The epithelium is hyperplastic and hyperkeratotic, especially around the orifice of the duct where there is a concentration of inflammatory cells.

The lesion has two components – hyperkeratosis and inflammatory swelling of minor mucous glands. Either may predominate, but typically, white thickening of the palatal mucosa is associated with small umbilicated swellings with red centres (Fig. 15.6). The white plaque is sometimes distinctly tessellated (pavement-like).

Microscopy

The white areas show hyperorthokeratosis and acanthosis with a variable inflammatory infiltrate beneath. The diagnostic feature is the swollen, inflamed mucous glands with hyperkeratosis extending up to the duct orifice (Fig. 15.7).

Management

The clinical appearances, history and ease of management are so distinctive that biopsy should not be necessary. If the patient can be persuaded to stop smoking the lesion resolves within weeks.

Key features are summarised Box 15.1.

Box 15.1 Pipe smoker's keratosis ('stomatitis nicotina')

- Affects mucosa exposed to smoke (mainly the hard palate)
- Areas protected by denture unaffected
- Palate is white (keratotic) with umbilicated swellings with red centres (inflamed mucous glands)
- Responds rapidly to abstinence from pipe smoking
- Statistically, a raised risk of oral cancer but not in the hyperkeratinised (palatal) area (Ch. 16)

Epidemiological evidence suggests that pipe smoking raises the risk of cancer, but when oral cancer develops in association with pipe smoking, it typically appears not in the keratotic area on the palate (one of the least common sites for cancer) but low down in the mouth, often in the lingual retromolar region. This may be the result of carcinogens pooling and having their maximal effect in drainage areas of the mouth. It also suggests that there are different causes for the hyperkeratosis and any carcinomatous change.

THRUSH

Thrush (acute candidosis, Ch. 12) is readily distinguishable from other white lesions. The patches can easily be wiped off and Gram-stained smears show a mass of long hyphae.

In a young adult, thrush in the absence of obvious predisposing cause strongly suggests HIV infection.

HIV-ASSOCIATED HAIRY LEUKOPLAKIA → Summary p. 278

Patients with HIV infection may develop a clinically and histologically distinctive white lesion. Hairy leukoplakia is an important manifestation of HIV infection with a low CD4+ count and, though not entirely unique to it, is otherwise exceedingly rare.

Clinical features

Hairy leukoplakia usually has a vertically corrugated or shaggy surface. The plaque is soft, usually painless and most frequently affects the lateral borders of the tongue (Fig. 15.8). Men who have sex with men are predominantly affected.

Pathology

Hairy leukoplakia shows hyperkeratosis or parakeratosis, or both, with a ridged or shaggy surface or, rarely, hair-like extensions of keratin. Secondary invasion of the surface by candidal hyphae is relatively common, but there is little or no inflammatory infiltration in the submucosa. More important is the presence of koilocyte-like cells, which are vacuolated and ballooned prickle cells with shrunken, dark (pyknotic) nuclei surrounded by a clear halo (Fig. 15.9).

Fig. 15.8 **Hairy leukoplakia in a patient with early symptomatic HIV infection.** The surface of the lesion is corrugated, accentuating the normal anatomy of the lateral border of the tongue.

The infiltrate consists of CD8+ lymphocytes exclusively and no difference has been found between the lesion and lesion-free sites, suggesting a lack of local immune activity, despite the rise in viral load that precedes the lesion's development. Epstein–Barr virus (EBV) capsid antigen can be identified by in-situ hybridisation in the epithelial cell nuclei (Fig. 15.9). Viral particles resembling EBV can be seen by electron microscopy. This finding appears to be unique to hairy leukoplakia.

Management

Biopsy confirmation of the diagnosis is essential. The likelihood that the EBV is the cause is suggested by the fact that hairy leukoplakia responds to treatment with antiherpetic drugs such as valaciclovir. However, in the absence of symptoms, treatment of hairy leukoplakia is probably not justified especially as it has a remittent course and can regress spontaneously. Also, use of antiherpetic drugs in this situation carries the risk of development of resistance, which may be disastrous for later more severe infections. Hairy leukoplakia is not premalignant but it indicates advanced immunodeficiency, a more rapid progression to AIDS and a poor prognosis.

Fig. 15.9 **Hairy leukoplakia.** (A) There is thickening of the epithelium and a thick superficial layer of parakeratin, below which the pale-staining layer of 'koilocyte-like' cells lies. Because this patient is severely immunosuppressed, there is no inflammatory reaction to the numerous candidal hyphae which are present in the surface layers of the epithelium. (B) In-situ hybridisation using probes complementary to the Epstein–Barr virus. The presence of viral DNA is shown by the dark brown staining in the upper prickle cells and koilocyte-like cells. Details of this technique are included in Chapter 1.

Fig. 15.10 **White sponge naevus.** The keratosis is irregular and folded and extends into areas which are not subject to friction.

Fig. 15.11 **White sponge naevus.** The epithelium is acanthotic and the prickle cell layer is composed of large vacuolated cells.

Key features are summarised in Box 15.2.

Box 15.2 **Hairy leukoplakia: key features**

- Usually a sign of HIV infection in male homosexuals
- Typically forms soft, corrugated, painless plaques on lateral borders of tongue
- Diagnosis by biopsy
- Histologically, koilocyte-like cells in prickle cell layer are typical
- Epstein–Barr virus antigens detectable in epithelial cell nuclei by in-situ hybridisation
- Indicates advanced immunodeficiency and poor prognosis but not premalignant
- May regress spontaneously or with HAART treatment (Ch. 24)

Hairy leukoplakia in the absence of HIV infection

Hairy leukoplakia has rarely been seen in immunodeficient, and even more rarely in immunocompetent, patients. In such patients it appears to resolve spontaneously.

WHITE SPONGE NAEVUS → Summary p. 278

White sponge naevus is a developmental anomaly inherited as an autosomal dominant trait, caused by mutation in keratin genes.

Clinical features

The appearance is distinctive. The affected mucosa is white, soft and irregularly thickened (Fig. 15.10). The abnormality is usually bilateral but only ever affects the lining. There are no defined borders and the edges fade imperceptibly into normal tissue. The anus and vagina can also be affected.

Pathology

The epithelium is hyperplastic, with uniform acanthosis and the rete ridges have a smooth lower border. Shaggy hyperparakeratosis and intracellular oedema with abnormally prominent epithelial cell membranes produce a so-called basket-weave appearance (Fig. 15.11). There is no dysplasia and inflammatory cells in the corium are typically absent.

Management

The appearance is readily recognised, particularly when there is widespread mucosal involvement. A positive family history is virtually confirmatory. If there is any doubt, biopsy confirms the diagnosis. The main requirement is to reassure the patient of the benign nature of the condition.

Key features are summarised in Box 15.3.

Box 15.3 **White sponge naevus: key features**

- Genetic – autosomal dominant trait
- Shaggy whitish thickening can involve entire oral mucosa
- White areas lack sharp borders
- Histologically, epithelial hyperplasia with basket-weave appearance
- No dysplasia or inflammation
- No treatment other than reassurance

CHRONIC MUCOCUTANEOUS CANDIDOSIS SYNDROMES → Summary p. 220

These syndromes are all rare, but difficult to manage. There are four main types (Box 15.4).

Box 15.4 **Chronic mucocutaneous candidosis syndromes**

> **Box 15.4** **Chronic mucocutaneous candidosis syndromes**
>
> - Familial (limited) type
> - Diffuse-type (Candida 'granuloma')
> - Endocrine candidosis syndrome
> - Late-onset (thymoma syndrome)

Chronic mucocutaneous candidosis is sometimes classed as an immunodeficiency disease, but an immune defect cannot always be found. In others it is limited to failure to respond to *C. albicans* or secondary to persistent antigenic stimulation. However, there are more profound defects in the diffuse and late-onset types, while the endocrine candidosis syndrome is part of an autoimmune disease.

Familial (limited) mucocutaneous candidosis

Inheritance is usually as an autosomal recessive trait. The onset is in infancy with persistent thrush in childhood. Later, the oral lesions become indistinguishable from those of sporadic cases of chronic hyperplastic candidosis (Figs 15.12 and 15.13).

Fig. 15.12 Chronic mucocutaneous candidosis. There are extensive red and white patches affecting much of the oral mucosa and severe angular stomatitis.

Fig. 15.13 Damage to the fingernails as seen here is typical of the more severe types of mucocutaneous candidosis.

There may be mild cutaneous involvement and sideropenia is characteristically associated.

Diffuse-type mucocutaneous candidosis

Most cases are sporadic. This is the most severe type and was earlier termed 'monilial granuloma' because of the extensive, warty and often disfiguring overgrowths on the skin. Nevertheless, there is no granuloma formation microscopically. Instead, the lesions are produced by epithelial proliferation and an extreme expression of the same process that produces oral epithelial plaques in response to candidal invasion.

These patients are usually also abnormally susceptible to bacterial diseases, particularly pulmonary and superficial suppurative infections.

Endocrine candidosis syndrome

In this variant, chronic mucocutaneous candidosis is associated with multiple glandular deficiencies and organ-specific autoantibody production. Nevertheless, there is no direct cause-and-effect relationship between the candidosis and the endocrine deficiency. Candidal infection can precede the onset of endocrine deficiency by as long as 15 years but, occasionally, this sequence is reversed. Treatment of the candidosis does not affect the endocrine deficiency and vice versa.

Endocrine candidosis syndrome is a manifestation of type I chronic polyendocrinopathy (Ch. 31). Addison's disease and hypoparathyroidism are most frequently associated and other glandular deficiencies can develop, but candidosis is sometimes so mild as to pass unnoticed. Hypoplastic dental defects are frequently also present.

Adrenal failure is the main threat to life in candida endocrinopathy syndrome, but is usually now treated effectively.

Late-onset mucocutaneous candidosis

This syndrome has a clear immunological basis, in that there is a persistent defect of cell-mediated immunity produced by a thymoma. In the full syndrome, myasthenia gravis and pure red cell aplasia are associated. Death from the thymoma or red cell aplasia is the main hazard.

Management of mucocutaneous candidosis syndromes

Microscopic confirmation of chronic candidosis is required (Fig. 15.14 and Ch. 16), but precise categorisation of these syndromes may have to await development of other features, such as endocrine deficiency or elucidation of a relevant family history.

Immunological investigation, apart from detection of autoantibodies to glandular tissues in the endocrine candidosis syndrome, is not generally helpful, though detection of impaired or absent cell-mediated immunity to *C. albicans* strongly suggests that the patient has a mucocutaneous candidosis syndrome rather than limited oral hyperplastic candidosis.

Fig. 15.14 Chronic hyperplastic candidosis. At high power the thick parakeratin layer at the surface of this lesion is seen to be invaded by numerous fungal hyphae.

Fig. 15.15 Oral keratosis of renal failure. The white lesions are symmetrical, soft and wrinkled.

The principles of management are therefore to treat the candidal infection with antifungal drugs such as itraconazole and to deal with associated disorders as appropriate. Antibacterial chemotherapy is necessary in diffuse-type chronic mucocutaneous candidosis (CMCC) and endocrine replacement is essential in endocrine candidosis.

Unlike 'idiopathic' chronic hyperplastic candidosis, chronic mucocutaneous candidosis appears to have little potential for malignant change (see Chs 12 and 16).

Key features are summarised in Box 15.5.

> **Box 15.5 Chronic mucocutaneous candidosis syndromes: key features**
>
> - Onset typically in infancy as persistent thrush
> - Gradual transformation into leukoplakia-like lesions
> - Ungual and/or mild cutaneous candidosis sometimes associated
> - Immune deficiency sometimes present
> - Pulmonary and superficial suppurative infections associated in diffuse CMCC with gross candidal epithelial proliferation
> - In endocrine candidosis syndrome, early-onset Addison's disease and/or hypoparathyroidism is associated but oral candidosis frequently mild
> - In late-onset CMCC, thymoma causes defective cell-mediated immunity. Myasthenia gravis and pure red cell aplasia may be associated

---

PSORIASIS

Psoriasis is a common skin disease estimated to affect 2% of the population. Oral psoriatic plaques are rare, but there may be an association between erythema migrans of the tongue (geographical tongue) or other mucosae and cutaneous psoriasis.

The diagnosis should only be considered when there is cutaneous psoriasis. The appearance of the oral lesions varies from translucent plaques to that of erythema migrans. Lesions may be asymptomatic.

Diagnosis is confirmed by biopsy, but the histological appearances of psoriasis and erythema migrans (Ch. 14) are sometimes very similar.

ORAL KERATOSIS OF RENAL FAILURE

Leukoplakia-like oral lesions are a rare and unexplained complication of longstanding renal failure.

Clinically, the plaques are soft, have a crenated surface and are typically symmetrically distributed (Fig. 15.15).

Pathology

The features may not be sufficiently distinctive to allow diagnosis without knowledge of the underlying disease. There is irregular acanthosis with mild atypia of the epithelial cells and moderate parakeratosis. The appearances are somewhat similar to those of hairy leukoplakia, but Epstein–Barr virus antigen is absent. Biopsy is useful also to exclude adherent bacterial plaques, which may also develop in patients with renal failure (Fig. 15.16).

Effective dialysis or renal transplantation cause resolution of the lesion. No local treatment is necessary or likely to be effective.

VERRUCIFORM XANTHOMA

Verruciform xanthoma is a rare proliferative lesion which can have a white, hyperkeratotic surface.

Clinically, verruciform xanthoma is most common in the fifth to seventh decades. It is usually found on the gingiva but can form in almost any site in the mouth. It can be white or red in colour, sessile, have a warty surface, and range in size from one to several centimetres across. It may be mistaken for a papilloma, leukoplakia or carcinoma clinically, but is readily

Fig. 15.16   Oral keratosis of renal failure. Microscopy shows acanthosis and a picture somewhat similar to hairy leukoplakia.

Fig. 15.17   Verruciform xanthoma. The epithelium is thin and parakeratotic and forms a series of spiky folds.

recognisable histologically. Verruciform xanthoma is benign and has no known associations with diseases such as hyperlipidaemia or diabetes mellitus associated with cutaneous xanthoma formation.

Pathology

The warty surface is due to the much infolded epithelium which, in white variants, is hyperkeratinised or parakeratinised. In haematoxylin and eosin stained sections, the parakeratin layer stains a distinctive orange colour. The elongated rete ridges are uniformly elongated and extend to a straight, well-defined lower border (Fig. 15.17).

Fig. 15.18   Verruciform xanthoma. At higher power, dermal papillae within the folded epithelium can be seen to contain many large rounded cells with foamy or vacuolated cytoplasm.

The diagnostic feature is the large, foamy, xanthoma cells which fill the connective tissue papillae but extend only to the lower border of the lesion (Fig. 15.18). These cells contain lipid and PAS-positive granules.

Simple surgical excision is curative.

Fig. 15.19   Skin graft. A skin graft placed on the right posterior hard palate appears as a scar-like, pale patch. Hair follicles occasionally survive transplantation to the mouth.

SKIN GRAFTS

A skin graft may be placed in the mouth to cover a raw area left after excision of, for example, a chronic white lesion.

Skin grafts typically appear sharply demarcated, smooth and paler than the surrounding mucosa and occasionally contain hairs (Fig. 15.19). However, grafts on the dorsum of the tongue may become corrugated and less easy to differentiate from a recurrence of leukoplakia (Fig. 15.20).

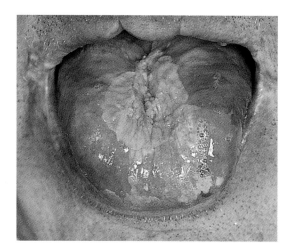

Fig. 15.20 Skin graft. This graft placed on the anterior dorsum of the tongue has contracted to produce an irregular margin and surface and might be mistaken for leukoplakia.

SUGGESTED FURTHER READING

Cawson RA, Langdon JD, Eveson JW 1996 Surgical pathology of the mouth and jaws. Wright, Oxford

Cawson RA, Binnie WH, Barrett AW, Wright JM 2001 Oral disease, 3rd edn. Mosby-Wolfe, London

Eisenberg E, Krutchkoff D, Yamase H 1992 Incidental oral hairy leukoplakia in immunocompetent persons. A report of two cases. Oral Surg Oral Med Oral Pathol 74:332–333

Epstein JB, Fatahzadeh M, Matisic J, Anderson G 1995 Exfoliative cytology and electron microscopy in the diagnosis of hairy leukoplakia. Oral Surg Oral Med Oral Pathol 79:564–569

Higgs JM, Wells RS 1974 Classification of chronic muco-cutaneous candidosis. Clinical data and therapy. Hautartz 25:159–165

Ravina A, Ficarra C, Chiodo M et al 1996 Relationship of circulating CD4+ T-lymphocytes and p24 antigenemia to the risk of developing AIDS in HIV-infected subjects with hairy leukoplakia. J Oral Pathol Med 25:108–111

Oral premalignancy

Various oral mucosal lesions, particularly red lesions (erythroplasias) and some white lesions (leukoplakias), have a potential for malignant change (Table 16.1). In some of them, such as chronic hyperplastic candidosis, the risk may be very low. By contrast, the risk with erythroplasia is exceedingly high.

In general, the most common white lesions have the lowest risk of malignant transformation. Practitioners will see many oral white lesions, but few carcinomas. However, they must be able to recognise lesions at particular risk and several features help to assess the likelihood of malignant transformation. The accuracy of such predictions is low, but the process of identifying 'at risk' lesions is fundamental to diagnosis and treatment planning. Important factors are listed in Box 16.1 and information on each of these should be sought.

The best predictor of the potential for malignant transformation is the degree of dysplasia seen histologically. For this reason, and because a few lesions will already be malignant, biopsy of red and white patches is mandatory. The term dysplasia (literally, abnormal growth) is given to the cytological abnormalities seen in both malignant and premalignant cells (Box 16.2). Premalignancy is distinguished from malignancy only by the latter's invasiveness and release of metastases.

Box 16.1   Risk factors for malignant change in white lesions

History
- Betel quid usage
- Tobacco smoking or topical tobacco habit[a]
- High alcohol intake
- Genetic disorders (see Ch. 17)

Clinical aspects
- Advanced age
- Female gender[b]
- Areas of reddening in the lesion
- Areas of speckling in the lesion
- Nodular or verrucous areas or ulceration
- High-risk site:
    - posterolateral tongue
    - floor of mouth
    - retromolar region
    - anterior pillar of fauces
- Large lesions
- Lesions present for long periods
- Enlargement or change in character of pre-existing lesion

Special investigations
- Degree of dysplasia on biopsy

[a]Nevertheless, surveys indicate that the risk of malignant change in white lesions is higher in non-smokers
[b]Surveys indicate that malignant change in white lesions is more frequent in women

---

Table 16.1   Lesions with potential for malignant change

Lesion/condition	Aetiology	Risk of malignant change*	Prevalence in the UK
Dysplastic leukoplakia	Unknown	High, but can regress	Uncommon
Erythroplasia	Idiopathic/smoking	Very high	Rare
Speckled leukoplakia	Idiopathic/smoking	High	Rare
Tertiary syphilis	*Treponema pallidum*	Very high	No longer seen
Oral submucous fibrosis	Betel quid chewing	High	Uncommon
Dyskeratosis congenita	Genetic	High	Rare
Pipe smoker's keratosis	Pipe smoking	Low and not in the keratotic area	Becoming uncommon
Snuff-dippers' keratosis	Smokeless tobacco	Low	Uncommon
Chronic candidosis	*Candida albicans*	Low	Uncommon
Lichen planus	Idiopathic	Low	Common
Discoid lupus erythematosus	Autoimmune	Unclear (mainly lip)	Uncommon

*Risks of malignant change are difficult to determine accurately and vary with many factors discussed below. If more than 25% of lesions become malignant in 5 years this is considered an exceptionally high risk. Malignant change in 2–3% of lesions in 5 years is considered a relatively low risk. Note that the highest risk lesions are uncommon. Common lesions appear in between 1 and 5% of the population.

SOFT TISSUE DISEASE

CHAPTER
16

> **Box 16.2** Epithelial dysplasia: histological features
>
> • Drop-shaped rete ridges
> • Nuclear hyperchromatism
> • Nuclear pleomorphism and raised nuclear/cytoplasmic ratio
> • Excess mitotic activity
> • Loss of polarity of cells
> • Deep cell keratinisation
> • Disordered or loss of differentiation
> • Loss of intercellular adherence

It must be emphasised that the implications of epithelial dysplasia are quite different from fibrous dysplasia, in which there is no risk of carcinomatous change.

Nuclei stain more densely due to greater nucleic acid content. They are variable in size, out of proportion to that of the cell, so that there may be little surrounding cytoplasm. Mitoses may be frequent and at superficial levels. Loss of polarity refers to the fact that basal cells in particular may lie higgledy-piggledy at angles to one another. Deep cell keratinisation (dyskeratosis) refers to individual cells which start to keratinise before the surface is reached and show eosinophilic change deeply within the epithelium. As differentiation is lost, organisation of the individual cell layers deteriorates and clearly-defined basal and spinous cell layers cannot be identified. Drop-shaped rete ridges are regarded as a particularly adverse feature. With loss of intercellular adherence, the cells become separated.

A lymphoplasmacytic infiltrate of highly variable intensity is usually present in the corium.

Dysplasia is usually graded as mild, moderate and severe as a guide to patient management (Figs 16.1–16.4). Carcinoma-in-situ is a term sometimes used for the most severe dysplasia where the abnormalities extend throughout the thickness of the epithelium, a state sometimes graphically called 'top-to-bottom change'. In such a lesion, all the cellular abnormalities characteristic of malignancy may be present; only invasion is absent. The significance of this grading is discussed below, but the histological assessment of oral epithelial dysplasia is notoriously unreliable because it is subjective and changes are not reliably correlated with behaviour.

PREMALIGNANT LESIONS AND CONDITIONS

Premalignant lesions are those lesions in which carcinoma may develop. Premalignant conditions are associated with a risk of carcinoma at some site within the mouth, not necessarily marked by a pre-existing lesion.

ERYTHROPLASIA ('ERYTHROPLAKIA') → Summaries pp. 277, 279

Erythroplasias are red patches. The surface is frequently velvety in texture and the margin may be sharply defined. Lesions of this type typically do not form plaques (hence the term

'erythroplakia' is misleading) but, instead, they are flat or depressed below the level of the surrounding mucosa (Fig. 16.5). Erythroplasia is uncommon in the mouth but carries the highest risk of malignant transformation and almost half of lesions turn out to be malignant on first biopsy.

Fig. 16.1 **Mild dysplasia.** In this lesion there is a thin layer of parakeratin and the structure, maturation and orderly differentiation of the epithelial cells is largely unaffected. However, there is a degree of irregularity of basal cells with variation in size and hyperchromatism.

Fig. 16.2 **Mild dysplasia.** In this lesion there is prominent orthokeratosis and a keratohyaline layer immediately below it. Dysplasia is more prominent than in the previous figure, with enlarged hyperchromatic and bizarre cells in the basal and lower prickle cell layers.

Pathology

Erythroplastic lesions usually show epithelial dysplasia which may be severe. In other cases, there may be micro- or frankly invasive carcinoma. The epithelium is atrophic and this, together with inflammation, accounts for the red colour seen clinically.

SPECKLED LEUKOPLAKIA → Summary p. 277

This term applies to lesions consisting of white flecks or fine nodules on an atrophic erythematous base (Figs 16.6 and 16.7). They can be regarded as a combination of or transition

Fig. 16.5 Erythroplasia. This slightly depressed, well-defined red patch on the dorsolateral tongue showed squamous carcinoma on biopsy.

Fig. 16.3 Moderate dysplasia. The dermal papillae extend close to the surface and there are elongated rete processes, some of which are broader deeply. Enlarged and hyperchromatic cells are visible at this low power in rete processes and in most of the prickle cell layer.

Fig. 16.6 Speckled leukoplakia. A poorly-defined speckled leukoplakia on the cheek of an elderly female. Carcinoma was present at the first biopsy.

Fig. 16.4 Severe dysplasia. This rete process is composed almost entirely of cells with dark and irregularly shaped nuclei. Only the most superficial layers of cells show maturation to squamous cells and the orderly maturation and differentiation of epithelial cells has been lost.

Fig. 16.7 Premalignant lesion in a betel quid chewer. The classical appearance of a speckled leukoplakia such as this is almost always associated with either severe dysplasia or invasive carcinoma. Note also the brown betel quid staining on the teeth.

between leukoplakia and erythroplasia. Speckled leukoplakia also more frequently shows dysplasia than lesions with a homogeneous white surface. The histological characteristics are usually, therefore, intermediate between leukoplakia and erythroplasia.

Many cases of chronic candidosis have this appearance.

IDIOPATHIC LEUKOPLAKIA → Summaries pp. 277, 278

Leukoplakia is defined as a white patch which cannot be wiped off the mucosa or ascribed to any specific disease process. Although the term is often used loosely for any white patch, it should be reserved for idiopathic lesions. If investigations fail to reveal any cause, the term may be appropriate.

The most extensive follow-up studies on white patches suggest that idiopathic leukoplakia now has the highest risk of developing cancer, especially now that late-stage syphilis forms a negligibly small group. Nevertheless, the malignant transformation rate of leukoplakia is relatively low, around 1–2% in 5 years and, even in smokers, the vast majority of leukoplakias show no dysplasia histologically and carry no risk of malignant transformation.

Clinical features

Idiopathic leukoplakias and dysplastic lesions do not have any specific clinical appearance, but are tough and adherent and typically form plaques whose surface is slightly raised above the surrounding mucosa. The surface is usually irregular. Small and innocent-looking white patches are as likely to show epithelial dysplasia as large and irregular ones (Figs 16.8 and 16.9). However, lesions with red, nodular or verrucous areas (Fig. 16.10) should be regarded with particular suspicion. The most common sites are the posterior buccal mucosa, retromolar region, floor of mouth and tongue.

Fig. 16.8 Homogeneous leukoplakia. There is a bright, white, sharply-defined patch extending from the gingiva on to the labial mucosa. The surface has a slightly rippled appearance and no red areas are associated.

Pathology

The histopathology is highly variable, but there is always parakeratosis or orthokeratosis, or both in different areas, and the two may alternate along the length of the specimen. The keratin gives the lesion its white appearance. The epithelium ranges from thinner than normal (atrophic) to much thicker (acanthotic) (see Figs 16.1 and 16.2).

Most leukoplakias show no dysplasia histologically. A minority display a range of dysplasia from mild to severe and treatment is planned partly on this basis. An inflammatory reaction of lymphocytes and plasma cells induced by the abnormal dysplastic cells is often present in the underlying connective tissue.

Fig. 16.9 An innocent-looking, poorly-defined inconspicuous white patch which showed dysplasia on biopsy. Despite excision, malignant transformation followed several months later.

Fig. 16.10 White patch with dysplasia. This post-commissural lesion is poorly defined and comprises both red and white areas. Lesions at this site are frequently due to candidosis.

SUBLINGUAL KERATOSIS

The term 'sublingual keratosis' is applied to white lesions on the floor of mouth and ventral tongue. Whether this lesion is a different entity from other leukoplakias is unclear. Malignant change was reported in an unusually high proportion of cases (30%) in one series, but this has not been widely confirmed. Probably the risk of malignant transformation is less than 10% and possibly much lower.

Clinical features

Sublingual keratosis is a white, soft plaque, usually with a finely wrinkled surface, an irregular but well-defined outline and sometimes bilateral with a butterfly shape. The plaque typically extends from the anterior floor of the mouth to the undersurface of the tongue (Figs 16.11 and 16.12). There is usually no associated inflammation.

Pathology

Sublingual keratosis is not distinctive histologically and the appearances are those described above for leukoplakia.

PROLIFERATIVE VERRUCOUS LEUKOPLAKIA

This is a rare and rather poorly defined clinical presentation of multiple white lesions with a very high risk of transformation. Lack of specific features makes it impossible to make the diagnosis confidently until many years have passed or carcinoma develops. In order for the diagnosis to have any value, it is important that the criteria are strictly applied. Not all verrucous leukoplakias are proliferative verrucous leukoplakia.

Clinical features

Patients are elderly and mostly female. Many are non-smokers. They develop flat leukoplakias that, over a period of decades, develop a verrucous surface and progress inexorably to verrucous or squamous carcinoma. Common sites affected are buccal mucosa, gingiva and tongue. It is common for several separate primary carcinomas to develop over many years. Lesions are difficult or impossible to eradicate surgically and recur or spread to new sites.

Pathology

The histological features of the lesions are those of idiopathic leukoplakia, with or without dysplasia.

PIPE SMOKER'S KERATOSIS → Summary p. 277

As noted earlier (Ch. 15), palatal keratosis due to pipe-smoking is benign. Any carcinomas related to pipe-smoking appear in another site in the mouth and may not be preceded by keratosis.

SMOKELESS TOBACCO-INDUCED KERATOSES

The majority of tobacco used worldwide is dried, cured and smoked in cigarettes or cigars. However, many cultures have traditional tobacco habits that use snuff or crude tobacco applied topically to the oral mucosa, termed smokeless tobacco habits. A dedicated smokeless tobacco user can consume several kilogrammes of tobacco each year in this way. Most smokeless tobacco habits have a limited geographic spread, but international travel and immigration have brought them

Fig. 16.11 Sublingual keratosis. This white patch involving the entire ventral tongue and floor of mouth has a uniformly wrinkled appearance. No red areas are associated but the site alone may possibly indicate a high risk of malignant transformation.

Fig. 16.12 Sublingual keratosis. This more irregular white patch is associated with some reddening in the floor of the mouth.

Table 16.2 Smokeless (topical) tobacco habits

Name	Habit	Where used	Carcinogenicity in oral mucosa
Chewing tobacco ('spit' tobacco)	Chewing a damp plug of cured leaf tobacco or loose strips of leaf. Often flavoured or sweetened	Historically widely used in Europe and USA, now mainly in the USA	Moderate to low for oral cancer
Snuff dipping with dry snuff	Placing a pinch of dry snuff in the buccal sulcus	South-eastern USA and Scandinavia	Relatively low. Associated with verrucous rather than squamous carcinomas
Betel quid (pan masala; paan) with tobacco	Areca nut, slaked lime, betel vine leaf with or without tobacco, sweeteners, flavourings and spices	Indian subcontinent, SE Asia, Phillipines, New Guinea and China	Very high when tobacco is included. Areca nut is associated with submucous fibrosis in addition
Nass	Tobacco, ash, cotton oil quid held in sulcus	Central Asia and Pakistan	High
Khaini	Tobacco and lime quid placed in sulcus	India and Pakistan	High
Dry (nasal) snuff	Dry snuff inhaled through nose	Now used mainly in Africa	Low, associated with nasal and sinus carcinoma
Gutka	Commercially prepared powder of areca nut, tobacco, lime and other flavourings and sweeteners	Indian subcontinent, SE Asia	Probably high, also risk of submucous fibrosis
Toombak	Rolled ball of tobacco and sodium bicarbonate placed in sulcus or floor of mouth	Sudan	High
Snus (moist snuff sachets; Scandinavian snuff)	Teabag-like pouch of moist unfermented snuff, sometimes with flavouring. Also some rolled leaf products	Originally Scandinavia but now prevalent in the USA	Thought to be low or very low. See section on harm reduction

to new populations and use is increasing dramatically in the USA, with 6% of males being users. Betel quid is widely used in the UK by immigrant communities and further details are given in the section on oral submucous fibrosis. Some smokeless tobacco habits are listed in Table 16.2.

Clinical features

Application of tobacco to the mucosa induces mostly hyperkeratotic lesions. Those that use betel quid frequently also may develop erosive lesions or erythroplakia. Lesions are limited to the site where the tobacco is held, usually in the buccal sulcus, and lesions do not have sharply defined margins. These changes seem to take prolonged periods to develop and, in the early stages, there is only erythema and mild, whitish thickening of the epithelium. Later there is extensive white thickening and wrinkling of the mucosa. Betel quid or areca nut users may also develop some localised fibrosis so that the lesions gradually become firm on palpation or submucous fibrosis. Before developing carcinoma, the mucosa will usually show varying degrees of dysplasia on biopsy, but even a non-dysplastic lesion signifies a risk of carcinoma.

Malignant change follows at the site of tobacco placement and only after many years of use. Most habits induce squamous

cell carcinoma, but snuff dippers develop verrucous carcinomas (Ch. 17) much more frequently but after a longer exposure. If these remain untreated, invasive squamous carcinoma may develop. Smokeless tobacco products also expose the oesophagus and pharynx to carcinogens and carcinoma may also develop at these sites.

Lesions associated with *snus*, moist snuff sachets, are characteristic. Unlike other habits, the site is often the upper buccal sulcus. The mucosa is greatly thickened, wrinkled and appears oedematous with a keratotic surface.

Pathology

The main changes are thickening of the epithelium with varying degrees of hyperorthokeratosis or parakeratosis. Regular and heavy users develop subepithelial fibrosis in the area where the tobacco is held and atrophy of underlying salivary glands. Later, there may be surface epithelial atrophy and the features of dysplasia may eventually be seen. Some lesions show carcinoma on first biopsy.

Management

Diagnosis is based on the history of smokeless tobacco use and the lesion in the area where the tobacco is held. It is important to ascertain exactly what type of tobacco is used and how it is prepared. Biopsy is required to exclude dysplasia or early malignant change. The most effective and important intervention is to stop the tobacco habit by patient education. Lesions that are dysplastic may not resolve completely but may regress, though there is a risk of delayed progression and malignant transformation. Non-dysplastic lesions in snuff dippers will resolve on stopping the habit even after 25 years of use. If the habit continues, regular follow-up and biopsies are required. Most smokeless tobacco users also smoke and this also needs to be addressed with smoking cessation advice.

Harm reduction for smokers Scandinavian moist snuff sachets (snus) have a lower carcinogen content than other tobacco products. This is because the tobacco is cured in steam and is not fermented, unlike the kiln-dried tobacco for cigarettes. The risk of developing carcinoma from these products appears very small, some claim negligible.

This has led to the proposal that smokers could reduce their risk of smoking-induced disease by switching to this type of smokeless tobacco. Statistically this makes some sense. The risk of lung and laryngeal carcinoma, of cardiovascular disease and other risks of inhaled tobacco are abolished and replaced by a low risk that affects a more readily examined site. Smokers also find this type of tobacco more acceptable than nicotine patches (and even nicotine patches have adverse health effects).

Opponents of this view point out that no tobacco product is safe, no use should be encouraged and that this is not a safe alternative to smoking. They worry that children and adolescents will develop this habit and progress to become smokers, though the Swedish experience suggests the opposite. There is no doubt that these products are still addictive and should never be recommended outside a smoking cessation programme with regular oral examination.

The concept of promoting a harmful product as an alternative to an even more harmful one has generated intense argument, similar to that which still surrounds the use of methadone for heroin users. This is a difficult ethical area and the interpretation of the evidence is still a matter of debate. Certainly there is a risk of sending conflicting messages to the public. Use of such products is rising dramatically in the USA but they are banned, though readily available, in Europe outside Sweden.

CHRONIC HYPERPLASTIC CANDIDOSIS (CANDIDAL LEUKOPLAKIA) → Summaries pp. 220, 277, 278

Chronic oral candidosis produces a tough adherent plaque, distinguishable only by biopsy from other leukoplakias.

Clinical features

Adults, typically males of middle age or over, are affected. The usual sites are the dorsum of the tongue and the post-commissural buccal mucosa. The plaque is variable in thickness and often rough or irregular in texture, or nodular with an erythematous background (speckled). Angular stomatitis may be associated, is sometimes continuous with intraoral plaques and suggests the candidal nature of the lesion (Figs 16.13 and 16.14).

Pathology

Unlike thrush, the plaque cannot be wiped off, but fragments can be detached by firm scraping. Gram or periodic acid–Schiff (PAS) staining then shows candidal hyphae embedded in clumps of detached epithelial cells.

Like thrush, the plaque of chronic candidosis is parakeratotic, but more coherent because it is not widely infiltrated by inflammatory exudate. In haematoxylin and eosin stained sections, hyphae form only faint tracks through the epithelium and are difficult to see. PAS stain clearly shows the hyphae growing (as in thrush) through the full thickness of the keratin to the prickle cell layer where the inflammatory cells tend to be more concentrated (Fig. 16.15).

Electron microscopy shows *Candida albicans* to be an intracellular parasite growing within the epithelial cytoplasm

Fig. 16.13 Chronic hyperplastic candidosis. This white localised patch and its associated erythema are the result of candidal infection alone; no dysplasia was present despite the speckled clinical appearance.

Fig. 16.14 Chronic hyperplastic candidosis. The typical site is the post-commissural buccal mucosa. This florid example is white and slightly nodular.

(Fig. 16.16). The hyphae, therefore, grow in relatively straight lines and do not follow a tortuous path along the intercellular spaces.

Induction of epithelial proliferation by *Candida albicans* infection has been demonstrated experimentally and in candidal plaques there is often rete hyperplasia with rounded down-growths and acanthosis. Dysplasia may be present, especially in speckled lesions.

The chronic inflammatory infiltrate in the corium is variable and a fibrinous inflammatory exudate may be seen at the basement membrane.

Management

After confirmation of the diagnosis by histology, treatment should be with a systemic antifungal drug such as fluconazole, but this may have to be continued for several months. Other factors likely to perpetuate candidal infection should be controlled. Stopping the patient from smoking and elimination of

Fig. 16.15 Chronic hyperplastic candidosis. Many hyphae are growing down through the epithelial plaque. (PAS stain.)

Fig. 16.16 Electron micrograph showing two candidal hyphae (very dark) growing through superficial keratinocytes of the oral mucosa. Note how they penetrate the cells and do not grow around them.

candidal infection from under an upper denture are important. Any iron deficiency should also be treated.

Excision of candidal plaque alone is of little value, as the infection can recur in the same site even after skin grafting. Vigorous antifungal therapy is therefore essential, but sometimes some residual (uninfected) plaque may persist after treatment and lesions often recur and require long-term intermittent antifungal therapy.

A potential for malignant change exists. The level of risk is controversial but low.

ORAL SUBMUCOUS FIBROSIS

Oral submucous fibrosis is an important and readily recognised condition in which the oral mucosa becomes fibrotic, immobile and contracts progressively causing limitation of opening (Chap. 13). More significantly, oral submucous fibrosis undergoes malignant transformation in 4–8% of cases and makes a significant contribution to the high incidence of oral cancer in the Indian subcontinent and in Asian immigrant populations.

The main immediate cause of oral submucous fibrosis has long been known to be the chewing of betel quid (*paan* or *pan*). The relative risk for users is almost 100× and betel quid is an extremely potent carcinogen. The simplest quid comprises chopped or grated areca nut mixed with slaked lime (CaOH) and wrapped in a leaf from the betel vine. There are enormous regional variations in additional ingredients, which include tobacco, spices and flavourings. The quid is folded tightly or tied, held in the buccal sulcus and occasionally chewed.

Areca nut contains alkaloids and the habit is addictive. However, it also has cultural significance, is associated with tradition and religious rituals and is regarded as a general tonic with beneficial medicinal effects. Similar mixtures of ingredients may be used as toothpastes. For these reasons, the habit is often acquired young, between the age of 5 and 12 in India and 10–20 in the UK. In London in 2001, 77% of Asian children had acquired the habit or depended on areca nut chewing. A heavy user may consume 20 or 30 quid each day and some will sleep with a quid in the mouth. Betel quid use is prevalent throughout the Indian subcontinent, SE Asia, Malaysia, the Phillipines, Taiwan and parts of China as well as in their emigrants.

The two main adverse effects of betel quid use are oral cancer and submucous fibrosis. However, other risks include carcinoma of the pharynx and oesophagus and possibly diabetes. A distinction must be drawn between quid containing tobacco, which causes cancer, and areca nut alone, which seems to carry the highest risk for submucous fibrosis.

In the UK and USA, it appears that most users add tobacco to the quid, even though they develop the habit using tobacco-free quid. Particularly worrying is the emergence of cheap commercially prepared quid ingredients and *gutka*, a flavoured and sweetened product aimed at children that can be imported legally into the UK.

Clinical features

Clinically, users of all types of quid show some common features. The teeth are typically stained dark red by a dye extracted from the nut by the lime. At the site of quid placement there is usually erythema and sometimes erythroplasia or leukoplakia. Long-term users have periodontitis and recession of the adjacent teeth. When red or white lesions are present they are treated as similar lesions in non-users but recognising that the risk of malignant transformation is much higher.

Only a very small proportion of users develop submucous fibrosis, but the consequences are dramatic. Symmetrical fibrosis develops in the buccal mucosa, soft palate or inner aspects of the lips. In the earliest stages, there may be a vesiculating stomatitis but, in established cases, the mucosa initially appears normal. Fibrosis and loss of vascularity cause extreme pallor of the affected area which then appears almost white. The fibrosis starts below the epithelium but extends to deeper tissues until they eventually become so hard that they cannot be indented with the finger (Fig. 16.17). Muscles of mastication are eventually involved. At this stage, the epithelium appears smooth, thin and atrophic (Figs 16.17 and 16.18). Ultimately, opening may become so limited that eating and dental treatment become increasingly difficult and tube feeding may become necessary.

Fig. 16.17   Oral submucous fibrosis. Typical appearance in a relatively advanced case with pale fibrotic bands of scarring running across the soft palate and down the anterior pillar of the fauces. Similar fibrous bands were present in the buccal mucosa bilaterally.

Fig. 16.18   Oral submucous fibrosis. There is fibrosis (A) extending from the epithelium down into the underlying muscle (B), which is replaced by hyalinised fibrous tissue.

If tobacco is included in the quid, erythroplasia and leukoplakia may develop (see Fig. 16.7) and the epithelium may show dysplasia on biopsy. Later, there is a very high risk of carcinoma and, if these changes develop when opening is limited, they may easily be missed.

Oral submucous fibrosis produces changes similar to those of scleroderma but limited to the oral tissues. There are no immunological findings to suggest any relationship to progressive systemic sclerosis. Scleroderma should be readily differentiated by the dermal and visceral involvement, the less severe oral changes and its autoantibody profile.

Pathology

It appears that the minority of areca users that develop submucous fibrosis are genetically predisposed. Occasionally there is a familial incidence. Those that are most susceptible can develop the disease in childhood after only a very few exposures to areca. Others develop more limited fibrosis over a period of many years. Cases have been reported in 11-year-olds in the UK.

The cause is unknown. Experimentally, an alkaloid component of areca nut, arecoline, can induce fibroblast proliferation and collagen synthesis and may penetrate the oral mucosa to cause progressive cross-linking of collagen fibres. It is also possible that insoluble collagen results from a collegen metabolic disorder.

The cause of the carcinomas and dysplastic lesions is presumed to be the same tobacco carcinogens that cause lesions in smokers. Similar molecular changes have been identified in the DNA of epithelial cells in quid users and non-users. The epithelial atrophy and relative avascularity may also play a role.

Histologically, the subepithelial connective tissue becomes thickened, hyaline and avascular and there may be infiltration by modest numbers of chronic inflammatory cells. The epithelium usually becomes thinned and may show atypia. Underlying muscle fibres undergo progressive atrophy and replacement by dense fibrous tissue (see Fig. 16.18).

Management

Treatment is largely ineffective. Patients must stop the causative habit but no regression usually follows; only stabilisation of the trismus can be expected and trismus often progresses despite cessation. Intralesional injections of corticosteroids may be tried in association with muscle stretching exercises or a 'trismus screw' between the teeth forcibly to stretch the bands of scar tissue, but these require dedication in use and the benefit is not usually great. Wide surgical excision of the affected tissues including the underlying buccinator muscle together with skin grafting can be carried out, but is likely to be followed by relapse.

The most important measure is to slow progression and reduce the risk of malignant progression by stopping the betel quid habit. Regular follow-up and biopsy of red or white lesions is essential but, even so, the risk of malignant change is reported to be about 5–8%. In severe cases, examination under anaesthetic or using endoscopy may be required.

LICHEN PLANUS

It has been estimated that 1–4% of patients with oral lichen planus develop carcinomas after 10 years. However, these rates are clearly wrong. Lichen planus is so common that this transformation rate would generate more cases of oral carcinoma than actually arise. As noted previously, this is an area of great controversy and there are often doubts about the original diagnosis of lichen planus.

Despite this uncertainty, it is clear that leukoplakia and dysplastic lesions often mimic lichen planus clinically and that the histological diagnosis is based on relatively non-specific features that overlap with those of dysplasia. Therefore, apparent lichen planus with unusual features, such as lesions in the floor of mouth or soft palate, late onset or unusual red areas should be regarded with suspicion, submitted for biopsy and followed up closely.

If lichen planus is truly premalignant, the transformation rate seems unlikely to exceed 0.05% in 10 years.

LUPUS ERYTHEMATOSUS

Lupus erythematosus is an uncommon connective tissue disease (Chs 12 and 23). There is a small risk of malignant change in cutaneous lupus, especially in lesions of the lower lip.

DYSKERATOSIS CONGENITA

Dyskeratosis congenita is a rare heritable recessive or dominant trait. The main features are dysplastic white or red lesions of the oral mucosa, cutaneous pigmentation, dystrophies of the nails and haematological abnormalities. Many patients may also be immunodeficient or have other abnormalities.

Causes of death include cancers of the mouth or other sites, bleeding (gastrointestinal or cerebral), but in 50% from infections, which are frequently opportunistic.

SYPHILITIC LEUKOPLAKIA

Leukoplakia of the dorsum of the tongue is a characteristic complication of tertiary syphilis, but is of little more than historical interest. Before effective treatment for syphilis, leukoplakia was a feared complication because of its very high malignant transformation rate.

Clinical features

Syphilitic leukoplakia has no distinctive features, but typically affects the dorsum of the tongue and spares the margins. The lesion has an irregular outline and surface. Cracks, small erosions or nodules may prove on histology to be foci of invasive carcinoma (Fig. 16.19). Carcinoma developing near the centre of the dorsum of the tongue is typically a sequel to syphilitic leukoplakia and, as a consequence of the great decline in late-stage syphilis, is exceedingly rare in this site now.

Pathology

In addition to hyperkeratosis and acanthosis, often with dysplasia, the characteristic late syphilitic chronic inflammatory changes, with plasma cells predominating, may be seen. Giant cells and, rarely, granulomas may be present. Endarteritis of small arteries is particularly characteristic. However, distinctive features of a syphilitic tissue reaction may be lacking.

Behaviour and management

The diagnosis is confirmed mainly by the serological findings. However, even if positive, biopsy is still essential, as minute areas of malignant change may be found, and the management is affected accordingly. In particular, the presence of syphilitic endarteritis may be a contraindication to radiotherapy.

Antibiotic treatment of syphilis does not cure the leukoplakia, which persists and can undergo malignant change even after serology has become negative.

EARLY CARCINOMA

Occasionally, an early carcinoma produces surface keratin and appears as a white patch (see Fig. 17.4). It should not be interpreted as malignant change in a leukoplakia.

MANAGEMENT OF DYSPLASTIC LESIONS

As will be noted in Chapter 17, the prognosis in oral carcinoma is good only when the diagnosis is made early and the tumour is small. The first principle of management is therefore early diagnosis and recognition of potentially malignant diseases is essential. Have a high index of suspicion that an oral

Fig. 16.19 Syphilitic leukoplakia. Carcinoma has developed in a patch of leukoplakia on the tongue of a patient who had had tertiary syphilis for many years. (Taken before the advent of colour photography.)

lesion may be premalignant and investigate appropriately. Red or white lesions in the mouth should never be ignored. They may turn out to be innocuous, but must be assessed with the possibility of premalignancy and malignancy borne in mind.

The best predictor of malignant potential is the presence of dysplasia on biopsy. However, even this is rather poorly correlated with behaviour and is not highly reproducible and rather subjective. Even when severe dysplasia is diagnosed, the risk of developing carcinoma may still be less than 20% and there is also the risk of inadequate sampling of large lesions, missing a small focus of carcinoma. Nevertheless, biopsy of a suspicious lesion is mandatory.

The level of risk cannot be reliably assessed from the histopathology alone and the clinical features listed in Box 16.1 should be used to help gauge the risk. Treatment options must be based on this clinical assessment and the dysplasia grade.

In the most extensive study based on no fewer than 782 cases of histologically unspecified oral white lesions followed for an average of 12 years, 2.4% underwent malignant change in 10 years and fewer than 5% after 20 years. However, even this low rate represents a risk of malignant change 50–100 times that in the normal mouth. It was also conspicuous that in this and in other studies the rate of malignant change in oral leukoplakias has been up to 10 times higher in non-smokers than in smokers and more frequent in women. Other, smaller, series have suggested rates of malignant change of 30% or more in unspecified types of white lesions, though in many cases no time scale has been indicated. The wide variation in the rate of malignant change in these different series suggests that the findings have been significantly affected by selection of cases.

It must be emphasised that these large follow-up studies have been on oral keratoses that had not been histologically assessed. Because of the rarity of dysplastic oral lesions, there are very few studies, and none on a large scale, that have followed their progress for adequate periods. In a study of 45 patients with oral dysplastic lesions, followed for up to 8 years, 11% underwent malignant change in this period and up to 30% of them regressed or even ultimately disappeared spontaneously.

The principles of the management of dysplastic lesions are summarised in Box 16.3. The management of dysplastic oral lesions remains controversial as their relative rarity has made it impossible as yet to accumulate enough data to make reliable predictions or evaluate treatment. It has to be assumed that dyplasia represents an early stage in the development of

carcinoma and provides an opportunity to treat carcinoma at an exceptionally early and potentially curative preinvasive stage.

Unfortunately, these assumptions are not well supported by clinical evidence. Lesions which are excised appear more likely to become frankly malignant, though this may reflect selection of the highest risk cases for surgery.

If lesions are of manageable size, it is tempting to excise them; this should presumably do no harm, but it is essentially a treatment of hope rather than certainty. An alternative approach is to observe the lesions for signs of deterioration, in the hope of detecting carcinoma as early as possible. Once carcinoma develops the treatment options are much more clear-cut.

A dysplastic lesion is associated with a higher risk of developing lesions elsewhere in the mouth and of developing more than one oral carcinoma. This process is sometimes described as 'field change' to convey the idea that large areas of the oral epithelium are predisposed to malignancy. Regular examination of the whole mouth is therefore essential.

Some dysplastic lesions regress spontaneously and surveys suggest that dysplastic lesions may regress as frequently as they undergo malignant change. However, disappearance of a white lesion does not necessarily indicate resolution of dysplasia and continued observation may still be indicated. Photographs or video records of lesions are an invaluable aid to long-term observation of lesions and should be used for high-risk lesions.

In practice, an attempt is usually made to remove lesions with moderate or severe dysplasia or high-risk clinical features (Box 16.4).

Box 16.4 **Options for management of premalignant lesions**

- Observation for early detection of carcinoma
- Surgical excision with grafting, if required
- Laser excision or vaporisation
- Topical chemotherapy
- Retinoids

Cryotherapy is generally considered inappropriate

Surgical excision is the most common approach. It provides an excision biopsy specimen which can be examined for the extent of the dysplasia and for possible carcinoma. Unfortunately, lesions in the highest risk areas in the posterior floor of mouth are technically difficult to excise and large lesions may require grafting.

The effectiveness of other treatments has not yet been assessed on any adequate scale.

After cryotherapy ablation, the area heals rapidly to leave an apparently normal mucosa. However, there is suspicion of a greater risk of invasive carcinomas subsequently arising in these sites and this treatment should not be promoted. Carbon dioxide laser ablation has also been advocated, but the same objections may apply. Topical chemotherapeutic agents such as bleomycin have also been used experimentally. Treatment with

---

Box 16.3 **Principles of management of dysplastic lesions**

- Stop any associated habits, e.g. betel quid or smoking
- Treat candidal infection and/or iron deficiency if present
- Biopsy to assess dysplasia
- Assess risk of premalignant change on clinical and histological findings
- Consider ablation of individual lesions (see Box 16.4)
- Maintain observation for signs of malignant change

systemic or topical retinoids has also been tried. Topical retinoids are largely ineffective and, though a proportion of white lesions resolve with systemic treatment, toxic effects are usually unacceptable. Further, lesions which resolve with treatment recur on withdrawal of the drugs and it is not clear that the risk of carcinoma is reduced.

With all such treatments, the lesion is not available for histological examination and multiple biopsy before treatment is required to ensure that malignant change is not already present. They may be of value in those for whom surgery is not practical because of, for instance, unfitness for anesthesia.

In summary, frequent clinical observation, preferably with photographic records, and immediate biopsy of any areas that are suspicious or change in appearance, is generally the best option. Selected lesions with clinical features of high risk or severe dysplasia on biopsy are probably best excised.

A number of as yet unproven investigations are available that are claimed to identify risk in dysplastic lesions or aid diagnosis of carcinoma. Tolonium chloride rinsing and brush biopsy are considered in Chapter 17 with oral cancer screening. Some 'visualisation' techniques claim to make dysplastic lesions more readily identifiable on examination. Some illuminate the mucosa with a wavelength of light that is normally absorbed but reflected by abnormal epithelium. Others use autofluorescence patterns or more complex laser reflectance. These techniques are sometimes used in conjunction with dyes. None has yet been proved effective in appropriately designed trials.

Ploidy analysis is claimed to be a more accurate predictor of malignant transformation than identifying the grade of dysplasia. Nuclei from the biopsy are stained with a DNA binding dye that allows the total DNA content of each cell to be measured. It is well known that dysplastic and malignant cells show chromosomal instability; their chromosomes have numerous deletions and duplications, sometimes of whole chromosomes. These changes can even be detected in epithelium that does not show dysplasia on routine light microscopic examination (Fig. 16.20). Though ploidy analysis has a more solid biological basis than previously mentioned techniques, its value is unproven.

SMOKING CESSATION

About 1 in 4 adults in the UK smoke, half the number that smoked in the 1970s. However, this reduction is mostly among older smokers; the number of young new smokers has remained stable and most start as teenagers. As half of cigarette smokers will eventually be killed by their habit, it is not surprising that almost three-quarters would like to stop.

Nicotine is powerfully addictive, having dopaminergic effects similar to cocaine. Even those who have had a laryngectomy or are dying of lung cancer will continue to smoke. Only 3% of smokers can quit smoking by willpower alone and smokers are encouraged to seek professional support to help them quit.

Dentists are well placed to help. They screen a large proportion of the UK population and oral adverse effects of smoking

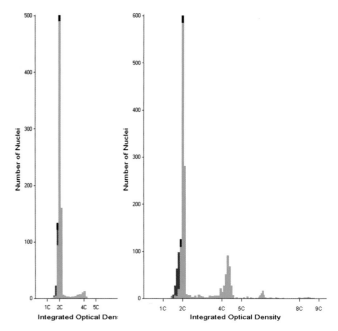

Fig. 16.20 **Ploidy analysis of normal and dysplastic epithelium.** Each graph shows the number of cells on the Y axis and the DNA content of each cell on the X axis. In normal mucosa (left graph) epithelial cells (green) almost all have a normal diploid DNA content (2c = equivalent to 2 sets of chromosomes or diploid) with a few cells having doubled their DNA content because they are about to divide (small peak at 4c). Lymphocytes (red) and fibroblasts (blue) act as a normal control. Dysplastic epithelium (right graph, green) has peaks at abnormal DNA content (main peak between 4c and 5c) and many cells with grossly abnormal DNA content, up to 9c. Such a lesion may carry a high risk of malignant transformation.

Box 16.5 **Oral adverse effects of smoking**

- Lip, oral and oropharyngeal squamous carcinoma
- Oral premalignant lesions
- Predisposition to periodontitis
- Increased risk of implant failure
- Predisposition to candidal infection
- Staining of teeth
- Taste impairment
- Halitosis

Recurrent aphous stomatitis may worsen on smoking cessation

---

enable them to raise the issue with patients (Box 16.5). Smoking cessation in dental practice is as effective as in medical primary care. Three minutes' advice will help an additional 2% to quit and 10 minutes' advice a further 6%. These may seem small proportions, but they represent a significant health benefit for individuals.

Smoking cessation advice must be provided as part of a structured programme to be effective. A simple approach is to *Ask* about smoking at every consultation, *Advise* on oral and health effects, *Assist* with health promotion material and offer support and *Arrange* follow-up or referral for specialist advice. A team approach is most effective at reinforcing the message. Smoking cessation literature should be available in the waiting room.

Some patients find nicotine replacement helpful in weaning themselves off tobacco. Chewing gum, skin patches, nasal spray, inhaler, tablets and lozenges are available. When used as part of an individualised cessation plan, nicotine replacement increases the success rate to 1 in 6. Such products are available over the counter and may be provided in dental surgeries. Bupropion (Zyban) may also help some patients.

SUGGESTED FURTHER READING

Abbey LM, Kaugars GE, Gunsolley JC et al 1995 Interexaminer and intraexaminer reliability in the diagnosis of oral epithelial dysplasia. Oral Surg Oral Med Oral Pathol Oral Radiol Endod 80:188–191

Axell T, Pindborg JJ, Smith CJ et al 1996 Oral white lesions with special reference to precancerous and tobacco-related lesions: conclusions of an international symposium held in Uppsala, Sweden, May 18–21 1994. J Oral Pathol Med 25:49–54

Barnard NA, Scully C, Eveson JW, Cunningham S, Porter SR 1993 Oral cancer development in patients with oral lichen planus. Oral Pathol Med 22:421–424

Barrett AW, Kingsmill VJ, Speight PM 1998 Frequency of fungal infection in biopsies of oral mucosal lesions. Oral Dis 4:26–31

Baudet-Pommel M, Janin-Mercier A, Souteyrand P 1991 Sequential immunopathologic study of oral lichen planus treated with tretinoin and etretinate. Oral Surg Oral Med Oral Pathol 71:197–202

Borle RM, Borle SR 1991 Management of oral submucous fibrosis: a conservative approach. J Oral Maxillofac Surg 49:788–791

Carr AB, Ebbert JO 2006 Interventions for tobacco cessation in the dental setting. Cochrane Database of Systematic Reviews: Reviews 2006 Issue 1. John Wiley & Sons, Ltd Chichester, UK DOI: 10.1002/14651858.CD005084.pub2

Cawson RA 1966 Chronic oral candidiasis and leukoplakia. Oral Surg Oral Med Oral Pathol 22:582–591

Cawson RA 1973 Induction of epithelial hyperplasia by Candida albicans. Br J Dermatol 89:497–503

Cawson RA, Binnie WH 1980 Candida leukoplakia and carcinoma: a possible relationship. In Mackenzie IC, Debelsteen E, Squier CA eds. Oral premalignancy. Proceedings of the first Dow Symposium. University of Iowa, Iowa, 59–66

Cawson RA, Rajasingham KC 1972 Ultrastructural features of the invasive phase of Candida albicans. Br J Dermatol 87:435–443

Cooke BED 1956 Leukoplakia buccalis and oral epithelial naevi. Br J Dermatol 68:151–174

Daniels TE, Hansen LS, Greenspan JS et al 1992 Histopathology of smokeless tobacco lesions in professional baseball players. Associations with different types of tobacco. Oral Surg Oral Med Oral Pathol 73:720–725

Davidson HR, Connor JM 1988 Dykeratosis congenita. J Med Genet 25:843–846

Einhorn J, Wersall J 1967 Incidence of oral carcinoma in patients with leukoplakia of the oral mucosa. Cancer 20:2184–2193

Eisen D, Ellis CN, Duell EA, Griffiths CEM, Voorhees JJ 1990 Effect of topical cyclosporine rinses on oral lichen planus. A double blind analysis. N Engl J Med 323:290–294

Eveson JW 1983 Oral premalignancy. Cancer Surveys 2:403–424

Farrand P, Rowe RM, Johnston A et al 2001 Prevalence, age of onset and demographic relationships of different areca nut habits among children in Tower Hamlets, London. Brit Dent J 190:150–154

Field EA, Field JK, Martin MV 1989 Does candida have a role in epithelial neoplasia. J Med Vet Mycol 27:277–294

Garewal HS, Katz RV, Meyskens F et al 1999 β-carotene produces sustained remissions in patients with oral leukoplakia. Results of a multicenter prospective trial. Arch Otolaryngol Head Neck Surg 125:1305–1310

Ho VC, Gupta AK, Ellis CN, Nickoloff BJ, Vorrhees JJ 1990 Treatment of severe lichen planus with cyclosporine. J Am Acad Dermatol 22:64–68

Holmstrup P 1992 The controversy of a premalignant potential of oral lichen planus is over. Oral Surg Oral Med Oral Pathol 73:704–706

Holmstrup P, Thorn JJ, Rindum J, Pindborg JJ 1988 Malignant development of lichen planus-affected oral mucosa. J Oral Pathol Med 17:219–225

Janthi V, Probert CSJ, Sher KS, Mayberry JF 1992 Oral submucosal fibrosis – a preventable disease. Gut 33:4–6

Karjalainen TK, Tomich CE 1989 A histopathologic study of oral mucosal lupus erythematosus. Oral Surg Oral Med Oral Pathol 67:547–554

Kaugars GE 1992 The prevalence of oral lesions in smokeless tobacco users and an evaluation of risk factors. Cancer 70:2579–2585

Kaugars GE, Silverman S, Lovas JGL et al 1996 Use of antioxidant supplements in the treatment of human oral leukoplakia. Review of the literature and current studies. Oral Surg Oral Med Oral Pathol Oral Radiol Endod 81:5–14

Kramer IRH, El-Labban N, Lee KW 1978 The clinical features and risk of malignant transformation in sublingual keratosis. Br Dent J 144:171–176

Larrson A, Axéll T, Andersson G 1991 Reversibility of snuff dippers' lesion in Swedish moist snuff users: a clinical and histologic study. J Oral Pathol Med 20:258–264

Laskaris G, Laskaris M, Theodoridou M 1995 Oral leukoplakia in a child with AIDS. Oral Surg Oral Med Oral Pathol 79:570–571

Lippman SM, Batsakis JG, Toth BT et al 1993 Comparison of low-dose isotretinoin with beta carotene to prevent oral carcinogenesis. N Engl J Med 328:15–20

McGrath JA 1999 Dyskeratosis congenita: new clinical and molecular insights into ribosome function. Lancet 353:1204–1205

Maher R, Lee AJ, Warnakulasuriya KAAS 1994 Role of areca nut in the causation of oral submucous fibrosis: a case-control study in Pakistan. J Oral Pathol Med 23:65–69

Mincer HH, Coleman SS, Hopkins KP 1972 Observations on the clinical characteristics of oral lesions showing histologic epithelial dysplasia. Oral Surg 33:389–399

Murti PR, Bhonsle RB, Pindborg JJ et al 1985 Malignant transformation rate in oral submucous fibrosis over a 17-year period. Community Dent Oral Epidemiol 13:340–341

Murti PR, Daftary DK, Bhonsle RB et al 1986 Malignant potential of oral lichen planus: observations in 722 patients from India. J Oral Pathol 15:71–77

O'Grady JF, Reade PC 1992 Candida albicans as a promotor of oral neoplasia. Carcinogenesis 13:783–786

Pillai R, Balaram P, Reddiar KS 1992 Pathogenesis of oral submucous fibrosis. Relationship to risk factors associated with oral cancer. Cancer 69:2011–2020

Pindborg JJ, Roed-Petersen B, Renstrup G 1972 Role of smoking in floor of the mouth leukoplakias. J Oral Pathol 1:22–27

Shibuya H, Amagasa T, Seto K-I, Ishibashi K, Horiuchi J-I 1986 Leukoplakia-associated multiple carcinomas in patients with tongue carcinoma. Cancer 57:843–846

Sigurgeirsson B, Lindelöf B 1991 Lichen planus and malignancy. An epidemiologic study of 2017 patients and a review of the literature. Arch Dermatol 127:1684–1688

Silverman S, Gorsky M 1997 Proliferative verrucous leukoplakia: a follow-up study of 54 cases. Oral Surg 84:154–157

Silverman S, Bhargava R, Mani NJ, Smith LW, Malaowalla AM 1976 Malignant transformation and natural history of oral leukoplakia in 57 518 industrial workers in Gujerat, India. Cancer 38:1790–1795

Silverman S, Gorsky M, Lozada F 1984 Oral leukoplakia and malignant transformation. A follow-up study of 257 patients. Cancer 53:563–568

Voute ABE, de Jong WFB, Schulten EAJM, Snow GB, van der Waal I 1992 Possible premalignant character of oral lichen planus; the Amsterdam experience. J Oral Pathol Med 21:326–329

Yavalzyilmaz E 1992 Oral-dental findings in dyskeratosis congenita. J Oral Pathol Med 21:280–284

Zain RB, Ikeda N, Gupta PC et al 1999 Oral mucosal lesions associated with betel quid, areca nut and tobacco chewing habits: consensus from a workshop held in Kuala Lumpur, Malaysia, November 25–27, 1996. J Oral Pathol Med 28:1–4

Zakrzewska JM, Lopes V, Speight P et al 1996 Proliferative verrucous leukoplakia: a report of ten cases. Oral Surg 82:396–401

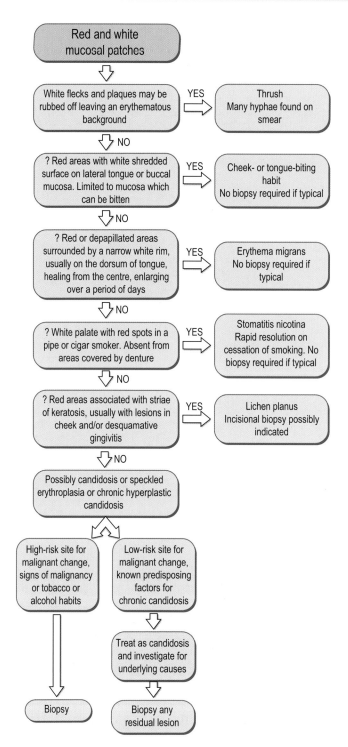

Summary chart 16.1 Differential diagnosis and management of the common causes of red and white patches of the oral mucosa.

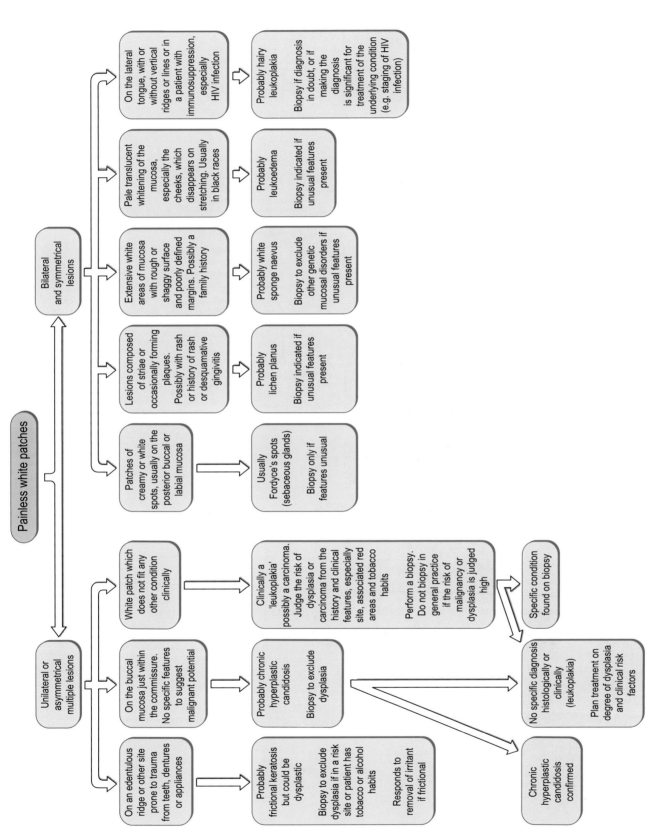

Painless white patches

Bilateral and symmetrical lesions

Patches of creamy or white spots, usually on the posterior buccal or labial mucosa

→ Usually Fordyce's spots (sebaceous glands). Biopsy only if features unusual

Lesions composed of striae or occasionally forming plaques. Possibly with rash or history of rash or desquamative gingivitis

→ Probably lichen planus. Biopsy indicated if unusual features present

Extensive white areas of mucosa with rough or shaggy surface and poorly defined margins. Possibly a family history

→ Probably white sponge naevus. Biopsy to exclude other genetic mucosal disorders if unusual features present

Pale translucent whitening of the mucosa, especially the cheeks, which disappears on stretching. Usually in black races

→ Probably leukoedema. Biopsy indicated if unusual features present

On the lateral tongue, with or without vertical ridges or lines or in a patient with immunosuppression, especially HIV infection

→ Probably hairy leukoplakia. Biopsy if diagnosis in doubt, or if making the diagnosis is significant for treatment of the underlying condition (e.g. staging of HIV infection)

Unilateral or asymmetrical multiple lesions

On an edentulous ridge or other site prone to trauma from teeth, dentures or appliances

→ Probably frictional keratosis but could be dysplastic. Biopsy to exclude dysplasia if in a risk site or patient has tobacco or alcohol habits. Responds to removal of irritant if frictional

On the buccal mucosa just within the commissure. No specific features to suggest malignant potential

→ Probably chronic hyperplastic candidosis. Biopsy to exclude dysplasia

White patch which does not fit any other condition clinically

→ Clinically a 'leukoplakia' possibly a carcinoma. Judge the risk of dysplasia or carcinoma from the history and clinical features, especially site, associated red areas and tobacco habits. Perform a biopsy. Do not biopsy in general practice if the risk of malignancy or dysplasia is judged high

→ Specific condition found on biopsy

→ No specific diagnosis histologically or clinically (leukoplakia). Plan treatment on degree of dysplasia and clinical risk factors

→ Chronic hyperplastic candidosis confirmed

Summary chart 16.2 Summary of the key features of the common and important oral white patches.

275

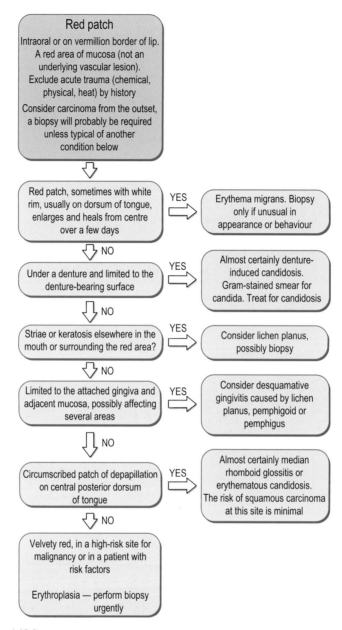

Summary chart 16.3 Differential diagnosis of common and important red patches affecting the oral mucosa.

Oral cancer

Over 90% of malignant neoplasms (cancers) of the mouth are squamous cell carcinomas arising from mucosal epithelium. Most of the remainder are adenocarcinomas of minor salivary glands: only a few are undifferentiated or metastases.

EPIDEMIOLOGY

Oral carcinoma accounts for only about 2% of all malignant tumours in such countries as the UK and the USA. In most countries where reliable data are available, the incidence of cancer of the mouth, though variable, is low. India and Sri Lanka are, however, exceptional, and cancer of the mouth accounts for approximately 40% or more of all cancer there, though the incidence varies widely in different parts of this subcontinent.

Approximately 2000 cases of intraoral and lip carcinoma are registered each year in the UK. For the last 50 years the incidence of oral cancer has declined but, though it is rare, cases are now more frequently seen in those aged 30–50.

Age and gender incidence

Oral cancer is an age-related disease and 98% of patients are over the age of 40. While the overall incidence in the population is only about 1 in 20 000, this rises to 1 in 1100 in males of 75 and over. There is a sharp and virtually linear rise in mouth cancer with age, as with carcinoma in many other sites.

Cancer of the mouth is considerably more common in men than women in most countries, and carcinoma of the lip is at least eight times as common in men as in women in Britain. Intraoral cancer used to be several times more frequent in men than women, but the male to female ratio is overall about 3:2 and, in south-east England, recent figures show little difference in incidence between the genders. The change is the result of the progressive decline in oral cancer in men, but a low, static rate in women.

The incidence of oral cancer rises steeply with age and, with an ageing population, oral cancer will become more common.

AETIOLOGY

It has not been possible to prove conclusively a causative association between specific aetiological factors and oral cancer.

This is partly because the quality of cancer statistics is very variable and partly because the aetiology of malignancy is complex and multifactorial. Causative factors operate over a long period and the process of malignant change is so slow that there is a prolonged lag period before it becomes evident. This has been shown strikingly in Japan, where cancers were still developing half a century after the radiation exposure from atomic bombs.

Significant or speculative risk factors for oral squamous cell carcinoma are summarised in Box 17.1.

Box 17.1 Possible aetiological factors for oral cancer

- Possible carcinogens
    Tobacco
    Alcohol
    Betel quid habit
- Sunlight (lip only)
- Infections
    Syphilis
    Candidosis
    Viruses
- Mucosal diseases
    Oral epithelial dysplasia
    Lichen planus
    Oral submucous fibrosis
- Genetic disorders (rare)
    Dyskeratosis congenita
    Fanconi's anaemia

Tobacco use

The earliest recorded tobacco-related death was in 1621 when a Thomas Herriot, who introduced clay pipe smoking to England, died (appropriately) of lip cancer. It was not thought at the time that pipe smoking had anything to do with Herriot's death.

The effects of tobacco on the mouth depend on the way it is used and this varies in different countries. In Westernised countries, cigarette smoking predominates and pipe smoking has declined. In some countries, notably in India, the southern states of the USA and Sweden, tobacco chewing or snuff-dipping (unsmoked tobacco held in the mouth for prolonged periods) is a habit. Methods of processing tobacco before use also vary widely, so that its products released into the mouth differ considerably in their effect.

Cigarette smoking

Smoking is considered to be a major aetiological factor, particularly in association with alcohol, and its importance is that it is preventable. However, it is difficult to demonstrate a direct causal link between cigarette smoking and oral cancer. In the UK, data have shown that oral cancer in males steadily declined over a period of more than three-quarters of a century while cigarette consumption grew steadily. Also, there is some evidence that the incidence of oral cancer in males may be rising again despite the fact that males are now smoking less.

Equally difficult to explain is the fact that mouth cancer in women has remained at a steady low level despite their widespread adoption of cigarette smoking. The escalation of their cigarette consumption is shown by the fact that the lung cancer rate in women has risen to nearly equal that of men in the USA.

Unlike pipe smoking or smokeless tobacco use, there is no specific oral lesion related to cigarette smoking, though heavy cigarette smokers develop patchy mucosal pigmentation.

Nevertheless, many studies have closely linked smoking, particularly in association with alcohol, to oral carcinoma. In case-control studies which take account of the amount and duration of tobacco consumption, the specific site and other factors such as alcohol, cigarette smoking has been shown to be closely associated and carry a significant relative risk. The risk of developing a second primary carcinoma is also closely linked to smoking and alcohol. Thus, smoking cigarettes infrequently appears to carry a very low risk, whereas the relative risk rises dramatically in heavy smokers.

Marijuana smoking is widespread and the smoke contains many of the carcinogens and co-carcinogens as tobacco smoke. It is suspected that it may be a more potent carcinogen than tobacco alone but this has not been confirmed in satisfactory studies.

Pipe smoking

Epidemiological evidence has associated oral cancer with pipe smoking, but the habit has steadily declined in most Westernised countries and has never become popular with women. Pipe smokers are also likely to develop stomatitis nicotina of the palate (Ch. 15), a white patch with no malignant potential.

Smokeless tobacco and betel quid

Smokeless tobacco habits are considered in Chapter 16. Betel quid usually contains tobacco and this habit is one of the most carcinogenic known. Areca nut without tobacco is also carcinogenic. For all smokeless tobacco habits, carcinomas tend to arise at the site in the mouth where the tobacco is habitually held and carcinomas are often preceeded by red or white lesions or dysplasia. However, carcinogens are also swallowed and the pharynx and oesophagus are also at risk.

The risk varies with the habit. In the southern USA, the habit of 'snuff dipping' causes extensive hyperkeratotic plaques and, after decades of continuous use, may lead to verrucous carcinoma (see below) as well as squamous carcinoma. However, this is a very slow process and cancers develop later in users than in non-users. Scandinavian moist snuff appears to carry a very low risk.

Most smokeless tobacco users also smoke.

Alcohol

Alcohol consumption has steadily risen in Britain, particularly in the past half-century when oral cancer was declining. However, as noted above, the incidence may now be rising. In some countries, such as Denmark, there is good epidemiological evidence to link alcohol intake with oral carcinoma and, in the Bas Rhin area of France, alcohol is held to be responsible for the highest oral and pharyngeal cancer incidence in Europe. The low incidence of mouth cancer among Mormons and Seventh Day Adventists, who neither drink nor smoke, supports this idea.

It is generally considered that the combination of smoking and drinking is the most important aetiological factor for mouth cancer and, as noted above, many oral cancer patients smoke and drink heavily. The relative risks for alcohol and tobacco consumption are shown in Figure 17.1.

Alcoholic drinks are not usually allowed to reside in the mouth for long periods and there is no specific alcohol-related oral lesion. The mechanism by which alcoholic drinks might cause carcinomas is unclear and may not be their ethanol content. Drinks with the highest content of congeners, such as raw home-brewed spirits, appear to have the closest association with carcinoma. By contrast, evidence from the USA suggests that beer-drinking is associated with a greater risk. It is also possible that alcohol might predispose to carcinoma through its action on the liver and some studies have found a correlation between mouth cancer and cirrhosis. As with smoking, the total consumption is probably a critical factor.

Concern over the possible carcinogenic effects of alcohol has led to a proposal that it should be banned from mouthwashes, some of which contain more than 25% alcohol. There is as yet no conclusive link between mouthwash use and oral carcinoma.

Infections and immunological factors

The oncogenic potential of viruses is well recognised and some evidence has been produced to suggest that the human papillomavirus (particularly HPV 16) genomes can be found to be incorporated into mouth cancer cells. The importance of this finding remains unclear, especially as HPV is equally frequently found in normal mucosa. Screening exfoliated mucosal cells for the presence of HPV DNA has not proved to be useful as a screening test. If HPV played a significant role in oral carcinogenesis, it would be expected that the immunosuppressed, who suffer enhanced HPV infection, would be at greater risk of oral carcinoma. However, though uterine cervical and anal cancer in patients with AIDS is HPV-associated, oral carcinoma is

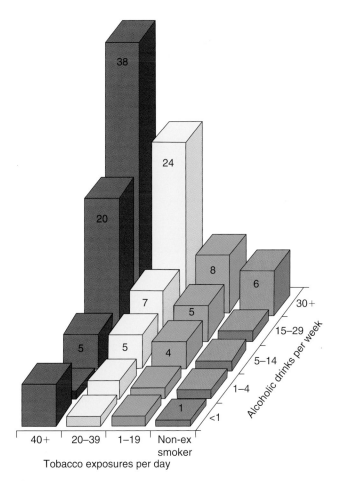

Fig. 17.1 **Relative risks of developing oral cancer in consumers (males in a Western population) of tobacco and alcohol.** The relative risk for a non-smoker and non-alcohol consumer is taken as one. A smoker consuming 30 cigarettes a day and 20 alcoholic drinks a week is seven times more likely to develop carcinoma.

uncommon and usually associated with other risk factors such as heavy tobacco or alcohol use. There is also no evidence of any greater susceptibility to intraoral cancer among patients who are deeply immunosuppressed therapeutically, though many are HPV carriers. Such patients have high rates of lip cancer, but only if exposed to strong sunshine.

There is better evidence that HPV plays a role in tonsil and oropharyngeal carcinoma. At these sites, up to 10% of carcinomas can be shown to contain HPV DNA integrated into the genome, but its precise contribution remains unclear and the focus of considerable research interest.

Syphilis

Syphilitic leukoplakia held pride of place as an infectious precancerous disease, in that the suggested rate of malignant change was between 30 and 100%. However, tertiary syphilis has become so rare that investigation of possible mechanisms has now become impossible and, even in developing countries,

syphilitic leukoplakia is no longer a significant risk factor (Ch. 16).

Chronic candidosis

Chronic candidosis can lead to formation of hyperkeratotic plaques or speckled leukoplakias with epithelial dysplasia. There have been isolated reports of malignant change in such lesions but, overall, this accounts for a very small proportion of cases (Ch. 16)

Malnutrition

There is a high incidence of mouth as well as oesophageal cancer in Paterson–Kelly syndrome, in which iron deficiency is a feature. However, this disease is no longer a significant risk factor.

Epidemiologically, a low vitamin A intake has been associated with oral carcinoma, but deficiency of beta-carotene has now been dismissed as contributing to cancer. In India, malnutrition is widespread and may contribute, together with betel quid chewing, to the high incidence. However, there appears to be no comparably high frequency of mouth cancer in other areas, such as many parts of Africa, where malnutrition is at least as severe.

Oral sepsis

Oral sepsis has traditionally been regarded as contributing to mouth cancer. The latter is most common in low socioeconomic groups, which tend to have the most neglected mouths. Oral cancer also progressively declined in frequency in Britain, where a slow but steady improvement in oral health is well documented.

Despite such considerations, the aetiological role of oral sepsis in mouth cancer remains unproven.

Sunlight

Exposure to the ultraviolet component of sunlight is a risk factor, with the result that lip cancer is predominantly a disease of outdoor workers, particularly farmers and fishermen. As with other skin cancers, fair-skinned persons are at most risk. There may be multiple lesions in the most severely affected.

The relationship between exposure to sunlight and lip cancer has been clearly shown in hot countries such as Australia and the USA with large immigrant, fair-skinned populations of European origin. In the USA, for example, the risk of lip cancer approximately doubles for every 250 miles nearer the equator to the site of residence.

Dysplastic lesions caused by sunlight may precede the carcinoma and sun-damaged lip may be identified clinically by its loss of elasticity and atrophic epithelium. Changes due to sunlight are preventable and dentists should encourage the need to wear a high-factor sun-block when exposed to strong sunlight.

Genetic factors

There are a few genetic disorders, notably dyskeratosis congenita (Ch. 16), of which oral cancer is a frequent feature, but such disorders are rare. Mice with a high susceptibility to oral cancer have also been bred. However, the genetics of oral cancer are highly complex and causative genes have not been identified in humans.

Precancerous lesions

Several premalignant lesions are recognised (Ch. 16). In general, the risk of malignant transformation in the more common white lesions is very low, but the risk from speckled leukoplakia and erythroplasia is high. However, it is not known what proportion of carcinomas arise in clinically recognisable premalignant lesion.

Key features of cancer of the mouth are summarised in Box 17.2.

Box 17.2   Cancer of the mouth: key features

- Account for approximately 2% of all cancers in the UK, but one of the most common cancers in the Indian subcontinent
- Males more frequently affected
- Most patients are over 40 and incidence rises rapidly with age
- Lower lip is the most common site and related to actinic damage
- Tongue, posterolaterally, is the most common site within the mouth
- Some arise in pre-existing white or red lesions
- Heavy tobacco smoking and alcohol consumption tend to be associated
- In the Indian subcontinent and South-east Asia, betel (areca nut) habit may be more important

---

EARLY SQUAMOUS CELL CARCINOMA → Summaries
pp. 247, 278, 279

In their earliest stages, carcinomas appear as painless red, speckled or white patches and only a minority are ulcerated (Figs 17.3 and 17.4). As noted in Chapter 16, a high proportion of erythroplasias and speckled leukoplakias are already malignant on first biopsy. The similar appearances of early carcinoma and premalignant lesions result from the processes of keratinisation and epithelial dysplasia and do not necessarily indicate that the carcinoma has arisen in a pre-existing lesion.

As a carcinoma enlarges, it may develop into a raised nodule or become ulcerated. Induration results from inflammation and fibrosis and infiltration of the tissues. By the time a carcinoma has formed an indurated ulcer with the typical rolled border, it will have been present for some time (Fig. 17.5). As noted below, diagnosis at this late stage is associated with a very poor prognosis and every attempt must be made to identify carcinomas as early as possible.

Ulceration may be associated with soreness, or stinging pain when sharply flavoured food is eaten. Pain is of no value in

Fig. 17.2   **High-risk sites for development of oral carcinoma.** The shaded U-shaped area accounts for only about 20% of the whole area of the interior of the mouth, but is the site of over 70% of oral cancers.

Fig. 17.3   Squamous carcinoma of the soft palate and mucosa posterior to the tuberosity appearing as a speckled leukoplakia.

the diagnosis of carcinoma, but is typically severe in the late stages. Bleeding, either spontaneously or to mild trauma, is also a late feature.

ORAL CANCER SITES

The lower lip is the most frequent site of oral cancer overall, while the tongue is the most frequently affected site within the mouth. In the oral cavity, the majority of cancers are concentrated in the lower part of the mouth, particularly the lateral borders of the tongue, the adjacent floor of the mouth and lingual aspect of the alveolar margin, forming a U-shaped area extending back towards the oropharynx (Fig. 17.2). This accounts for only about 20% of the whole area of the interior of the oral cavity, but 70% of oral cancers are concentrated there. This distribution may be due to the likelihood that

Fig. 17.6   Squamous carcinoma of lip. There is an indurated, crusted ulcer with keratosis at one margin in the centre of the lower lip.

Fig. 17.4   Early squamous carcinoma. Despite its inconspicuous appearance, this small white patch on the lateral border of the tongue was found to be a squamous carcinoma on biopsy.

Fig. 17.5   Advanced squamous carcinoma. The classical ulcer with a rolled border and central necrosis is a late presentation. Note the surrounding areas of keratosis and erythema which had been present for many years before the carcinoma developed.

carcinogens could pool and concentrate in the lower mouth before swallowing. Possibly for the same reason, the hard palate and central dorsum of tongue are very rarely affected.

Carcinoma of the lip

The lip is the most common single site for oral cancer but infrequently seen in dental practice. Being visible, it is often recognised at a very early stage and so has a better prognosis than intraoral cancer. The usual site is the vermilion border of the lower lip to one side of the midline. Men of middle age or over are predominantly affected.

An area of thickening, induration, crusting or shallow ulceration of the lip, less than a centimetre in diameter, is a common early presentation (Fig. 17.6). Advanced, neglected tumours

Fig. 17.7   Advanced carcinoma of lip. There is extensive ulceration and necrosis and distortion. Nowadays such extensive lesions are unusual. (Taken before the advent of colour photography.)

(Fig. 17.7) are unlikely to be seen now. Spread to lymph nodes tends to be slow. The submental nodes are usually the first to be affected.

Carcinoma of the tongue and floor of mouth

The anterior part of the tongue, particularly the lateral border, and the adjacent ventral tongue and floor of mouth are frequently involved. Presentation is often late with an ulcer 2 cm or more in diameter. Approximately 60% or more patients with localised lesions less than 2 cm in diameter survive for 5 or more years after treatment. In more advanced disease, the usual picture is of a typical malignant ulcer several centimetres in diameter, hard in consistency, with rolled or irregular, raised edges and a rough infected floor which bleeds readily. As growth proceeds, the carcinoma becomes fixed to surrounding tissues and infiltrates the tongue, which becomes progressively stiffer and more painful. Eating, swallowing and talking become difficult. By this time, pain is usually the main symptom and may radiate widely. The lymph nodes also become involved.

Affected lymph nodes are enlarged and hard, the surface becomes irregular and they become fixed to deeper tissues and skin. The growth has spread beyond the tongue when the majority of patients are first seen. In such circumstances the prognosis is poor. Only one patient in six survives for 5 years or longer. In the late stages, local spread of the growth causes gross destruction of adjacent parts with widespread sloughing. The tongue becomes fixed; pain is severe and persistent; swallowing and speech are difficult. Affected lymph nodes may ulcerate through the skin. The combination of pain, infection and difficulty in eating cause loss of weight, anaemia and deterioration of general health. This state (malignant cachexia) is ultimately fatal. In other patients, aspiration of septic material from the mouth causes bronchopneumonia, and in a few haemorrhage from the growth is the cause of death.

A small, but possibly growing, proportion of patients survive treatment of the primary growth but die later from distant metastases.

Carcinoma of the alveolar ridge, cheek and palate

These show essentially the same features as carcinoma elsewhere. Carcinoma of the buccal mucosa is particularly associated with betel quid chewing. Carcinoma of the alveolar ridge and palate are more likely to erode bone at an earlier stage, making treatment more complex.

PATHOLOGY

The essential features of carcinoma are invasion of surrounding tissues by the malignant epithelial cells and, if untreated, spread to lymph nodes and distant sites. The invading cells grow into the tissues, forming irregular branching processes, the tips of which are often cut off in a section to give the appearance of separate islands of tumour (Fig. 17.8). In the more infiltrative, higher grade carcinomas, single cells and small clusters of cells detach along the invasive front of the lesion. Tumour cells invade deeper tissues regardless of their nature (Fig. 17.9). Muscle, fat, nerves and eventually bone are infiltrated and destroyed. Invading cancer cells excite an inflammatory reaction and become surrounded by lymphocytes and plasma cells.

Fig. 17.8 A small squamous carcinoma. At low power, the epithelium is seen to invade deeply into the connective tissue and underlying muscle. At this early stage there is no ulceration.

Fig. 17.9 Squamous carcinoma. Higher power shows strands of malignant epithelium invading the connective tissue.

The individual cells show the features of malignancy. Large and irregularly shaped nuclei, darkly stained nuclei (hyperchromatism), frequent and sometimes abnormal mitoses and loss of the well-ordered architecture of epithelium are seen (Fig. 17.10). These are essentially the same changes as are seen in dysplastic epithelium (Ch. 16).

Squamous carcinoma is graded according to its degree of differentiation, that is the degree to which the malignant cells differentiate to form prickle cells and keratin. In well-differentiated tumours, the cells have cytoplasm which stains palely with eosin or may form concentric layers of keratin (cell-nests or keratin pearls (Fig. 17.11). In poorly-differentiated

Fig. 17.10 **Squamous carcinoma.** At high power, a group of tumour cells shows typical cytologic irregularity. Surrounding and beneath the tumour, muscle fibres are being destroyed.

Fig. 17.12 **Squamous carcinoma.** In this poorly-differentiated carcinoma there is little or no keratin formation and the malignant cells show great pleomorphism with variably-sized nuclei, many of which are hyperchromatic, and frequent mitotic figures.

Fig. 17.11 **Squamous carcinoma.** In this moderately well-differentiated tumour many of the neoplastic epithelial cells are forming keratin pearls.

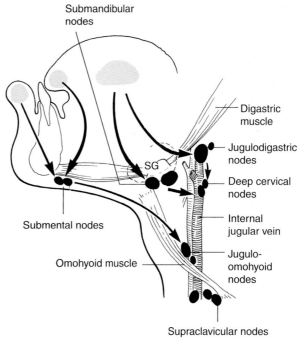

Fig. 17.13 Typical routes of lymphatic spread from lip and intraoral squamous carcinomas (SG, submandibular salivary gland).

tumours, the cells tend to be more irregular and darkly staining and show little evidence of a squamous pattern. In the most poorly-differentiated carcinomas, the cells have little cytoplasm and may not be recognisable as epithelial cells by routine microscopy (Fig. 17.12). Poorly-differentiated carcinomas tend to infiltrate more widely at an early stage, are more likely to metastasise and carry a poorer prognosis.

Spread of oral carcinoma

Carcinoma invades adjacent tissue by direct extension. Bone initially forms a barrier but is eventually destroyed, usually by superficial erosion, so that it can invade along the medullary cavity.

Perineural infiltration and vascular invasion are less common (Figs 17.13 and 17.14) but highly significant. Carcinomas that spread along nerves are less likely to be excised and more likely to recur because of their unpredictable outline. Those with vascular invasion are more likely to metastasise.

Metastatic spread is primarily via the lymphatics to the regional lymph nodes. The specific sites of metastasis depend on the drainage of the tumour site but, because most carcinomas arise posteriorly in the lower mouth, the submandibular and jugulodigastric nodes are most frequently involved. Lymphatic drainage from the tip of the tongue is to the submental nodes and then to the jugulo-omohyoid group, low down in the neck. From the dorsum and sides of the tongue, drainage is to the submandibular nodes and then to the jugulodigastric group (Fig. 17.15). Lip and floor-of-mouth carcinomas may

Fig. 17.14 Squamous carcinoma. In this carcinoma, malignant epithelium is invading around nerve sheaths. Although this is infrequent, occasionally carcinoma may spread some distance from the main tumour mass along nerve trunks.

Fig. 17.15 Squamous carcinoma. Less frequent than perineural invasion is vascular invasion. Here a cluster of poorly-differentiated malignant epithelial cells have eroded the wall of the vessel and entered the circulation.

spread bilaterally. Spread of cancer may be by an abnormal route and all the lymph nodes of both sides of the neck must be examined. One in five carcinomas of the tongue generates 'fast track' metastases, resulting from spread directly to deep cervical nodes at level 3, without involving submental or submandibular nodes first.

Oral cancer spreads progressively down the jugular lymphatic chain and it is unusual for it to involve supraclavicular lymph nodes until a late stage. Although these patterns of spread are relatively predictable overall, there is great difficulty in identifying and predicting metastatic spread to the neck when planning treatment for an individual case.

Metastatic carcinoma is initially limited to the affected node but, in time, spreads through the capsule into the tissues of the neck. Excision is then difficult and the chances of survival are diminished. This extracapsular spread is evident clinically as fixation of the node. Metastatic carcinoma forms a solid mass when small but, in larger masses, the central areas become necrotic and may break down so that the metastasis becomes cystic and fluctuant clinically.

Bloodstream spread is an uncommon, late feature of the disease and often after several episodes of treatment.

Key features are summarised in Box 17.3.

Box 17.3   Oral cancer: clinicopathological features and behaviour

- Early cancers appear as white or red patches or shallow ulcers and are painless or only slightly sore
- Later carcinomas appear as ulcers with prominent rolled edges and induration and become painful
- Over 70% or oral cancers form on the lateral borders of the tongue and adjacent alveolar ridge and floor of mouth
- Over 95% are well- or moderately well-differentiated squamous cell carcinomas
- Spread is by direct invasion of surrounding tissues and by lymphatic metastasis
- The submandibular and jugulodigastric nodes are most frequently involved
- The prognosis deteriorates sharply with local spread and nodal involvement

---

MANAGEMENT

Early diagnosis is critical if patients are to be cured. Treatment and survival are highly dependent on tumour size. Even so, patients are usually recommended to have the most aggressive treatment that they can accept. There is usually only one chance to cure a patient; recurrence is often the start of a prolonged course that ends in death.

Management is complex and depends on the age and medical condition of the, usually elderly, patient, as well as its exact site, degree of spread (stage) and histological type. An appropriate treatment protocol must be selected for each individual, taking these features into account. Oral carcinomas are not normally treated according to standardised protocols unlike carcinomas at other body sites. The great variation between tumour extent and general health factors makes the effectiveness of treatment very difficult to ascertain. There have been very few large-scale trials of surgical and multimodality treatment and a sound evidence base for treatment of individual cases is often lacking.

Preoperative assessment

The first stages in management are to identify the type, spread and stage of the carcinoma and to evaluate comorbidity.

Spread is assessed by clinical examination and imaging. Palpation is not always effective in delineating the outline of a tumour. Well-differentiated carcinomas containing much keratin are usually firm and readily identified, but dispersed lesions, particularly those in the posterior tongue, may be impalpable. Clinical signs, such as nerve palsies, also indicate extent of spread. Imaging involves computerised tomography (CT), magnetic resonance imaging (MRI) and positron emission tomography (PET), often in combination. Extension to the base of skull, prevertebral fascia, large areas of skin or around the carotid sheath usually render tumours inoperable. Extension to the posterior tongue risks aspiration of food and saliva postoperatively and may necessitate laryngectomy with consequent loss of voice. Imaging includes the neck and chest to identify or exclude lymph node and blood-borne metastases.

Many patients are heavy smokers or alcoholic. They often have systemic cardiovascular or respiratory, neurological or liver disease that will pose an anaesthetic risk or compromise recovery from surgery. Nutritional status may need to be improved before treatment. The patient's psychological fitness for possible disfiguring surgery, and future difficulty in speaking and swallowing must also be assessed. These and other complications of surgery must be understood by patients if they are to make properly informed choices and consent to treatment.

Biopsy of the carcinoma provides information on the degree of differentiation and pattern of spread. Carcinomas with dispersed or perineural invasion are more difficult to identify accurately at operation and more likely to be incompletely excised. Those with vascular invasion are at risk of blood-borne distant metatsases.

Actual and potential dental infection in the mouth must be dealt with before starting treatment, particularly if this is to be by irradiation. Dental infection or extractions may lead to extensive osteomyelitis in irradiated bone because of its poor vascularity and this osteoradionecrosis is very resistant to treatment. The sockets should be healed, as nearly as possible, before radiotherapy is begun. In practice, teeth with extensive caries or periapical lesions for which rapid successful treatment cannot be guaranteed are usually extracted because of the need to start treatment quickly.

Once all the information necessary is available, all patients should have an individual treatment plan defined by a multidisciplinary team in a cancer centre. The team includes at least one surgeon, medical oncologist and radiotherapist, nurse specialist, pathologist, dietitian, speech therapist and other specialties. Staging according to the TNM classification (Table 17.1) is the major determinant of possible treatments. The team will propose either a curative or palliative care plan for the patient to discuss and will review the patient's progress and plan treatment for any recurrence. Because head and neck surgery and radiotherapy have significant morbidity, the patient's view of these adverse effects is often the major consideration in the final treatment plan.

Treatment

In practice, most intraoral carcinomas are treated by surgery combined with radiotherapy ('multimodality therapy'). Surgery alone is preferred for small carcinomas of the tongue that may be easily excised, for those involving bone because of the risk of later radionecrosis, and for verrucous carcinoma. Irradiation provides a more acceptable cosmetic and functional result than major surgery but involves considerable discomfort during a

Table 17.1 TNM staging for oral carcinoma

T	N	M
T1 <2cm greatest dimension	N0 No regional lymph node metastases	M0 No distant metastases
T2 2–4 cm greatest dimension	N1 One ipsilateral node <3 cm diameter	M1 Distant metastasis (e.g. liver, lung)
T3 >4 cm greatest dimension	N2 Ipsilateral or contralateral nodes 3–6 cm diameter	
T4 extending to adjacent structures, e.g. bone, sinus, skin	N3 Lymph node metastasis >6cm diameter	
Stage 1 T1 N0 M0 Stage 2 T2 N0 M0 Stage 3 T3 N0 M0 Stage 4 any T4 any N2 or N3 any M1		

long course of treatment and has unwanted effects in the long term (Box 17.4).

Box 17.4 Unwanted effects of radiotherapy to the oral region

During treatment
- Severe xerostomia
- Mucositis and ulceration
- Acute candidosis
- Skin erythema

Long term
- Xerostomia
- Mucosal and skin atrophy
- Risk of osteomyelitis (osteoradionecrosis)
- Scarring and fibrosis of tissues
- Cataract if eye irradiated (e.g. antral carcinoma)
- Risk of late radiation-induced malignancy

When surgery is used it is usually performed first, unless there has been a poor response to, or recurrence after, irradiation (salvage surgery). The aim is to excise the carcinoma with as wide a margin as possible, ideally 1 cm or more. Modern surgical methods allow excision, reconstruction, grafting or bypassing of almost any structure in the oral regions. However, a margin of more than a few millimetres is rarely achieved in practice, because carcinomas have unpredictable irregular outlines or extend close to important anatomical structures. Also, wider excision may make reconstruction difficult. Reconstructive surgery is normally performed at the same operation as excision, to provide a better cosmetic and functional result and utilises a range of donor tissue sites. Excision by a few millimetres is insufficient to guarantee removal of the carcinoma, which may recur at the original site and postoperative radiotherapy is usually recommended.

Radiotherapy usually involves exposure to beams of X-rays or gamma-rays from X-ray generators or radioactive isotopes such as cobalt (external beam radiotherapy or teletherapy). Ionising radiation damages normal as well as neoplastic tissue, so that treatment planning is critical. The lesion is accurately localised by imaging techniques and a dose, usually in the region of 60 Gy for oral lesions, is given. Damage to surrounding tissues is limited by fractionating the dose over many visits (perhaps 30 daily fractions) and by applying external beams from many angles, but avoiding radiosensitive tissues such as the eye and bone. For teletherapy, a mask is made to fit the patient's head to allow reproducible beam angulation between visits. Radiotherapy planning and mask construction are complex and involve a short delay before treatment can start. Alternatively, implantation of radioactive materials, either as needles or grains, into and around the carcinoma (brachytherapy) is undertaken in some centres and is particularly useful for small lingual carcinomas. Development of radiation-induced sarcoma is a risk that has been estimated to be 1.6% after 10 years.

When surgery is to be recommended and no cervical lymph nodes appear involved, a decision must be made whether or not to perform a neck dissection. Neck dissection removes all the cervical lymph nodes along the jugular chain from the base of skull to the clavicle, together with those in the submandibular and submental triangles and posterior triangle of the neck. Depending on the type of resection, the sternomastoid muscle, internal jugular vein and accessory nerve may also be sacrificed. Even when no metastasis is detectable, small deposits of carcinoma may already have spread to lymph nodes. If left in place, they will grow over a period of months or years to form a recurrence, from which further cervical metatsases or distant metastases may seed. Performing an elective neck dissection in such cases removes these microscopic occult metastases, but its value is a matter of controversy. For tongue carcinoma, many surgeons prefer to perform an elective neck dissection.

Chemotherapy is less widely used in the UK than in Europe. Alone it gives good initial control but relapse will always occur without surgery or radiotherapy. For best effect it is carried out *concomitantly* with radiotherapy and gives approximately a 10% improvement in survival at best. The usual agents are the alkylating agent cisplatin with 5-fluorouracil, though many apparently equally effective regimens are in use including taxols. All regimens have significant adverse effects, particularly with mucositis and immunosuppression and these are compounded by radiotherapy. Only the fittest patients are able to tolerate concomitant chemotherapy. *Neoadjuvant* chemotherapy is given before surgery or radiotherapy and *adjuvant* chemotherapy after, both reducing adverse effects but being less effective. Chemotherapy agents act by radiosensitisation as well as their direct effects on cancer cells.

Treatment failure

Approximately half the patients suffer treatment failure and recurrence, either at the primary site, in lymph nodes or in distant sites such as lung, liver or bone.

Primary site recurrence usually signifies a poor prognosis because either a full course of radiotherapy or as large an excision as practical will already have been performed. Recurrence in lymph nodes usually appears within 2 years after treatment. The metastases probably arise from microscopic deposits of carcinoma already in the lymph nodes at the time of initial therapy (occult metastases). They may be treated surgically by neck dissection or by radiotherapy and do not necessarily indicate failure of treatment and further treatment is often curative.

Recurrent carcinoma is often less well differentiated and more aggressive. It invades more widely and unpredictably in the tissues, particularly if previously irradiated, and is difficult to localise. Re-excision is often impossible.

Primary and recurrent disease have been treated more aggressively in recent years and more patients now succumb to distant blood-borne metastases than previously. Distant metastases are usually multiple and there is no effective treatment.

Palliative care

Palliative treatment is given to patients who have advanced tumours or for treatment failures. Radiotherapy is the most practical method for palliative care, but surgery is occasionally used when a large tumour compromises the airway or becomes grossly necrotic.

Novel treatments

A wide range of new treatments is under trial.

In sentinel node biopsy, a radioisotope is injected around the tumour the night before surgery, followed by a blue dye at the time of surgery. These drain via lymphatics to the *sentinel* lymph nodes, those that are first in the drainage pathway and are most likely to be involved by metastasis. These nodes are identified at surgery using a radiosensitive probe and by their blue colour, removed and examined either immediately by frozen section or the following day. If no metastasis is present, the rest of the neck is probably uninvolved and a neck dissection and its adverse effects can be avoided. If metastasis is present, a neck dissection is performed separately. As metastasis is confirmed in only about 80% of therapeutic neck dissections and 33% of elective (apparently metastasis-free) radical neck dissections, this technique holds great promise. It is useful in breast carcinoma and melanoma, but is, as yet, unproven for oral carcinoma.

In photodynamic therapy, a light-sensitising drug is administered and permeates the whole body. Exposure of the tumour to light of an appropriate wavelength triggers a photochemical reaction which should kill the cancer cells. This technique shows promise for superficial lesions and management of recurrence in palliative care, but requires long-term assessment of its value.

Up to 90% of head and neck cancers, including oral carcinomas, overexpress epidermal growth factor receptor (EGFR). EGFR controls cell cycle and apoptosis and has indirect effects in invasion and metastasis. Novel agents that inhibit the receptor include antibodies such as Cetuximab and small molecule tyrosine kinase inhibitors such as Iressa. These agents have shown promise in early trials. Farnesyl transferase inhibitors inhibit expression of the RAS oncogene, also mutated or amplified in about one-third of oral carcinomas. Early trials suggest they may be useful.

OncoVex is an engineered herpes simplex virus that can grow in, and thus lyse, tumour but not normal cells that is currently under trial. There is intense research activity to identify the molecular basis of oral carcinoma now that gene targeted and gene therapy treatments are available.

Intensity modulated radiotherapy is available in a few UK centres. It allows the radiation dose and shape of the beam to be controlled much more precisely, allowing a higher dose to be given to the tumour while reducing adverse effects.

SURVIVAL FROM ORAL CANCER

Duration of survival after treatment depends on many factors (Box 17.5). In comparison with malignant neoplasms at other body sites, oral carcinoma has a poor prognosis. The quality of life in the terminal stages is also poor.

Box 17.5   **Some factors adversely affecting survival from oral cancer**

- Delay in treatment
- Advanced age
- Male gender
- Poor general health, usually smoking-related diseases
- Tumour size
- Posterior location
- Lack of histological differentiation (high histological grade)
- Lymph node spread

The poorer survival of older people is probably because they are less able to withstand radiotherapy or surgery. The reason for the poorer survival rates for males is uncertain, although later presentation is a possibility. Tumour stage at the start of treatment depends both on its growth rate and on delay in diagnosis. Because the stage of disease is critical to survival, it is used to plan treatment and every oral carcinoma patient should be staged according to the TNM staging system (see Table 17.1). Each carcinoma is given a score for size (T), lymph node metastasis (N) and distant blood-borne metastasis (M). These are combined together to give a score between stage 0 (premalignancy) and IV. Unfortunately, most patients with oral carcinoma present at Stage III or IV (Fig. 17.16).

However, some small (early) carcinomas are fast-growing and aggressive, but large tumours, even if slow-growing, are more difficult to manage. In either case, delay in treatment allows further tumour spread and poorer chances of long-term survival.

The highest mortality from oral cancer is in the first 2 years, the disease then continues to claim victims but at a slower rate, and those few that survive for 10 years have a reasonable

Fig. 17.16   Neglected cancer of the buccal mucosa about to ulcerate through the cheek.

chance of having been cured. As a guide to survival rates, nearly 90% of males with early-stage disease survive the first year, about 65% survive for up to 5 years, while just under 55% survive for 10 years. Of males with late-stage disease well under 45% survive the first year, about 16% survive for 5 years, and 12% survive for 10 years.

As to the site of the growth, the extremes are seen in cancer of the lip, where the 5-year survival rate for males is over 77%. For cancer of the tongue it is 26% and, in the mesopharynx, it is only 17.6%. Tumours, particularly of the posterior third of the tongue, are not readily detectable and more difficult to excise. In general, therefore, the more posterior the tumour is, the poorer the survival.

Role of the dentist

Early diagnosis is critical if patients are to be cured. Small carcinomas are more easily excised, less likely to have metastasised and have the best prognosis. Unfortunately, most carcinomas present at a relatively late, incurable stage and health care workers, including dentists, frequently either fail to make the diagnosis or have actively delayed referral.

Dentists must be alert to the possibility of carcinoma even though they may encounter it only once or twice in a practising lifetime. The nature of a chronic ulcer, white or red lesion, or swelling of the mucous membrane must be confirmed by biopsy. Indecision about taking a biopsy or trying the effect of local measures or antibiotics can prove fatal.

Any high-risk premalignant lesion or suspected carcinoma should be referred the same day to a specialist treatment centre. An appropriately worded referral letter should state the urgent nature of the referral and the suspected malignant nature of the lesion. It is better if the biopsy is performed by the cancer management team. Never perform an *excisional* biopsy of a possible small carcinoma. Once the biopsy site has healed, there may be no clue to its site or size, making further treatment difficult. Survival is reduced in such circumstances.

The dental practitioner is likely to see more patients with white mucosal patches. As noted in Chapter 15, the vast majority of such lesions are benign and may be biopsied in a practice setting. However, it is inadvisable to perform a biopsy of a high-risk lesion (for instance an erythroplasia or speckled leukoplakia) because the practitioner may be forced into the unenviable position of having to tell the patient that they have cancer, a task for which most dentists are not trained.

Although much of a patient's treatment has to be performed in hospital, patients may continue to see their practitioner after treatment. The dental practitioner is also ideally placed for the prevention of oral cancer and can contribute in other ways (Box 17.6).

Box 17.6 Role of the dental practitioner in cancer prevention and diagnosis

Prevention
- Actively discourage smoking and betel quid use
- Encourage moderation of alcohol intake
- Health promotion and education on oral carcinoma
- Provide check-ups for the edentulous and/or institutionalised elderly and other high-risk non-attenders

Early diagnosis
- Be vigilant and suspicious
- Always examine mucosa as well as the teeth
- Monitor low-risk premalignant lesions
- Refer all high-risk lesions on discovery
- Perform biopsy appropriately

After treatment
- Manage simple denture problems after surgery
- Alleviate the effects of post-irradiation dry mouth, e.g. preventing caries (Ch. 3)
- Monitor for recurrence, new premalignant lesions and second primary tumours
- Monitor for cervical metastasis
- Maintain morale of and provide additional support to patients and their relatives

---

ORAL CANCER SCREENING

Screening is the process of applying a rapid test or examining a population to identify a group at risk from a disease. This group can then be referred for accurate and earlier diagnosis. An example is the national cervical carcinoma screening scheme using the cervical smear test. Oral carcinoma screening should be possible because the tumour is so accessible and because those at most risk (elderly persons, particularly those who smoke and drink alcohol) are readily identified. A simple effective screening test is an examination of the mouth for red and white lesions.

Because screening is not an accurate diagnostic test, it may be performed by appropriately trained health care workers in the community. Such oral cancer screening schemes have proved successful in several countries with a high incidence. In the UK, such a scheme would have the advantage that it might reach the highest risk individuals who tend to be irregular dental attenders. It would also provide an opportunity for preventive advice to the same group.

Although a national screening scheme for the UK has been widely discussed, it has only been applied on a limited scale and is currently considered not to be cost effective. In the meantime, oral cancer screening continues to fall within the remit of the general dental and medical practitioner.

Screening and detection aids

Several tests are marketed, some without a clear distinction as to whether they are for screening or diagnosis, the latter demanding a much higher reliability.

Tolonium chloride (toluidine blue) rinsing

Toluidine blue is a dye which binds to nucleic acids and can be used as an oral rinse in the hope of staining carcinoma and dysplastic lesions blue. The technique was extensively evaluated many decades ago and is now the subject of a resurgence of interest. It may be of value when deciding which part of an extensive lesion should be biopsied or when the clinician does not feel confident about a clinical diagnosis.

However, the technique is not an accurate test for either carcinoma or premalignancy and is no more than an adjunct to clinical diagnosis. If used indiscriminately on white lesions, lichen planus and ulcers, the technique has a high false-positive rate. Also, toluidine blue is itself mutagenic and it seems inadvisable to use it as a general screening test. The general rule should be that any suspicious lesion must be subjected to biopsy as soon as possible, regardless of the pattern of staining with toluidine blue.

Brush biopsy

This technique is relatively non-invasive and therefore attractive for screening or long-term follow-up. It uses a round stiff-bristle brush to collect cells from the surface and subsurface layers of a lesion by vigorous abrasion. The brush is rotated in the fingers in one spot until bleeding starts, to ensure a sufficiently deep sample, but there is little or no pain, minimal bleeding and no need for sutures. The cells collected are transferred to a microscope slide and the smear is scanned in an image analyser to identify abnormal cells, which are examined for diagnosis.

A high degree of sensitivity and specificity for carcinoma is claimed, but studies have shown widely varying accuracy. There is a significant false-positive rate for identification of dysplasia and occasional false-negatives make it mandatory that incisional biopsies be carried out when there is any doubt. This technique requires fuller evaluation in properly controlled trials before it can be recommended.

Saliva tests

The attractive possibility that oral cancer might be diagnosed by a simple saliva test has reached the newspapers. Examples of such investigations include detecting tumour RNA, aberrant DNA sequence or expression of mutated p53 gene, loss of heterozygosity or microsatellite instability, concentrations of both albumin and alpha amylase, interleukin 6 and 8 levels, microarray analysis levels of expression of multiple genes, and assay for numerous markers including cytokines and even the oral flora. Despite claims for high sensitivity, diagnosis of oral cancer by saliva examination therefore remains little more than an attractive possibility.

VERRUCOUS CARCINOMA

This variant of squamous cell carcinoma is a low-grade neoplasm. In the UK, it is more frequent in the elderly, particularly males, and has a characteristic white, warty appearance, forming a well-circumscribed mass raised above the level of the surrounding mucosa (Fig. 17.17). If small, it may easily be mistaken for a papilloma. Verrucous carcinoma is particularly associated with the habit of snuff dipping (see above).

Pathology

Verrucous carcinoma consists of close-packed papillary masses of well-differentiated squamous epithelium which is heavily keratinised. The lower border of the lesion is well defined and formed by blunt rete processes which indent but do not invade the underlying tissues. There is typically chronic inflammation in the stroma (Fig. 17.18).

Verrucous carcinoma is slow-growing and spreads laterally rather than deeply. It can be excised relatively easily unless it is

Fig. 17.17 **Verrucous carcinoma.** An extensive lesion covering most of the buccal mucosa and starting to involve the skin at the commissure. Such longstanding lesions are likely to develop invasive squamous carcinoma and may then metastasise. By kind permission of Professor SJ Challacombe.

Fig. 17.18 **Verrucous carcinoma.** The epithelium is thickened and thrown into a series of folds with a spiky parakeratotic surface. Deeply, the carcinoma retains a broad pushing front.

extensive. If left untreated for a period of years, a focus within verrucous carcinoma may progress to invasive squamous carcinoma and release metastases. The neoplasm must then be treated as a conventional squamous carcinoma.

SUGGESTED FURTHER READING

Al-Bakkal G, Ficarra G, McNeill K et al 1999 Human papilloma virus type 16 E6 gene expression in oral exophytic epithelial lesions as detected by rtPCR. Oral Surg Oral Med Oral Pathol Oral Radiol Endod 87:197–200

Anderson DL 1971 Cause and prevention of lip cancer. J Can Dent Assoc 37:138–143

Caniff JP, Harvey W, Harris M 1986 Oral submucous fibrosis: its pathogenesis and management. Br Dent J 160:429–434

Cawson RA, Langdon JD, Eveson JW 1996 Surgical pathology of the mouth and jaws. Wright, Oxford

Cawson RA, Binnie WH, Barrett AW, Wright M 1998 Lucas's pathology of tumors of the oral tissues. Churchill Livingstone, Edinburgh

Cawson RA, Binnie WH, Barrett AW, Wright JM 2001 Oral disease, 3rd edn. Mosby-Wolfe, London

Franceschi S, Munoz N, Snijders PJF 2000 How strong and how wide is the link between HPV and oropharyngeal cancer? Lancet 356:871–872

Girod SC, Pfahl M 1996 Retinoid actions and implications for prevention and therapy of cancer. Int J Oral Maxillofac Surg 25:69–73

Goldberg HI, Lockwood SA, Wyatt SW, Crosset LS 1994 Trends and differentials from cancers of the oral cavity and pharynx in the United States, 1973–1987. Cancer 74:565–572

Hogewind WFC, van der Waal I, van der Kwast WA, Snow GB 1989 The association of white lesions with oral squamous cell carcinoma. A retrospective study of 212 patients. Int J Oral Maxillofac Surg 18:163–164

Hopper C 1996 The role of photodynamic therapy in the management of oral cancer and precancer. Oral Oncol Eur J Cancer 32B: 71–72

Kusama K, Okutso S, Takeda A et al 1996 p53 gene alterations and p53 protein in oral epithelial dysplasia and squamous cell carcinoma. J Pathol 178:415–421

Link JO, Kaugars GE, Burns JC 1992 Comparison of oral carcinomas in smokeless tobacco users and nonusers. J Oral Maxillofac Surg 50:452–455

Lukinmaa P-L, Hietanen J, Söderholm A-L, Lindquist C 1992 The histologic pattern of bone invasion by squamous cell carcinoma of the mandibualr region. Br J Oral Maxillofac Surg 30:2–7

Murti PR, Bhonsle RB, Pindborg JJ, Daftary DK, Gupta PC, Mehta FS 1985 Malignant transformation rate in oral submucous fibrosis over a 17-year period. Community Dent Oral Epidemiol 13:340–341

Ogden GR, Kiddie RA, Lunny DP, Lane DP 1992 Assessment of p53 protein expression in normal, benign and malignant oral mucosa. J Pathol 166:389–394

Shah JP 1990 Patterns of cervical lymph node metastases from squamous cell carcinomas of the upper aerodigestive tract. Am J Surg 160:405–409

Shah JP, Batsakis JG, Johnson NW 2002 Oral cancer. Taylor & Francis, London

Shahnavaz SA, Regezi JA, Bradley G et al 2000 p53 gene mutations in sequential oral epithelial dysplasias and squamous cell carcinomas. J Pathol 190:417–422

Warnakulasuriya A 2000 Lack of molecular markers to predict malignant potential of oral cancer. J Pathol 190:407–409

Woolgar JA, Scott J 1995 Prediction of cervical lymph node metastasis in squamous cell carcinoma of the tongue/floor of mouth. Head Neck 17:463–472

Neoplastic and non-neoplastic diseases of salivary glands

Normal function and health of the mouth depend on normal secretion of saliva by the major and minor glands. Failure of salivary secretion causes a dry mouth which is both distressing and promotes oral infections.

OBSTRUCTION → Summaries pp. 172, 314

Salivary calculi

A stone can form in a salivary gland or duct. At least 80% of calculi form in the submandibular gland, about 6% in the parotid and about 2% in the sublingual and minor salivary glands.

Clinical features

Adults are mainly affected – males twice as often as females. Calculi are usually unilateral. The classical symptom is pain when the smell or taste of food stimulates salivary secretion. Alternatively, duct obstruction can lead to infection, pain and swelling of the gland.

Occasionally there are no symptoms until the stone passes forward and can be palpated in the duct or seen at the duct orifice

(Fig. 18.1). Alternatively, the stone may be seen in a radiograph. However, about 40% of parotid and 20% of submandibular stones are not radiopaque and sialography may be needed to locate them.

Calculi are not a cause of dry mouth.

Pathology

Salivary calculi usually form by deposition of calcium salts around a nidus of organic material and have a layered structure. The roughness of their surface may cause the duct lining to undergo squamous metaplasia (Fig. 18.2). An adherent layer of microbial flora often grows on stones and this, together with obstruction, usually triggers inflammation and fibrosis around the duct.

Management

The stone should be identified by plain radiography and the degree of damage to the gland from ascending infection and sialadenitis assessed by sialography.

Fig. 18.1   Salivary calculus. This stone has impacted just behind the orifice of the submandibular duct forming a hard nodule. The yellow colour of the stone is visible through the thin mucosa.

Fig. 18.2   Salivary calculus in a duct. To the left is the salivary calculus which has a lamellar structure and an irregular surface. On the surface is a thick layer of microbial flora filling the space between the stone and the epithelial lining. In the surrounding wall, there is an infiltrate of lymphocytes and plasma cells and neutrophils are migrating through the duct epithelium into the lumen.

If sufficiently far forward in the duct, a stone may sometimes be milked forward and manipulated out of the orifice without difficulty. If this fails, or the stone is distally placed, treatment should start with the least invasive method likely to succeed. Lithotripsy uses an ultrasonic shock wave applied extraorally and focused on the stone. A series of repeated treatments may be enough to fracture the stone into small pieces that will pass out of the duct orifice. If this fails, stones in the duct but outside the gland can be removed using a 'basket' of fine wire manipulated down the duct and around the stone. Alternatively, microendoscopy can be combined with laser disruption of the stone. These conservative techniques are often successful and, perhaps surprisingly, the gland will often recover normal function despite repeated attacks of chronic sialadenitis.

If conservative measures fail and the stone is within the duct, the duct has to be opened. An incision, usually under local anaesthesia, is made along the line of the duct just long enough to release the mass. A temporary suture should be put around the duct behind the calculus to prevent it from slipping backwards. The papilla should be left unsutured or the margins of the opening are sutured to the mucosa on either side to prevent subsequent scarring and fibrous obstruction.

When stones are within the gland or a sialogram reveals that the gland is severely damaged by recurrent infection and fibrosis, it will probably have to be excised.

Key features of salivary calculi are summarised in Box 18.1.

Box 18.1   Salivary calculi: key features

- Adult males mainly affected
- Usually (80%) in submandibular gland
- Usually form by accretion of calcium salts round organic nidus
- Typically cause pain by obstructing food-related surge of salivary secretion
- Occasionally asymptomatic until palpable in the mouth or seen in routine radiograph
- Do not cause dry mouth
- Should be removed by manipulation or incision of duct

Parotid papilla and duct strictures → Summary p. 314

The usual cause of strictures at the papilla is chronic trauma (from such causes as projecting clasps, faulty restorations or sharp edges of broken teeth) leading to fibrosis. Fibrosis makes the duct papilla difficult to find and may prevent insertion of a probe.

Strictures of the duct are almost always caused by fibrosis resulting from ulceration and inflammation round a calculus or scarring following inadequate surgery.

Sialography should show the degree of narrowing of the duct or papilla and dilatation behind. Once the cause has been removed, treatment depends on the site of the obstruction. The papilla may have to be excised and the duct lining sutured to the oral mucosa on either side. Alternatively, the duct may be dilated with bougies.

Salivary fistula

Salivary fistula, a communication between the duct system or gland with the skin or mucous membrane, is uncommon. Internal fistulae drain into the oral cavity and cause no symptoms. By contrast, parotid fistula on the skin is troublesome and often persistent. It may be the result of an injury to the cheek or a complication of surgery. Infection often becomes superimposed and persistent leakage of saliva prevents healing. The treatment is primarily by surgical repair but is difficult, especially because of the risk of damage to branches to the facial nerve.

Mucoceles and cysts

The most common type of salivary and soft-tissue cyst is the extravasation mucocele of minor glands. It is not a true cyst as it has no epithelial lining. Retention cysts are far less common. Mucoceles mainly affect the minor salivary glands, particularly of the lip. The cause is usually damage to the duct of a mucous gland. This may be caused by a blow on the lip, as might happen to a football referee holding a whistle in his mouth.

Clinical features

Mucoceles most often form in the lower lip but, occasionally, on the buccal mucosa or floor of the mouth (ranula). They are usually superficial and rarely larger than 1 cm in diameter. In the early stages, they appear as rounded fleshy swellings. Later, they are obviously cystic, hemispherical, fluctuant and bluish due to the thin wall (Fig. 18.3). A mucocele cannot be distinguished from a retention cyst clinically, but this is of little practical importance. A similar mass in the upper lip is much more likely to be a salivary neoplasm.

Fig. 18.3   Mucous extravasation cyst. The typical presentation at the commonest site: a rounded bluish, translucent cyst in the lower lip.

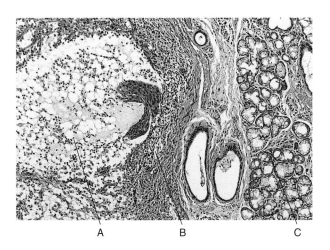

Fig. 18.4 **Extravasation mucocele.** To the left is a cavity of spilt mucin with the remnants of the ruptured duct lining epithelium at its edge. To the right is the associated minor mucous salivary gland. A, saliva and macrophages; B, compressed connective tissue wall; C, minor salivary gland.

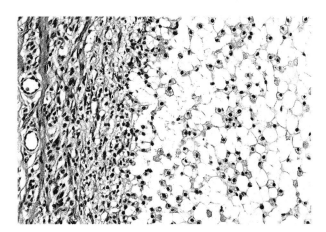

Fig. 18.5 **Extravasation mucocele.** Higher power showing the lining of the mucin-filled space. Macrophages are migrating into the mucin and in phagocytosing it develop a foamy or vacuolated cytoplasm.

Pathology

Preceding the formation of a mucocele, saliva leaking from a damaged duct into the superficial surrounding tissues excites an inflammatory reaction (Figs 18.4 and 18.5). The pools of saliva gradually coalesce to form a rounded collection of fluid, surrounded by compressed connective tissue without an epithelial lining.

Less frequently, the duct may become obstructed but less severely damaged so that saliva does not escape into the surrounding tissues. A retention cyst thus forms with a lining of compressed duct epithelium (Fig. 18.6).

Treatment

A small superficial mucocele should be excised with the underlying gland. The latter is usually found to have been removed with the cyst but if not, recurrence is likely.

Key features are summarised in Box 18.2.

Fig. 18.6 **Mucous retention cyst.** Remnants of the minor mucous salivary glands are visible, together with their dilated duct, the epithelium of which is continuous with the epithelial lining of the cyst (above).

Fig. 18.7 **Ranula.** A large bluish, translucent swelling in the floor of the mouth caused by a mucous extravasation or retention cyst.

Box 18.2 **Mucoceles and cysts: key features**

- Most common soft tissue cyst
- Most frequently on lower lip
- Usually caused by damage to duct and extravasation of saliva
- Saliva leaking into surrounding tissues causes mild inflammation
- Saliva eventually pools up to form a mucocele with connective tissue lining
- Rarely due to duct obstruction and dilatation forming a retention cyst with epithelial lining

---

Ranula

A ranula is an uncommon type of salivary cyst arising from the sublingual or submandibular salivary glands.

The structure is usually the same as other salivary retention cysts. Ranulae are usually unilateral and 2 or 3 cm in diameter (Fig. 18.7). Occasionally, they extend across the whole of the floor of the mouth. They are soft, fluctuant and bluish. They are typically painless but may interfere with speech or mastication. Treatment is preferably by marsupialisation with removal of the related gland. A simple incision leads to recurrence. Enucleation is difficult because of the very thin wall.

SIALADENITIS

Mumps → Summary p. 316

Mumps is due to a paramyxovirus (the mumps virus) and causes painful swelling of the parotids and sometimes other glands. It is highly infectious and is the most common cause of acute parotid swelling.

Clinical features

Children are mainly affected. An incubation period of about 21 days is followed by headache, malaise, fever and tense, painful and tender swelling of the parotids. Permanent nerve deafness or, rarely, meningitis are possible complications. Adults who contract mumps may develop orchitis or oophoritis and may have severe and prolonged malaise. After an attack immunity is long-lasting.

The diagnosis is usually obvious from the history and clinical findings, especially in a child. However, mumps may be mistaken for a dental infection or bacterial sialadenitis, if unilateral. Rarely, when the submaxillary or sublingual glands are affected, mumps may have to be differentiated from lymphadenitis. In cases of doubt, a history of mumps earlier in life usually excludes this diagnosis. If necessary, the diagnosis can be confirmed by a rise in titre of complement-fixing antibodies. Afterwards, antibodies to the S antigen disappear relatively quickly, and their presence indicates recent mumps. The V antibody is persistent and indicates infection at some time previously.

Mumps vaccination is provided as the measles-mumps-rubella (MMR) vaccination, introduced in 1988. Before this there were epidemics every three years. Recent patient concern about the MMR has reduced uptake to below the level required to prevent epidemics and there have been recent outbreaks, notably in 2005 among university students who had not been immunised. Immunisation is not completely effective in preventing the disease, but the acute episode is milder and, particularly in adults, may take atypical forms.

MMR vaccination is given at around 1 and 4 years of age. It is a live virus and a small minority of recipients develop a mild presentation of mumps with salivary gland swelling 3 weeks after the first dose.

Suppurative parotitis

Suppurative parotitis traditionally affected debilitated patients, particularly postoperatively, as a result of xerostomia secondary to dehydration. Currently, suppurative parotitis is more commonly seen in ambulant patients with severe xerostomia, particularly Sjögren's syndrome, and as an uncommon complication of tricyclic antidepressant treatment. Important bacterial

Fig. 18.8 Suppurative parotitis – pus is leaking from the parotid papilla.

causes include *Staphylococcus aureus*, streptococci and anaerobes. Typical clinical features are pain in one or both parotids with swelling, redness and tenderness and often increasing malaise and fever. The regional lymph nodes are enlarged and tender, and pus exudes or can be expressed from the parotid duct (Fig. 18.8). The progress of the infection depends largely on the patient's underlying physical state.

Pathology

An intense acute inflammatory infiltrate extends along and dilates the ducts. Inflammation also extends into the periductal tissues and to a varying degree into acini. If neglected, abscesses form and there are varying degrees of acinar destruction.

Treatment

Treatment can be started with flucloxacillin, but only after pus has been obtained for culture and sensitivity testing. The antibiotic can be changed if the bacteriological findings dictate and drainage is rarely necessary.

Tuberculous sialadenitis

Mycobacterial parotitis is frequently a feature of advanced AIDS but, occasionally, also develops in immunocompetent adults. The chronic inflammatory swelling typically resembles a tumour and the diagnosis is only made after histological detection of non-caseating granulomas and identification of *M. tuberculosis* by PCR.

Chronic sialadenitis → Summary p. 314

Chronic sialadenitis is usually a complication of duct obstruction. It is usually unilateral and asymptomatic or with intermittent painful swelling of the gland. Sialography may show dilatation of ducts behind the obstruction.

Fig. 18.9 **Chronic sialadenitis resulting from obstruction.** The ducts contain casts of mucin and neutrophils and are surrounded by a layer of fibrosis. There is severe acinar atrophy and the space previously occupied by acinar cells now contains infiltrates of lymphocytes and plasma cells.

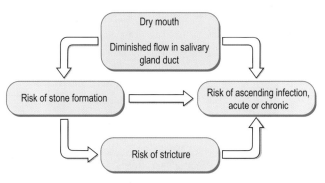

Fig. 18.10 **Interrelationships between dry mouth, calculi and their complications.** Note: dry mouth may promote stone formation, but stones do not cause dry mouth.

calculi and ascending infection and the relationships between these conditions are shown in Fig. 18.10.

Box 18.3 **Causes of xerostomia**

Organic causes
- Sjögren's syndrome
- Irradiation
- Mumps (transient)
- HIV infection
- HCV infection
- Sarcoidosis
- Amyloid
- Iron deposition (haemochromatosis, thalassaemia)

Functional causes
- Dehydration
- Fluid deprivation or loss
- Haemorrhage
- Persistent diarrhoea and/or vomiting
- Psychogenic
   Anxiety states
   Depression
- Drugs

Drugs
- Diuretic overdosage
- Drugs with antimuscarinic effects
   Atropine, ipratropium, hyoscine and other analogues
   Tricyclic and some other antidepressants
   Antihistamines
   Antiemetics (including antihistamines and phenothiazines)
   Neuroleptics, particularly phenothiazines
- Some older antihypertensives (ganglion blockers and clonidine)
- Drugs with sympathomimetic actions
   'Cold cures' containing ephedrine, etc.
   Decongestants
   Bronchodilators
   Appetite supressants, particularly amphetamines

Pathology

There are varying degrees of destruction of acini, duct dilatation and a scattered chronic inflammatory cellular infiltrate, predominantly lymphoplasmacytic (Fig. 18.9). Extensive interstitial fibrosis and, sometimes, squamous metaplasia in the duct epithelium follow. Calculus formation may be seen in the dilated ducts.

If possible, the obstruction should be removed but, more often, the gland has to be excised and the mass examined histologically to exclude a neoplasm.

DRY MOUTH (XEROSTOMIA)

Many patients with severe xerostomia make no complaint of dry mouth, though they may, for instance, admit that they have difficulty in eating dry food. Some complain of an unpleasant taste in the mouth. Conversely, some who complain of dry mouth have normal salivary flow rates on objective testing and the problem is neurotic in nature. Salivary flow studies are valuable when patients complain of dry mouth. Important causes are summarised in Box 18.3. Patients may suffer xerostomia,

SJÖGREN'S SYNDROME → Summary p. 316

In 1933, Sjögren noticed the association of dryness of the mouth and dryness of the eyes. Later, he found that there was a significant association with rheumatoid arthritis. These combinations of complaints are caused by two closely related but distinct diseases.

Primary Sjögren's syndrome (sicca syndrome) comprises dry mouth and dry eyes not associated with any connective tissue disease. 'Sicca syndrome' is also sometimes used for organic causes of dry mouth that lack the immunological anomalies of Sjögren's syndrome.

Secondary Sjögren's syndrome comprises dry mouth and dry eyes associated with rheumatoid arthritis or other connective tissue disease.

Clinical features

Females are affected nearly 10 times as frequently as males. Sjögren's syndrome affects 10–15% of patients with rheumatoid arthritis, possibly 30% of patients with lupus erythematosus and

Fig. 18.11 Sjögren's syndrome. The mucosa is dry, red, atrophic and wrinkled and sticks to the fingers or mirror during examination. These changes are common to all causes of xerostomia.

Fig. 18.12 Tongue in Sjögren's syndrome. Longstanding dry mouth and repeated candidal infection produce this depapillated but lobulated tongue.

Fig. 18.13 Sjögren's syndrome. Extensive cervical caries is a frequent complication of dry mouth. In addition to the lack of saliva, patients may attempt to stimulate salivary flow with sweets or chewing gums.

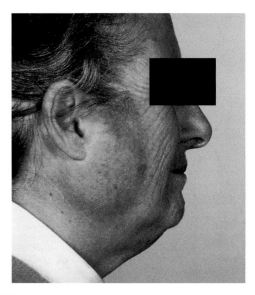

Fig. 18.14 Salivary gland swelling in primary Sjögren's syndrome. The outline of the parotid gland is clearly demarcated.

a variable proportion of patients with or without other connective tissue diseases. Sjögren's syndromes are therefore relatively common. In the absence of drug treatment or radiotherapy, they are the main cause of dry mouth, but their most serious consequence is damage to the eyes and the risk of lymphoma. Primary Sjögren's syndrome tends to cause more severe oral and ocular changes and has a higher risk of lymphomatous change than secondary.

Major oral effects of Sjögren's syndrome are summarised in Box 18.4.

In the early stages, the mucosa may appear moist, but salivary flow measurement shows diminished secretion. In

---

Box 18.4   Oral effects of Sjögren's syndrome

- Discomfort
- Difficulties with eating or swallowing
- Disturbed taste sensation
- Disturbed quality of speech
- Predisposition to infection

---

established cases, the oral mucosa is obviously dry, often red, shiny and parchment-like (Fig. 18.11). The tongue is typically red, the papillae characteristically atrophy and the dorsum becomes lobulated with a cobblestone appearance (Fig. 18.12). With diminished salivary secretion, the oral flora changes and candidal infections are common. The latter are the main cause of soreness of the mouth in Sjögren's syndrome and cause generalised erythema of the mucosa, often with angular stomatitis. Plaque accumulates and there may be rapidly progressive dental caries (Fig. 18.13). The most severe infective complication is suppurative parotitis.

Swelling of the parotids is not common, but a history of swelling at some stage may be obtained in about 30% of patients. Swelling due to the syndrome itself shows no inflammation and is rarely painful (Fig. 18.14). A hot, tender parotid swelling with red, shiny overlying skin indicates suppurative parotitis. Parotid swelling appearing years after the onset strongly suggests lymphomatous change (below).

Drug allergies may be a feature. In particular, a curious feature is allergy to trimethoprim which can cause a syndrome of fever, headache, backache and meningeal irritation.

The association of dry mouth, which can destroy appetite, together with the pain of rheumatoid arthritis persisting over many years is a deeply distressing condition. Depression is a common consequence. These patients need support and reassurance as well as efforts to overcome the symptoms.

Sjögren's syndrome can have serious ocular effects (Box 18.5).

Box 18.5   Ocular effects of Sjögren's syndrome

- Failure of tear secretion
- Failure of clearance of foreign particles from the cornea and conjunctiva (keratoconjunctivitis sicca)
- Gritty sensation in the eyes and inflammation
- Risk of impairment or loss of sight

Aetiology and pathology

Sjögren's syndrome is an autoimmune (connective tissue) disease which shows a corresponding variety of immunological abnormalities (Table 18.1). A retrovirus or other virus is as yet unconfirmed as a cause. The disease is systemic and affects all exocrine glands including those of the skin, vagina, lung and pancreas, though these rarely cause significant problems.

Histological changes are shown in Box 18.6. Lymphocytes infiltrate the glands and cluster around ducts, replacing acinar cells (Fig. 18.15). The mechanisms of acinar cell destruction are unclear; they do not appear to be the target of direct lymphocyte killing. Over a period of years, the lymphocytic infiltrates

---

Box 18.6   Histological changes in salivary glands in Sjögren's syndrome

- Polyclonal infiltration mainly by CD4 lymphocytes
- Infiltrate initially periductal
- Progressive spread of infiltrate through the glandular tissue
- Progressive destruction of secretory acini
- Proliferation of some duct tissue as epimyoepithelial islands

---

Table 18.1   Typical patterns of autoantibodies in primary and secondary Sjögren's syndromes

Autoantibodies	Primary SS	Secondary SS
Salivary duct antibody	10–36%	67–70%
Rheumatoid factor	50%±	90%±
SS-A (Ro) antibodies	5–10%	50–80%
SS-B (La) antibodies	50–75%	2–5%
Rheumatoid arthritis precipitin	5%±	75%±

---

enlarge and replace more of the gland. The ductal cells proliferate, possibly in response to cytokines released by the lymphocytes to form islands and sheets of cells around the ducts. Although myoepithelial cells are not a feature, the islands are often called myoepithelial islands (Fig. 18.16) and the overall appearance is sometimes called myoepithelial sialadenitis.

The final result is destruction of acini and replacement of the whole gland by a dense lymphocytic infiltrate (Fig. 18.16). However, the infiltrate remains confined within the gland capsule and does not cross the intraglandular septa.

Diagnosis

Other causes of xerostomia must be excluded (see Box 18.3). Diagnostic tests in Sjögren's syndrome are summarised in Box 18.7.

Normal salivary flow is between 1 and 2 ml per minute but may be reduced to 0.5 ml/min or less. Pathological changes

Fig. 18.15   Sjögren's syndrome. The histological appearance is typical. Dense, well-defined foci of lymphocytes surround the larger ducts in the centre of the lobules. In the area occupied by the lymphocytes, there is complete acinar atrophy and a rim of residual salivary parenchyma remains around the periphery of the lobule.

Fig. 18.16   Sjögren's syndrome. In late disease no salivary acini remain and the gland is replaced by a confluent infiltrate of lymphocytes. A few ducts remain and proliferate to form the epimyoepithelial islands. Such extensive changes sometimes suggest that there has been progression to a low-grade lymphoma.

in labial salivary glands correlate closely with those in the parotids and lip biopsy avoids the risks of damage to the facial nerve or a parotid fistula inherent in parotid gland biopsy. A snowstorm appearance on sialography (so-called sialectasis) is due to leakage of contrast material through the duct walls (Fig. 18.17). However, in a patient who is not taking xerostomia-inducing drugs, but with rheumatoid arthritis or other connective tissue disease and *objectively confirmed diminished salivary flow*, further investigation seems hard to justify.

Management

Many aspects need to be taken into account (Box 18.8), but the combination of painful arthritis and dryness of the mouth in secondary Sjögren's syndrome can reduce life to prolonged misery.

Ophthalmological examination is particularly important to exclude keratoconjunctivitis sicca, which is symptomless in its early stages. Anaemia should be excluded, particularly when there is rheumatoid arthritis.

Dryness of the mouth can be relieved to some degree by providing artificial saliva (Box 18.9). Cholinesterase inhibitors, such as pilocarpine, are sometimes recommended to stimulate salivary secretion, but any benefits may be counterbalanced by side-effects such as nausea, diarrhoea and bradycardia.

Dryness of the eyes is treated with artificial tears, such as methyl cellulose solution. In dentate patients, sweet-eating

should be prohibited, a high standard of oral hygiene maintained and frequent dental checks are necessary. Topical fluorides should be applied regularly and 0.2% chlorhexidine mouth rinses may help to reduce plaque formation. Soreness of the mouth, due to infection by *Candida albicans*, can be treated with nystatin or amphotericin mixture, not tablets. Ascending parotitis should be treated as described earlier.

In view of the risk of malignant lymphoma, immunosuppressive treatment or irradiation to reduce the size of swollen

Fig. 18.17 **Sjögren's syndrome.** The sialogram shows the typical snowstorm appearance of blobs of contrast medium that have leaked from the duct system. Emptying and clearance of the contrast medium are also much delayed because of the reduced salivary flow.

glands is contraindicated. In any case, such measures have no lasting benefit in Sjögren's syndrome.

Key features are summarised in Box 18.10.

> **Box 18.10 Sjögren's syndromes: key features**
>
> - Middle-aged or elderly women mainly affected
> - Rheumatoid arthritis or other connective tissue disease associated in secondary Sjögren's syndrome
> - Dry mouth
> - Dry eyes
> - Polyclonal infiltration of salivary glands by CD4 lymphocytes with acinar destruction
> - Multiple autoantibodies particularly Ro (SS-A) and La (SS-B)
> - Significant risk of salivary gland and extrasalivary lymphomas
> - Depression often

Lymphoma in Sjögren's syndrome → Summary p. 316

This, the most serious complication, is unpredictable and estimated to develop in nearly 6%. Persistent swelling, particularly in longstanding disease, is suggestive, as is sudden enlargement of previously swollen glands. As well as parotid swelling, the cervical lymph nodes may be involved. Fever and night sweats may be associated and suggest the development of lymphoma. The tumour is typically a MALT lymphoma (see Chapter 22 and below).

Benign lymphoepithelial lesion

Benign lymphoepithelial lesion is a term that has been used to describe salivary gland swelling with the histological features of Sjögren's syndrome. Other features of Sjögren's syndrome were thought to be absent but this appears to have been due to inadequate investigation. Benign lymphoepithelial lesion is a misleading term which should be avoided as there is a high risk of lymphomatous change and it is probably not a separate entity from Sjögren's syndrome.

IRRADIATION DAMAGE

Salivary tissue is highly sensitive to ionising radiation. Irreversible destruction of acini and fibrous replacement can result from therapeutic radiation of the head and neck. Troublesome xerostomia with its attendant complications, such as rampant dental caries, is the typical result.

The management of dry mouth is as described earlier. However, it is especially important to control dental caries and its sequelae because of the danger of irradiation-associated osteomyelitis (Ch. 6) secondary to periapical infection or extractions.

HIV-ASSOCIATED SALIVARY GLAND DISEASE →
Summaries pp. 315, 316

Chronic parotitis in children is said to be almost pathognomonic of HIV infection. In adults, xerostomia, sometimes with cystic parotid gland swellings, may develop and be associated with generalised lymphadenopathy (Ch. 22). Young males are predominantly affected.

Pathology

The histological features are essentially similar to those of Sjögren's syndrome, apart from gross cyst formation. Also, the infiltrate is by CD8 lymphocytes and autoantibodies typical of Sjögren's syndrome are lacking. As in Sjögren's syndrome, lymphomatous change is a hazard.

HIV salivary gland cysts respond to highly active retroviral therapy.

SJÖGREN-LIKE SYNDROME IN GRAFT-VERSUS-HOST DISEASE

A disease similar to primary Sjögren's syndrome develops in about a third of all cases of graft-versus-host disease (GVHD), particularly when severe. The histological changes in lip biopsies are the same as in Sjögren's syndrome and serve to distinguish GVHD from salivary gland damage secondary to irradiation used for immunosuppression before marrow transplantation.

HYPERSALIVATION (PTYALISM)

True ptyalism is not a significant complaint as any excess of saliva can readily be swallowed. 'False ptyalism' is more common and is either delusional (a disturbed patient may suddenly become alarmed at 'water' continually appearing in the mouth) or due to faulty neuromuscular control that leads to drooling despite normal salivary flow (Box 18.11).

> **Box 18.11 Causes of ptyalism**
>
> **Local reflexes**
> - Oral infections (e.g. acute necrotising ulcerative gingivitis)
> - Oral wounds
> - Dental procedures
> - New dentures
>
> **Systemic**
> - Nausea
> - Acid regurgitation (reflux oesophagitis)
>
> **Toxic**
> - Iodine. Heavy metal poisoning
>
> **'False ptyalism' (drooling)**
> - Psychogenic
> - Bell's palsy
> - Parkinson's disease
> - Stroke

SALIVARY GLAND NEOPLASMS → Summary p. 315

Salivary gland tumours comprise a significant proportion of oral tumours and are the next most common neoplasms of the mouth after squamous cell carcinoma. However, tumours of the minor intraoral salivary glands are less common than in the parotids. The incidence of salivary gland cancers in Europe is estimated to be about 1.2 per 100 000 and, in England and Wales, about 600 salivary gland cancers are registered each year. However, over 75% of salivary gland tumours are benign, so that the total number (benign and malignant) seen annually in Britain may be approximately 2400. Women are slightly more frequently affected. About 70% of salivary gland tumours develop in the parotid and a few affect the submandibular glands. Tumours in the sublingual glands are a rarity but usually malignant (Fig. 18.18).

Little is known of the aetiology of salivary gland tumours except that they can result from irradiation to the head area. In survivors of the atomic blasts at Hiroshima and Nagasaki, there has been an excess of salivary gland tumours. Similarly, these tumours can follow therapeutic irradiation of, for example, the thyroid and, it is suggested, multiple dental diagnostic radiographs.

Classification

The classification of salivary gland tumours is complex and histological diagnosis is recognised to be difficult. The current World Health Organization lists 24 malignant and 13 benign tumours and still more are recognised. However, many are rarities and a simplified classification of the commoner and more important entities is shown in Box 18.12. The full classification with notes and a brief note on each entity is shown in Appendix 18.1.

> **Box 18.12** Salivary gland neoplasms (simplified classification, see also Appendix 18.1)
>
> **Epithelial tumours**
> *Adenomas*
> - Pleomorphic adenoma ('mixed tumour') and myoepithelioma
> - Warthin's tumour
> - Oncocytoma (oxyphilic adenoma)
> - Basal cell adenoma
>
> *Carcinomas*
> - Mucoepidermoid carcinoma
> - Acinic cell carcinoma
> - Adenoid cystic carcinoma
> - Polymorphous low-grade adenocarcinoma
> - Salivary duct carcinoma
> - Epithelial-myoepithelial carcinoma
> - Adenocarcinoma NOS
> - Undifferentiated carcinoma
> - Carcinoma ex pleomorphic adenoma (malignant mixed tumour)
>
> **Non-epithelial tumours**
> - Lymphomas
> - Metastases to parotid lymph nodes

General clinical features of salivary gland tumours

Adults are predominantly affected. The usual intraoral site is the palate, often at the junction of the hard and soft palate (Fig. 18.19), or occasionally the cheek or lip. Typical clinical features

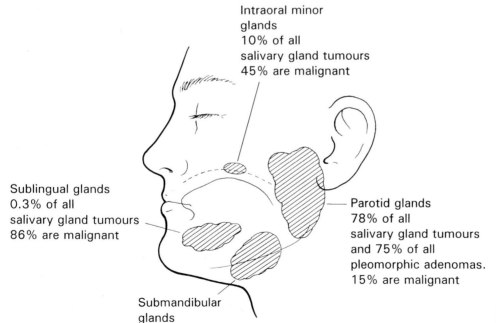

Intraoral minor glands
10% of all salivary gland tumours
45% are malignant

Sublingual glands
0.3% of all salivary gland tumours
86% are malignant

Parotid glands
78% of all salivary gland tumours
and 75% of all pleomorphic adenomas.
15% are malignant

Submandibular glands
12% of all salivary gland tumours
30% are malignant

Fig. 18.18 The distribution of salivary gland neoplasms showing the approximate overall frequency of tumours in different sites and the relevant frequency of benign and malignant tumours by site.

Fig. 18.19 **Pleomorphic adenoma.** The junction of hard and soft palates is a common intraoral site; the tumour usually feels rubbery and lobulated on palpation.

Table 18.2 Typical clinical features of salivary gland tumours	
Benign salivary gland tumours	**Malignant salivary gland tumours**
Slow-growing	Sometimes fast-growing and painful
Soft or rubbery consistency	Sometimes hard consistency
Comprise 85% of parotid tumours	Comprise 45% of minor gland tumours
Do not ulcerate	May ulcerate and invade bone
No associated nerve signs	May cause cranial nerve palsies*
*Malignant parotid tumours can cause facial palsy in particular. Adenoid cystic carcinoma can cause multiple cranial nerve lesions especially lingual, facial or hypoglossal.	

of benign and malignant salivary gland tumours are shown in Table 18.2. However, in their early stages, benign and malignant salivary gland tumours cannot be distinguished clinically.

Pleomorphic adenoma → Summary p. 315

Pleomorphic adenomas ('mixed tumours') account for about 75% of parotid tumours (Fig. 18.20), but a lower proportion of intraoral salivary gland tumours. They arise mainly from duct epithelium or myoepithelial cells. A wide variety of structures may be seen (Box 18.13).

Box 18.13 Important histological features of pleomorphic adenomas
• Capsule – never complete
• Ducts
• Sheets or strands of dark-staining epithelial cells
• Squamous metaplasia and foci of keratin
• Fibrous and elastic tissue
• Myxoid tissue
• Cartilage, sometimes calcified. Rarely, true bone formation

Fig. 18.20 **Pleomorphic adenoma.** This slowly enlarging lump in the lower pole of the parotid gland is caused by a pleomorphic adenoma, but the appearance is not specific and any benign and some low-grade malignant neoplasms could appear the same.

These varied tissues are completely disordered in arrangement and the proportions of the different components also vary widely (Figs 18.21–18.24). The fibrous, myxoid, or cartilaginous mesenchymal elements are due to the pluripotential properties of myoepithelial cells. Some tumours are predominantly myxoid and can burst at operation, if not gently handled, and then recur. Myoepithelial cells cannot be identified by light microscopy and can appear dark and angular, spindle-shaped or resemble plasma cells. However, immunohistochemistry shows their typical double staining with epithelial (cytokeratin) markers and mesenchymal markers, particularly S-100 protein, vimentin and actin. Myoepithelial cells may occasionally predominate or are the only cells present. Such a tumour is termed a *myoepithelioma*.

Growth of pleomorphic adenomas is slow and may take several years to reach an inch (2.5 cm) in diameter. They form

Fig. 18.21 **Pleomorphic adenoma.** The histological appearances are very varied. In this typical area there are clusters of ducts containing eosinophilic material surrounded by stellate cells lying in a mucinous stroma.

Fig. 18.24 **Pleomorphic adenoma.** At the margins of pleomorphic adenomas there are often extensions of the tumour into and beyond the capsule, rendering enucleation an ineffective treatment.

Fig. 18.22 **Pleomorphic adenoma.** In this area there has been maturation of the mucinous stroma to form a cartilage-like material within which there are more cellular islands with ducts.

Fig. 18.25 This excised pleomorphic adenoma is 3 cm across and the lobular shape is clearly seen.

Fig. 18.23 **Plemorphic adenoma.** In this lesion there is formation of true cartilage which is undergoing calcification.

rubbery, often lobulated swellings (Fig. 18.25). When close under the mucosa, the tumour may appear bluish. The swelling is typically attached to the overlying mucosa but mobile on the deeper tissues. If neglected, pleomorphic adenomas can grow to a great size and occasionally undergo malignant change.

Treatment is by wide excision: recurrence is otherwise inevitable. The reputation of the pleomorphic adenoma for recurrence is due to the great surgical difficulties of complete removal of tumours from the parotid (the common site), where the facial nerve, in particular, makes dissection hazardous. Pleomorphic adenomas have an unusually strong tendency to seed and recur in the incision scar if opened at operation or if incompletely excised. In the case of parotid tumours, therefore, recurrences are prevented only by removing the gland with the tumour intact. The recurrence rate is low in skilled hands, but recurrences are typically multifocal and difficult to eradicate.

Warthin's tumour (adenolymphoma) → Summary p. 315

Warthin's tumour arises in the parotid glands and accounts for about 9% of tumours there. It has a highly characteristic histological appearance consisting of tall, eosinophilic columnar cells which form a much-folded layer covering dense lymphoid tissue, including many germinal centres (Fig. 18.26).

Fig. 18.26 **Warthin's tumour.** At higher power the tall columnar epithelial cells are readily identified and beneath them the lymphoid tissue.

Fig. 18.27 **Warthin's tumour.** Tall columnar cells surround lymphoid tissue and line a convoluted cystic space.

These structures line and form papillary projections into cystic spaces (Fig. 18.27).

Warthin's tumour is benign and responds to enucleation but is sometimes multiple.

Oncocytoma

Oncocytoma is a rare benign tumour that virtually only affects the parotids, particularly in the elderly. It consists of large eosinophilic cells with small compact nuclei ('oncocytes'), which are typically arranged in solid cords.

Oncocytosis is the term given to replacement or transformation of acinar cells of the parotid (or rarely other glands) by cells having the same appearance as those of an oncocytoma but without loss of the normal lobular architecture. Oncocytosis is usually an age-related change and when widespread the gland becomes swollen and soft.

Other adenomas

Other adenomas lack the connective tissue components of the pleomorphic adenoma and may have a uniform cellular

Fig. 18.28 **Mucoepidermoid carcinoma.** The mucous cells surround microcysts. Underlying the mucous cells are the epidermoid (squamous) cells.

structure, often with a tubular or trabecular pattern. Canalicular adenomas particularly affect the upper lip and consist of small darkly-staining cells in a tubular or trabecular pattern but sometimes resembling an adenoid cystic carcinoma.

Adenomas other than pleomorphic adenoma respond to enucleation or simple excision.

MALIGNANT SALIVARY GLAND TUMOURS →
Summary p. 315

Mucoepidermoid carcinoma

Mucoepidermoid carcinomas account for between 3 and 9% of salivary gland neoplasms.

Histologically, they consist of two cell types, namely large, pale mucus-secreting cells surrounded by epidermoid (squamous) cells. Either may be predominant. If mainly mucoid, the tumour tends to be cystic; if mainly epidermoid, the tumour is solid and often then more aggressive (Figs 18.28 and 18.29). There is no well-defined capsule, but the tumour usually grows slowly.

Despite benign cytological appearances, mucoepidermoid carcinomas can be invasive and occasionally metastasise. Those which are obviously malignant microscopically are uncommon, but more likely to metastasise.

Treatment is by wide excision, but the tumour may recur.

Acinic cell carcinoma

Acinic cell carcinomas are rare and account for about 1% of salivary gland tumours. Their behaviour is also unpredictable from their histological appearance.

Fig. 18.29 Mucoepidermoid carcinoma. At higher power the finely granular mucous cells are seen to the right with the underlying epidermoid cells to the left.

Fig. 18.30 Acinic cell carcinoma. The tumour is composed of granular acinar-type cells, sometimes arranged in acinus-like clusters and sometimes forming irregular sheets. Cytological atypia is uncommon.

Fig. 18.31 Adenoid cystic carcinoma. There is an ulcerated mass arising from a minor gland in the palate. The clinical appearance would be the same as other malignant salivary neoplasms.

Fig. 18.32 Adenoid cystic carcinoma. The small darkly staining cells of the adenoid cystic carcinoma form cribriform islands with large holes which have been likened, rather inappropriately, to Swiss cheese.

Histologically, they show an almost uniform pattern of large cells, similar to serous cells, with granular basophilic cytoplasm, often in an acinar arrangement (Fig. 18.30). A characteristic feature is scattered round 'holes', thought to be entrapped secretion. Sometimes these are so numerous as to give the tumour a lace-like appearance.

Despite apparently benign histological appearances, acinic cell carcinomas can be invasive and occasionally metastasise. More obviously malignant variants with nuclear pleomorphism and hyperchromatism are also occasionally seen microscopically.

Adenoid cystic carcinoma

Adenoid cystic carcinoma usually has a highly characteristic histological pattern consisting of rounded groups of small darkly-staining cells of almost uniform size, surrounding multiple small clear spaces (cribriform or 'Swiss cheese' pattern) (Figs 18.31 and 18.32). Adenoid cystic carcinomas usually grow relatively slowly, but tend to infiltrate along nerve sheaths. When they reach and spread along bony canals their extent is considerably greater than radiographs show. Metastases usually appear late. The prognosis is poor unless the tumour is vigorously treated by early wide excision at the earliest possible stage, often combined with radiotherapy.

Polymorphous low-grade adenocarcinoma

Polymorphous low-grade adenocarcinoma arises in minor glands, particularly of the palate. It consists of cytologically benign-looking pale-staining cells in lobular, papillary or papillary cystic, cribriform or trabecular configurations (Fig. 18.33). It is invasive and can spread along nerve sheaths but rarely metastasises.

Fig. 18.33 **Polymorphous low-grade adenocarcinoma.** (A) Targetoid pattern; (B) cribriform area; (C) surviving acini inside the tumour; (D) papillary cystic area.

Salivary duct carcinoma

This aggressive carcinoma resembles high-grade breast carcinoma and metastasises early. The prognosis is poor. Lesions arise mainly in the parotid but can develop in all glands.

Epithelial-myoepithelial carcinoma

Epithelial-myoepithelial carcinoma is a tumour of major glands. It consists of ducts or trabeculae of benign-looking dark-staining cells with an outer layer of clear cells. The latter sometimes predominate and the tumour has to be distinguished from other clear cell tumours, most of which are malignant.

Adenocarcinomas

Adenocarcinomas of the salivary glands show a variety of appearances. A few show attempts at duct formation typical of adenocarcinomas, while others have a papillary cystic pattern. Some are so poorly differentiated that their glandular origin is difficult to discern. When a salivary carcinoma does not fall into any definable category, as happens fairly frequently, it is classified as adenocarcinoma NOS ('not otherwise specified').

Fig. 18.34 **Carcinoma arising in a pleomorphic adenoma.** In longstanding pleomorphic adenomas, the stroma may become hyalinised, dense and acellular. In such tumours, there is a risk of transformation to carcinoma, as shown here by clusters of cells showing cytological atypia.

Undifferentiated carcinomas

These usually consist of closely set, small, darkly-staining cells with little cytoplasm. Rapid spread and metastasis is typical. Some types are caused by Epstein–Barr virus infection, particularly those in patients from Mongoloid races.

Fig. 18.35   Haemangioma of the parotid. (A) The lobular structure of the gland is seen to be preserved, with a small lobule of normal parotid centrally. (B) The tissue that replaces the lobules, closely packed small capillary vessels with a few scattered residual serous acini (arrowed).

Malignant change in pleomorphic adenoma

Pleomorphic adenoma is one of the few benign tumours that can undergo malignant change. Clinically, this is sometimes suggested by a sudden spurt in growth or development of pain or facial palsy.

Histologically, malignant change in pleomorphic adenoma is shown by obviously carcinomatous features adjacent to the benign cellular picture of the remainder of the tumour (Fig. 18.34). This is typically a late phenomenon, usually only after the tumour has been present for many years or in recurrences after inadequate excision.

Secondary tumours

Carcinomas and, occasionally, other tumours can metastasise to the salivary glands, particularly the parotid. Such secondaries can sometimes resemble primary salivary gland carcinomas:

renal cell carcinoma metastases in particular can closely resemble epithelial-myoepithelial carcinoma. Diagnosis may depend on finding a primary elsewhere but, usually, the prognosis is almost hopeless in view of the dissemination of the tumour.

Non-epithelial tumours

Lymphoma

The most common non-epithelial tumours of salivary glands are lymphomas. They can arise in the lymph nodes that lie within the gland, in which case they are identical to lymphomas arising in the cervical lymph nodes and nodes elsewhere. These will usually be high-grade B-cell lymphomas or Hodgkin's disease and may be the first sign of widespread disease.

Alternatively, lymphomas may arise in the gland parenchyma and are typically MALT (mucosa-associated lymphoid tissue) lymphomas. These are described in more detail in

Chapter 22. The majority arise as a complication of Sjögren's syndrome and development of lymphoma is indicated by a persistent painless swelling of the gland, particularly in patients with longstanding disease.

MALT lymphomas are usually low grade and indolent, but high-grade types can also arise in salivary glands.

Diagnosis is difficult because of the difficulty in identifying the early stages of low-grade lymphomas.

Haemangioma of the parotids

Haemangioma is a rare tumour which may be present at birth or first seen in childhood. Girls are more frequently affected. It forms a soft, sometimes bluish, swelling.

Histologically, the parotid structure is largely replaced by angiomatous tissue among which glandular elements can be found (Fig. 18.35). This angiomatous proliferation may occasionally be so vast as to form an arteriovenous fistula.

Sometimes these tumours regress spontaneously but, if this has not happened by the age of 10 years, excision may be required. Corticosteroids may delay tumour growth and facilitate later surgery. In adults, the tumours have the typical histology of haemangiomas of other tissues.

Intraosseous salivary gland tumours

Ectopic salivary gland tissue is occasionally present in the mandible, either in a cavity in the bone near the angle (Stafne bone cavity) or, occasionally, in other sites. Rarely, salivary gland tumours of any type can develop within the jaw (presumably from this ectopic salivary tissue) and may be mistaken by an unsuspecting pathologist for odontogenic tumours. However, they are most frequently mucoepidermoid carcinomas.

Radiographically, intraosseous salivary tumours produce cyst-like or poorly circumscribed areas of radiolucency. The diagnosis can only be made histologically. Wide excision is required.

TUMOUR-LIKE SALIVARY SWELLINGS

Necrotising sialometaplasia

This tumour-like lesion mainly affects the minor glands of the palate. It is of unknown cause. Middle-aged males are predominantly affected and are often cigarette smokers.

Typically, a relatively painless, ulcerated swelling 15–20 mm in diameter, forms on the hard palate often in the first molar region (Fig. 18.36). The margins are irregular and heaped-up or everted. Clinically, it resembles a carcinoma, for which it has sometimes also been mistaken histologically.

Pathology

There is chronic inflammation of minor salivary glands and necrosis of acini. The duct tissue undergoes squamous metaplasia and proliferates to produce a pseudo-carcinomatous appearance (Fig. 18.37).

Necrotising sialometaplasia is often excised for diagnosis, but usually heals spontaneously after 8–10 weeks.

Fig. 18.37 Necrotising sialometaplasia. The histological features may also be mistaken for malignancy. There is necrosis of all the acinar cells and only hyperplastic ducts showing squamous metaplasia remain.

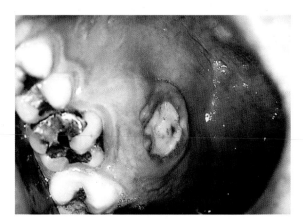

Fig. 18.36 Necrotising sialometaplasia. The clinical appearances are similar to those of a malignant salivary neoplasm.

Fig. 18.38 Sialadenosis. In this case of idiopathic sialadenosis there is conspicuous swelling of the parotid glands producing a characteristic appearance.

SIALADENOSIS → Summary p. 316

Sialadenosis is a non-neoplastic, non-inflammatory enlargement of salivary glands, most noticeably of the parotids, due to
a variety of causes (Fig. 18.38 and Box 18.14). Histologically,
there is hypertrophy of serous acini and oedema of interstitial
connective tissue.

<table>
<tr><td colspan="2">Box 18.14   Important causes of sialadenosis</td></tr>
<tr><td>

- Alcoholism
- Diabetes mellitus
- Other endocrine diseases
- Pregnancy
- Drugs (e.g. sympathomimetics)
- Bulimia
- Idiopathic

</td></tr>
</table>

SUGGESTED FURTHER READING

Barnes L, Rao U, Krause J, Contis L, Schwartz A, Scalamonga P 1994
Salivary duct carcinoma. Part I. A clinicopathologic evaluation and
DNA analysis of 13 cases with review of the literature. Oral Surg Oral
Med Oral Pathol 78:64–73

Barnes L, Eveson JW, Reichart P 2005 Pathology and genetics of head
and neck tumours. WHO Classification of Tumours, Volume 9. IARC
Press, Lyon

Brook I 1992 Diagnosis and management of parotitis. Arch Otolaryngol
Head Neck Surg 118:469–471

Brookstone M, Huvos AG 1992 Central salivary gland tumors of the
maxilla and mandible: a clinicopathologic study of 11 cases with an
analysis of the literature. J Oral Maxillofac Surg 50:229–236

Callender DL, Frankenthaler RA, Luna MA, Lee SS, Goepfert H 1992
Salivary gland neoplasms in children. Arch Otolaryngol Head Neck
Surg 118:472–476

Cawson RA, Langdon JD, Eveson JW 1996 Surgical pathology of the
mouth and jaws. Wright, Oxford

Cawson RA, Binnie WH, Barrett AW, Wright JM 1998 Lucas's
pathology of tumors of the oral tissues. Churchill Livingstone,
Edinburgh

Cawson RA, Binnie WH, Barrett AW, Wright JM 2001 Oral disease, 3rd
edn. Mosby-Wolfe, London

Delgado R, Vuitch F, Albores-Saavedra J 1993 Salivary duct carcinoma.
Cancer 72:1503–1512

Ellis GL, Corio RL 1983 Acinic cell adenocarcinoma. A
clinicopathologic analysis of 294 cases. Cancer 52:542–549

Epstein JB, Stevenson-Moore P, Scully C 1992 Management of
xerostomia. Can Dent Assoc J 58:140–143

Eveson JW, Cawson RA 1986 Warthin's tumor (cystadenolymphoma) of
salivary glands. A clinicopathologic investigation of 278 cases. Oral
Surg Oral Med Oral Pathol 61:256–262

Falzon M, Isaacson PG 1991 The natural history of benign
lymphoepithelial lesion of the salivary gland in which there is a
monoclonal population of B cells. A report of two cases. Am J Surg
Pathol 15:59–65

Gleeson MJ, Bennett MH, Cawson RA 1986 Lymphomas of salivary
glands. Cancer 58:699–704

Gleeson MJ, Cawson RA, Bennett MH 1986 Benign lymphoepithelial
lesion: a less than benign disease. Clin Otolaryngol 11:47–51

Hamper K, Brugmann M, Koppermann R et al 1989 Epithelial-
myoepithelial duct carcinoma of salivary glands: a follow-up and
cytophotometric study of 21 cases. J Oral Pathol Med 18:299–304

Hamper K, Lazar F, Dietel M et al 1990 Prognostic factors for adenoid
cystic carcinoma of the head and neck: a retrospective evaluation of
96 cases. J Oral Pathol Med 19:101–107

Hickman RE, Cawson RA, Duffy SW 1984 The prognosis of specific
types of salivary gland tumors. Cancer 54:1620–1624

Holliday RA, Cohen WA, Schinella RA et al 1988 Benign
lymphoepithelial parotid cysts and hyperplastic cervical
lymphadenopathy in AIDS-risk patients: a new CT appearance.
Radiology 168:439–441

Labrouyie E, Merlio JPH, Beylot-Barry M et al 1993 Human
immunodeficiency virus type I replication within cystic
lymphoepithelial lesion of salivary glands. Am J Clin Pathol
100:41–46

Lewis JE, Olsen KD, Weiland LH 1991 Acinic cell carcinoma.
Clinicopathologic review. Cancer 68:172–179

McCluggage G, Sloan J, Cameron S, Hamilton P, Toner P 1995 Basal
cell adenocarcinoma of the submandibular gland. Oral Surg Oral Med
Oral Pathol 79:342–350

O'Connell JE, George MK, Speculand GB, Pahor AL 1993
Mycobacterial infection of the parotid gland: an unusual cause of
parotid swelling. J Laryngol Otol 107:560–564

Qureshi AA, Gitelis A, Templeton AA, Piasecki PA 1994 'Benign'
metastasizing pleomorphic adenoma. A case report and review of the
literature. Clin Orthopaed Rel Res 308:192–198

Raad II, Sabbagh MF, Caranasos GJ 1990 Acute bacterial sialadenitis: a
study of 29 cases and review. Rev Infect Dis 12:591–601

Seifert G, Miehlke A, Haubrich J, Chilla R 1986 Diseases of the salivary
glands. Georg Thieme Verlag, Stuttgart

Takeichi N, Hirose F, Yamamoto H, Ezaki H, Fujikura T 1983 Salivary
gland tumors in atomic bomb survivors, Hiroshima, Japan. II
Pathologic study and supplementary epidemiologic observations.
Cancer 52:377–385

Toynton SC, Wilkins MJ, Cook HT, Stafford NDS 1994 True malignant
mixed tumour of a minor salivary gland. J Laryngol Otol 108:76–79

Van der Wal JE, Snow GB, van der Waal I 1990 Intraoral adenoid
cystic carcinoma. The presence of perineural spread in relation to
site, size, local extension and metastatic spread in 22 cases. Cancer
66:2031–2033

Vincent SD, Hammond HL, Finkelstein MW 1994 Clinical and
therapeutic features of polymorphous low-grade adenocarcinoma.
Oral Surg Oral Med Oral Pathol 77:41–47

Vitali C, Bombardieri S, Jonsson R et al 2002 Classification criteria
for Sjögren's syndrome: a revised version of the European criteria
proposed by the American–European Consensus Group. Ann Rheum
Dis 61:554–558

Waldron CA, Koh ML 1990 Central mucoepidermoid carcinoma of the
jaws: report of four cases with analysis of the literature and discussion
of the relationship to mucoepidermoid, sialodontogenic and glandular
odontogenic cysts. J Oral Maxillofac Surg 48:871–877

Wolvius EB, van der Valk P, van der Wal JE et al 1996 Primary non-
Hodgkin lymphoma of the salivary glands. An analysis of 22 cases. J
Oral Pathol Med 25:177–181

WHO classification of salivary gland tumours 2005

Malignant epithelial tumours	
Acinic cell carcinoma	See text of Chapter 18
Mucoepidermoid carcinoma	See text of Chapter 18
Adenoid cystic carcinoma	See text of Chapter 18
Polymorphous low-grade adenocarcinoma	See text of Chapter 18
Epithelial myopepithelial carcinoma	See text of Chapter 18
Clear cell carcinoma NOS[1]	Composed of clear cells and with no features of other tumours. Usually intraoral minor glands, especially the palate. Low-grade malignancy, prognosis good
Basal cell adenocarcinoma	Appear like basal cell adenomas but infiltrative. Recur locally but rarely metastasise
Sebaceous carcinoma	Very rare, usually in parotid and the elderly. High grade
Sebaceous lymphadenocarcinoma	Extremely rare low-grade malignancy
Cystadenocarcinoma	Low-grade malignancy of parotid gland and introral glands. Recurs locally and may metastasise
Low-grade cribriform cystadenocarcinoma	Very rare, resembles breast ductal carcinoma, usually in the parotid and the elderly
Mucinous adenocarcinoma	Very rare high-grade malignancy of elderly, usually palate and sublingual glands
Oncocytic carcinoma	Very rare high-grade carcinoma, usually in parotid, fewer in submandibular
Salivary duct carcinoma	See text of Chapter 18
Adenocarcinoma NOS	See text of Chapter 18
Myoepithelial carcinoma	The malignant variant of myoepithelioma, high grade with recurrence and frequent metastasis, arise in all glands but particularly the parotid
Carcinoma ex pleomorphic adenoma	See text of Chapter 18
Carcinosarcoma	A highly malignant neoplasm containing both carcinoma, of any pattern, with a sarcoma, usually chondrosarcoma or osteosarcoma. Survival is very poor
Metastasising pleomorphic adenoma	Very rare. An apparently benign pleomorphic adenoma that metastasises, to bone, lung or lymph node. Arise in the parotid, submandibular and palatal glands
Squamous cell carcinoma	Rare, resemble mucosal squamous carcinomas. Metastasis to a parotid node could be mistaken for a salivary primary. Parotid and submandibular glands, wide age range
Small cell carcinoma Large cell carcinoma	Very rare neuroendocrine carcinomas. Metastasis to a parotid node could be mistaken for a salivary primary
Lymphoepithelial carcinoma	Common in Japan, SE China and in Inuit races, but otherwise very rare. Associated with Epstein–Barr virus infection. Usually parotid or submandibular glands, wide age range. Respond well to radiotherapy
Sialoblastoma	Very rare high-grade lesion, often congenital arises in first 2 years of life. High grade but respond well to excision
Benign epithelial tumours	
Pleomorphic adenoma	See text of Chapter 18

Myoepithelioma	Similar to pleomorphic adenoma but without the varied histological appearances, formed of sheets of epithelial cells of various shapes.
Basal cell adenoma	Rare lesions of parotid glands composed of sheets of small dark cells. Some types present with multiple lesions in the same or more than one gland
Warthin's tumour	See text of Chapter 18
Oncocytoma	See text of Chapter 18
Canalicular adenoma	Similar to basal cell adenoma but with characteristic histology. Usually upper lip and buccal glands of the elderly
Sebaceous adenoma	Very rare lesion, wide age range, sheets of squamous epithelium with sebaceous differentiation
Lymphadenoma, sebaceous and non-sebaceous	Very rare lesions of the parotid and the elderly
Ductal papillomas, inverted, intraductal and sialadenoma papilliferum	Develop in or, often, near the opening of minor gland ducts, wide age range
Cystadenoma	Rare lesion of numerous duct-like cysts, arise in any gland and in middle age and the elderly
Soft tissue tumours	
Haemangioma	See text of Chapter 18
Lymphoma	
Hodgkin lymphoma	See text of Chapter 22
Diffuse large B-cell lymphoma	See text of Chapter 22
Extranodal marginal B-cell lymphoma ('MALT lymphoma')	See text of Chapter 22
Secondary tumours	

[1]NOS indicates 'not otherwise specified'

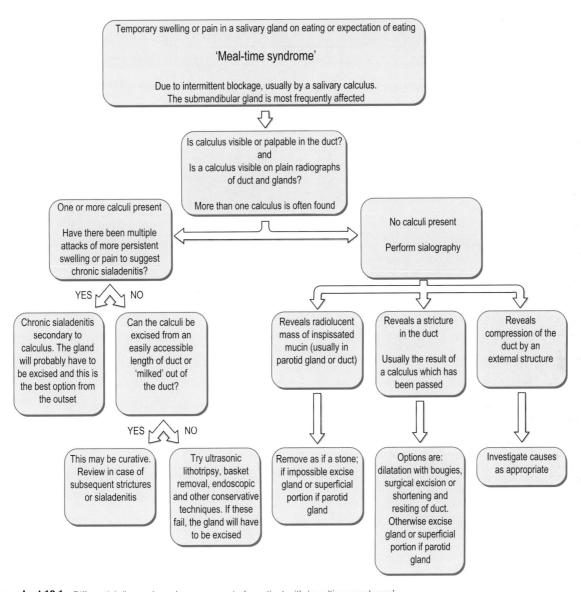

Summary chart 18.1 Differential diagnosis and management of a patient with 'mealtime syndrome'.

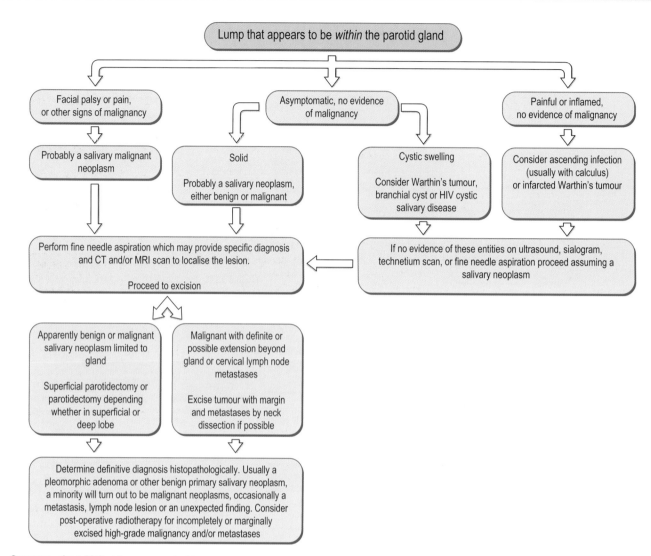

Summary chart 18.2 Management decisions and treatment for a lump in the parotid gland.

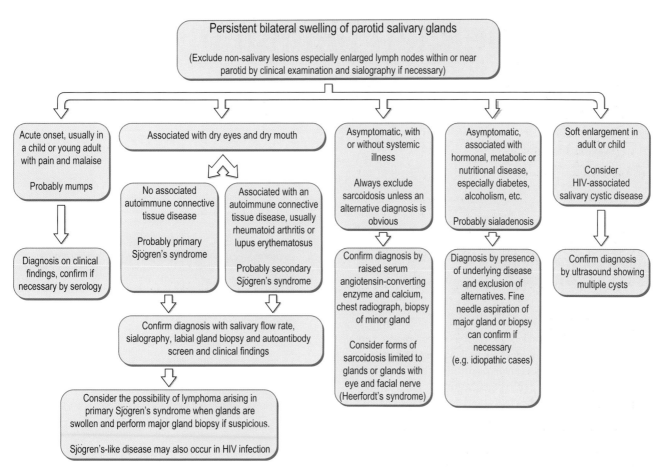

Summary chart 18.3 Summary of the diagnosis of persistent bilateral swelling of the parotid glands.

CHAPTER 19

Common benign mucosal swellings

FIBROUS POLYPS, EPULIDES AND DENTURE-INDUCED GRANULOMAS → Summary p. 323

Fibrous nodules are the most common soft-tissue swellings of the mouth. They are not neoplasms but hyperplastic swellings that develop in sites subject to chronic minor injury and/or low-grade infection (Box 19.1). Fibromas are not recognised as an entity and, in any case, cannot be distinguished from fibrous hyperplasia. The term epulis (literally, 'on the gingiva') refers only to the site. It has no implications for the cause or histology but, in practice, most epulides are fibrous.

Box 19.1   Fibrous nodules: practical points

- The most common oral tumour-like swellings
- Most frequently form at gingival margins (fibrous epulis) or in relation to a denture
- They are hyperplastic responses to chronic irritation
- Should be excised complete and sent for histological examination

---

Irritation of the gingival margin by the sharp edge of a carious cavity or by calculus may lead to the formation of a fibrous epulis; irritation of alveolar or palatal mucosa by a rough area on a denture may provoke development of a denture granuloma. Though different names are given to these lesions they are similar in origin and structure.

Clinical features

A fibrous epulis is most common near the front of the mouth on the gingiva between two teeth (Fig. 19.1). Fibrous polyps can also form on the buccal mucosa (Fig. 19.2). Denture-induced hyperplasias ('denture granulomas') often form at the edge of dentures (Fig. 19.3). These swellings are pale and firm but may be abraded and ulcerated, and then inflamed.

'Leaf fibroma' is another fibrous overgrowth which forms under a denture but has become flattened against the palate (Fig. 19.4). It may be difficult to see until lifted away from its bed.

Fig. 19.1   Fibrous epulis. This lesion, arising from the gingival margin between the lower central incisors, is firm, pink and not ulcerated.

Fig. 19.2   Fibrous polyp. This lesion on the buccal mucosa has arisen as a result of cheek biting and is a firm, painless polyp covered by mucosa of normal appearance.

Pathology

These nodules consist of irregular interlacing connective tissue fibres without encapsulation but covered by epithelium, which is usually hyperplastic (Fig. 19.5).

314

Fig. 19.3 **Denture-induced granuloma.** Fibrous hyperplasia at the posterior border of this upper partial denture has resulted in a firm mucosal swelling moulded to fit the denture.

Fig. 19.5 **Fibrous polyp.** The lesion is composed of mature fibrous tissue covered by hyperplastic epithelium with spiky rete processes. A few inflammatory cells are present near the base.

Fig. 19.4 **'Leaf fibroma'.** Flat lesions formed between the denture and mucosa are often termed leaf fibromas because of their shape. Raising this example with a probe reveals its pedunculated shape.

Bone formation is sometimes seen in a fibrous epulis (Fig. 19.6). In American texts, a fibrous epulis containing bone is termed (in an apparent desire to cause confusion) a 'peripheral ossifying fibroma', even though it has no relation to the ossifying fibroma of bone and is not a fibroma.

Fibrous nodules should be excised together with the small base of normal tissue from which they arise. In the case of a fibrous epulis, the underlying bone should be curetted. There should be no recurrence if this is done thoroughly and the source of irritation is removed.

Histological examination is needed to confirm that an epulis is fibrous and not a giant-cell lesion, pyogenic granuloma or a malignant tumour, which can very rarely form on the gingival margin and simulate a non-neoplastic epulis.

Giant-cell fibroma

This variant is distinguished microscopically by large, mononucleate, stellate, darkly-staining cells (quite unlike the

Fig. 19.6 **Fibrous epulis with ossification.** Much of the surface of this pedunculated nodule is ulcerated and hyperplastic epithelium covers the margins. Centrally, the lesion is very cellular, partly as a result of inflammatory infiltrate, and trabeculae of woven bone are being deposited and maturing into lamellar bone. The presence of bone in a fibrous epulis appears to be of no clinical significance.

multinucleate cells of a giant-cell granuloma) and less conspicuous multinucleate cells, scattered between short, coarse fibrous tissue bundles. Clinically, giant-cell fibromas are typically pedunculated and usually arise from the gingivae or tip of tongue. The surface is frequently verrucous.

The treatment is the same as for a fibrous epulis.

Fig. 19.7 **Papillary hyperplasia of the palate.** A small leaf fibroma is also present in the anterior palate.

Fig. 19.8 **Papillary hyperplasia.** There are nodules, each similar to a fibrous polyp and the subepithelial inflammatory infiltrate indicates probable candidal infection.

Fig. 19.9 **Papillary hyperplasia.** Higher power view of an uninflamed lesion after antifungal treatment. The mucosa is thrown into a series of convoluted folds covered by hyperplastic epithelium.

Fig. 19.10 **Pyogenic granuloma.** A bright red polypoid swelling. The gingiva is a common site.

PAPILLARY HYPERPLASIA OF THE PALATE

Nodular overgrowth of the palatal mucosa is occasionally seen, particularly under dentures in older persons in whom low-grade trauma or infection exacerbates the proliferation (Fig. 19.7). Candidosis is sometimes superimposed but is not the cause. Mild palatal papillary hyperplasia is also occasionally seen in non-denture wearers.

Histologically, palatal papillary hyperplasia shows close-set nodules of vascular fibrous tissue with a variable chronic inflammatory infiltrate and a covering of hyperplastic epithelium (Figs 19.8 and 19.9).

There is no justification for stripping palatal papillary hyperplasia. Dentures should be kept clean and not worn overnight. Any superimposed candidal infection should be treated with an antifungal drug.

PYOGENIC GRANULOMA AND PREGNANCY EPULIS
→ Summary p. 323

Pyogenic granuloma is relatively uncommon. Clinically, it is usually red and relatively soft (Fig. 19.10). Microsopically, it consists of many dilated blood vessels in a loose oedematous connective tissue stroma (Fig 19.11). There is typically a dense acute inflammatory infiltrate, but this may be scanty or absent. A pregnancy epulis has the same histological appearances and can only be distinguished by the nature of the patient and, usually, an associated pregnancy gingivitis (see also Fig. 31.9).

Fig. 19.11 **Pyogenic granuloma.** Lobular nodule of granulation tissue. Differences from a fibrous polyp (Fig. 19.5) include the ulcerated surface.

Fig. 19.12 **Giant-cell epulis.** Small lesion with a maroon colour in a child. Courtesy of Mrs H Pitt-Ford.

Fig. 19.13 **Giant-cell epulis.** Larger lesion showing the blue-purple colour.

Fig. 19.14 **Giant-cell epulis.** At high magnification clusters of giant cells in vascular fibrous tissue may be seen lying immediately below the covering epithelium.

GIANT-CELL EPULIS → Summary p. 323

The giant-cell epulis, like the fibrous epulis, is probably hyperplastic, but less common.

Clinically, a giant-cell epulis is usually found on the gingival margin between teeth anterior to the permanent molars. Its development may therefore be related to the resorption of deciduous teeth. The swelling is rounded, soft, and typically maroon or purplish (Figs 19.12 and 19.13).

Histologically, numerous multinucleate cells lie in a vascular stroma of plump spindle-shaped cells. The appearance is similar to that of a giant-cell granuloma of the jaw, but for the fact that the epulis is just below the stratified squamous epithelium (Fig. 19.14). Very rarely, a giant-cell epulis is a manifestation of hyperparathyroidism, in which case changes in blood chemistry confirm the diagnosis (Ch. 10).

A giant-cell epulis should be excised, together with its gingival base, and the underlying bone curetted. Adjacent teeth need not be extracted if they are healthy and, if treatment is thorough, there should be no recurrence.

PAPILLOMAS → Summary p. 323

These benign lesions have spiky exophytic or rounded cauliflower-like shapes up to a centimetre or so in diameter. Probably all are caused by human papillomavirus (HPV) even though it cannot be detected in some lesions.

Human papillomaviruses are ubiquitous and almost all individuals harbour some of the over 100 types as commensals. HPV types tend to infect particular anatomic sites. However, this is not absolute and oral lesions containing types 6 and 11 and rounded non-keratinised papillomas (condylomas) are not necessarily infections transmitted from genital warts. Though some HPV types are associated with tonsil and oropharyngeal carcinoma, the oral papillomas are not premalignant.

Oral papillomas respond to local excision.

Oral papillomas of all types are occasionally multiple but, if numerous or confluent, HIV infection or other cause of immunodeficiency should be suspected. Extensive lesions in the immunosuppressed are difficult or impossible to eradicate.

Squamous cell papilloma

Papillomas mainly affect adults and have a distinctive, clinically recognisable, cauliflower-like or branched structure of finger-like processes (Fig. 19.15).

Histologically, the papillae consist of stratified squamous epithelium supported by a vascular connective tissue core (Fig. 19.16). Most are keratinised and so appear white.

Human papillomavirus (HPV) of various subtypes are associated, but koilocytes (keratinocytes with crumpled nuclei,

Fig. 19.15 **Squamous papilloma arising on the alveolar ridge.** Note the spiky white surface.

Fig. 19.16 **Papilloma.** The lesion consists of thickened fingers of epithelium. Slender vascular cores of connective tissue support each frond. The fronds are keratinised and so appear white clinically.

perinuclear space and condensed cytoplasm) are seen in only a minority. It is possible that some oral papillomas are true benign epithelial neoplasms, though this does not match their limited growth potential. Alternatively, papillomavirus may be present but cannot be detected or has disappeared from the lesion.

Fig. 19.17 **Focal epithelial hyperplasia.** Multiple pale pink slightly raised rounded nodules on the labial mucosa. Courtesy of Dr Braz Campos Durso.

Infective warts (verruca vulgaris)

Lesions caused by autoinoculation from warts on the hands are uncommon but seen particularly in children. The lesions may appear identical to squamous papillomas, be more rounded or even only slightly raised.

Histologically, the structure is generally similar to that of papillomas, but there are typically large clear cells (koilocytes) with pyknotic nuclei and prominent keratohyaline granules in the superficial layers of the prickle cells. There is also positive staining of the nuclei with peroxidase-labelled antiserum to HPV.

Focal epithelial hyperplasia

Focal epithelial hyperplasia or Heck's disease causes numerous rounded mucosal nodules up to a centimetre across, usually clustered on the labial, buccal mucosa and tongue mucosa (Fig. 19.17). These may be confluent, producing raised plaques or a cobblestone appearance.

Children, adolescents and young adults are affected, often with familial clusters. The condition is an infection by human papillomavirus types 13 and 32 which spread easily between family members under close living conditions.

Unlike most other papillomas, the surface is smooth or slightly nodular without keratin so that the lesions appear pink rather than white. No treatment is required and there is usually resolution, though only after many years. If appearance dictates, individual lesions are readily excised or removed by laser.

OTHER BENIGN NEOPLASMS

Intraoral adenomas arise from minor salivary glands. They typically form smooth, round or lobulated, painless firm swellings and are most frequently found on the palate (Ch. 18).

Neoplasms such as neurofibroma and lipoma, which are occasionally found in the mouth, are discussed in the following chapter.

SUGGESTED FURTHER READING

Abbey LM, Page DG, Sawyer DR 1980 The clinical and histopathologic features of a series of 464 oral squamous cell papillomas. Oral Surg 49:419–427

Anneroth G, Sigurdson A 1983 Hyperplastic lesions of the gingiva and alveolar mucosa. A study of 175 cases. Acta Odontol Scand 41:75–86

Carlos R, Sedano HO 1994 Multifocal papilloma virus epithelial hyperplasia. Oral Surg 77:631–635

Cawson RA, Langdon JD, Eveson JW 1996 Surgical pathology of the mouth and jaws. Wright, Oxford

Cawson RA, Binnie WH, Barrett AW, Wright JM 1998 Lucas's pathology of tumors of the oral tissues. Churchill Livingstone, Edinburgh

Cawson RA, Binnie WH, Barrett AW, Wright JM 2001 Oral disease, 3rd edn. Mosby-Wolfe, London

Ellis GL, Jensen JL, Reingold IM, Barr RJ 1977 Malignant neoplasms metastatic to the gingivae. Oral Surg Oral Med Oral Pathol 44:238–245

Giansanti JS, Waldron CA 1969 Peripheral giant cell granuloma: Review of 720 cases. J Oral Surg 27:787–791

Hirshberg A, Leibovich P, Buchner A 1993 Metastases to the oral mucosa: analysis of 157 cases. J Oral Pathol Med 22:385–390

Houston GD 1982 The giant cell fibroma. A review of 464 cases. Oral Surg 53:582–587

Zain RB, Fei YJ 1990 Fibrous lesions of the gingiva: a histopathologic analysis of 204 cases. Oral Surg Oral Med Oral Pathol 70:466–470

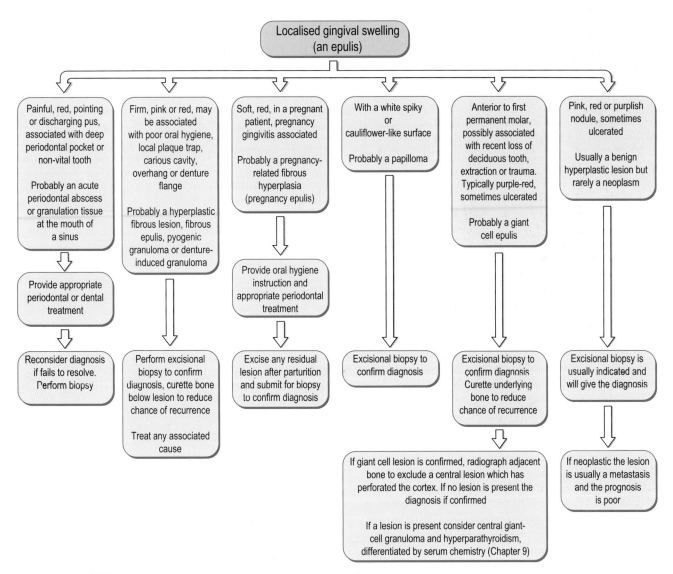

Summary chart 19.1 Differential diagnosis and management of the common localised gingival swellings.

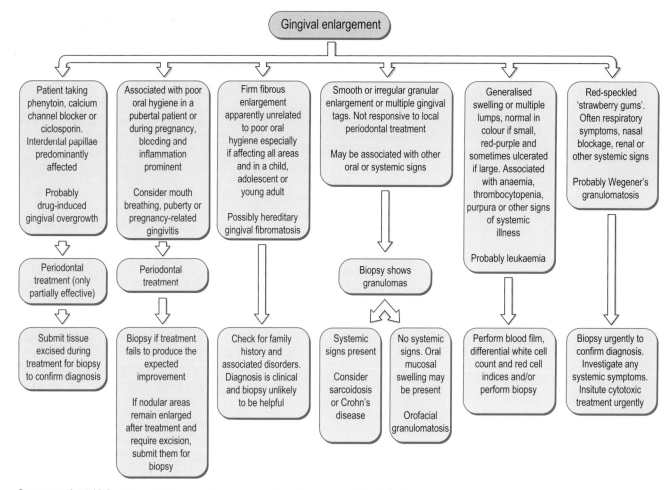

Summary chart 19.2 Differential diagnosis of common and important causes of gingival enlargement.

CHAPTER 20
Soft tissue (mesenchymal) neoplasms

BENIGN TUMOURS

Neurofibromas

These uncommon tumours arise from nerve sheaths. They form smooth, painless lumps in the mouth. When seen in the mouth, neurofibromatosis should be suspected.

Histologically, neurofibromas are cellular with plump nuclei separated by fine, sinuous collagen fibres among which mast cells can usually be found. Excision is curative.

Neurilemmomas

Neurilemmomas arise from axon sheaths and are also uncommon. They also form painless smooth swellings.

Histologically, the appearance is distinctive with multiple rounded masses of elongated spindle cells with palisaded nuclei (Antoni A tissue – Fig. 20.1). There is also a variable amount of unorganised loose connective tissue with scanty cells, sometimes with pleomorphic nuclei (Antoni B tissue). Excision is curative.

Lipoma and fibrolipoma

Lipomas can occasionally grow, particularly from the buccal fat pad, as soft, sometimes yellowish, swellings, which may be pedunculated (Fig. 20.2). They grow slowly and cause no symptoms unless bitten, or become conspicuous because of their size.

Histologically, lipomas consist of apparently normal fat (Fig. 20.3) comprising adipocytes with single large cytoplasmic

Fig. 20.2 Lipoma of the cheek. The tumour forms a pale, very soft yellowish swelling.

Fig. 20.3 Lipoma. The lobular structure of the fat is visible.

Fig. 20.1 Neurilemmoma. Antoni A tissue showing striking palisading of nuclei.

fat vacuoles. The fat cells are supported by thin fibrous tissue septa and usually surrounded by a variable thin fibrous capsule (Fig. 20.4). When fibrous tissue forms a large part of the tumour it is called a fibrolipoma. Lipomas should be excised.

Granular cell tumour

Clinically, granular cell tumours typically form painless smooth swellings. The tongue is the most common site.

Histologically, large granular cells form the bulk of the lesion. Electron microscopy suggests that the granular cells originate from Schwann cells. However, in the light microscope, all stages of apparent transition between striated muscle cells and granular cells are found at the periphery and are a striking histological feature (Fig. 20.5). Centrally, the granular cells are large, with clearly defined cell membranes and filled with eosinophilic granules that are lysosomes, with cell debris, mitochondria and degenerate cell membrane.

The granular cell tumour can induce striking pseudoepitheliomatous (pseudocarcinomatous) hyperplasia of the overlying epithelium (Figs 20.6 and 20.7). Though only present in a minority, this may be florid such that granular cell tumours have been mistaken histologically for carcinomas with resulting overtreatment. Simple excision should, however, be curative.

Congenital (granular cell) epulis

The rare congenital epulis is typically present at birth as a smooth but prominent soft nodule usually on the alveolar ridge (Fig. 20.8). Females are predominantly affected and, occasionally, the mass is so large as to obstruct respiration.

Fig. 20.4 **Lipoma.** The fat cells are closely packed between septa of fibrous tissue and often only partially encapsulated at the margin.

Histologically, large pale granular cells with sharply defined cell membranes are covered by epithelium with lacks pseudoepitheliomatous hyperplasia. Immunohistochemistry suggests that the origin is myogenous. Excision is curative but spontaneous regression is also seen.

Haemangiomas → Summary p. 337

Haemangiomas are mostly vascular malformations. Vascular neoplasms (apart from Kaposi's sarcoma) are rare.

Haemangiomas may be localised, but are occasionally diffuse and associated with similarly affected areas of the face. Rarely, the meninges are also involved, causing epilepsy and mental defect (Sturge–Weber syndrome). Isolated haemangiomas form purple, flat or nodular lesions which blanch on

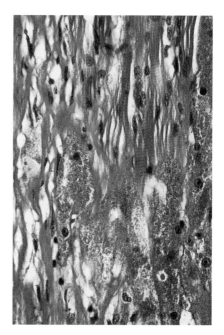

Fig. 20.5 **Granular cell tumour.** At high power, the granular cells apparently merging with muscle fibres are characteristic and indicate the diagnosis.

Fig. 20.6 **Granular cell tumour.** The irregular proliferation of the overlying epithelium (pseudoepitheliomatous hyperplasia), which is very florid in this example, may mimic a squamous carcinoma in superficial biopsy specimens.

pressure (Fig. 20.9). Histologically, haemangiomas comprise either capillary, cavernous or both types of vessels. The capillary type consists of innumerable minute blood vessels and vasoformative tissue – mere rosettes of endothelial cells

(Fig. 20.10). The cavernous type consists of large blood-filled sinusoids.

Excision of mucosal haemangiomas should be avoided unless trauma causes repeated episodes of bleeding. Cryosurgery may allow removal of a haemangioma without excessive bleeding.

Lymphangioma

These uncommon tumours usually form pale, translucent, smooth or nodular elevations of the mucosa. However, they may be noticed because they suddenly swell and become dark purple due to bleeding into the lymphatic spaces. Rarely, lymphangiomas are diffuse and extensive and cause generalised enlargement of the tongue (macroglossia) or lip.

Histologically, lymphangiomas consist of thin-walled, vascular spaces containing pinkish amorphous material as a result of fixation of lymph (Fig. 20.11).

Fig. 20.7 High power of a superficial area in Figure 20.6 showing the small irregular islands of epithelium that appear to invade the fibrous tissue and superficial muscle. Some show keratin formation similar to keratin pearls in squamous carcinoma. Granular cells are only present along the lower edge of the figure.

Fig. 20.8 Congenital epulis. A firm pink non-ulcerated nodule on the alveolar ridge of a neonate is the typical presentation.

Fig. 20.9 Cavernous haemangioma of the cheek. The colour is deep purple and the structure, a mass of thin-walled blood sinuses, is visible through the thin epithelium. A mass engorged with blood and as prominent as this is liable to be bitten and bleed profusely.

Fig. 20.10 Capillary haemangioma. Numerous large and small closely packed capillary vessels extend from the epithelium into the deeper tissues.

Fig. 20.11 Lymphangioma. There is a localised aggregation of cavernous lymphatics which form a pale superficial swelling. Bleeding into these lesions causes them suddenly to become purple or almost black.

Localised lymphangiomas can be excised, but this is more difficult in the diffuse type where the operation may have to be done in stages.

MALIGNANT CONNECTIVE TISSUE TUMOURS

Sarcomas of virtually any type can affect the oral soft tissues, but most are rare. Kaposi's sarcoma has become the most common type, but among HIV-negative persons, rhabdomyosarcoma is the most common. Sarcomas tend to affect a considerably younger age group than carcinomas and rhabdomyosarcomas, in particular, may be seen in children. Sarcomas grow rapidly, are invasive, destroy surrounding tissues and usually spread by the bloodstream. Many sarcomas are clinically indistinguishable from one another, but others, such as Kaposi's sarcoma and malignant melanoma, are pigmented and must be differentiated from benign pigmented lesions.

Rhabdomyosarcoma

Rhabdomyosarcomas show striated muscle differentiation and are the most common oral sarcomas in HIV-negative children or young adults. They form rapidly growing soft swellings, usually centred around the maxilla or in the orbit and arise in young children and adolescents. Two main forms are recognised, alveolar and embryonal.

Genetics

Alveolar rhabdomyosarcomas show a characteristic cytogenetic abnormality, namely a chromosomal translocation t(2;13) which is of diagnostic value. Specific gene transcripts can be identified in biopsy material and some confer a significantly worse prognosis. Embryonal rhabdomyosarcomas do not show these fusion products.

Histologically, the embryonal type, which more frequently affects children, consists of cells of variable shape and size. Some are strap- or tadpole-shaped, like rhabdomyoblasts in the early embryo, and more differentiated muscle-like cells with cross-striations are difficult to find. The alveolar type consists of slit-like spaces into which hang tear-shaped, darkly-staining cells attached to the walls. These alveoli are separated by a fibrous stroma. Diagnosis is aided by immunostaining for markers of muscle differentiation including the transcription factors myoD1 and myogenin.

Treatment is by excision and combination chemotherapy, but the prognosis is poor.

Fibrosarcoma

Fibrosarcomas consist of broad interlacing bands of fibroblasts with a streaming or herring-bone pattern (Fig. 20.12). Some produce abundant collagen; others are highly cellular with close-packed nuclei among which there are often mitoses.

Treatment is by radical excision. Local recurrence and spread are common but metastasis is rare.

Kaposi's sarcoma → Summary p. 337

Classical (sporadic) Kaposi's sarcoma was described in 1872 in Central Europe among elderly persons of Mediterranean or Jewish origin, as a multiple pigmented sarcoma of the skin. It is predominantly cutaneous, mainly affects the lower extremities, and visceral lesions are rarely clinically apparent. Head and neck involvement in this sporadic form is exceedingly rare. Kaposi's sarcoma with broadly similar characteristics is also common in Africa, particularly in Zaire, where it formed about 12% of all malignant tumours in the pre-AIDS era.

Since the outbreak of AIDS, Kaposi's sarcoma has become the most common type of intraoral sarcoma. It mainly affects male homosexuals with AIDS and, rarely, intravenous drug addicts or haemophiliacs who have acquired HIV infection from blood products. Kaposi's sarcoma rarely also develops in deeply immunosuppressed, HIV-negative patients. The cause in immunosuppressed patients is infection with human herpesvirus 8 (HHV-8). The mechanism of HHV-8's power of sarcomagenesis is unclear, but it appears to interfere with internal cell signalling pathways, dysregulating the cell cycle.

Within the mouth, the palate is the most frequent site and the tumour appears as a purplish area or nodule which bleeds readily

Fig. 20.12 Fibrosarcoma of the tongue. There are streams of neoplastic fibroblasts, but the striking feature is the spindle-shaped, darkly staining nuclei and their variation in size and mitoses.

(Fig. 20.13). In any male below the age of about 50, with such a lesion, Kaposi's sarcoma must be excluded since (in the absence of immunosuppressive treatment) it is pathognomonic of AIDS. Kaposi's sarcoma is occasionally the first manifestation of HIV infection, but usually associated with a low CD4 count and opportunistic infections such as candidosis, hairy leukoplakia or HIV-associated gingivitis. Human herpes-virus 8 DNA can be found in Kaposi's sarcoma cells and patients with both HIV and HHV-8 infection appear to have a high risk of developing Kaposi's sarcoma. This tumour may be the cause of early symptoms but, when first seen, is usually multifocal, with lesions affecting skin, lymph nodes and viscera.

Histologically, Kaposi's sarcoma is a vascular tumour in which factor VIII antigen (a marker for endothelial cells) can be identified. The early 'pre-sarcomatous' lesion consists of a mass of capillary-size blood vessels, sometimes with mononuclear cell cuffing. It resembles granulation tissue, particularly in the mouth where superficial lesions can be traumatised and become secondarily inflamed. Later, there is increasingly widespread angiomatous proliferation and, in some areas, the vessels may be slit-shaped when obliquely sectioned. There is also proliferation of angular or spindle-shaped interstitial cells (Fig. 20.14). Ultimately, the latter predominate and show increasing numbers of mitoses. Central necrosis may develop and extravasation of red cells can leave deposits of haemosiderin. Immunocytochemistry to detect HHV-8 is diagnostic (Fig. 20.15).

Associated HIV infection is usually suggested by other clinical manifestations (such as opportunistic infections) and lymphopenia in the blood picture.

The clinical differential diagnosis is from oral purpura, bacillary angiomatosis and pyogenic granulomas, from which it can be distinguished by microscopy. Primary intraosseous Kaposi's sarcoma is rare but two cases have been reported. Gingival Kaposi's sarcoma causing severe periodontal bone loss is also uncommon but has also been documented.

Transmission of HHV-8 is clearly important for developing Kaposi's sarcoma. Sexual transmission, particularly among men who have sex with men, and non-sexual transmission occur; both routes implicate saliva. However, oral HHV-8 shedding has no predictive value either for the development of Kaposi's sarcoma or survival. Oral HHV-8 may be shed at any time and independently of the patient's immune state and carries with it the risk of transmitting Kaposi's sarcoma.

Management

Almost all oral Kaposi's sarcoma is in HIV-infected patients. Before the introduction of highly active antiretroviral treatment (HAART), Kaposi's sarcoma was controlled by chemotherapy and radiotherapy. These were sufficiently effective to give good control and death usually followed HIV-associated opportunistic infections.

The picture is now greatly changed. HAART given for control of HIV replication has greatly reduced the incidence of Kaposi's sarcoma and has become the first-line treatment.

Fig. 20.13 **Kaposi's sarcoma.** Lesions are red, maroon or bluish and highly vascular. They may be flat or form tumour masses and the gingivae or palate are characteristic sites. Courtesy Prof WH Binnie.

Fig. 20.14 **Kaposi's sarcoma.** The tumour is composed of spindle and plump cells with cytological atypia and frequent mitoses. Many of the small holes visible are the result of formation of capillaries by the tumour cells.

Fig. 20.15 **Kaposi's sarcoma.** Immunocytochemistry for human herpes-virus 8 reveals numerous infected cell nuclei (dark brown) confirming the diagnosis.

Nevertheless, HAART has not proved to be completely effective for long-term control and cannot be tolerated by some patients.

Many Kaposi lesions are relatively indolent and may not require aggressive treatment. Localised lesions in the mouth may be amenable to local excision complemented by chemotherapy for more widespread involvement. Radiation is widely used in other parts of the body, but is usually avoided in the mouth because of adverse effects. Currently, the most effective chemotherapy regimens are interferon alpha with didanosine for slowly progressing disease or pegylated liposomal doxorubicin and HAART simultaneously, the latter inducing remission in 80% of cases. However, Kaposi's sacoma remains a disease that is controlled rather than cured.

Key features of Kaposi's sarcoma are summarised in Box 20.1.

Box 20.1   Kaposi's sarcoma: key features

- The most common type of oral sarcoma
- Most common in male homosexuals with AIDS
- Due to Herpes-virus 8
- Appears clinically as a flat or nodular purplish area
- Consists histologically of minute, proliferating blood vessels
- Good response to HAART, but long-term control may be difficult
- May be widely disseminated when oral lesions appear
- Death more frequently from associated opportunistic infections

---

Other sarcomas of oral soft tissues

Neurofibrosarcomas, liposarcomas, leiomyosarcomas and even soft-tissue osteosarcomas and chondrosarcomas may be seen, but all are rare. Sarcoma is a complication of therapeutic irradiation. Lymphomas are discussed in Chapter 22.

SUGGESTED FURTHER READING

Cawson RA, Langdon JD, Eveson JW 1996 Surgical pathology of the mouth and jaws. Wright, Oxford

Cawson RA, Binnie WH, Barrett AW, Wright JM 2001 Color atlas of oral disease, 3rd edn. Mosby-Wolfe, London

Chen S-Y, Thakur A, Miller AS, Harwick RD 1995 Rhabdomyosarcoma of the oral cavity. Report of four cases. Oral Surg Oral Med Oral Pathol Oral Radiol Endod 80:192–201

Damm DD, Cibull ML, Geissler RH et al 1993 Investigation into the histogenesis of congenital epulis of the newborn. Oral Surg Oral Med Oral Pathol 76:202–212

DiCerbo M, Sciubba JJ, Sordill WC, DeLuke DM 1992 Malignant schwannoma of the palate: a case report and review of the literature. J Oral Maxillofac Surg 50:1217–1221

El Naggar AK, Batsakis JG, Ordonez NG et al 1993 Rhadomyosarcoma of the adult head and neck: a clinicopathological and DNA ploidy study. J Laryngol Otol 107:716–720

Geist JR, Gander DL, Stefanac SJ 1992 Oral manifestations of neurofibromatosis types I and II. Oral Surg Oral Med Oral Pathol 73:376–382

Greager JA, Reichard K, Campana JP, Das Gupta TK 1994 Fibrosarcoma of the head and neck. Am J Surg 167:437–439

Hajdu SI 1993 Peripheral nerve sheath tumours. Histogenesis, classification and prognosis. Cancer 72:3549–3552

Herdier BG, Kaplan LD, McGrath MS 1994 Pathogenesis of AIDS lymphomas. AIDS 8:1025–1049

Hirshberg A, Leibovich P, Buchner A 1993 Metastases to the oral mucosa: analysis of 157 cases. J Oral Pathol Med 22:385–390

Kraus DH, Dubner S, Harrison LB et al 1994 Prognostic factors for recurrence and survival in head and neck soft tissue sarcomas. Cancer 74:697–702

Mark RJ, Sercarz JA, Tran L, Selch M, Calcaterra TC 1991 Fibrosarcoma of the head and neck. Arch Otolaryngol Head Neck Surg 117:396–401

Meehan S, Davis V, Brahim JS 1994 Embryonal rhabdomyosarcoma of the floor of the mouth. A case report. Oral Surg Oral Med Oral Pathol 78:603–606

Noel J-C, Hermans P, Andre J et al 1996 Herpesvirus-like DNA sequences in Kaposi's sarcoma. Cancer 77:2132–2136

Peszkowski MJ, Larsson A 1990 Extraosseous and intraosseous oral traumatic neuromas and their association with tooth extraction. J Oral Maxillofac Surg 48:963–967

Regezi JA, MacPhail LA, Daniels TE et al 1993 Oral Kaposi's sarcoma: a 10-year retrospective histopathologic study. J Oral Pathol Med 11:292–297

Shapiro SD, Abramovitch K, Van Dis ML 1984 Neurofibromatosis: oral and radiographic manifestations. Oral Surg Oral Med Oral Pathol 58:493–498

Stewart CM, Watson RE, Eversole LR et al 1988 Oral granular cell tumors: a clinicopathologic and immunocytochemical study. Oral Surg Oral Med Oral Pathol 65:427–435

Tran LM, Mark R, Meier R, Calcaterra TC, Parker RG 1992 Sarcomas of the head and neck. Cancer 70:160–177

Weiss SW, Goldblum JR 2001 Enzinger and Weiss's soft tissue tumors, 4th edn. Mosby, St Louis

Zuker RM, Buenchea R 1993 Congenital epulis: review of the literature and report of a case. J Oral Maxillofac Surg 51:1040–1043

Melanoma and other pigmented lesions

Melanoma is a highly malignant oral tumour. It usually appears as a pigmented patch which must be distinguished from many other pigmentations listed in Box 21.1.

LOCALISED MUCOSAL PIGMENTATION →
Summary p. 337

Physiological and racial pigmentation

This is the most common cause of oral pigmentation. The gingivae are particularly affected (Fig. 21.1). The inner aspect of the lips is typically spared. Intraoral pigmentation is commoner in those with a dark skin. However, light-skinned individuals have up to an average of 30 cutaneous local pigmented lesions of various types and occasionally one will be present in the mouth.

Post-inflammatory pigmentation

Inflammation interferes with the synthesis of melanin by melanocytes and its transfer to keratinocytes. Melanosomes

escape from the epithelium into the underlying connective tissue where they are taken up by macrophages, a process known as melanin 'drop out'. Accumulation of this subepithelial melanin gives rise to post-inflammatory pigmentation. The process is commoner in dark-skinned races. Intraorally, the most common inflammatory condition to become pigmented is lichen planus (Fig. 21.2) and it can become very dark. Pigmentation may also develop in other inflamed sites and scars. This type of pigmentation is also seen diffusely through the mouth of heavy cigarette smokers.

Fig. 21.1   **Racial pigmentation.** The distribution of melanotic mucosa around the gingival margin is characteristic.

Fig. 21.2   **Pigmented lichen planus.** Inflammatory conditions may become pigmented, especially in dark-skinned races. Here melanin delineates mucosa affected by lichen planus.

Amalgam tattoo → Summary p. 337

Fragments of amalgam frequently become embedded in the oral mucosa and form the most common pigmented patches which may simulate melanomas clinically. They are usually close to the dental arch and typically 5 mm or more across (Fig. 21.3). Dense tattoos may be radiopaque.

Pathology

Amalgam is seen as brown or black granules deposited particularly along collagen bundles and around small blood vessels (Fig. 21.4). There may be no inflammatory reaction or there may be a foreign body reaction with amalgam granules in the macrophages or giant cells.

Excision is necessary to exclude a melanoma.

Fig. 21.3 Amalgam tattoo. Typical appearance and site; however, the lower second premolar from which the amalgam probably originated has been crowned.

Fig. 21.4 Amalgam tattoo. There are large fragments of amalgam surrounded by foreign body giant cells and macrophages and smaller particles dispersed in fibrous tissue. Silver leaching from the smaller fragments has stained the adjacent collagen brown.

Peutz–Jeghers syndrome → Summary p. 337

Peutz–Jeghers syndrome, a rare heritable disease, is characterised by multiple mucocutaneous pigmented macules and intestinal polyposis. The pigmented macules typically develop during the first decade of life and can be widespread, affecting the hands and feet and perioral skin as well as the oral mucosa. Cutaneous macules usually fade after puberty but the oral macules persist (Fig. 21.5).

Clinically, the oral macules resemble other melanotic macules and affect the lips, buccal mucosa, tongue and palate.

The intestinal polyps mainly affect the small intestine, are regarded as hamartomatous and rarely undergo malignant change. Colon cancer is a hazard but the risk for breast and gynecological cancers is particularly high. Multiple oral melanotic macules may therefore indicate the need for cancer screening.

Histologically, the oral macules show slight acanthosis and melanin in the basal layer. The melanocytes may have elongated dendritic processes.

The genetic locus of this syndrome is the mutated gene LKB1(STK11) on chromosome 19p. This was the first gene to be found that predisposes to cancer by disabling protein kinase activity.

Oral melanotic naevi → Summary p. 337

Pigmented naevi are benign lesions of melanocytes which form circumscribed brown to black patches about 5 or 6 mm across (Fig. 21.6). They are somewhat more frequent in white females, possibly because of overuse of sunbeds. They are asymptomatic but should be excised and sent for microscopy to exclude early malignant melanoma.

Pathology

The main features are modest numbers of pigmented melanocytes in the basal cell layer but many clumps of melanocytes in

Fig. 21.5 Peutz–Jehgers syndrome. There are multiple flat, pigmented patches on the palate. Those on the lips are most characteristic but fade with age.

the corium (Fig. 21.7). Rarely, intraepithelial foci of proliferating melanocytes project into the corium and appear to be dropping off the basal layer (junctional activity). Equally rarely, junctional activity is associated with circumscribed nests of melanocytes in a limited area of the upper corium (compound naevus).

Blue naevus

The epithelium is normal, but beneath and separate from it is a focus of spindle-shaped pigmented melanocytes.

All these types of naevi should be excised and sent for histology to exclude malignant melanoma

Oral melanotic macules associated with HIV infection

Oral and labial melanotic macules may develop in up to 6% of patients with HIV infection. This is approximately twice the frequency seen in HIV-negative persons. Also, oral melanotic macules appear to become more numerous as HIV infection advances. Increasing numbers of oral melanotic macules may be a sign of HIV infection and can appear in growing numbers long before HIV infection is recognised.

Histologically, there are increased numbers of melanocytes in large clusters or spread throughout the epithelium. Excess melanin deposition is present in the basal cell layer and upper part of the lamina propria.

Excision biopsy of melanotic macules is necessary for diagnosis but, unlike those in HIV-negative persons, these macules are more likely to enlarge and to recur after excision. Oral melanotic macules which enlarge or recur after excision may therefore be a sign of HIV infection.

MALIGNANT MELANOMA → Summary p. 337

Intraoral melanomas are rare but have an appallingly poor prognosis. Their long asymptomatic period, and the fact that they are less readily seen than cutaneous melanomas, causes their diagnosis to be made undesirably late.

UV exposure, fair complexion and sun sensitivity are well recognised aetiological factors for cutaneous melanoma. No aetiological factors for mucosal melanoma apart from ethnic differences have been identified.

Mucosal melanomas are more common in India, Africa and Japan, but cutaneous melanomas are less frequent in these countries. Oral melanomas may account for up to 12% of all melanomas in Japan as opposed to 0.2–8% in Europe and the USA.

The peak age incidence is between 40 and 60 years; children are exceedingly rarely affected, but melanoma has been found even in a 3-month-old child. Men are slightly more frequently affected (58%). The most frequent sites are the palate and upper alveolar ridge (Fig. 21.8). The tongue is rarely affected and a few melanomas develop in sites scattered about within

Fig. 21.6 Melanocytic naevi. These flat, pigmented patches are occasionally found on the lip and intraorally.

Fig. 21.7 Intramucosal naevus. A cluster of naevus cells lies in the connective tissue separated from the epithelium by a layer of normal fibrous tissue.

Fig. 21.8 Melanotic patch. There is poorly-demarcated pigmentation of varying density in the palate. All pigmented lesions such as this should be treated with the utmost suspicion and biopsied to exclude melanoma.

the mouth. They are usually dark brown or black, but 15% of oral melanomas may be non-pigmented and typically red or reddish brown.

Oral melanomas may be flat but are usually raised or nodular and may ulcerate. They are typically firm and rubbery but asymptomatic at first. Hence, melanomas may go unnoticed until they cause soreness, bleeding or a neck mass. Pigment may be so readily shed that rubbing the surface with a gauze stains the latter black or dark brown. Later, nodular growth, pain, ulceration, bleeding or loosening of teeth may develop.

Melanomas grow in a predictable fashion. Initially, the malignant melanocytes grow only within the epithelium, spreading laterally. This preinvasive or *in situ* stage is called the radial or horizontal growth phase and lesions of this type rarely metastasise. Later, the melanocytes extend out of the epithelium into the connective tissue in the vertical growth phase. This stage is associated with metastases. In the skin, lesions are often detected in the radial growth phase, but this is rare in the mouth where almost all melanomas are invasive on diagnosis. Because of their rapid growth, most oral melanomas are at least a centimetre across before being noticed and approximately 50% of patients have metastases at presentation, most commonly as cervical lymphadenopathy. In addition to the regional lymph nodes, metastases can involve the lungs, liver, brain and bones.

About 30% of melanomas are preceded by an area of hyperpigmentation, often by many years. These lesions are either dysplasia of melanocytes or melanoma in the radial growth phase. Early diagnosis by biopsy is essential if there is to be a chance of surgical removal before metastasis.

Pathology

Melanomas consist of neoplastic melanocytes often surrounded by clear halos, both within the epithelium and invading deeper tissues. These cells are round to spindle-shaped and typically speckled or intensely pigmented with melanin (Figs 21.9 and 21.10). However, in amelanotic melanomas, the absence of pigment makes these cells more difficult to recognise.

Malignant melanocytes invade both epithelium and connective tissue. In the radial growth phase, the malignant melanocytes cluster along the basement membrane forming nests of *in situ* melanoma. In the invasive vertical growth phase, melanoma spreads into and within the supporting connective tissue. In most advanced lesions, a combined pattern of invasive neoplasm with radial component is seen.

Atypical melanocyte nuclei are hyperchromatic and angular. The neoplastic cells can assume a variety of shapes including spindled, plasmacytoid and epithelioid. Other melanoma cells can be small or clear cells, with a signet ring appearance.

Invasion of blood vessels is common and may be responsible for early metastatic spread. Another feature is lack of an inflammatory reaction. Mitotic activity may be prominent, but absence of mitotic activity does not exclude malignant melanoma.

Immunohistochemistry

Diagnosis is greatly helped by immunohistochemistry, which is often essential for confident diagnosis because of the very varied histological appearances of melanocytes. Immunomarkers used include S-100 and HMB-45 and MelanA, currently regarded as being more specific. However, oral malignant melanomas can react variably with the usual immunochemical markers, so that it has been suggested that they may be a separate entity from cutaneous melanomas.

Key features are summarised in Box 21.2.

Box 21.2   Malignant melanoma: key features

- Peak incidence between 40 and 60 years
- Usually appear as black or brown patches
- Amelanotic melanomas appear red
- Later cause soreness and bleeding
- Histologically consist of neoplastic melanocytes often surrounded by clear halos, within the epithelium and invading deeper tissues
- Neoplastic melanocytes are round to spindle-shaped and typically speckled or intensely pigmented with melanin
- Should be widely excised but median survival probably not longer than 2 years

---

Fig. 21.9   Superficial spreading melanoma. Numerous pigmented and atypical melanocytes form nests and clusters along the basement membrane and are present within the epithelium and superficial connective tissue.

Fig. 21.10   Melanoma. Malignant spindled and round melanocytes, often with bizarre nuclei and some with melanin pigment, invading deep tissue.

Amelanotic melanomas

These tumours are most likely to cause difficulties in clinical diagnosis. They appear pink, red or reddish brown rather than the usual grey-black of melanotic melanomas. The presence of melanin can be confirmed with special stains such as Masson-Fontana and immunocytochemistry (as described above) should be confirmatory when pigment is absent. Probably because of greater delay in diagnosis, the prognosis is appreciably worse than for pigmented melanomas. In such cases, the diagnosis is rarely made until a biopsy and immunohistochemistry has been carried out.

Treatment

Oral melanomas are highly malignant and have a high mortality. Early diagnosis is critical to survival so that early biopsy of all oral pigmented lesions is essential.

The results of different forms of treatment are variable. Wide excision with, if possible, a 2 to 5 cm margin (often with a simultaneous neck dissection) followed by radical radiotherapy or chemotherapy or both is recommended.

Up to 50% of oral melanomas involve regional lymph nodes at presentation. The 5-year survival for node-negative patients may be 30%, but 20% for node-positive patients. Many chemotherapeutic regimens and gene therapy are under trial.

Immunotherapy with, for example, interferon, remains of uncertain value.

Advanced and otherwise untreatable malignant melanomas in other sites have been treated with temazolomide, an oral alkylating agent, and cisplatin with apparent success.

MELANOTIC NEUROECTODERMAL TUMOUR OF INFANCY

One of these tumours (Ch. 9) may rarely show through the palatal mucosa as an ill-defined pigmented area in a neonate or infant.

DIFFUSE MUCOSAL PIGMENTATION →
Summary p. 337

The most important cause of diffuse pigmentation is Addison's disease (Ch. 31), but it is rare. Racial pigmentation is common and though most obvious on the gingivae is typically widespread. Other rare causes are drugs (such as chlorhexidine and phenothiazines, but many others) and cancer of the lung can occasionally cause pigmentation of the soft palate.

SUGGESTED FURTHER READING

Barrett AW, Bennett JH, Speight PM 1995 A clinicopathological and immunohistochemical analysis of primary oral malignant melanoma. Oral Oncol Eur J Cancer 31B:100–115
Boardman LA, Thibodeau SN, Schaid DJ et al 1998 Increased risk for cancer in patients with the Peutz–Jeghers syndrome. Ann Intern Med 128:896–899
Buchner A, Hansen LS 1980 Amalgam pigmentation (amalgam tattoo) of the oral mucosa: a clinicopathological study of 268 cases. Oral Surg Oral Med Oral Pathol 49:139–147
Buchner A, Hansen LS 1987 Pigmented nevi of the oral mucosa: a clinicopathologic study of 36 cases and review of 155 cases from the literature. Oral Surg Oral Med Oral Pathol 63:566–572
Cawson RA, Langdon JD, Eveson JW 1996 Surgical pathology of the mouth and jaws. Wright, Oxford
Cawson RA, Binnie WH, Barrett AW, Wright JM 2001 Color atlas of oral disease, 3rd edn. Mosby-Wolfe, London
Eisen D, Voorhees JJ 1991 Oral melanoma and other pigmented lesions of the oral cavity. J Am Acad Dermatol 24:527–537
Ficarra G, Shillitoe EJ, Adler-Storthz K et al 1990 Oral melanotic macules associated with HIV. Oral Surg Oral Med Oral Pathol 70:301–307
Gazit D, Daniels TE 1994 Oral melanocytic lesions: differences in expression of HMB-45 and S-100 antigens in round and spindle cells of malignant and benign lesions. J Oral Pathol Med 23:60–64
Kaugars GE, Heise AP, Riley WT, Abbey LM, Svirsky JA 1993 Oral melanotic macules. A review of 353 cases. Oral Surg Oral Med Oral Pathol 76:59–61
Langford A, Pohle HD, Gelderblom H et al 1989 Oral hyperpigmentation in HIV-infected patients. Oral Surg Oral Med Oral Pathol 67:301–307
Patton LL, Brahim JS, Baker AR 1994 Metastatic malignant melanoma of the oral cavity. A retrospective study. Oral Surg Oral Med Oral Pathol 78:51–56
Strauss JE, Strauss SI 1994 Oral malignant melanoma: a case report and review of literature. J Oral Maxillofac Surg 52:972–976
Umeda M, Shimada K 1994 Primary malignant melanoma of the oral cavity – its histological classification and treatment. Br J Oral Maxillofac Surg 32:39–47

Oral discoloration, pigmentation or pigmented lesion

Exclude extrinsic causes of pigmentation

Black, dark brown or bluish-brown pigment, radiopaque, usually adjacent amalgam restorations, lesions usually in gingivia or hard palate

Pigment is amalgam or other foreign material. Biopsy is diagnostic but clinical and radiographic diagnosis may be adequate

Decorative tattooing

Chlorhexidine staining

Black or dark brown/blue line around gingival margin and periodontal pockets

Pigment may be lead or other heavy metal sulphides. Check for occupational exposure, drugs such as cisplatin. Analysis of serum or biopsy may be helpful

Black or dark brown pigment localised to the dorsum of the tongue with or without overgrowth of filiform papillae

Pigment probably bacterial in origin (black hairy tongue). Check history for possible associations: radiotherapy, drug treatment, recent period of ill-health. Biopsy and microbiology unhelpful, diagnosis clinical

Consider blood and blood-derived pigmentation

Haemangioma or varix. Check for haemangiomas elsewhere and exclude extension into bone radiographically if overlying jaw. Consider risks of haemorrhage before biopsy or excision. Cryotherapy, arteriography and embolisation may be of value

Localised lesion which blanches on pressure

Discoloration is due to blood in vessels

Red, blue, brown or yellow-brown pigmentation or vascular appearance but no blanching on pressure

Pigment is extravascular blood-derived pigment and/or blood in very small vessels

Consider a bruise or haemorrhage, Kaposi's sarcoma (check for other signs of immunosuppression), pyogenic granuloma, capillary haemangioma, benign and malignant vascular neoplasms. Biopsy indicated. Consider risk of haemorrhage before biopsy or excision

Melanin pigment

Black, brown or bluish-grey discoloration

Racial pattern pigmentation

Dark-skinned races, gingiva especially involved. Diagnosis clinical. Biopsy not indicated unless diagnosis unclear

Inflammatory pigmentation

Pigmentation follows the distribution of an inflammatory condition, e.g. lichen planus and is in a dark-skinned patient. Biopsy usually required for pigmentation and underlying condition

Addison's disease

Neither inflammatory nor racial pattern. Check for history, signs and symptoms of Addison's disease. Biopsy will require steroid cover

Drug-induced pigmentation

Increased mucosal pigmentation due to smoking.

Diagnosed by excluding other causes. Biopsy may be helpful

Generalised diffuse or patchy pigmentation

Associated with a tumour mass

Pigmented neuroectodermal tumour of infancy

Pigmented swelling on the gingiva of a neonate. Biopsy indicated

Melanoma

Most likely cause of pigmented tumour. Check for signs of malignancy. Consider possibility of a metastasis, search for a primary lesion and check history for pre-existing lesion. Biopsy indicated

Discrete flat pigmented patches

Benign melanotic macule

Single or a few. No signs of malignancy. Often freckles also on the facial skin. Impossible to differentiate from melanoma (much less likely) clinically. Biopsy indicated

Multiple lentigenes syndromes

Very large numbers of melanotic macules on face periorally or possibly intraorally. Often diagnosed in child or adolescent. Consider Peutz-Jehgers, LEOPARD and other syndromes and investigate for other signs and family history. Biopsy a lesion to exclude other causes

Melanoma and melanoma in situ

Most frequently on the palate. May be signs of malignancy. Early lesions are unremarkable pigmented patches that cannot be distinguished from benign pigmentation. Be suspicious of enlargement, ulceration and in older patients. Biopsy all suspicious intraoral pigmented patches

Summary chart 21.1 The common causes of oral pigmented lesions.

Self-assessment questions and learning guides

These self-assessment questions and learning guides are based on the material of the previous section, but may also link to material covered elsewhere. They are not intended to be comprehensive, but give an indication of the understanding and problem solving abilities expected at an undergraduate level. You will not find all the information you require to answer these questions in this textbook of essential facts. Use these questions to guide your additional reading and learning.

CHAPTER 12

- What features of oral ulcers would suggest viral infection as the cause?
- What tests are available to identify the presence of viral infection? For which orofacial infections might they be diagnostic?
- What treatment and advice would be appropriate for the parent of a child with primary Herpes simplex infection?
- What are the significant complications of Herpes zoster infection of the head and neck?
- A child has small ulcers on the palate suggestive of viral infection. How would you investigate them? Should they be advised to take time off school?
- Are universal infection control procedures sufficient for a patient with oral primary syphilis?
- Why do candidal infections tend to recur?
- A patient presents with angular stomatitis. How should they be investigated and treated and what would you do if treatment failed?

CHAPTER 13

- How may a traumatic ulcer be differentiated from squamous cell carcinoma?
- How would you investigate a patient with recurrent aphthous stomatitis to exclude underlying predisposing causes?
- What treatments are available for recurrent aphthous stomatitis? What are their advantages and disadvantages?
- What questions would you ask a patient if you were considering making the diagnosis of Behçet's disease?

- Which chronic mucosal diseases cause persistent ulcers?
- How may lichen planus and lichenoid reactions be differentiated?
- What is the value of biopsy in the diagnosis of lichen planus?
- How would you investigate a patient with desquamative gingivitis to differentiate the possible causes?
- What are the similarities and differences between the lesions of lupus erythematosus and lichen planus?
- How may the chronic ulcers of vesiculo-bullous diseases be differentiated from those in lichen planus?
- What special precautions are required when taking a biopsy for the diagnosis of pemphigus or pemphigoid?
- Primary herpetic gingivostomatitis and severe erythema multiforme may present with similar lesions. How would you differentiate these two conditions?

CHAPTER 14

- Which laboratory investigations may aid diagnosis for a patient with a sore but apparently normal tongue?
- What conditions would you consider as possible causes of a sore red tongue?
- How many distinctive oral presentations of candidosis can you identify?
- Why is a smear for microscopy a better diagnostic test than microbiological culture in candidal infection?

CHAPTER 15

- List the white patches that affect the oral mucosa. How may they be differentiated?
- Would any special precautions be necessary to undertake a biopsy of suspected oral hairy leukoplakia?

CHAPTER 16

- Which white lesions of the oral mucosa carry a risk of malignant transformation?
- Which white lesions of the oral mucosa carry no significant risk of malignant transformation?

- What diseases cause red patches of the oral mucosa?
- Which conditions presenting as red patches carry a risk of malignant transformation?
- What investigations would be appropriate for a patient presenting with an oral white lesion?
- Why is a biopsy considered mandatory for all oral white lesions?
- How does biopsy aid the diagnosis and management of risk of malignant transformation?
- What are the earliest signs of oral squamous carcinoma and how do they differ from those in the later stages of the disease?
- What interventions would be appropriate for a patient with a dysplastic oral lesion?
- How would you select the appropriate area of a red or white patch for biopsy?
- How would you decide whether a red or white lesion was suitable for biopsy in a general practice setting?
- What information about a red or white lesion should be provided to the histopathologist?

CHAPTER 17

- What public health measures might reduce the incidence of oral carcinoma? Why are they so difficult to implement?
- What is the difference between staging and grading of carcinomas?
- How is oral squamous carcinoma staged and what is the importance of the stage for treatment and survival?
- How can the general dental practitioner contribute to the management of a patient with oral squamous carcinoma?
- How may the dental practitioner contribute to the prevention of oral carcinoma?
- Why does oral squamous carcinoma have such a high mortality?
- How does the growth and spread of oral carcinoma determine treatment?
- How does the growth and spread of oral carcinoma cause death?

CHAPTER 18

- What are the causes of 'meal-time syndrome'?
- What investigations aid the differentiation of salivary calculi from salivary duct strictures?
- What other lesions may resemble a mucous extravasation in the lower lip?
- What investigations aid the diagnosis of mumps? For how long is the condition infectious?
- How would you identify possible causes of dehydration in a patient with dry mouth?
- Does the clinical presentation of dry mouth aid the differential diagnosis of its possible causes?
- What combination of laboratory investigations would be required to make a diagnosis of Sjögren's syndrome?

- What is the role of the general dental practitioner in management of dry mouth?
- What is the role of the hospital dental specialties in the management of Sjögren's syndrome?
- What is the importance of sudden salivary swelling in a patient with Sjögren's syndrome? How would you investigate a patient with this complaint?
- What are the potential complications of an incisional biopsy of the parotid gland?
- A young adult presents with bilateral salivary gland swelling. What features in the history, examination and special investigations aid your differential diagnosis?
- How would you answer the previous question if the parotid mass were unilateral?
- Which salivary gland swellings should be subjected to incisional biopsy and which may not? Explain why.
- What alternative investigations might you consider when a biopsy of a salivary gland is contraindicated?
- What features of a salivary neoplasm would suggest that it is malignant?
- A 35-year-old male presents with an ulcerated mass on the palate. Discuss the differential diagnosis and appropriate investigations.
- How is a sialogram performed? What information can a sialogram provide?
- How may ultrasound aid the diagnosis of swellings of the head and neck?

CHAPTER 19

- What are the common causes of lesions of the attached gingiva?
- How do fibrous hyperplastic lesions mature if left untreated?
- How would you differentiate a pyogenic granuloma from a Kaposi's sarcoma?

CHAPTER 20

- Why is it important to know about the pathology of the granular cell tumour?
- Does a lymphangioma differ from a cystic hygroma?
- How might you check a lesion for potentially dangerous vascularity before biopsy?

CHAPTER 21

- Which features in the history, examination and investigations would allow the differential diagnosis of oral pigmented lesions?
- Which oral pigmented lesions should be subjected to biopsy and why?
- What features of an oral pigmented lesion suggest melanoma?

THE MEDICALLY COMPROMISED PATIENT

Anaemias, leukaemias and lymphomas

Haematological disease is common and can cause serious complications or oral symptoms (Box 22.1).

Haemoglobin estimation and routine indices are informative and should be carried out when any patient has suspicious signs in the mouth or has to undergo oral surgery.

Box 22.1   Important effects of haematological diseases

- Anaesthetic complications
- Oral infections
- Prolonged bleeding
- Mucosal lesions

ANAEMIA

Causes and important types are summarised in Table 22.1.

Table 22.1   Types and features of important anaemias

Type of anaemia	Causes or effects
1. Iron deficiency (microcytic, hypochromic anaemia)	Usually due to chronic blood loss
2. Folate deficiency (macrocytic)	Pregnancy, malabsorption, alcohol*, phenytoin-induced etc.
3. Vitamin B_{12} deficiency (macrocytic anaemia)	Usually due to pernicious anaemia, occasionally to malabsorption
4. Leukaemia and aplastic anaemia (normochromic normocytic)	Raised susceptibility to infection and bleeding tendency often associated
5. Sickle cell disease (normocytic anaemia)	Genetic. Sickle cells seen in special preparations
6. Beta-thalassaemia (hypochromic, microcytic)	Genetic. Many misshapen red cells
7. Chronic inflammatory disease (normochromic, normocytic)	Rheumatoid arthritis is a common cause
8. Liver disease (usually normocytic)	Haemorrhagic tendency may be associated

*Alcoholism should always be excluded when macrocytosis in the absence of anaemia is found – it is a characteristic sign of alcoholism.

Iron deficiency (microcytic) anaemia is the most common type and usually results from chronic menstrual blood loss. Women of child-bearing age or over, or men with peptic ulcer or haemorrhoids are mainly affected.

Pernicious anaemia chiefly affects women of middle age or over and is the main cause of macrocytic anaemia. Unlike other anaemias, it can cause neurological disease, particularly subacute combined degeneration of the spinal cord.

Folate deficiency also causes a macrocytic anaemia, often in younger patients, particularly in pregnancy. It must be firmly differentiated from pernicious anaemia because administration of folate to the latter can worsen neurological disease.

Leukaemia is an uncommon but frequently lethal cause of normocytic anaemia, but should be suspected in an anaemic child.

Sickle cell trait is most common in immigrants from the West Indies. Sickle cell anaemia is relatively uncommon.

Thalassaemia is mainly seen in immigrants from the Mediterranean area.

Clinical features

Anaemia, irrespective of cause, produces essentially the same clinical features (Box 22.2), particularly if severe, but some anaemias have distinctive features.

Box 22.2   General clinical features of anaemia

- Pallor
- Fatigue and lassitude
- Breathlessness
- Tachycardia and palpitations
- Glossitis or other mucosal lesions

The complexion is a poor indicator of pallor. The conjunctiva of the lower eyelid, the nail beds and, sometimes, the oral mucosa, are more reliable. Cardiovascular signs (tachycardia or oedema of the ankles) result from severe anaemia. Glossitis and other mucosal diseases (Box 22.3) by contrast, can be the earliest signs as discussed below.

Fig. 22.1 **Iron deficiency anaemia.** The tongue is slightly reddened, smooth and depapillated. There is also angular cheilitis as a result of candidal infection.

Box 22.3 **Features of anaemia important in dentistry**

Mucosal disease
- Glossitis
- Angular stomatitis
- Recurrent aphthae
- Infection, particularly candidosis

Risks from general anaesthesia
- Shortage of oxygen can be dangerous

Lowered resistance to infection
- Apart from candidosis, this is seen only in severe anaemia or when due to leukaemia

---

Mucosal disease

Glossitis

Anaemia is the most important, though not the most common, cause of a sore tongue. Soreness *can precede a fall in haemoglobin levels*, particularly when resulting from vitamin B_{12} or folate deficiency, and can be their first sign. Later, there may be obvious inflammation and atrophy of the filiform papillae (Fig. 22.1). Variants of sore tongue have been discussed in Chapter 14, but it is emphasised again that this symptom always requires careful haematological investigation, initially by means of a haemoglobin level and routine indices. Serum iron, ferritin and red cell folate levels may be required. Even though the haemoglobin may be within normal limits, enlarged erythrocytes (mean corpuscular volume [MCV] >96 fl) frequently indicate pernicious anaemia. If any deficiency is found, the underlying cause, such as gastrointestinal disease, must be investigated.

Fig. 22.2 **Acute osteomyelitis in an anaemic patient.** Widespread bone destruction followed straightforward extraction of the posterior teeth. The patient was found to have a haemoglobin level of 4 g/dl.

Recurrent aphthae

Aphthae are sometimes secondary to haematological deficiency, particularly of vitamin B_{12} or folate, in patients whose aphthae start or worsen late in life.

Candidosis and angular stomatitis

Iron deficiency, in particular, is a predisposing factor for candidosis (Ch. 12). Angular stomatitis is also a classical sign of iron deficiency anaemia and due to candidosis.

Dangers of general anaesthesia

Any reduction of oxygenation can precipitate irreparable brain damage or myocardial infarction when there is significant anaemia. General anaesthesia should therefore be given in hospital. The dangers are particularly great in sickle cell disease, as discussed later.

Lowered resistance to infection

Oral candidosis is the main example but, in the past particularly, osteomyelitis could follow extractions in severe anaemia (Fig. 22.2). Currently, sickle cell disease is more important in this context.

SICKLE CELL DISEASE AND SICKLE CELL TRAIT

Sickle cell anaemia mainly affects people of African, Afro-Caribbean, Indian, Mediterranean or Middle Eastern origin. About 5000 persons in Britain are estimated to have sickle cell disease (homozygotes), but many more have sickle cell trait (heterozygotes). The defect in sickle cell disease is an abnormal haemoglobin (HbS) with the risk of haemolysis, anaemia and other effects. In heterozygotes, sufficient normal haemoglobin (HbA) is formed to allow normal life with only rare complications.

Sickle cell disease

The complications arise from polymerisation of deoxygenated HbS, which is less soluble than HbA. This forms long fibres which deform the red cells into sickle shapes and makes them vulnerable to haemolysis. Chronic haemolysis causes chronic anaemia, but patients, under normal circumstances, typically feel well, as HbS more readily releases its oxygen content to the tissues than HbA. Exacerbation of sickling raises blood viscosity, causing blocking of capillaries and sickling crises (Boxes 22.4 and 22.5).

Box 22.4   **Factors that can precipitate sickling crises**

- Hypoxia, particularly from poorly conducted anaesthesia
- Dehydration
- Infections (including dental)
- Acidosis and fever

Box 22.5   **The main types of sickling crises**

- Painful crises
- Aplastic crises
- Sequestration crises

These patients are also abnormally susceptible to infection, particularly pneumococcal or meningococcal, and osteomyelitis.

Painful crises are caused by blockage of blood vessels and bone marrow infarcts. Painful crises can affect the jaws, particularly the mandible, and mimic acute osteomyelitis clinically and radiographically. The infarcted tissue forms a focus susceptible to infection, and *Salmonella* osteomyelitis is a recognised hazard.

Aplastic crises are caused by human parvovirus B19 infection and require immediate transfusion.

Sequestration crises result from sickle cells pooling in the spleen, liver or lungs. An acute chest syndrome, with pain, fever and leucocytosis, is the most common cause of death.

Dental aspects of sickle cell trait and disease

Sickling trait should be suspected, particularly in those of Afro-Caribbean origin, and investigated if anaesthesia is anticipated. If the haemoglobin is less than 10 g/dl, the patient is probably a homozygote with sickle cell disease. Screening tests depend on the lower solubility of HbS which produces turbidity when a reducing agent is added. Confirmation is by electrophoresis.

In those with sickle cell trait, the main precaution is that general anaesthesia should be carried out with full oxygenation. In sickle cell disease, the oral mucosa may be pale or yellowish due to haemolytic jaundice. Radiographic changes can be seen in the skull and sometimes the jaws (Ch. 10).

Occasionally, crises may be precipitated by dental infections such as acute pericoronitis. Prompt antibiotic treatment is therefore important. Painful bone infarcts should be treated with nonsteroidal anti-inflammatory analgesics and fluid intake should be increased. Admission to hospital is required for severe painful crises not responsive to analgesics. Rigorous routine dental care is necessary because of the susceptibility to infection.

THE THALASSAEMIAS

Alpha-thalassaemias mainly affect Asians, Africans and Afro-Caribbeans, while beta-thalassaemias mainly affect those from the Mediterranean littoral such as Greeks (thalassaemia – literally, 'sea in the blood').

Thalassaemias result from diminished synthesis of one or more of the globin chains of haemoglobin. The resulting relative excess of either the alpha or beta globin chains, which are unstable, causes them to precipitate in the red cells. Haemolysis can result.

The severity of the disease depends on the numbers of alpha or beta globin genes affected. In simplified terms, the diseases are *thalassaemia minor* in heterozygotes and *thalassaemia major* in homozygotes.

Thalassaemia minor causes mild but persistent microcytic anaemia but is otherwise asymptomatic apart, sometimes, from splenomegaly. Iron therapy is ineffective and leads to iron deposition in the tissues.

Thalassaemia major (usually homozygous beta-thalassaemia) causes severe hypochromic, microcytic anaemia, great enlargement of liver and spleen and skeletal abnormalities (Ch. 10) due to marrow expansion. There is failure to thrive and early death if regular transfusions are not given. They are life-saving, prevent the development of bony deformities, but lead to progressive iron deposition in the tissues. Haemosiderosis is the main cause of complications in survivors and leads to dysfunction of glands and other organs. Xerostomia can result from iron deposition in the salivary glands. Desferrioxamine, a chelating agent, may reduce iron overload, and folic acid treatment may ameliorate the haemolytic anaemia.

LEUKAEMIA

The effect of leukaemic overproduction of white cells is to suppress other cell lines of the marrow (Box 22.6). Leukaemia can affect virtually any of the white cell series, but different types of acute leukaemia cannot be distinguished clinically.

Box 22.6   **Major effects of acute leukaemia**

- Anaemia due to suppression of erythrocyte production
- Raised susceptibility to infection due to deficiency or abnormalities of granulocytes
- Bleeding tendency (purpura) due to suppression of platelet production

---

Acute leukaemia → Summary p. 324

Acute lymphoblastic leukaemia is the most common leukaemia in children (usually between 3 and 5 years), while acute myeloblastic anaemia is the most common type in adults.

Splenomegaly or hepatomegaly, or both, and lymphadenopathy, particularly in lymphoblastic leukaemia, are usually associated. Mucosal pallor or abnormal gingival bleeding, particularly in a child, strongly suggests acute leukaemia (Box 22.7). Diagnosis depends on the peripheral blood picture and marrow biopsy.

Box 22.7   **Oral and perioral effects of acute leukaemia**

- Gingival swelling
- Mucosal ulceration
- Leukaemic deposits
- Purpura
- Anaemia
- Cervical lymphadenopathy

Gingival swelling results from lack of healthy, mature white cells to counter low-grade gingival infection. The gingivae become packed and swollen with leukaemic cells, particularly in acute myelogenous leukaemia in adults. The gingivae are often purplish and may become necrotic and ulcerate (Figs 22.3 and 22.4).

Mucosal ulceration is often a combined effect of immunodeficiency and cytotoxic drugs, such as methotrexate. Herpetic infections and thrush are common and ulceration may be caused by a variety of opportunistic microbes. Also as a result of the immunodeficiency, the first sign of acute leukaemia may occasionally be an infection such as acute osteomyelitis following routine extractions.

Leukaemic deposits are tumour-like masses of leukaemic cells which may occasionally form in the mouth or salivary glands (Fig. 22.5).

Purpura can appear as excessive gingival bleeding, purplish mucosal patches, blood blisters, or prolonged bleeding after surgery. Leukaemic infiltration of an extraction socket can delay healing (Fig. 22.6).

Anaemia can cause mucosal pallor and is an important sign in children among whom anaemia is otherwise uncommon.

Cervical lymphadenopathy is particularly common in lymphocytic leukaemia but may be seen in other types or be secondary to opportunistic infections in the mouth.

Management

Biopsy of gingival swelling unresponsive to conventional treatment may lead to the diagnosis of leukaemia.

Fig. 22.4   Acute leukamia. The gingivae and bone marrow of the interdental bone contain a confluent infiltrate of leukaemic cells.

Fig. 22.5   Myeloid leukaemia. An ulcerated tumour mass formed by leukaemic cells emigrating into the tissues.

Fig. 22.3   Acute myelocytic leukaemia. The gingivae are grossly swollen and purplish; in addition there is ulceration along the palatal aspect of the anterior teeth resulting from the increased susceptibility to infection.

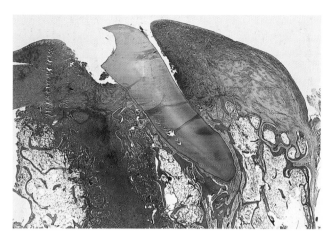

Fig. 22.6 Acute myelogenous leukaemia. Leukaemic cells have densely infiltrated the swollen gingiva and the extraction socket, which has been prevented from healing.

Fig. 22.7 High-grade non-Hodgkin lymphoma. Neoplastic lymphocytes with large vesicular nuclei are packed in confluent sheets. Mitotic figures are numerous.

Ideally, patients with leukaemia or any others having cytotoxic treatment, should have meticulous oral hygiene to control the bacterial population, before complications develop (see Fig. 5.32).

Mouth rinses (0.2% chlorhexidine or tetracycline and amphotericin) will often control severe gingival changes and superficial infections. Mucosal ulceration by Gram-negative bacilli or anaerobes may need specific antibiotic therapy, which is also necessary for systemic spread of infection.

Oral ulceration caused by methotrexate may be controlled by giving folinic acid. Extractions should be avoided because of the risks of severe infections, bleeding, or anaemia. If unavoidable, blood transfusion and generous antibiotic cover are required.

Chronic leukaemia

Chronic leukaemia is a slowly progressive disease of adults. Chronic lymphocytic leukaemia can be completely asymptomatic and may not even shorten life.

Oral manifestations (Box 22.8) are relatively uncommon or mild.

Box 22.8 Possible oral effects of chronic leukaemia

- Mucosal pallor
- Gingival or palatal swelling
- Purpura
- Oral ulceration (ulceration may be due to infection or cytotoxic drugs or both)

Management

Routine dentistry can usually be carried out with normal care. If there is significant anaemia, bleeding tendencies, or susceptibility to infection, similar precautions need to be taken to those for acute leukaemia.

LYMPHOMAS

Lymphomas, unlike leukaemias, are solid tumours, though lymphocytic lymphoma can be accompanied by lymphocytic leukaemia.

Lymphomas can arise from any type of lymphocyte, but more frequently from B cells. They are all malignant. They comprise Hodgkin's disease and the more common non-Hodgkin lymphoma.

Lymphomas involve the cervical lymph nodes relatively frequently, but are rare in the mouth. However, in AIDS, lymphomas may account for 2% of oral neoplasms.

Non-Hodgkin lymphomas

The risk of developing a lymphoma is raised in the following conditions:

1. some of the primary immunodeficiency diseases
2. cytotoxic immunosuppressive treatment
3. AIDS
4. connective tissue diseases, especially rheumatoid arthritis and Sjögren's syndrome.

Adults are predominantly affected and, within the mouth, lymphomas form non-descript, usually soft, painless swellings, which may become ulcerated by trauma.

Histologically, lymphomas frequently present difficulties of precise diagnosis. Non-Hodgkin lymphomas may be diffuse and appear as solid sheets of lymphocytes which may be predominantly small or large. Alternatively, they may have a *follicular* pattern. Most follicular lymphomas are low grade and have a better prognosis. The neoplastic lymphocytes show varying degrees of differentiation from mature small cells to large immunoblasts which may resemble histiocytes (Fig. 22.7). Most are of B-cell origin (Fig. 22.8).

Invasion of adjacent tissues may be seen and helps to confirm the malignant nature of these tumours (Fig. 22.9). If traumatised,

Fig. 22.8 High-grade lymphoma. Immunocytochemistry for a B-cell marker produces a ring of positive brown stain on the membrane of virtually every tumour cell, indicating its B-cell origin.

Fig. 22.9 High-grade non-Hodgkin lyphoma. Small darkly staining lymphoma cells infiltrating through muscle and fat.

inflammatory cells can obscure the lymphomatous nature of the tumour. However, lymphoma cells are monoclonal and this can be recognised by immunohistochemistry by production of kappa or lambda light chains only (Ch. 1).

Management

As well as biopsy, staging is necessary to determine the extent of spread. In general, localised disease is treated by irradiation while disseminated disease (the majority of patients) is treated by combination chemotherapy. Oral complications of treatment, such as ulceration and infection, are common.

Burkitt's lymphoma

This was the first lymphoma where an association with the Epstein–Barr virus (EBV) was shown. It is predominantly extranodal. It is unusual in that its onset is in childhood and it is endemic in East Africa. It is also unusual in that the jaw is the single most common initial site and spread to the parotid glands is common. Over 95% of cases respond completely to single-dose chemotherapy.

Fig. 22.10 Burkitt's lymphoma. Small darkly staining neoplastic lymphocytes form sheets in which the macrophages containing cellular debris form round, pale holes (starry sky appearance).

Histologically, Burkitt's lymphoma is a small-cell lymphoma containing scattered pale histiocytes which give the dark sheets of cells a so-called 'starry sky' appearance (Fig. 22.10). Lymphomas resembling Burkitt's lymphoma microscopically can also be a complication of immunosuppressive treatment or AIDS but do not behave like African Burkitt's lymphoma.

Hodgkin's disease

The cervical lymph nodes are frequently affected, but lesions are exceptionally uncommon in the mouth. They are not clinically distinguishable from non-Hodgkin lymphoma.

Histologically, the characteristic features are the mixed cellular picture and occasional Reed-Sternberg giant cells with paired (mirror-image) nuclei.

Permanent cure of some types of Hodgkin's disease is possible as a result of irradiation of localised disease or combined chemotherapy and the overall 5-year survival rate may be up to 80%.

MALT lymphoma

MALT (mucosa-associated lymphoid tissue) lymphomas develop from the marginal zone lymphocytes and arise in extranodal sites such as the stomach, small intestine, thyroid and lung rather than in lymph nodes. MALT lymphomas account for 10% of all non-Hodgkin lymphomas. Marginal zone lymphocytes (so called because they are found in the marginal zone of tonsils and Peyer's patches) home to mucosa and are involved in mucosal immunity.

MALT lymphomas are unusual. They are mostly low grade and indolent and survival is excellent even in disseminated disease. Very few patients die from low-grade MALT lymphoma and it may even regress spontaneously. MALT lymphomas of the stomach develop in the presence of *Helicobacter pylori* infection and are of interest because elimination of *H. pylori* can lead to complete regression of the tumour. MALT lymphomas also arise in autoimmune diseases, in the thyroid in Hashimoto thyroiditis and in salivary glands as a complication of Sjögren's syndrome. Salivary MALT lymphoma usually presents as persistent painless swelling and complicates primary rather than secondary Sjögren's syndrome. Most patients are 50–65 at diagnosis.

Mikulicz syndrome is bilateral swelling of salivary and lacrimal glands sometimes due to sarcoidosis (see Fig 28.9), but in the original patient the appearance was caused by a MALT lymphoma.

Histologically, the MALT lymphomas consist predominantly of marginal-zone B cells which range from a lymphocyte-like to monocyte-like appearance. The monocytoid B cells have a rim of clear cytoplasm. These neoplastic cells infiltrate and destroy the ductal epithelium, which proliferates in response to form much larger islands. The islands of epithelium containing numerous lymphocytes are called lymphoepithelial ('myoepithelial') lesions. The MALT lymphoma is centred on these islands, but the remainder of the gland is replaced by non-neoplastic lymphocytes and these can form lymphoid follicles so that the gland develops a resemblance to lymph node.

Management

Any patient with primary Sjögren's syndrome and persistently swollen glands must be followed up and investigated with MALT lymphoma in mind.

Diagnosis requires tissue, usually a tail of parotid biopsy. Fine needle aspirate cannot be used for diagnosis unless the lymphoma is high grade. Even histologically, the diagnosis is not always evident because there is overlap with the histological appearances of Sjögren's syndrome. Definitive diagnosis requires molecular analysis to prove that the lymphocytes in the gland are clonal. This is done by polymerase chain reaction analysis of the immunoglobulin chain genes and it is often assumed that finding clones of lymphocytes indicates lymphoma. However, lymphocytes' normal function is to generate clones of cells in response to antigenic challenge and, at least in the early stages, any clones of lymphocytes may be physiological. Identifying early MALT lymphoma with certainty remains difficult. Cytogenetic changes, including trisomy 3, may aid diagnosis in later disease.

The management of MALT lymphoma is also highly controversial. Patients tend to be treated by radiotherapy or chemotherapy even though evidence suggests that many lymphomas do not progress without treatment. Some untreated patients have remained well for 30 years after diagnosis. Despite this indolent behaviour, MALT lymphoma can spread to other mucosal sites ('homing') and can progress to high-grade lymphoma. All patients require long-term follow-up because these developments require more aggressive treatment.

Nasopharyngeal (T-cell and NK-cell) lymphomas
(Box 22.9)

These lesions, which for a long time were not recognised as lymphomas, produce their initial symptoms in the nasal cavity and are discussed in Chapter 28.

Fig. 22.11 Nasopharyngeal lymphoma. Typical slight anterior swelling and ulcer due to perforation of the palate by the tumour.

Fig. 22.12 Nasopharyngeal lymphoma. Neoplastic infiltration of a vessel wall simulating vasculitis.

Box 22.9   Key features of nasopharyngeal T-cell lymphoma

- Onset typically indistinguishable from Wegener's granulomatosis
- Downward extension may cause central ulceration or necrosis of the palate enabling early diagnosis (Fig. 22.11)
- Histologically, the cellular picture is pleomorphic but damage to blood vessels mimics vasculitis (Fig. 22.12)
- T-cell or NK-cell markers confirm the diagnosis
- Spread of disease is similar to that of other lymphomas and, usually, a fatal outcome
- Spread may be limited or delayed by radiotherapy

LEUCOPENIA AND AGRANULOCYTOSIS

Leucopenia is a deficiency of white cells (fewer than 5000/μL with many possible causes (Box 22.10). It is a peripheral blood manifestation of actual or incipient immunodeficiency.

Box 22.10   Important causes of leucopenia

- Leukaemia
- Aplastic anaemia
- Drugs (Box 22.12)
- Autoimmune
- HIV infection

Leucopenia can be a chance haematological finding and may cause no symptoms until it becomes so severe as to impair defences against infection. Thus, lymphopenia in an apparently healthy person may be a sign of HIV infection.

Agranulocytosis

Agranulocytosis is the term given to the clinical effects of severe neutropenia, namely fever, prostration and mucosal ulceration, particularly of the gingivae and pharynx.

Drug-induced leucopenia

Management

Box 22.11   Leukopenia: principles of general and dental management

General
- Stop any drug which may be causative
- Give antibiotics
- Give blood transfusions if necessary

Dental
- Optimise oral hygiene
- Control oral infections (as for acute leukaemia)
- Avoid extractions
- Antibiotic cover and transfusions if necessary if surgery is unavoidable

Aplastic anaemia

Aplastic anaemia is failure of production of all bone marrow cells (pancytopenia). The systemic and oral effects are not unlike those of acute leukaemia (purpura, anaemia and susceptibility to infection). Aplastic anaemia may be of unknown cause but is probably autoimmune. Otherwise, drugs (Box 22.12) are the main cause.

Box 22.12   Important causes of drug-induced leucopenia

- Analgesics, especially phenylbutazone*
- Antibacterial drugs, especially chloramphenicol or (rarely) co-trimoxazole
- Phenothiazine antipsychotic drugs
- Antithyroid drugs such as thiouracil
- Cytotoxic drugs

*Use now restricted as a consequence.

The management is to stop any drugs that may be responsible and to give antibiotics and transfusions. Nevertheless, approximately 50% of patients die within 6 months, usually from infection or haemorrhage, but marrow transplantation has occasionally been successful. Dental management is as for acute leukaemia.

Cyclic neutropenia

In cyclic neutropenia, there is a fall in the number of circulating neutrophils at regular intervals of 3–4 weeks. There have been only about 40 reported cases in 70 years and undue emphasis has been placed on the fact that cyclic neutropenia occasionally, but not necessarily, causes oral ulceration or rapidly progressive periodontitis.

SUGGESTED FURTHER READING

Bahler DW, Swerdlow SH 1998 Clonal salivary gland infiltrates associated with myoepithelial sialadenitis (Sjogren's syndrome) begin as nonmalignant antigen-selected expansions. Blood 91:1864–1872

Banerjee AK, Layton DM, Rennie JA et al 1991 Safe surgery in sickle cell disease. Br J Surg 78:516–519

Cranfield T, Bunch C 1995 Acute leukaemias. Medicine (UK) 23:503–509

Field EA, Speechley JA, Rugman FR 1995 Oral signs and symptoms in patients with undiagnosed vitamin B_{12} deficiency. J Oral Pathol Med 24:468–470

Gregory G, Olujohungbe A 1994 Mandibular nerve neuropathy in sickle cell disease. Local factors. Oral Surg Oral Med Oral Pathol 77:66–69

Hatton C, Mackie PH 1996 Haemoglobinopathies and other congenital haemolytic anaemias. Medicine Int 24:14–19

Higgs DR 1993 The thalassaemia syndromes. Q J Med 86:559–564

Jordan RC, Speight PM 1996 Lymphoma in Sjogren's syndrome. From histopathology to molecular pathology. Oral Surg 81:308–320

Luker J, Scully C, Oakhill A 1991 Gingival swelling as a manifestation of aplastic anaemia. Oral Surg Oral Med Oral Pathol 70:55–56

O'Connor N, Bunch C 1995 Laboratory diagnosis in haematology. Medicine Int 23:489–494

O'Rourke C, Mitropoulous C 1990 Orofacial pain in patients with sickle cell disease. Br Dent J 169:130–132

Pippard MJ, Heppleston AD 1996 Microcytic and macrocytic anaemias. Medicine Int 24:4–10

Podlesh SW, Boyden DK 1996 Diagnosis of acute bone/bone marrow infarction of the mandible in sickle haemoglobinopathy. Report of a case. Oral Surg Oral Med Oral Pathol Oral Radiol Endod 81:547–549

Sansevere JJ, Miles M 1993 Management of the oral and maxillofacial patient with sickle cell disease and related haemoglobinopathies. J Oral Maxillofac Surg 51:912–916

Haemorrhagic diseases

Purpura (usually due to platelet defects) and clotting defects are the main causes of haemorrhagic disorders.

INVESTIGATION OF A HISTORY OF EXCESSIVE BLEEDING

A careful history (Box 23.1) is absolutely essential and is as important as the blood tests.

Box 23.1 Information required about haemorrhagic tendencies

- Results of previous dental operations? Have simple extractions led to prolonged bleeding?
- Has bleeding persisted for more than 24 hours?
- Has admission to hospital ever been necessary for dental bleeding?
- Have other operations or injuries caused prolonged bleeding?
- Is there a family history of prolonged bleeding?
- Are anticoagulants or other drugs being taken?
- Is there any medical cause such as leukaemia or liver disease?
- Does the patient carry a warning card or hospital letter about bleeding tendencies?

Most of the severe haemorrhagic diseases, such as haemophilia, are hereditary and a positive family history should be carefully evaluated. Bleeding for up to 24 hours after an extraction is usually due to local causes or a minor defect of haemostasis manageable by local measures. More prolonged bleeding is significant. Even a *mild* haemophiliac can bleed for weeks after a simple extraction.

Clinical examination

Signs of anaemia and purpura should be looked for. Examination of the mouth shows how any operation should be planned. In the case of haemophilia, all essential extractions should be carried out at a single operation with factor VIII cover. Radiographs should be taken to anticipate possible difficulties with the extractions.

Laboratory investigations

Details of investigations are decided by the haematologists, but summarised in Box 23.2.

Box 23.2 Important investigations in haemophilia

- Haemoglobin level and blood picture
- Assessment of haemostatic function, particularly the
    Bleeding time
    Prothrombin time (expressed as the INR)
    Activated partial thromboplastin time (APTT)
    Thrombin time
- Blood grouping and cross-matching

It is essential to look for anaemia. It is an almost inevitable result of repeated bleeding and worsened by any further bleeding as a result of surgery. Anaemia increases the risks of general anaesthesia and should be treated before any surgery. Anaemia is also an essential feature of some haemorrhagic diseases, particularly acute leukaemia.

Blood grouping is required as transfusions may be needed before operation to improve haemostasis or afterwards, if blood loss is severe.

PURPURA

Purpura is typically the result of platelet disorders (Box 23.3) and relatively rarely caused by vascular defects. The bleeding time is prolonged but clotting functions are normal. An exception is von Willebrand's disease, where there is an associated deficiency of a clotting factor.

Box 23.3 Causes of purpura

Platelet disorders
- Idiopathic thrombocytopenic purpura
- Connective-tissue diseases (especially SLE)
- Acute leukaemias
- Drug-associated
- HIV infection

Vascular disorders
- Von Willebrand's disease
- Corticosteroid treatment
- Ehlers–Danlos syndrome
- Infective
- Nutritional
- Hereditary haemorrhagic telangiectasia

General features of purpura

Purpura (bleeding into the skin or mucous membranes, causing petechiae or ecchymoses or 'spontaneous bruising') also causes prolonged bleeding after injury or surgery. Unlike haemophilia, haemorrhage immediately follows the trauma but, usually, bleeding in purpura ultimately stops spontaneously as a result of normal coagulation.

Many women will say that they bruise easily, but such bruises are usually only a few millimetres across. The most informative test of platelet function is the *bleeding time*, supplemented as necessary by tests of platelet aggregations and adhesion. Deficiency of platelets (fewer than $100\,000/mm^3$) is termed thrombocytopenia, but spontaneous bleeding is uncommon until the count falls below $50\,000/mm^3$.

A typical site of oral purpura is the palate where the posterior border of a denture presses into the mucosa. Excessive gingival bleeding or blood blisters are other signs (Fig. 23.1).

Idiopathic thrombocytopenic purpura

The immediate cause is IgG autoantibodies which bind to platelets. The number of platelets in the peripheral blood is greatly reduced.

(A)

(B)

Fig. 23.1 **Systemic purpura.** (A) The lesions are due to spontaneous bleeding into the tissues and often form at sites of trauma. (B) Lesions on the tongue.

The disease may affect children or young adult women and the first sign may be profuse gingival bleeding or post-extraction haemorrhage. More often there is spontaneous bleeding into the skin.

Management

Thrombocytopenic purpura frequently responds, at least in the short term, to corticosteroids which can be used for urgently needed surgery. Long-term use of corticosteroids is associated with their usual hazards. Some cases resolve spontaneously, but persistent cases may respond to splenectomy. However, 10–20% of cases are unresponsive to any form of treatment and, now that haemophilia is a manageable disease, such cases have become one of the most troublesome of the haemorrhagic diseases. For operative treatment, transfusions of platelet concentrates can be given, but immunosuppressive drugs may also have to be given to prevent platelet destruction by antibodies. As with other platelet disorders, aspirin and other anti-inflammatory analgesics should be avoided.

AIDS-associated purpura

Autoimmune thrombocytopenia can complicate HIV infection and can be an early sign. Purpuric patches in the mouth, particularly in a young male, should suggest this possibility and also need to be distinguished from oral Kaposi's sarcoma by tests of haemostasis and, if necessary, biopsy.

Drug-associated purpura

Many drugs, particularly aspirin, interfere with platelet function (Box 23.4). Others act as haptens and cause immune destruction of platelets or suppress marrow function causing pancytopenia (aplastic anaemia) of which purpura is typically an early sign. The most frequent cause of aplastic anaemia in Britain has been phenylbutazone.

Box 23.4 Important causes of drug-associated thrombocytopenia
• Chloramphenicol • Phenylbutazone • Indomethacin • Thiazide diuretics • Quinine and quinidine

Other drugs affecting thrombus formation include the antiplatelet drugs, such as clopidogrel, and glycoprotein inhibitors. These drugs may affect the activated partial prothrombin time and may complicate major surgical procedures.

Fibrinolytic drugs, such as streptokinase, used in the acute treatment of myocardial infarction are potential causes of bleeding tendencies so that dental surgery is possibly hazardous.

If purpura develops, the drug should be stopped but, in the case of aplastic anaemia, the process may be irreversible and fatal.

Infections

Tropical infections are increasingly brought into Britain on aircraft. Fortunately, the viral haemorrhagic fevers have not been brought here. They include Ebola, Lassa fever, Congo Crimea haemorrhagic fever – there was an epidemic of the last recently in Afghanistan.

Bleeding from every orifice is the main feature of these diseases and probably first starts from the gingival margins. Platelet dysfunction is the main cause and the mortality is high.

Nutritional disorders

Scurvy is the only cause of vitamin deficiency-related bleeding. It is now of little more than historical interest. The defect is in the impaired connective tissue support for blood vessels together with a platelet disorder due to vitamin C deficiency.

Gingival bleeding is typically the first sign. The gingivae become engorged and swollen and, as mentioned earlier, the disease was so severe among the Crusaders that the Christian knights had to have their grossly swollen gingivae cut back to enable them to eat.

Hereditary haemorrhagic telangiectasia

This is an uncommon autosomal dominant disorder with telangiectases particularly of the skin, but also of the oral mucosa and gastrointestinal tract due to fragility of vessel walls. Significant haemorrhage is rarely a problem, but intracranial or visceral bleeding can be dangerous. Oral surgery is generally safe, but regional anaesthetic blocks should be avoided because of the risk of deep bleeding into the soft tissues.

Cryosurgery or argon laser treatment can obliterate the telangiectases, but is only required for lesions which have bled significantly or recurrently, or for cosmetic concerns about the skin lesions.

Localised oral purpura

Blood blisters occasionally appear in the oral mucosa after minor or unnoticed trauma, but there is no haemostatic defect. Such blisters may form in the throat and cause a choking sensation ('angina bullosa haemorrhagica'). Rupture of a blood blister leaves an ulcer (Figs 23.2–23.4).

Systemic purpura should be excluded by haematological examination and the patient can be reassured.

Von Willebrand's disease

Von Willebrand's disease is characterised both by a prolonged bleeding time and deficiency of factor VIII. It is usually inherited

Fig. 23.2 **Localised oral purpura.** An intact blood blister on the soft palate and fauces.

Fig. 23.3 **Localised oral purpura.** A ruptured blood blister has formed a large ulcer on the soft palate.

Fig. 23.4 **Localised oral purpura.** A blood-filled space lies immediately below the epithelium in this intact bulla.

as an autosomal dominant: both males and females are therefore affected.

The deficiency of factor VIII is usually mild compared with the platelet defect, so that purpura is the more common manifestation. However, some patients have factor VIII levels low enough to cause a significant clotting defect. The platelet defect is usually correctable with desmopressin, which may also be sufficient to correct any significant factor VIII deficiency. In unusually severe cases, the deficiency of factor VIII is such that surgery has to be managed as for haemophilia A. However, factor VIII remains active in the blood for a considerably longer period.

Disseminated intravascular coagulation

This disorder, also known as consumption coagulopathy or defibrination syndrome, is an uncommon and complex disorder of haemostasis. Precipitating causes include incompatible blood transfusions, severe sepsis, burns and severe trauma. Up to 57% of head injuries can trigger this disorder and the risk of ischaemic brain damage.

Bleeding results from consumption of platelets and of clotting factors internally and from activation of the fibrinolytic system. Purpura and bleeding, particularly from the gastrointestinal tract, are typical features. Clotting in capillaries can damage the kidneys, liver, adrenal glands and brain in particular.

Because of the varied effects of this disorder, management is difficult but urgent. Relief of the underlying cause is important. Depending on the haematolological findings, treatment may include heparinisation, replacement of clotting factors and/or platelets or antifibrinolytic treatment. However, no individual form of treatment is completely reliable.

CLOTTING DISORDERS

Important causes are shown in Box 23.5.

> **Box 23.5** Important causes of coagulation defects
>
> **Heritable deficiencies of plasma factors**
> * Haemophilia A (by far the most important cause)
> * Haemophilia B
> * Von Willebrand's disease with low factor VIII levels
>
> **Acquired clotting defects**
> * Vitamin K deficiency
> * Anticoagulant treatment
> * Liver disease

Haemophilia A

Haemophilia is the most common and severe clotting disorder. Haemophilia A (factor VIII deficiency) affects approximately 6 per 100 000 of the population and is about 10 times as common as haemophilia B (Christmas disease, factor IX deficiency). In the past, extractions in haemophiliacs have been fatal, and extractions are still common emergencies or occasions when haemophiliacs need specific treatment.

Severe haemophilia typically causes effects in childhood, usually as a result of bleeding into muscles or joints after

Fig. 23.5 Haemophilia. This was a mild and unsuspected haemophiliac who had never had any previous serious bleeding episodes. This enormous haematoma developed after a submucous injection for extirpation of an incisor pulp. (By kind permission of Mr AJ Bridge.)

minor injuries. By contrast, mild haemophilia (factor VIII level over 25%) may cause no symptoms until an injury, surgery or a dental extraction precipitates prolonged bleeding. This may not happen until adult life. Severe and prolonged bleeding deeply into the soft tissues can also follow local anaesthetic injections. Inferior dental blocks are most dangerous because of the rich plexus of veins in this area from which blood can lead down to the glottis. Even a submucous infiltration can occasionally have severe consequences (Fig. 23.5).

Clinical features

As mentioned earlier, a positive family history is always significant. However, over 30% of haemophiliacs have a negative family history and, occasionally, haemophilia is discovered only as a result of post-extraction haemorrhage. By contrast, it is certain that a patient who has had extractions or tonsillectomy without serious bleeding is not haemophiliac.

Typically, bleeding starts after a short delay as a result of normal platelet and vascular responses which provide the initial phase of haemostasis. There is then persistent bleeding which, if untreated, can continue for weeks or until the patient dies. Pressure packs, suturing, or local applications of haemostatics are ineffective.

Haemarthroses are well-recognised complications of uncontrolled haemophilia, but most dangerous is intracranial haemorrhage. Deep tissue bleeding can also occasionally spread down from the neck and obstruct the airway. Many haemophiliacs are carriers of HBV, HBC or HIV infection as a result of receiving untreated blood products. Formation of antibodies to factor VIII is another complication.

Principles of management

Box 23.6   Principles of dental management of haemophilia

- History
- Laboratory findings
    Prolonged activated partial thromboplastin time
    Normal prothrombin time
    Normal bleeding time
    Low factor VIII levels
- Regular meticulous dental care to avoid the need for extractions
- Preoperative planning of unavoidable extractions or other surgery
- Preoperative replacement therapy
- Postoperative precautions

Before surgery, radiographs should be taken to forestall any complications resulting from unsuspected disease and to decide whether any other extractions are necessary. Arrangements must usually be made for admission to hospital. The number of occasions when replacement therapy has to be given should be kept to a minimum. When replacement therapy has been given, as much surgical work as possible should be done in that session. It is always wise to plan treatment with the possibility in mind that the next time the patient needs surgery, he may be in a place where replacement therapy is unobtainable or has developed antibodies to factor VIII.

A factor VIII level between 50 and 75% is necessary for dental extractions and factor VIII requirement depends on the serum level and the expected severity of the surgical trauma. It is usual also to give tranexamic acid or desmopressin to reduce the amount of factor VIII needed.

Postoperatively, an antibiotic such as oral penicillin (250 mg four times a day for 7 days) is usually given to reduce the chance of wound infections and secondary haemorrhage. The risks of bleeding are greatest on the day of operation and again from 4 to 10 days postoperatively. If bleeding starts at any time after the operation, factor VIII must be given or may be given prophylactically on the fourth or fifth postoperative day. Administration of tranexamic acid is usually continued for 10 days. Aspirin and related analgesics should be avoided.

For routine dentistry, relative analgesia is preferable for sedation, to avoid the risk from accidental damage to a vein. Now that haemophiliacs have a personal stock of factor VIII for use in emergencies, these problems have greatly declined. However, it may be necessary to check that the factor VIII has been taken.

Extractions in mild haemophilia may be managed by giving antifibrinolytic drugs, particularly tranexamic acid or desmopressin rather than factor VIII. For those with antibodies to factor VIII, factor VIII inhibitor bypassing fraction may be given.

Christmas disease (haemophilia B)

Christmas disease is inherited in the same way as, and is clinically identical to, haemophilia A. However, factor IX is more stable than factor VIII. Dried factor IX fraction is given for replacement.

Factor IX remains active in the blood for more than 2 days, so that replacement therapy can be given at longer intervals than for haemophilia A. All other aspects of management of haemophilia A and B arc the same.

Acquired clotting defects

Overall, these are more common than the inherited defects (Box 23.7).

Box 23.7   Important acquired clotting disorders

- Vitamin K deficiency
- Anticoagulants
- Liver disease

Vitamin K deficiency

Causes include obstructive jaundice or, less commonly, malabsorption. Important causes of obstructive jaundice are hepatitis, gall stones and carcinoma of the pancreas.

Extractions or other surgery should preferably be delayed until haemostasis recovers. In emergency, vitamin K can be given, preferably by mouth, and its effectiveness checked by the prothrombin time. If the latter does not return to normal within 48 hours, there is probably parenchymal liver disease.

Anticoagulant treatment

Coumarin anticoagulants, such as warfarin, are used for thromboembolic disease which can complicate atrial fibrillation or insertion of prosthetic heart valves. The underlying condition may therefore influence dental management more than the treatment. Anticoagulation should be checked regularly to maintain the prothrombin time. This is reported as the INR (International Normalised Ratio), at 2 to 3 in most cases, but at 3 to 4.5 for those with prosthetic valves. Dental extractions can usually be carried out safely with an INR of 2 to 3, but the INR alone is not a completely reliable guide to haemostatic function.

As a precaution, only a few teeth should be extracted at one session, trauma should be minimal and the sockets can be sutured over a layer of oxidised cellulose. Because of the risk of rebound thrombosis, anticoagulation should not be stopped. For more major surgery, anticoagulant treatment may have to be stopped if the physician agrees. If serious bleeding starts, tranexamic acid can be given but, if otherwise incontrollable, vitamin K may be needed.

Short-term anticoagulation with heparin is given before renal dialysis. Heparin is effective only for about 6 hours.

Extractions or other surgery can therefore be delayed for 12–24 hours after the last dose of heparin when the benefits of dialysis are also maximal.

Liver disease

Haemorrhagic tendencies can result either from obstructive jaundice (infective hepatitis also has an obstructive component) or from extensive liver damage. In obstructive jaundice, vitamin K absorption may be severely impaired. Viral hepatitis or alcoholism are important causes of liver failure which results in inability to metabolise vitamin K and to produce most clotting factors. Haemorrhage can be severe and difficult to control. In mild liver disease, vitamin K may be effective. In more severe cases it is valueless, but tranexamic acid and fresh plasma infusions may control bleeding.

MANAGEMENT OF PROLONGED DENTAL BLEEDING

Patients returning with prolonged bleeding from an extraction socket are a relatively common problem. It is not usually a real emergency, except in so far as the patient and friends or relatives are alarmed. Only a little blood diluted with saliva can give the impression of significant blood loss.

The essential measures are to reassure the patient and accompanying persons, who should be coaxed out of the surgery. The patient should then be given a local anaesthetic and the mouth cleaned up to identify the source of bleeding. Any rough edges of the socket should be tidied up, the margins squeezed together and the soft tissue margins neatly sutured over it. A small piece of Surgicel or fibrin gauze can be put in the socket mouth beforehand, but suturing is the essential measure.

When all is calm, enquiry should be made into any family history of bleeding tendencies, or any other cause of haemorrhagic disease as discussed earlier.

The patient should be kept under observation to make sure that bleeding has been completely controlled. But continued oozing of blood from beneath the sutured tissues suggests some haemorrhagic disease and this, or a family history of this, are indications for referring the patient to hospital, as prolonged dental bleeding is a recognised way in which haemophilia is sometimes first recognised.

SUGGESTED FURTHER READING

Ascher LF, Ord RA 1992 Pseudothrombocytopenia in maxillofacial surgery patients: a report of two cases. J Oral Maxillofac Surg 50:1108–1110

Association of Haemophilia Clinic Disorders of Canada 1995 Haemophilia and von Willebrand's disease: 2. Management. Can Med Ass J 153:147–157

Beatty C 1995 The patient with easy bruising and bleeding. Medicine UK 23:514–517

Capitano AM, Sacco R, Mannucci PM 1991 Pseudopathologies of haemostasis and dental surgery. Oral Surg Oral Med Oral Pathol 71:184–186

Chesterman CN, Chong BH 1995 Acquired haemostatic failure. Medicine UK 23:518–524

Durham TM, Hodges ED, Harper J et al 1993 Management of traumatic oral-facial traumatic injury in the hemophiliac patient with inhibitor. Paediatr Dent 15:282–287

Giles AR, Lilicrap DP 1995 Haemophilia A and related disorders. Medicine Int 23:525–530

Lethagen SR 1995 Pathogenesis, clinical picture and treatment of von Willebrand's disease. Ann Med 27:641–651

Ludlum CA, Steel CM 1993 Haemostasis: von Willebrand's variants. Lancet 341:997

McLaughlin P, Chen S, Phillips JG 1994 Disseminated intravascular coagulation presenting as perioral haemorrhage. Br J Oral Maxillofac Surg 32:94–95

Manabe M, Tsujimaki M, Kakuta S, Nagumo M 1993 Acquired factor X deficiency: an experience with multiple tooth extraction. J Oral Maxillofac Surg 51:922–924

Marshall DAS, Berry C, Brewer A 1993 Fatal disseminated intravascular coagulation complicating dental extraction. Br J Oral Maxillofac Surg 31:178–179

Morrison AE, Ludlam CA 1994 Acquired haemophilia and its management. Br J Haematol 89:231–236

Rakocz M, Mazar A, Varon D et al 1993 Dental extractions with bleeding disorders: the use of fibrin glue. Oral Surg Oral Med Oral Pathol 75:280–282

Saulnier J, Marey A, Horellou M-H et al 1994 Evaluation of desmopressin for dental extractions in patients with haemostatic disorders. Oral Surg Oral Med Oral Pathol 77:6–12

Steinberg MJ, Moores JF 1995 Use of INR to assess degree of antocoagulation in patients who have dental procedures. Oral Surg Oral Med Oral Pathol Oral Radiol Endod 80:175–177

Todd D, Galbraith D 1993 Management of an orthognathic surgery patient with factor XI deficiency: review and case report. J Oral Maxillofac Surg 51:417–420

Wahl MJ, Howell J 1996 Altering anticoagulant therapy: a survery of physicians. JADA 127:625–638

Wood GD, Deeble T 1993 Warfarin: dangers with antibiotics. Dent Update October: 350–353

Immunodeficiencies and HIV disease

Immune deficiencies can be primary or, more frequently, acquired (Box 24.1) and affect B- or T lymphocytes, or both. T lymphocytes regulate B-lymphocyte activity; T-cell defects may therefore impair antibody production as well as cell-mediated immunity. There can also be failures of production of individual immunoglobulins such as IgA, or of complement components.

Box 24.1   Important causes of immunodeficiency

Primary (genetic)
- T or B lymphocyte defects (Swiss-type agammaglobulinaemia, Di George's syndrome, etc.)
- IgA deficiency
- Complement component deficiencies
- Down's syndrome (multiple defects)

Secondary (acquired)
- Infections (HIV, other severe viral or bacterial infections, malaria, etc.)
- Drug-induced (immunosuppressive and anticancer treatment)
- Malnutrition (worldwide a major cause)
- Cancer (particularly lymphoreticular)
- Diabetes mellitus

Any patient who develops recurrent infections, particularly if they respond poorly to treatment or are caused by otherwise harmless microbes (opportunistic infections), is likely to be immunodeficient (Fig. 24.1).

The main causes of *severe* immunodeficiency are HIV infection and immunosuppressive treatment, particularly for organ transplants. Many cancer patients are also severely immuno-deficient as a result of both the neoplasm and cytotoxic drugs used for treatment. The severe primary immunodeficiencies are rare and, unless a marrow transplant can be given, are usually fatal in childhood.

Oral manifestations of immunodeficiencies

The main effect, as mentioned earlier, is abnormal susceptibility to infections, particularly candidosis or viral infections such as herpes zoster as in AIDS (see below). Resistance to treatment or recurrences of such infections strongly suggest immunodeficiency as do opportunistic infections by microbes which rarely affect normal persons. General oral manifestations of

Fig. 24.1 White patches of thrush and erythema in a patient on long-term immunosuppressive treatment.

Box 24.2   Important oral manifestations of immune deficiency states

Infections (some examples only)
- Herpes simplex, Herpes zoster
- Human herpes-virus 8
- Epstein–Barr virus
- Cytomegalovirus
- Candidosis
- Bacterial infections

Neoplasms
- Kaposi's sarcoma
- Lymphomas

Other possible manifestations
- Lymphadenopathy
- Hairy leukoplakia
- Thrombocytopenia
- Lupus erythematosus

---

immunodeficiencies are summarised in Box 24.2, but there is some variation in presentation between different causes.

SELECTIVE IGA DEFICIENCY

Selective IgA deficiency is common and potentially relevant for the mouth, as IgA is the only immunoglobulin secreted in the saliva. Selective IgA deficiency may affect about 1 in 600 of the population and has varied possible effects (Box 24.3).

Susceptibility to oral infections

Evidence regarding the effect of IgA deficiency on dental caries and periodontal disease is conflicting. Both high and low prevalences of dental caries have been reported. Compensatory secretion of other immunoglobulins into the mouth may explain these variable findings. Gingivitis may be less severe than normal, but even this may be the result of antibiotic treatment for respiratory infections. There is no clear evidence of any significant association between oral mucosal infection and IgA deficiency.

Atopic disease

IgA deficiency may facilitate absorption of allergens. Asthma, eczema or any of the related diseases may be the first sign. However, this has no oral effects unless allergic angio-oedema involves the floor of mouth or lips.

C1 ESTERASE INHIBITOR DEFICIENCY

The familial form of this disease, hereditary angio-oedema, is, pedantically speaking, an immunodeficiency, but there is no abnormal susceptibility to infection. There is also a rare acquired type associated mainly with lymphoproliferative diseases. They are discussed in Chapter 25, together with allergic angio-oedema, which it simulates clinically.

LEUKOPENIA AND AGRANULOCYTOSIS

Immunodeficiency disorders are frequently associated with deficiency of circulating leucocytes. A severe fall in the leucocyte count leads to abnormal susceptibility to infection. In agranulocytosis this is typically shown initially by oropharyngeal ulceration.

IMMUNOSUPPRESSIVE TREATMENT

Bone marrow transplantation

Bone marrow transplantation is used, if suitable donors can be found, for such conditions as some severe primary immunodeficiency diseases, some leukaemias, aplastic anaemia and some lymphomas and other neoplasms. Preoperatively, total immunosuppression by cytotoxic chemotherapy and, sometimes, total body irradiation is required to prevent graft rejection.

Oral sources of infection should be eliminated and the mouth brought to as near perfect health as possible. Elimination of oral infection (particularly periodontal disease) has a significant effect on lessening post-transplant complications and also lessens the need for dental treatment during the difficult post-transplant period.

Possible complications after transplantation are numerous (Box 24.4), particularly during the initial intensive phase of immunosuppression.

Graft-versus-host disease

This results from an attack on an immunosuppressed host by transplanted immunocompetent cells. It is, in effect, a graft rejection reaction in reverse. It most frequently follows bone marrow transplantation, both because of the deep immunosuppression and because of the many immunologically active cells in the implanted marrow.

The oral effects of graft-versus-host disease are lichen planus, a Sjögren-like syndrome with xerostomia, and a condition resembling systemic sclerosis (Ch. 25) with limited oral opening.

Graft-versus-host disease can be acute and self-limiting or responsive to treatment, or chronic. The last is the chief cause of morbidity and mortality.

Post-transplant management

The main considerations are maintenance of meticulous oral hygiene, use of fluorides to control caries and prompt treatment of any infections that develop.

In successful cases, deep immunosuppression is maintained for up to a year post-transplantation. The implanted marrow then takes over normal haematological and immune functions. Any oral surgery should preferably be postponed until this happens.

OTHER ORGAN TRANSPLANTS

Transplantation of other organs, most frequently kidneys, is associated with similar complications to those of bone marrow transplantation. The main differences are that immunosuppression is less complete but has to be maintained indefinitely.

The chief problems are therefore the enhanced susceptibility to infections and the greater risk of lymphomas. Gingival hyperplasia due to cyclosporin may be difficult to control and can lead to accelerated periodontal destruction.

THE ACQUIRED IMMUNE DEFICIENCY SYNDROME (AIDS)

A great variety of oral diseases can be features of the acquired immune deficiency syndrome (see Table 24.3). They sometimes form the first sign of the disease and some of them herald rapid deterioration and, sometimes, early death.

HIV disease has spread worldwide and is epidemic in parts of the USA and, particularly, Africa. More than 40 million adults, worldwide, are estimated to be infected. Innumerable children, particularly in Africa, have been orphaned by or have acquired the disease. The pandemic is most severe in sub-Saharan Africa where 25 million adults, approximately 9% of the population, are infected. As indicated in Table 24.1, it is estimated that by 2005 there were 2.4 million deaths from AIDS in sub-Saharan Africa alone.

In the former Soviet Union, cases have risen to 700 000, a jump of nearly 70% in one year and it is predicted that one million Russians will have become infected within two or three years. Worldwide, the numbers of persons already infected but who have not yet developed AIDS for some areas is suggested in Table 24.1. Overall, the numbers of children and adults newly infected is estimated to be 4.9 million and the global total of persons living with HIV is estimated to be 40.3 million. The total number of deaths by 2005 is estimated to be 3.1 million.

However, there may be little purpose in quoting such figures as the disease will have claimed many more victims by the time this is read.

AIDS is transmissible to health care personnel, particularly surgeons, dental surgeons and nurses, via needles or other sharp instruments. However, the risk of acquiring HIV infection by such means is considerably smaller than that of hepatitis B.

Aetiology

AIDS is caused by a retrovirus, the human immunodeficiency virus (HIV), mainly HIV-1. HIV-2 is prevalent in West Africa, from where it has spread to central Africa. HIV-2 infection may progress more slowly and cause less deep immunosupression

The chief mode of transmission in many parts of the world is by men who have sex with men. These used to account for over 80% of cases in Britain, but this figure has greatly declined in recent years. In the UK, 28% of cases of HIV infection are in men who have sex with men, 0.01% are in intravenous drug abusers and in 55% there has been heterosexual transmission. Heterosexual transmission is far less common in the Western World than in Africa. Nevertheless, as a result of spread of the virus in the population, heterosexual transmission has become more frequent. The great rise in the frequency of heterosexual transmission in the UK in recent years has been affected by a variety of factors. In most cases, this is the result of migration of individuals who have acquired the infection in high-risk areas. However, an increasing proportion of this heterosexual infection is acquired in the UK. Once infected, pregnant women can transmit the infection to the fetus directly or by breast feeding. Many haemophiliacs have acquired the disease from infected blood products but heat-treatment of clotting factor concentrates should have eliminated this risk and there appear to have been no cases among them or other transfusion recipients in the UK in recent years.

The incubation period of AIDS is highly variable. In men who have sex with men, the average is approximately 5 years, but is sometimes as long as 10 years. Testing of infected persons also shows deterioration of immune function long before clinically apparent disease and it is still not clear whether all those who have become infected will develop the full, lethal syndrome.

In 5–15% of cases, HIV infection shows no clinical progress for periods up to 10 years, possibly because of variations in pathogenicity of HIV strains, or stronger host immune responses.

Immunology

The human immunodeficiency virus directly infects lymphocytes and other cells, such as some macrophages, which carry the CD4 marker. However, the virus appears only to be able to fuse with and enter CD4 cells as a result of interaction between the gp120 envelope proteins and a CD4 binding site by means of a family of co-receptors. The virus kills T-helper (CD4) cells and reverses the ratio of helper to suppressor lymphocytes.

Antibody is produced in response to the virus but is not protective. Antibodies to HIV indicate only that infection has been acquired and all seropositive persons must be assumed to be capable of transmitting it.

The main effect of depletion of T-helper cells is deepening depression of cell-mediated immunity. Thus, there are declining responses of lymphocytes to antigens in vitro and impaired or absent delayed hypersensitivity responses long before any clinical signs of the disease appear. Apparently paradoxically, there is also polyclonal B-lymphocyte activation resulting in hypergammaglobulinaemia and autoantibody production. The main effect of the immunodeficiency and chief cause of death is infection by a great variety of microbes.

Table 24.1 Estimated number of adults and children newly infected and dying from HIV infection during 2005

	New infections during 2005	Total deaths 2005
Sub-Saharan Africa	3.2 million	2.4 million
North America	43 000	18 000
Western and Central Europe	22 000	12 000
Eastern Europe and Central Asia	270 000	62 000
South and South-East Asia	990 000	480 000

The human immunodeficiency virus also attacks the central nervous system, cells of which carry receptors for the virus.

Diagnosis

Clinical criteria of AIDS diagnosis are summarised in Box 24.5.

Confirmation of the diagnosis is by immunological methods, but testing can only be carried out with the clear consent

---

Box 24.5   CDC definition of AIDS in patients with laboratory evidence of HIV

A definite diagnosis of:
1. Bacterial infections, multiple or recurrent in a child <13 years
2. Disseminated coccidioidomycosis
3. HIV encephalopathy (HIV dementia or subacute encephalitis)
4. Disseminated histoplasmosis
5. Isosporiasis with diarrhoea for >1 month
6. Kaposi's sarcoma
7. Lymphoma of the brain (primary)
8. Non-Hodgkin lymphoma of B cell or unknown immunological phenotype and one of several specified types
9. Disseminated mycobacterial disease (other than *Mycobacterium tuberculosis*)
10. Extrapulmonary *Mycobacterium tuberculosis* involving at least one site outside the lungs
11. Recurrent *Salmonella* (non-typhoid) septicaemia
12. HIV wasting syndrome

Or a presumptive diagnosis of:
1. Candidosis of the oesophagus
2. Cytomegalovirus retinitis with loss of vision
3. Kaposi's sarcoma
4. Lymphoid interstitial pneumonia and/or pulmonary lymphoid hyperplasia in a child ≤13 years of age
5. Disseminated mycobacterial disease
6. *Pneumocystis carinii* pneumonia
7. Toxoplasmosis of the brain in a patient ≥1 month of age

The following conditions, in the presence of HIV infection, have been added to the definition of AIDS:
1. Cervical cancer
2. Two episodes of bacterial pneumonia in 12 months
3. Pulmonary tuberculosis

---

of the patient, explanation of the implications and reassurance ('counselling').

Detection of anti-HIV antibodies is often misnamed 'the AIDS test', but it cannot predict the development of symptomatic disease. It has been useful for detecting HIV-infected persons, particularly among blood donors, and provides a relatively simple means of initiating the confirmation of the diagnosis. Antibodies appear after about 6 to 8 weeks and most persist for life. A positive result indicates the presence of HIV infection, but must be confirmed by other methods of antibody detection.

In doubtful cases, detection of viral antigens, such as p24 protein, in the blood provides a more direct and reliable indicator of infection. HIV DNA can be quantified and several commercial assays are available. Indirect immunofluorescence to detect HIV-specific IgM may be needed in difficult cases. Haematological markers, indicating progression to AIDS, include viral antigens in the serum, high beta-2 microglobulin levels and failure of or greatly depressed antigen-induced interferon gamma production. T-helper (CD4) lymphocytes counts of less than $0.2 \times 10^9/l$ or a total lymphocyte count of less than $1 \times 10^9/l$ represent advanced disease.

Problems in diagnosis include the fact that a few patients fail to produce HIV-specific antibodies or lose them as the disease progresses. In such cases, HIV antigens or HNA nucleic acid may be detectable by reverse transcription polymerase chain reaction analysis which is highly sensitive.

For infants in poor countries where facilities are limited, saliva can be used for HIV detection and, in association with clinical assessment, is probably 90% effective.

Clinical indicators of a poor prognosis are oral thrush, Herpes zoster or other persistent or recurrent infections, hairy leukoplakia, unexplained constitutional symptoms, cutaneous anergy and lymphadenopathy. Approximately 20–70% of such patients can be expected to deteriorate within less than 5 years.

Clinical aspects

Possible major events after infection by HIV are shown in Figure 24.2 but, as mentioned earlier, it is still uncertain whether any symptomless carriers will ultimately remain healthy.

Usually, there is a latent period for several years before signs of immunodeficiency appear. Within 10 years, approximately 50% of infected persons will probably have developed AIDS and the remainder will usually have prodromal disease or laboratory markers of immune deficiency. Severe infectious complications are to be expected and are usually the chief cause of death.

The earliest clinical manifestation of HIV infection can be a transient illness resembling glandular fever, associated with

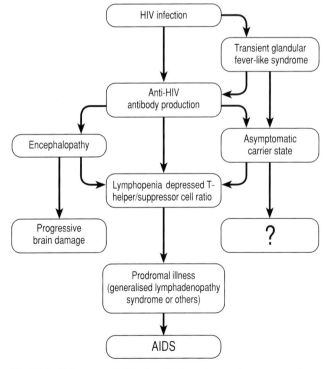

Fig. 24.2   Outcomes of HIV infection. The fate of currently asymptomatic carriers is unknown.

antibody production (seroconversion illness). Thereafter, in progressive cases, markers of declining cell-mediated immunity eventually become detectable and, later, various clinical syndromes.

Generalised lymphadenopathy syndrome (GLS), with widespread persistent enlargement of lymph nodes, is a typical early sign. However, the course of AIDS is highly variable and none of the prodromal symptoms appear to be inevitable.

The full syndrome of AIDS is characterised by multiple infections by bacteria, fungi, parasites and viruses. Many of these infections, such as *Pneumocystis carinii*[1] pneumonia, are opportunistic and almost unknown in immunocompetent persons. Sometimes the first clinical sign of AIDS can be *Pneumocystis carinii* pneumonia.

Though infections are the main cause of death, there is also a greatly raised incidence of tumours, particularly Kaposi's sarcoma and lymphomas, which frequently affect the oral or perioral tissues and may be the first signs of HIV infection. Plasmablastic lymphoma has a predilection for the oral cavity and is virtually only seen in HIV infection. In normal persons, these tumours are not merely uncommon or rare, but particularly rare in the mouth.

Neuropsychiatric disease in AIDS can range from depression to dementia and death. Opportunistic infections or tumours can also involve the central nervous system. These neurological disorders may be associated with, but can develop in the absence of, immunodeficiency.

A lesser manifestation of AIDS in some patients is autoimmune disease, particularly thrombocytopenic purpura or, less frequently, a lupus erythematosus-like disease.

Once AIDS has developed, the outcome is usually fatal within 2–3 years, though the course of the disease can be modified by highly active antiretroviral therapy (HAART).

In the terminal stages of AIDS, the patient may be emaciated, with persistent diarrhoea, suffering a multiplicity of infections, disfigured by skin disease, breathless from *Pneumocystis carinii* pneumonia, frequently with a malignant tumour, and sometimes also blind and demented.

HIV assessment and staging

Staging of HIV infection is important for selecting patients for treatment and assessing prognosis and for epidemiological studies. The Centers for Disease Control/World Health Organization classification (Table 24.2) takes both clinical and laboratory findings into account. The clinical categories correspond to progressively more severe infections. Category A includes asymptomatic cases and those with persistent generalised lymphadenopathy. Category B comprises those with previous thrush, hairy leukoplakia, zoster, idiopathic thrombocytopaenia and similar conditions. Category C includes a broad

Table 24.2 CDC/WHO laboratory classification of HIV infection

CD4 cells/μl	or Total lymphocyte count/μl	Clinical category		
		A	B	C
[1] >500	>2000	A1	B1	C1
[2] 200–499	1000–1999	A2	B2	C2
[3] <200	<1000	A3	B3	C3

range of 'AIDS-defining conditions' and severe infections such as Kaposi's sarcoma, lymphoma, *Pneumocystis* pneumonia, oesophageal candidosis and wasting.

General management of HIV/AIDS

The main principles are to confirm the diagnosis, control the many types of infection, to treat any tumours and to give highly active antiretroviral therapy (HAART).

Highly active antiretroviral therapy

The prognosis for AIDS has greatly improved since the introduction of HAART. The latter is the term given to the use of combinations of antiretroviral drugs, such as two nucleoside reverse transcriptase inhibitors (nRTIs) plus one or two protease inhibitors, or two nRTIs plus a non-nucleoside transcriptase inhibitor. All these drugs are capable of causing a wide variety of adverse effects and compliance may be unpredictable. Some important oral adverse effects from the drugs mentioned in Box 24.6 are indicated in brackets. However, new drugs are constantly being introduced and it is not yet clear whether one combination of these drugs is more effective than another.

Box 24.6 Antiretroviral drugs used for HAART

Nucleoside reverse transcriptase inhibitors
- Abacavir (Stevens–Johnson syndrome)
- Didanosine (dry mouth)
- Zalcitabine (oral ulcers)
- Stavudine
- Lamivudine
- Zidovudine

Nucleotide analogues
- Adefovir, Tenofovir

Non-nucleoside reverse transcriptase inhibitors
- Nevirapine (Stevens–Johnson syndrome)
- Efavirenz (Stevens–Johnson syndrome)

Protease inhibitors
- Indinavir (dry mouth, taste disturbance)
- Nelfinavir
- Ritonavir (taste disturbance, circumoral paraesthesia)
- Saquinavir (oral ulceration)

The benefits of highly active antiretroviral therapy are that levels of cirulating virions may be lowered to undetectable levels and that variable levels of immune recovery may be evident.

---

[1]This organism had long been thought to be a protozoan but, more recently, examination of its DNA appears to have shown that it is a fungus. Nevertheless, it is not treated with antifungal drugs.

The result can be a striking fall in the incidence of opportunistic infections and regression of Kaposi's sarcoma. CMV retinitis (causing blindness) has hitherto resisted treatment, but has responded well to HAART. In Britain, the mortality from AIDS has fallen by more than 40% since 1996.

A controversial issue in the application of HAART is whether treatment should start early or late after acquisition of HIV infection. In the UK, to minimise toxic effects in longer-term treatment, unlike the USA and most of Europe, the policy has been to delay treatment until after the CD4 count falls below 350 cells/mm^3, in an attempt also to delay the rising tide of drug-resistance due to long-term treatment. However, administration of HAART within 180 days of infection raises levels of HIV-specific CD4 cells and patients can stop treatment for up to a year and still suppress HIV levels in the blood.

Despite initial optimism, the long-term toxicity of these regimens is as yet unknown, compliance may be difficult to maintain and their cost is such that they are available only in more affluent communities. Worse is the finding that even the most vigorous of such treatments does not completely control HIV replication, even when there is a clear decline in morbidity and mortality. It is estimated that HAART fails in up to 50% of recipients each year, partly at least due to poor compliance with this demanding form of treatment.

Other problems are that resistance to HAART has developed and there has been a considerable rise in new cases of multi-drug-resistant HIV over the past 5 years. One consequence is that patients receiving HAART may feel that they are non-infective and transmit the disease to others. There are also as yet inaccessible reservoirs of infection. The latter are mainly inactive B cells which contain dormant HIV DNA.

Key features of AIDS are summarised in Box 24.7.

Box 24.7 AIDS: key features

- Caused by a retrovirus – usually HIV-1
- Transmitted sexually or by intravenous drug abuse and by blood or blood products
- Progressive deterioration mainly of cell-mediated immunity
- Immunodeficiency leads to opportunistic infections such as *Pneumocystis carinii* pneumonia
- Common oral lesions include candidosis and hairy leukoplakia
- Kaposi's sarcoma and lymphomas, often in oral regions
- Neurological and psychological disorders
- Deaths mainly due to opportunistic infections

In women, smoking negates some of the benefits of HAART in terms of such changes as poorer virological and immunological response, but overall there appears to be no significant difference between smokers and non-smokers in the risk of death due to AIDS.

ORAL LESIONS IN HIV/AIDS

More than 75% of patients with AIDS have orofacial disease (Table 24.3). Before the introduction of HAART, among 2235

Table 24.3 Oral disease in HIV infection

	More common diseases	Less common
Infections	*Fungal* Thrush and other forms of candidosis	*Deep mycoses* Cryptococcosis Histoplasmosis Aspergillosis Geotrichosis
	Viral Herpes simplex Varicella-zoster EB virus, including hairy leukoplakia	*Viral* Human papillomavirus Cytomegalovirus
	Bacterial HIV-associated gingivitis and periodontitis Necrotising gingivitis	*Bacterial* *M. tuberculosis* and non-tuberculous ('atypical') mycobacterioses *Klebsiella* pneumonia *S. enteritidis*, *E. coli* and *E. cloacae* infections Sinusitis Exacerbations of apical periodontitis Submandibular cellulitis
Tumours	Kaposi's sarcoma	Non-Hodgkin lymphoma (squamous cell carcinoma)
Other	Lymphadenopathy	*Neurological disease* Paraesthesiae Hyperaesthesia Facial palsy Dysphagia
Miscellaneous		Recurrent aphthae Progressive necrotising ulceration Delayed wound healing Purpura Pigmentation

HIV-positive, homosexual or bisexual men in San Francisco, the most frequent oral lesions were hairy leukoplakia (18.7%), thrush (6.6%) or erythematous candidosis (2.1%), Kaposi's sarcoma (1.6%) and oral ulcers (2%). Overall, the tongue is the reported site of oral manifestations and it has been found to be involved in 75% of patients dying from AIDS. Tongue lesions include any of those described below, but there may also be non-specific glossitis or melanotic pigmentation. However, the frequency of such lesions varies in other groups. Kaposi's sarcoma and hairy leukoplakia, for example, are disproportionately frequent in men who have sex with men.

With the use of HAART, the frequency of HIV-related oral lesions is declining. However, untreated and undiagnosed HIV disease is still likely to present with these infections.

Candidosis

Thrush or other forms of oral candidosis may be seen in over 70% of patients at some stage. It indicates declining immunity and that other infections may be associated or are likely to follow. The main risk factors are low CD4 counts and smoking. Approximately

Fig. 24.3 **Erythematous candidosis.** An extensive red patch on the palate without white flecks which appears as denture stomatitis but without any denture being worn. Such a presentation is characteristic of immunodeficiency.

Fig. 24.5 **Hairy leukoplakia.** Close-up view shows the corrugated surface and suggests the soft texture of the lesion.

Fig. 24.4 **Herpes simplex ulceration in immunodeficiency.** There is extensive ulceration along the midline of the dorsal tongue and separate ulcers towards the lateral margins. In immunodeficiency, the ulcers may be chronic and their clinical appearance may not suggest viral infection. Biopsy may be required for diagnosis.

Fig. 24.6 **Hairy leukoplakia.** The characteristic appearance on the lateral margin of the tongue. Posteriorly, the vertical ridging pattern of the lateral tongue is enhanced. (By kind permission of Professor WH Binnie.)

50% of patients with HIV-associated thrush are likely to develop AIDS within 5 years. As well as *Candida albicans*, other isolates such as *C. dubliniensis* can be responsible.

Most other types of candidosis, such as angular stomatitis, palatal erythema or hyperplastic candidosis, may also be seen (Fig. 24.3).

Candidosis is an important marker of immune failure in patients receiving HAART.

Viral mucosal infections

Herpetic stomatitis is less common than might be expected, but can cause atypical or chronic ulceration (Fig. 24.4). Severe orofacial zoster may indicate a poor prognosis.

Cytomegalovirus can be found in some oral ulcers. Severe and hitherto intractable cytomegalovirus infections, such as retinitis, have been reported to respond to valganciclovir which may be less toxic than ganciclovir.

The Epstein–Barr virus is the cause of hairy leukoplakia which is highly characteristic of HIV infection (Ch. 15) (Figs 24.5 and 24.6).

Papillomaviruses have been isolated from proliferative lesions, such as verruca vulgaris, condyloma acuminatum and focal epithelial hyperplasia.

Bacterial infections

Infections by bacteria which otherwise rarely involve the oral tissues, such as *Klebsiella pneumoniae*, *Enterobacter cloacae* and *Escherichia coli*, can develop. In the later stages, there may be oral lesions secondary to systemic infections, particularly mycobacterial ulcers.

Bacillary angiomatosis is a vascular proliferative disease caused by *Bartonella henselae* and should respond to antimicrobial therapy. However, it can mimic Kaposi's sarcoma clinically and, to some extent, histologically. It affects the skin more frequently than the oral cavity. Biopsy is essential to exclude Kaposi's sarcoma.

Systemic mycoses

Histoplasmosis or cryptococcosis can give rise to proliferative or ulcerative lesions. Histoplasmosis most frequently affects the palate, gingivae and oropharynx, and can be fatal.

Tumours

Nearly 50% of patients with AIDS have a malignant tumour at the time of presentation. By far the most frequent are Kaposi's sarcoma and non-Hodgkin lymphomas. Unlike non-AIDS patients, these tumours are particularly frequent in the head and neck region.

Kaposi's sarcoma → Summary p. 337

Among patients with AIDS, this is mainly seen in men who have sex with men and, in some areas of the USA, for example, it has become the most common malignant tumour of the oral cavity. It is also very occasionally seen in HIV-negative immunosuppressed organ transplant patients. AIDS-type Kaposi's sarcoma is associated with a high rate of second neoplasms, particularly lymphomas and clinical suspicion of the diagnosis of Kaposi's sarcoma is also strengthened by coexisting or a history of opportunistic infections.

Kaposi's sarcoma in the mouth, particularly in a young male who is not receiving immunosuppressive treatment, is virtually pathognomonic of AIDS. It is usually associated with a CD4 lymphocyte count of less than 200/µl and frequently associated with other effects of HIV infection such as candidosis, hairy leukoplakia or HIV-associated gingivitis.

Human herpes-virus 8 (HHV-8) DNA can be found in Kaposi's sarcoma cells and patients with both HIV and HHV-8 infection have a high risk of developing Kaposi's sarcoma. Though oral Kaposi's sarcoma may be the cause of early symptoms, the tumour is usually multifocal, with lesions affecting skin, lymph nodes and viscera. At autopsy most organs are frequently found to be involved.

The site may be oropharyngeal, cutaneous or in the cervical lymph nodes. Within the mouth, the palate is the most frequent site and the tumour typically produces a flat or nodular purplish lesion. The clinical differential diagnosis is from oral purpura, bacillary angiomatosis and pyogenic granulomas, from which it can be distinguished by biopsy (Ch. 20).

Lymphomas → Summary p. 364

These can develop in intraoral sites or salivary glands far more frequently than in HIV-negative persons. Typical sites within the mouth are the palate or gingiva, where the tumours form soft painless swellings which ulcerate when traumatised.

Microscopically, most lymphomas in AIDS are high-grade B-cell lymphomas of large cell or immunoblastic type. EBV is associated in about 50%.

Burkitt's lymphoma is 1000 times more common than in HIV-negative persons in the Western world. Plasmablastic

Fig. 24.7 **Purpura.** Patches such as these in AIDS can be mistaken for Kaposi's sarcoma.

lymphoma is seen virtually only in HIV-positive persons and has a strong predilection for the oral cavity.

Lymphadenopathy

Lymphadenopathy is characteristic of AIDS and its prodromes. Cervical lymphadenopathy is probably the most common head and neck manifestation of HIV infection.

Microscopy

Typical findings are smaller numbers of T-helper cells in the paracortical region associated with greater numbers of T-suppressor cells there and in the follicles. Follicles may initially be hyperplastic but later undergo involution. The lymph nodes become virtually or entirely functionless.

Enlarged cervical lymph nodes can also be due to lymphomas.

Autoimmune disease

The most common autoimmune phenomenon in AIDS is thrombocytopenic purpura (Fig. 24.7). This can give rise to oral purple patches which may be mistaken for Kaposi's sarcoma, petechiae or blood blisters. Other autoimmune diseases reported in AIDS are lupus erythematosus and a Sjögren-like salivary gland disease.

Gingivitis and periodontitis → Summary p. 364

HIV-related periodontal disease includes necrotising gingivitis and accelerated periodontitis (Ch. 5). Necrotising ulcerative periodontitis (NUP) indicates immunological deterioration and a poor prognosis. Spirochaetes such as *Borrelia* are involved (Fig. 24.8).

Types of gingivitis and periodontitis seen in HIV infection are summarised in Summary chart 24.1.

Fig. 24.8 **HIV-associated necrotising periodontitis.** Soft tissue and bone are lost virtually simultaneously and tissue destruction of the degree shown here can take only a few months. A low CD4 count and a poor prognosis are typically associated. (By kind permission of Professor WH Binnie.)

Gingivitis or periodontitis in HIV infection

Disease is more severe, though sometimes only slightly more so, than in immunocompetent patients

Pattern of disease similar to chronic adult periodontitis or rapidly progressive disease in immunocompetent patients

Diagnose periodontal disease exacerbated by immunosuppression

Unusual pattern of disease

Necrosis or ulceration, usually centred on the interdental papilla and often producing interdental cratering and 'reverse architecture'. Sometimes extends away from gingival margin to involve bone or deep - soft tissues

Band of erythema along gingival margin, often bright red, and sometimes involving whole width of attached gingiva or patchy punctate erythema of gingiva

Involving alveolar bone or soft tissue, often with extensive loss of attachment without significant pocketing

Diagnose necrotising periodontitis ('HIV-associated periodontitis')

Limited to gingival soft tissues

Diagnose necrotising (ulcerative) gingivitis (acute or chronic)

Consider and exclude the causes of desquamative gingivitis unrelated to immunodeficiency.
Exclude gingival candidosis

Treat as in immunocompetent patient

Review frequently for relapse in maintenance phase

Treat with oral hygiene instruction, debridement, povidone-iodine application or chlorhexidine gel, chlorhexidine mouthwash and systemic metronidazole or penicillin if necessary. Remove any small sequestra of bone after partial separation

Treat by oral hygiene measures

Fails to resolve

Biopsy indicated.

Consider lymphoma, viral infection (especially herpes viruses), deep mycoses and exotic opportunistic infections

Resolves (though may recur)

Diagnose necrotising gingivitis or periodontitis. Review frequently for relapse in maintenance phase

Resolves

Diagnose florid plaque-related gingivitis

Fails to resolve

Diagnose HIV-associated gingivitis or 'linear gingival erythema'

Summary chart 24.1 Types of gingivitis and periodontitis seen in HIV infection.

Salivary gland disease

Chronic parotitis in children, possibly due to Epstein–Barr virus or cytomegalovirus, is almost pathognomonic of HIV infection.

A Sjögren-like syndrome with xerostomia, but lacking the characteristic autoantibodies (particularly SS-A and SS-B), can affect adults. In children with HIV/AIDS, chronic parotid swelling or xerostomia is frequent and can be an early manifestation.

Parotid swellings due to lymphoepithelial lesions are frequently cystic, bilateral and identifiable by CT scanning or ultrasound.

Recognition of parotid cysts or microscopic diagnosis of Sjögren-like changes, particularly in a young adult male, are important indicators of HIV infection of which surgeons should be aware when dealing with a tumour-like lesion of salivary glands.

Tuberculous parotitis is relatively frequent in advanced AIDS.

Miscellaneous oral lesions

Mucosal ulcers

Major aphthae (Fig. 24.9) can be troublesome, interfere with eating and accelerate deterioration of health. They become more frequent and severe with declining immune function. Necrotising oral ulceration of an ill-defined nature and aphthae-like ulcers are common oral signs (Fig. 24.10). In the floor of these ulcers, cytomegalovirus can sometimes be seen.

Oral ulcers associated with HIV infection should always be biopsied as they may be amenable to treatment if specific agents such as herpes virus, cytomegalovirus or mycobacteria are identified. Major aphthae usually respond dramatically to thalidomide, but this should only be used when other causes have been excluded.

Oral hyperpigmentation → Summary p. 337

Occasionally, pigmentation may be secondary to Addison's disease due to fungal destruction of the adrenals. Alternatively, it may be a complication of treatment with zidovudine or due to unknown mechanisms.

Neurological disease

Orofacial effects include facial palsy and trigeminal neuropathy.

Oral adverse effects of HAART

Most of the protease inhibitors, such as sequinavir, can cause xerostomia, disturbed taste sensation and perioral paraesthesia. Many of these and other components of HAART can also cause erythema multiforme.

Risks of transmission of HIV infection to healthcare workers

All patients, even if not known to be HIV positive or receiving HAART, must be regarded as potentially infective and treated with full infection control as for hepatitis B. A few nurses and others have become infected as a result of needle-stick injuries causing accidental injection of a significant amount of infected blood. By contrast, many other needle-stick injuries where little blood has been transferred have failed to transmit the virus. In Brazil, where there is a high incidence of HIV infection, only four cases of occupational transmission have been documented for the period 1981–2004. All were due to percutaneous injuries. Most healthcare workers who have developed AIDS have not acquired it as a result of their occupation.

As to the risk to general surgeons, at least two in the Western world are known to have died from the disease, acquired at operation. By contrast, only one dental surgeon is known as

Fig. 24.9 HIV-associated aphthous stomatitis. Major aphthae typically become more frequent and severe as immune function deteriorates and can add considerably to the patient's disabilitites.

Fig. 24.10   Major aphthous ulcers are a complication of HIV infection and become more frequent and severe as immune function declines.

yet to have acquired the disease occupationally. He was working in New York (then by far the highest incidence area in the Western world), did not practice a high standard of infection control and had had many needle-stick injuries. No other dental surgeons, even in high-incidence areas, are known to have acquired the disease occupationally.

Infection control, as discussed earlier, and awareness of the patient's low resistance to secondary infection are then major management considerations.

General aspects of dental management

Possible oral and systemic features of this disease which may affect dental management have been discussed above.

Despite the possibility of acquiring infection from such patients or of transmitting it to others, however remote, it is unethical to refuse them treatment. However, strict adherence to infection control measures must be implemented and the operator should take particular care to avoid accidental self-injury with an instrument that may have been contaminated with serum or blood. However, the possibility of transmitting HIV infection during dental treatment inevitably causes anxiety, but the risk is considerably lower than that of acquiring viral hepatitis.

Oral infections and other features of AIDS or its prodromes may enable patients to be recognised. A young adult male who develops thrush for no apparent reason is likely to have HIV disease, but if he has oral Kaposi's sarcoma, it is virtually pathognomonic. However, there are many more patients with nothing to suggest that they are infective. At the time of writing, there are tens of thousands of antibody-positive, potentially infective persons in Britain, and the number rises each month.

In those who have lesions such as those just described but who are unaware of having HIV infection, it is important to inform patients of this infection and that, with their agreement, it should be confirmed by appropriate testing. In such negotiations the strictest confidence must be observed.

Post-exposure prophylaxis and needle-stick injury

Any healthcare worker suffering a needle-stick or other exposure to potentially HIV transmitting body fluids should be assessed to determine whether anti-retroviral drugs should be prescribed in an attempt to reduce the risk of transmission of HIV. All

NHS employers are required to have a procedure in place that allows post-exposure prophylaxis to be given within 24 hours. After that time the effectiveness is much reduced. Whether or not post-exposure prophylaxis with HAART is appropriate depends on the risk of transmission assessed by the type of injury and infectivity of the patient. If required, the drugs are selected to take into account any drug resistant HIV strains in the donor. The adverse effects of post-exposure prophylaxis are significant and treatment is usually continued for 4 weeks.

The immediate action for any injury potentially contaminated with infectious body fluids is to wash liberally with soap and water and encourage free bleeding. Wounds should not be sucked or scrubbed. Splashes to the mucous membranes, including conjunctivae, should be irrigated copiously with water. This should be done before and after removal of contact lenses. Saliva is considered infectious in the context of dental surgery because it is almost certainly contaminated with small amounts of blood.

HIV infection is transmitted by less than 3 in 1000 medical needle-stick injuries and less than 1 in 1000 exposures to mucous membranes. Post-exposure prophylaxis is considered approximately 80% effective in preventing transmission.

RESTRICTIONS ON TYPE OF WORK THAT MAY BE PERFORMED BY INFECTED DENTAL CLINICIANS

Current regulations require that dental clinicians who have become or think that they have become infected by HIV, hepatitis or other blood-borne viruses should seek counselling and appropriate medical supervision.

If infection is confirmed, changes to clinical practice may mean cessation of work involving exposure-prone procedures. The latter are those where there is a risk of exposing the patient's open tissues to the blood of the worker and include procedures where clinicians' gloved hands may come into contact with sharp instruments or tissues (spicules of bone or teeth) inside patients' open body cavities.

This may mean that infected clinicians may be restricted to carrying out prosthetic dentistry or cease the practice of dentistry. Whether current restrictions are too draconian is a matter of current debate.

SUGGESTED FURTHER READING

Barrett AP 1986 Oral complications of bone marrow transplantation. Aust NZ J Med 16:239–240
Berkowitz RJ, Strandford S, Jones P et al 1987 Stomatological complications of bone marrow transplantation in a pediatric population. Pediatr Dent 9:105–110
Carpenter CCJ, Cooper DA, Fischl M et al 2000 Antiretrovial therapy in adults. Updated recommendations of the International AIDS Society – USA Panel. JAMA 283:381–389
Chaushu G, Itzkovitz-Chaushu S, Yefenof E et al 1995 A longitudinal follow-up of salivary secretion in bone marrow transplant patients. Oral Surg Oral Med Oral Pathol Oral Radiol Endod 79:164–169

Dahllof G, Heimdahl A, Modeer T et al 1989 Oral mucous membrane lesions in children treated with bone marrow transplantation. Scand J Dent Res 97:268–277
D'Aquila R, Walker B 1999 Exploring the benefits and limits of highly active antiretroviral therapy. JAMA 282:1668–1669
DeSimone JA, Pomerantz RJ, Babinchak TJ 2000 Inflammatory reactions in HIV-1 infected persons after initiation of highly active antiretroviral therapy. Ann Intern Med 133:447–454
Grabar S, Le Moing V, Goujard C et al 2000 Clinical outcome of patients with HIV-1 infection according to immunologic and virologic

response after 6 months of highly active antiretroviral therapy. Ann Intern Med 133:401–413

Greenberg MS, Dubin G, Steward JCB et al 1995 Relationship of oral disease to the presence of cytomegalovirus DNA in the saliva of AIDS patients. Oral Surg Oral Med Oral Pathol Oral Radiol Endod 79:175–179

Greenspan D, Greenspan JS 1996 HIV-related oral disease. Lancet 348:729–733

Kline MW 1996 Oral manifestations of pediatric human immunodeficiency virus infection: a review of the literature. Pediatrics 97:380–388

Lin RY, Goodhart P 1993 The role of oral candidiasis in survival and hospitalization patterns: analysis of an inner city hospital human immunodeficiency virus/acquired immune deficiency registry. Am J Med Sci 305:345–353

Loder N 2000 Drug-resistant HIV shows a worrying increase in the UK. Nature 407:120

Patton LL, McKaig R, Straauss R et al. 2000 Changing prevalence of oral manifestations of human immunodeficiency virus in the era of protease inhibitor therapy. Oral Surg 90:299-304

Rosen FS, Cooper MD, Wedgwood RJP 1995 The primary immunodeficiencies. N Engl J Med 333:434–440

Schwartzlander B, Garnett G, Walker N et al 2000 AIDS in a new millennium. Science 289:64–67

Scully C, Laskaris G, Pindborg J et al 1991 Oral manifestations of HIV infection and their management. Oral Surg Oral Med Oral Pathol 71:158–171

Silverman S 1996 Color atlas of oral manifestations of AIDS, 2nd edn. Mosby, St Louis

Smaglik P 2000 Reservoirs dog AIDS therapy. Nature 405:270–272

Tappuni AR, Flemming GJ 2001 The effect of antiretroviral therapy on the prevalence of oral manifestations in HIV-infected patients: a UK study. Oral Surg 92:623-628.

Weinert M, Grimes RM, Lynch DP 1996 Oral manifestations of HIV infection. Ann Intern Med 125:485–496

Allergy and autoimmune disease

Many endocrine diseases are immunologically mediated and most of the immunologically-mediated diseases have some dental relevance (Box 25.1).

Box 25.1 Aspects of immunologically-mediated diseases affecting dental management

- Systemic effects affecting dental management
- Immunologically-mediated oral diseases
- Risks of abnormal reactions to drugs (e.g. penicillin anaphylaxis)

Immunologically-mediated diseases fall into two main groups (Box 25.2). By far the most common are atopic disease and contact dermatitis, which are abnormal reactions to exogenous antigens. The autoimmune diseases, by contrast, are mediated by antibodies directed against host tissues.

Box 25.2   Important immunologically-mediated diseases

Atopic disease and related allergies (reactions to exogenous antigens)
- Asthma; eczema; hay fever; urticaria; food allergies
- Some drug reactions
- Anaphylaxis and acute allergic angio-oedema
- Contact dermatitis

Autoimmune diseases (reactions to endogenous antigens causing autoantibody production)

Connective tissue diseases
- Rheumatoid arthritis
- Sjögren's syndromes*
- Lupus erythematosus*
- Systemic sclerosis*

Autoimmune diseases with specific autoantibodies
- Pernicious anaemia (chronic atrophic gastritis)*
- Idiopathic and drug-associated thrombocytopenic purpura*
- Drug-associated leucopenia*
- Autoimmune haemolytic anaemia
- Addison's disease*
- Hypothyroidism (Hashimoto's thyroiditis)*
- Hyperthyroidism
- Idiopathic hypoparathyroidism*
- Pemphigus vulgaris*
- Mucous membrane pemphigoid*

*Can give rise to characteristic oral changes

ATOPIC DISEASE

Atopic disease is the common type of allergy and affects approximately 10% of the population. It is mediated by IgE and susceptibility is genetically determined.

There are no oral manifestations of atopic disease itself and there is no such entity as oral eczema. However, acute angio-oedema (sometimes a drug reaction) can indirectly involve the mouth by causing oedematous swelling of the floor of the mouth or lips as discussed below.

Acute severe asthma has a significant mortality and is a potential cause of an emergency in the dental surgery. Drugs (Box 25.3) used to treat it and other atopic diseases may complicate dental treatment.

Box 25.3   Effects of drugs used for atopic disease

- Antihistamines (for minor allergies)
  - Drowsiness
  - Potentiation of sedating drugs
  - Dry mouth
- Corticosteroid inhalers
  - Oropharyngeal thrush
- Systemic corticosteroids for severe asthma (see Box 31.10)

Contact dermatitis

Contact dermatitis resembles eczema clinically, but is a cell-mediated (type 4) reaction. There is no convincing evidence of any oral counterpart to contact dermatitis (Figs 25.1 and 25.2). Contact dermatitis of the hands to dental materials is a hazard to dentists and especially to laboratory technicians. Methyl methacrylate monomer, in particular, is a sensitising agent, but contact dermatitis to it is a surprisingly rare occupational hazard of dentistry.

Latex allergy

Latex allergy is the main allergic disease affecting healthcare workers.

The necessity for gloving for all clinical work has resulted in a growing frequency of latex allergy. In one dental school,

the prevalence of latex allergy was 9%, while 22% complained of chronic glove dermatitis. Once latex allergy to gloves has been acquired, there are reactions to all rubber products such as rubber tubing, anaesthetic masks, catheters and tourniquets. Powdered latex gloves should no longer be used in the UK; the starch powder spread latex proteins into the environment. For those with latex allergy, gloves made from other plastics are required but, as yet, there is no completely satisfactory alternative. Despite this, some centres are phasing out latex gloves.

Patients exposed to latex through medical procedures are also at risk (Box 25.4).

> **Box 25.4 Individuals at risk of latex allergy**
>
> - Healthcare professionals
> - Atopic patients
> - Spina bifida
> - Urogenital anomalies
> - Latex industry workers
> - Those subject to multiple surgical procedures before the age of 7 years

Fig. 25.1 Allergic rash triggered by impression material. There is generalised facial erythema and slight oedema.

Fig. 25.2 Hypersensitivity to impression material. The same patient as in Figure 25.1, showing the site of the impression photographed at the same time. No allergic response is evident intraorally.

Latex allergy is important because it most frequently manifests as an urticarial contact reaction. In dentistry, this has the potential to put the airway at risk. More rarely, reactions to latex can be severe and have been fatal.

It is not always obvious that a medical or dental device may contain rubber, for instance bungs in local anaesthetic cartridges may contain latex. Even covered latex, such as a sphygmomanometer cuff, can shed latex proteins and trigger a reaction. For severe cases, it may be necessary to refer patients to a centre with a latex-free surgery. Less severe cases can be premedicated with methylpredisone and chlorpheniramine.

Allergy to mercury and other metals

The main sources of reactions are mercury in amalgam and nickel. Patients allergic to mercury are not prone to contact reactions in the oral mucosa which cannot mount contact dermatitis reactions. Amalgam restorations can safely be inserted, provided that no amalgam reaches the patient's skin.

Mucosal reactions, such as lichenoid-type lesions, have been reported, but evidence is conflicting as to whether these are true allergic reactions.

Fragments of amalgam lost in the submucosal tissues frequently do not cause any reaction histologically.

Nickel allergy is a less common source of allergic reactions. It may be present in bridges and crowns. Even in patients allergic to nickel, a nickel-containing appliance may cause no reaction in the mouth, but may affect the skin.

The dangers of mercury are either from systemic absorption, particularly of organic mercury compounds such as methyl mercury, or from the development of hypersensitivity (contact dermatitis). Mercury intoxication is frequently confused with allergy by the public and the media.

Hypersensitivity to mercury or its salts causes an inflammatory and sometimes vesiculating reaction when contacting skin. This can readily be confirmed by patch testing, but even those

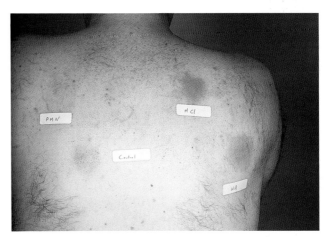

Fig. 25.3 Patch testing for dental materials. Four panels of 12 patches impregnated with different dental materials have been in contact with the skin for 48 hours. Erythema, oedema and a palpable nodule indicate reaction to mercury but amalgam restorations provoked no intraoral reaction.

with proven sensitivity can tolerate mercury amalgams in the mouth (Fig. 25.3). Nevertheless, in practical terms, it is usually simpler to use composite materials to obviate the precautions necessary to prevent mercury coming into contact with their skin. If a dentist develops sensitivity, gloving and covering the arms (as required for infection control) should provide adequate protection during preparation and insertion of amalgams.

Systemic mercury toxicity is another possible occupational hazard of dentistry. Mercury, and particularly methyl mercury, are neurotoxic. To what extent the metal is converted to organic compounds in the body is unclear, but care should be taken in handling mercury and preventing it from being spilt or scattered in fine particles during amalgam mixing. Drilling out old amalgams also gives off traces of mercury vapour if the bur is poorly cooled. Serious pollution arises from spilling a substantial quantity of mercury, particularly on to carpeted or wooden flooring. Indeed, such absorbent materials are no longer permissible in a clinical environment for this and infection control reasons. Decontamination can then be difficult. Even worse is when (as has happened) a dental surgery assistant spills mercury behind an autoclave but fails to report the accident. As a result of the rapid evaporation, mercury absorption by the dental staff can then rise to alarming levels. Encapsulated amalgam has rendered most of these risks of only historical interest.

Nevertheless, dentists have had decades of exposure to mercury and absorbed significant amounts, but do not appear to have been significantly harmed.

Though mercury, and particularly its organic compounds, are undoubtedly toxic, public anxiety about mercury-containing dental amalgams has been aroused by unscrupulous practitioners, scaremongers and others. It was conspicuous, for example, that the alleged dangers of mercury toxicity ('allergy') achieved sudden publicity when a new and expensive composite restorative material was introduced.

Minute traces of mercury can be absorbed through the oral mucosa from amalgams and may occasionally give rise to mucosal lichenoid reactions. Otherwise, there is no evidence that dental amalgams are toxic or the cause of vague symptoms such as poor memory, lassitude and depression from which most people seem to suffer from time to time. It has also been shown that patients who complain of vague symptoms from 'mercury allergy' tend also to suffer from a variety of complaints (such as irritable bowel syndrome) which have no clear organic basis. In one group of 20 patients complaining of amalgam-related symptoms, none was found to be hypersensitive to mercury. It also, incidentally, cannot be shown that alternative materials such as composites, of which there is much less experience, are necessarily safer. Some of them give off traces of formaldehyde, which can trigger allergic and irritant reactions and is a suspected carcinogen.

A few patients with multiple sclerosis have been persuaded that their disease had been caused by their amalgam restorations and demanded their replacement. There is no medical justification for so doing, apart from offering the patient some temporary emotional comfort.

Despite the high risks of litigation in the USA, the Council on Dental Therapeutics of the American Dental Association has stated that, 'there is insufficient evidence to justify claims that mercury from amalgam restorations has an adverse effect on the health of the patients'.

HEREDITARY AND ALLERGIC ANGIO-OEDEMA →
Summary p. 409

Hereditary angio-oedema is due to deficiency of C1 esterase inhibitor. Since C1 esterase inhibitor is an inactivator of the first complement component, its absence leads to uncontrolled activation of the classical pathway. In the process, C4 is consumed and its persistently low level in the serum during asymptomatic periods is a useful diagnostic test. Alternatively, serum C1 esterase inhibitor titration may be necessary for diagnosis of genetic variants.

As a result of stimuli such as minor injuries (including dental trauma), episodes of increased capillary permeability cause gross but localised oedematous swelling. Visceral angio-oedema can cause acute abdominal pain but, more important, oedema of the head and neck region can cause respiratory obstruction, and there is a significant mortality.

Similar angio-oedema may also be an effect of the angiotensin converting enzyme inhibitors.

Management

Treatment of an acute attack is with purified C1 esterase inhibitor concentrate. Prophylaxis and maintenance treatment is with the synthetic androgen stanozolol which, if taken daily, maintains C1 esterase inhibitor at normal levels.

Allergic angio-oedema is an IgE-mediated acute hypersensitivity reaction to an allergen. It can cause gross swelling of the lips, face and neck and can then also threaten the airway. Patients may have a history of allergic disease and, usually, raised IgE levels.

Intramuscular epinephrine should be given immediately if the airway is threatened by an attack of allergic angio-oedema.

THE AUTOIMMUNE DISEASES

This blanket term is used for a variety of diseases due to defective modulation of immune responses and production of autoantibodies which can damage host tissues. The autoimmune diseases have many features in common (Box 25.5). By no means are all of their mechanisms are clearly understood (Box 25.6). All of those listed in Box 25.2 are likely to show these features. Those with particular dental relevance have been discussed in other chapters and only the connective tissue diseases are described here.

is the main feature, but it is a multisystem disease. The temporomandibular joints are often involved in the more severe cases, but clinical effects are frequently insignificant (Ch. 11).

The chief importance of rheumatoid arthritis in dentistry is its association with Sjögren's syndrome. Drugs used for rheumatoid arthritis (particularly aspirin and other anti-inflammatory drugs, corticosteroids, antimalarials, gold and penicillamine) can also affect dental management or occasionally cause oral reactions. Many patients with rheumatoid arthritis are anaemic as a result of the disease itself, or as a result of gastric blood loss induced by analgesics.

Sjögren's syndromes

See Chapter 18.

Systemic lupus erythematosus

Systemic lupus erythematosus (SLE) can affect almost any body system, which may affect dental management. Oral mucosal lesions are seen in about 20%.

The most important of the many autoantibodies seen in SLE are antinuclear factors. Only antibodies against double-stranded DNA (anti-dsDNA) are peculiar to SLE, but many other antinuclear factors are found in other connective tissue diseases.

Clinically, the features vary according to the main organ systems affected (Table 25.1).

Joint pains and rashes are the most common manifestations, but the 'classical' picture of a young woman with a butterfly rash across the mid-face is uncommon and not peculiar to SLE. Corticosteroids and other immunosuppressives or antimalarials are the main forms of treatment.

Box 25.5 Typical features of autoimmune disease

- Significantly more common in women
- Onset often in middle age
- Family history frequently positive
- Levels of immunoglobulins (autoantibodies) usually raised
- Circulating autoantibodies frequently also detectable in unaffected family members
- Circulating autoantibodies to several tissues but not all attacked (e.g. antithyroid antibodies are common in Sjögren's syndrome)
- Often a higher risk of developing other autoimmune diseases (e.g. greater risk of patients with thyroiditis developing pernicious anaemia)
- Immunoglobulin and/or complement often detectable at sites of tissue damage (e.g. pemphigus vulgaris)
- Often associated with HLA-B8 and DR3
- Immunosuppressive treatment frequently limits tissue damage

---

Box 25.6 Types of autoimmune disease

Organ or cell-specific autoantibodies
- Hashimoto's thyroiditis
- Chronic atrophic gastritis (pernicious anaemia)
- Addison's disease
- Idiopathic hypoparathyroidism
- Pemphigus
- Pemphigoid
- Idiopathic thrombocytopenic purpura
- Autoimmune haemolytic anaemia
- Myasthenia gravis

Non-organ specific autoantibodies (the connective tissue diseases)
- Lupus erythematosus
- Rheumatoid arthritis
- Sjögren's syndrome
- Systemic sclerosis
- Primary biliary cirrhosis
- Dermatomyositis
- Mixed connective tissue disease

The connective tissue diseases

The main connective tissue diseases are rheumatoid arthritis, lupus erythematosus, systemic sclerosis, primary biliary cirrhosis and Sjögren's syndrome. The last can be associated with any of them or develop in isolation.

A characteric feature is the multiplicity of autoantibodies, none of which is specific to the tissues under attack and which frequently also are not specific to the disease either. Thus, in rheumatoid arthritis, the most constantly found autoantibody (rheumatoid factor) is not directed against the joint tissues but against an immunoglobulin. Moreover, rheumatoid factor is frequently detectable in other diseases of this group in the absence of arthritis. The connective tissue diseases are probably mediated by immune complex (type 3) reactions causing inflammation and tissue damage.

Rheumatoid arthritis

Rheumatoid arthritis is by far the most common connective tissue disorder and affects at least 3% of the population. Arthritis

---

Table 25.1 Organs and tissues affected in systemic lupus erythematosus

Organ/tissue	Clinical feature
Joints	Joint pains and arthritis
Skin	Rashes
Mouth	Stomatitis, Sjögren's syndrome
Serous membranes	Pleurisy, pericarditis
Heart	Endocarditis, myocarditis
Lungs	Pneumonitis
Kidneys	Nephritic syndrome
Central nervous system	Neuroses, psychoses, strokes, cranial nerve palsies
Eyes	Conjunctivitis, retinal damage
Gastrointestinal tract	Hepatomegaly, pancreatitis
Blood	Anaemia, purpura

Dental aspects

About 20% of patients with SLE develop oral lesions. These somewhat resemble lichen planus (Ch. 13). However, they are more difficult to treat and may not respond to the doses of systemic corticosteroids which control more major manifestations of the disease.

Antimalarials used in treatment can also cause oral lichen planus. Otherwise, dental management may be affected by the pattern of systemic involvement, but frequently the treatment is likely to affect dental management more than the disease itself. The chief dental considerations are summarised in Box 25.7.

> **Box 25.7** Features of lupus erythematosus affecting dental management
>
> - Corticosteroid and other immunosuppressive drugs
> - Painful oral lesions
> - Sjögren's syndrome
> - Bleeding tendencies (antiplatelet antibodies or anticoagulants)
> - Anaemia
> - Cardiac disease and risk of endocarditis

Discoid lupus erythematosus

Discoid LE mainly causes mucocutaneous lesions essentially similar to those of SLE but without the latter's serological changes and systemic disorders.

Systemic sclerosis (scleroderma)

Systemic sclerosis is rare, but causes subcutaneous and visceral fibrosis. It has a poor prognosis. The pathogenesis of the progressive fibrosis and stiffening of the skin and often the gastrointestinal tract, lungs, heart and kidneys is unclear. Inflammatory changes are minimal. Circulating antinuclear antibodies are detectable in about 50% of patients, but their role is also unclear.

Clinically, the most common early sign is Raynaud's phenomenon and joint pains. Later, the skin becomes thinned, stiff and pigmented and the facial features become smoothed-out and mask-like. Opening of the mouth may become limited (Ch. 11). Fibrosis of viscera is liable to cause dysphagia, dyspnoea and pulmonary hypertension. Later, there may be renal involvement, hypertension and cardiac failure.

Immunosuppressive drugs appear to be ineffective and the 5-year survival rate is only about 50%. Oral features are summarised in Box 25.8.

Localised scleroderma (morphoea)

Morphoea is characterised by localised fibrosis resembling that of scleroderma, but without the latter's systemic involvement of serological changes. The face is frequently the chief site and the area of fibrosis resembles the scar from a sabre cut (coup de sabre). Childhood morphoea is a possible cause of facial hemiatrophy.

> **Box 25.8** Possible oral features of systemic sclerosis
>
> - Sjögren's syndrome
> - Limited oral opening
> - Widened periodontal ligament shadow in 7%
> - Gross resorption of the jaws, rarely
> - Firm whitish-yellow fibrotic mucosal plaques, very rarely

SUGGESTED FURTHER READING

Black C 1994 Scleroderma (systemic sclerosis). Medicine UK 22:70–75

Field EA, Longman LP et al. 1998 The dental management of patients with natural rubber latex allergy. Br Dent J 185:65–69

Hall FC, Walport MJ 1994 Systemic lupus erythematosus. Medicine UK 22:58–64

Herrström P, Högstrom B 1993 Clinical study of oral galvanism: no evidence of toxic mercury exposure but anxiety disorder an important background factor. Scand J Dent Res 101:232–237

Katelaris CH, Widmer RP, Lazarus RM 1996 Prevalence of latex allergy in a dental school. Med J Aust 164:711–714

Mjör IA 1994 Side effects of dental materials. No evidence that dental restorations are hazardous to health (editorial). Br Med J 309: 621–622

Sim TC, Grant JA 1990 Hereditary angioedema: its diagnostic and management perspectives. Am J Med 88:656–665

Smart ER, Macleod RI, Lawrence CM 1992 Allergic reactions to rubber gloves in dental patients: report of three cases. Br Dent J 172:443–445

Walls RS 1996 Latex allergy: a real problem (editorial). Med J Aust 164:707–708

Cervical lymphadenopathy

Dental and periodontal infections are by far the most common causes of cervical lymphadenopathy (Fig. 26.1). However, other possible causes include life-threatening diseases such as carcinomatous metastases or lymphomas. In HIV infection, lymphadenopathy is one of its most common features. Cervical lymphadenopathy without an obvious local cause is therefore a warning sign that must not be ignored.

Important causes of cervical lymphadenopathy are summarised in Box 26.1, but many have been discussed in other chapters.

Box 26.1   Important causes of cervical lymphadenopathy

Infections
- Bacterial
    Dental, tonsils, face or scalp infections
    Tuberculosis
    Syphilis
    Cat-scratch disease
    Lyme disease
- Viral
    Herpetic stomatitis
    Infectious mononucleosis
    HIV infection
- Parasitic
    Toxoplasmosis
- Possibly infective
    Mucocutaneous lymph node syndrome (Kawasaki's disease)

Neoplasms
- Primary
    Hodgkin's disease
    Non-Hodgkin lymphoma
    Leukaemia – especially lymphocytic
- Secondary
    Carcinoma – oral, salivary gland or nasopharyngeal
    Malignant melanoma
    Other mesenchymal tumours

Miscellaneous
- Sarcoidosis
- Drug reactions
- Connective tissue diseases

Investigation

The most common cause of persistent cervical lymphadenopathy is a recent viral illness. Various clinical features provide

important guides as to the likely cause of lymphadenopathy (Box 26.2).

Box 26.2   Preliminary considerations

- Patient's age
- Localised or generalised lymphadenopathy
- Clinical characters of the nodes
- Duration of the swelling
- Associated signs or symptoms

A soft lymph node in an otherwise healthy child is unlikely to be of great significance. It is usually due to a recent viral infection and typically resolves spontaneously after a month or so. Cervical lymphadenopathy associated with generalised lymphadenopathy in a child with a sore throat and fever is likely to be

Fig. 26.1 Enlarged submandibular lymph node with incipient drainage to the skin.

due to infectious mononucleosis as discussed below. By contrast, persistent lymphadenopathy associated with anaemia in a child is likely to be due to lymphocytic leukaemia. In the older patient with a hard lymph node, a carcinoma must be suspected. Rarely, such a metastasis can form in the early stages of the disease when the primary is still small. Otherwise, a carcinoma in the anterior part of the mouth should be readily detectable by careful clinical examination. By contrast, a carcinoma of the posterior lateral border of the tongue may be difficult to visualise. Even more difficult to detect is a small primary in the nasopharynx. Various patterns of involvement of cervical lymph nodes can be produced by spread of carcinoma of the mouth (Ch. 17).

In a patient with Sjögren's syndrome, enlargement of cervical lymph nodes may be due to infection secondary to the dry mouth, but may alternatively be due to the development of lymphoma – a recognised hazard of this disease.

Investigations for cervical lymphadenopathy where the cause is not obvious are summarised in Box 26.3. The first-line investigation should always be fine needle aspiration (FNA). This will provide an accurate diagnosis of most lymphomas, metastases and many infections including tuberculosis. Inadequate specimens or failed diagnosis should therefore trigger a re-aspiration in the first instance.

In difficult cases or when FNA fails, biopsy provides the most reliable diagnosis. Biopsy is only justified if all other investigations have proved inadequate and must be done by an expert. Biopsy may spill infectious material or malignant cells into the neck as well as produce unsightly scarring.

TUBERCULOUS CERVICAL LYMPHADENOPATHY →
Summary p. 172

Tuberculous infection of the cervical lymph nodes is a primary infection which accounts for less than 10% of tuberculosis in Britain. *Mycobacterium tuberculosis* (human) accounts for over 90% of isolates. Patients are mostly adults, mainly immigrants of Asian or Afro-Caribbean origin. Non-tuberculous ('atypical') mycobacteria, particularly *M. avium intracellulare* or *M. scrofulaceum*, are now the major cause of cervical mycobacterial lymphadenitis in immunocompetent children. As discussed earlier, the incidence of mycobacterial infections is growing and multiply-resistant strains are becoming widespread.

Clinical features (Box 26.4)

Box 26.4   Typical clinical features of tuberculous lymph nodes

- Firm swelling, usually of a group of nodes
- Nodes typically become matted
- Abscess or sinus formation, if neglected
- Calcified nodes from past, healed disease (Fig. 26.2)

Box 26.3   Investigation of cervical lymphadenopathy

History
- Is there a history of a systemic illness?
- Has there been any contact with infectious disease (e.g. HIV or syphilis)?
- Has there been an animal scratch?
- Are there recurrent fever, lassitude, sweats or anaemia to suggest Hodgkin's disease?
- Do any symptoms (e.g. epistaxis or hoarseness) suggest a nasopharyngeal cause?
- Are any drugs (especially phenytoin) being taken?

Examination
- Check the temperature
- Identify the node and its drainage area
- Check carefully for dental, other oral, pharyngeal or skin causes in the area
- If a possible primary cause is found (e.g. an oral ulcer) it should be biopsied
- If no local cause is found, consider ENT referral for a nasopharyngeal cause
- Examine the other side of the neck. Bilateral lymphadenopathy suggests a systemic cause

Special investigations (as appropriate)
- Blood picture (leukaemia? glandular fever?)
- Chest radiograph for mediastinal nodes (e.g. Hodgkin's disease, sarcoidosis)
- Serology (glandular fever, toxoplasmosis, HIV)
- Angiotensin-converting enzyme and calcium levels (sarcoid)
- Mantoux test (tuberculosis)
- Fine needle aspiration (primary or metastatic neoplasm, tuberculosis)
- Thyroid scan and function tests for unsuspected thyroid tumour
- Blind biopsy of nasopharynx and tonsils if needle biopsy of the node shows malignancy
- Biopsy of node itself is a last resort. Send fresh material for mycobacterial culture

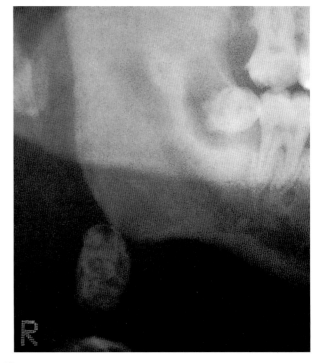

Fig. 26.2   Tuberculosis. Calcified cervical lymph node seen in a panoramic tomogram. Calcified nodes are often multiple and indicate past rather than active infection. (By kind permission of Mr EJ Whaites.)

Fig. 26.3 **Tuberculosis.** Numerous multinucleate Langhans giant cells are conspicuous in this granuloma.

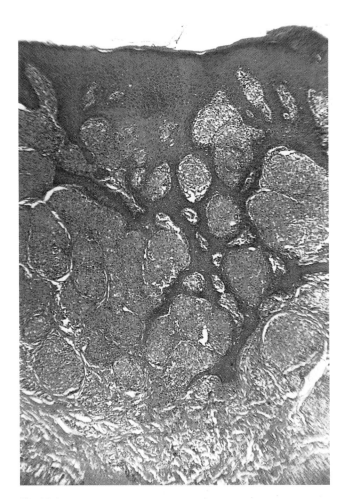

Fig. 26.4 **Leprosy, another granulomatous disease.** In the tuberculoid form, multiple compact non-caseating granulomas are present in the corium.

Pathology

Diagnosis depends on finding granulomas (Fig. 26.3) in which mycobacteria should be demonstrable by Ziehl–Neelsen staining or by immunofluorescence using auramine-rhodamine. However, infection by non-tuberculous mycobacteria, even in immunocompetent children, is likely to give rise to poorly-defined or irregular granulomas without palisading, or to ill-defined aggregates of epithelioid histiocytes. Caseation may be absent (Fig. 26.4), but there may be areas of necrosis with numerous neutrophils. Ziehl–Neelson staining is also negative.

Mycobacterial culture or detection of mycobacterial DNA is required. The tuberculin skin test should be positive, unless the patient is severely immunodeficient.

Management

The clinical picture is variable and the diagnosis is usually only made after fine needle aspiration or excision of a node. If a tuberculous ('cold') abscess and sinus form, incision is contraindicated and affected nodes should be excised intact. A course of isoniazid should also be given.

SYPHILIS

The cervical lymph nodes are enlarged, soft and rubbery when the primary chancre is in the mouth or on the lip. They are also involved in the widespread lymphadenopathy of the secondary stage.

In the primary stage, diagnosis is by finding *Treponema pallidum* in a direct smear from the oral lesion. Later, diagnosis depends on the serological findings (Ch. 12).

Management

Antibiotic treatment, usually with penicillin, is required.

369

CAT-SCRATCH DISEASE

This infection is common in the USA and, though uncommon, is increasingly frequently found in Britain.

Typical features are summarised in Box 26.5.

Box 26.5 Typical features of cat-scratch disease

- Children frequently affected
- Frequently a history of a scratch by a cat or other animal
- Formation of papule, which may suppurate, at the site of inoculation
- Mild fever, malaise and regional lymphadenitis 1–3 weeks after exposure
- Lymph nodes soften and typically suppurate
- Conjunctivitis may be associated. Encephalitis is a rare complication

---

Pathology

There is destruction of lymph node architecture, necrosis and lymphocytic infiltration, formation of histiocytic granulomas and central suppuration (Fig. 26.5).

These appearances can readily be mistaken for one of the systemic mycoses. However, it may be possible to show the usual causative organism, *Bartonella henselae*. It is a small Gram-negative bacillus demonstrable with a silver (Warthin–Starry) stain, but not with haematoxylin and eosin, at the site of inoculation or in the lymph nodes.

Management

Diagnosis depends on a history of a scratch, particularly by a cat, clinical features and exclusion of other causes for lymphadenopathy. The histological findings are confirmatory if *B. henselae* can be identified.

The disease is typically mild and self-limiting but may lead to suppuration and sinus formation. The response to antibacterials is variable. Trimethoprim-sulphamethoxazole has been recommended, but some cases resolve spontaneously.

LYME DISEASE

Lyme disease is caused by a spirochaete, *Borrelia burgdorferi*, which is transmitted by insects, particularly deer ticks. The disease is worldwide but far more common in the USA than in Britain.

Typical features are summarised in Box 26.6.

Box 26.6 Typical features of Lyme disease

- A rash spreading outwards from the insect bite
- Enlarged regional lymph nodes
- Fever and often other systemic symptoms
- Arthritis (the main chronic effect) particularly of the knees, rarely of the temporomandibular joints
- Neurological complications (in about 15% of patients) include facial palsy or other cranial nerve lesions

---

Management

Diagnosis is by the history and clinical picture. It is confirmed serologically or, sometimes, by demonstration of the spirochaete by silver staining of a skin biopsy.

The spirochaete is sensitive to penicillin or tetracycline which should be given as early as possible. However, joint pains may recur or destructive arthritis may develop later.

INFECTIOUS MONONUCLEOSIS

The Epstein–Barr virus (EBV) is the main cause of this self-limiting lymphoproliferative disease with polyclonal activation of B lymphocytes.

Typical features are summarised in Box 26.7.

Box 26.7 Typical features of infectious mononucleosis

- In children especially
  Generalised lymphadenopathy, typically with conspicuous enlargement of the cervical nodes
  Sore throat
  Fever
- In adolescents
  Lymphadenopathy often less conspicuous
  Vague illness with fever
- In the anginose type of disease
  Sore throat, tonsillar exudate and pharyngeal oedema
  Palatal petechiae (Fig. 26.6)

Fig. 26.5 Cat-scratch disease. There is necrosis in larger more irregular foci than tuberculosis (left) and giant cells.

The clinical features are usually distinctive but, rarely, there is more persistent lymphadenopathy which may mimic a lymphoma both clinically and histologically.

Fig. 26.6 Petechiae on the palate are frequently seen in infectious mononucleosis.

Management

The diagnosis is confirmed by a peripheral blood picture showing the atypical (monocyte-like) lymphocytes. A heterophil antibody (Paul–Bunnell) test and, if necessary, demonstration of a raised titre of EBV antibodies are confirmatory. If these tests are negative in an otherwise typical case, cytomegalovirus infection or toxoplasmosis should be considered. Acquisition of HIV infection frequently also gives rise to an illness resembling infectious mononucleosis.

There is no specific treatment, but infection is usually self-limiting.

Ampicillin or amoxycillin should be avoided. They are prone to cause irritating macular rashes unrelated to penicillin allergy.

THE ACQUIRED IMMUNE DEFICIENCY SYNDROME

Lymphadenopathy is one of the most frequent manifestations of HIV infection (Ch. 22). Soon after infection there may be a transient glandular fever-like illness. Later, there may be widespread and persistent lymphadenopathy (generalised lymphadenopathy syndrome: GLS), which is likely to progress to AIDS in over 50% within less than 4 years. Lymphadenopathy in AIDS may also be due to lymphomas.

TOXOPLASMOSIS

Toxoplasma gondii is a common intestinal parasite of many domestic animals, particularly cats. *T. gondii* is a low-grade pathogen but can affect previously healthy persons, particularly young women. Infection can be acquired by ingestion of oocytes and three main types of disease can result (Box 26.8).

Management

The diagnosis is confirmed serologically by a high or rising titre of antibodies or by other immunological methods.

Antimicrobial treatment is required only for severe infections and is with pyrimethamine and a sulphonamide.

MUCOCUTANEOUS LYMPH NODE SYNDROME (KAWASAKI'S DISEASE)

Kawasaki's disease is endemic in Japan and there have been outbreaks in Hawaii and the USA, where it has surpassed rheumatic fever as the leading cause of childhood-acquired heart disease. In Britain, it has caused approximately 100 deaths per annum.

The distribution of cases suggests an infectious cause, but no agent has been identified with certainty.

Typical clinical features are summarised in Box 26.9.

The overall mortality is 1–3%, from heart failure secondary to coronary artery disease or dysrhythmias secondary to myocardial ischaemia.

Management

The diagnosis usually depends on the clinical and, particularly, electrocardiographic findings.

Fig. 26.7 **Castleman's disease.** Hyaline vascular-type disease. There is gross hyperplasia of lymphoid follicles, with the lymphocytes forming tight concentric layers round blood vessels with swollen endothelial cells. (From Oral Disease 3rd edn by Cawson, Binnie, Barret and Wright, with permission from Mosby.)

There is no specific treatment, but aspirin, despite the possible risk of Reye's syndrome, is frequently given to lessen vascular damage and thromboses. However, a single large dose of intravenous gammaglobulin given with aspirin, in the early, acute stages appears to be the most effective means of reducing the risk of coronary artery damage.

LANGERHANS CELL HISTIOCYTOSIS

Cervical lymph nodes can be enlarged, sometimes massively, in isolation or more frequently in association with multisystem disease (Ch. 9).

GIANT (ANGIOFOLLICULAR) LYMPH NODE HYPERPLASIA: CASTLEMAN'S DISEASE

This uncommon disease usually affects the thorax but can, occasionally, cause a cervical mass resembling a lymphoma. There are unicentric and multicentric variants which, in turn, may be histologically hyaline vascular or a plasma cell variant.

Most cases of unicentric hyaline vascular Castleman's disease are benign, while the plasma cell variant, which is associated with high levels of interleukin-6 (IL6), tends to have systemic effects and is more common in multicentric disease. The latter is generally associated with HIV and HHV-8 infection and has become more common as a result.

Adolescents or young adults are most frequently and children rarely affected.

In the cervical region, the lesion usually consists of a single large mass. Systemic complications include fever, anemia, hypergammaglobulinaemia and autoimmune disease.

Multicentric Castleman's disease

Unlike localised Castleman's disease which is generally benign, multicentric Castleman's disease has systemic effects and can be lethal. Most cases are associated with human herpes-virus 8 in patients with HIV infection associated with high serum levels of HHV-8. The number of multicentric cases has risen as a result of the spread of HIV infection and their manifestations have changed. HHV-8 encodes a homologue of interleukin 6 (vIL6) which may mediate some of the systemic features. Occasionally, Castleman's disease and Kaposi's sarcoma have developed in HIV-negative immunosuppressed patients. HHV-8 appears to play a role in the pathogenesis of HIV-associated multicentric Castleman's disease and exacerbations in HIV-positive patients are correlated with high levels of HHV-8 viral load. HHV-8 has also been detected in HIV-negative patients with this disease, including one who developed Kaposi's sarcoma.

Multifocal Castleman's disease in children is rare but may have a more favourable course than in adults.

Pathology

In the head and neck region, 98% of these lesions are of the hyaline vascular type.

The main features are gross hyperplasia of lymphoid follicles, with the lymphocytes forming tight concentric layers round blood vessels with swollen endothelial cells which frequently proliferate (Fig. 26.7).

In the plasma cell type, there are hyperplastic germinal centres and sheets of plasma cells in the interfollicular areas. Dissolution of lymphoid follicles is a feature only of the HHV-8+ variant of plasma cell Castleman's disease in some patients.

In hyaline-vascular disease, there may be conspicuous hyperplasia of follicular dendritic cells. There are atrophic germinal centres, often populated by cytologically atypical follicular dendritic reticulum cells.

Management

Localised Castleman's disease is usually benign, but the mass may be so large that resection may be justified. This not merely confirms the diagnosis, but is usually curative. Otherwise, a short course of high-dose corticosteroids or a single other immunosuppressive drug is effective. Multicentric Castleman's disease is aggressive regardless of histological type, is frequently associated with other malignant tumours and tends to have a chronic or rapidly fatal course.

In some reports, the mortality has been 45%, despite the fact that all but one were receiving HAART. Chemotherapy, radiation and interferon-alpha may induce remission. Alleviation of the systemic manifestations by thalidomide and resolution of a case of AIDS-related Castleman's disease with anti-CD20 monoclonal antibodies have also been reported.

Successful treatment of Castleman's disease with HAART in HIV-infected patients has been reported, but its value is not yet clear.

Complications

Of the many possible complications of Castleman's disease, development of lymphoma and Kaposi's sarcoma, particularly in patients with HIV/AIDS, are two of the most important.

Possible manifestations of Castleman's disease in the maxillofacial region

The main maxillofacial manifestations are cervical lymphadenopathy as mentioned above and less frequently, a parotid gland swelling. The cervical lymphadenopathy is sometimes due to the development of a lymphoma. As a consequence of the frequency of HIV/AIDS associated with HHV-8 infection, Kaposi's sarcoma, which can appear as purplish oral mucosal lesions, can be associated with this disease.

Paraneoplastic pemphigus with severe oral ulceration is a recognised complication (see Ch. 13). Paraneoplastic pemphigus in a child or adolescent is rare and should in fact be regarded as a possible manifestation of Castleman's disease. The latter can sometimes precede the onset of paraneoplastic pemphigus by many years.

Activation of Behçet's disease with oral aphthae is another possible complication of multicentric HHV-8-associated Castleman's disease. Connective tissue diseases that may be associated include primary Sjögren's syndrome, lupus erythematosus, rheumatoid arthritis, scleroderma and less well-defined conditions. A rare cause of complications is bleeding due to autoimmune thrombocytopenia or infection secondary to autoimmune neutropenia.

In a particularly rare case, trigeminal neuropathy was associated with unicentric mesenteric Castleman's disease. The neuropathy resolved promptly after surgical removal of the mass.

However, the most uncommon maxillofacial manifestation of Castleman's disease to be seen is a lesion within the oral cavity.

PHENYTOIN AND OTHER DRUG-ASSOCIATED LYMPHADENOPATHIES

Lymphadenopathy is an occasional toxic effect of long-term treatment with the antiepileptic drug phenytoin. Phenytoin lymphadenopathy (unlike that caused by many other drugs) is not usually associated with serum sickness-like symptoms of fever, rashes and joint pains. Moreover, the histopathology of phenytoin-associated lymphadenopathy can mimic a lymphoma.

Lymphadenopathy frequently first affects the neck but usually becomes widespread.

Management

Substitution of phenytoin with another anticonvulsant such as carbamazepine should allow the lymphadenopathy to subside and confirm the diagnosis.

Other drugs which can cause lymphadenopathy include penicillin (rarely), phenylbutazone (limited use), some other non-steroidal anti-inflammatory drugs and some antimalarials. As mentioned earlier, lymphadenopathy with these drugs is typically associated with serum sickness-like features.

SUGGESTED FURTHER READING

Collip PJ 1992 Cat-scratch disease: therapy with trimethoprim-sulphamethoxazole. Am J Dis Child 146:397–399

Eisenkraft BL, Som PM 1999 The spectrum of benign and malignant etiologies of cervical node calcification. NJR 172:1433–1437

Evans MJ, Smith NM, Thornton CM et al 1998 Atypical mycobacterial lymphadenitis in childhood – a clinicopathological study of 17 cases. J Clin Pathol 51:925–927

Haberman TM, Steensma DP 2000 Lymphadenopathy. Mayo Clin Proc 75:723–732

Karcher AM, Zaman A, Brewis C et al 2000 Neck lumps: expect the unexpected. Lancet 355:1070

Mason WH, Takahashi M 1999 Kawasaki syndrome. Clin Infect Dis 28:169–187

CHAPTER
26

Ogden GR, Kerr M 1989 Mucocutaneous lymph node syndrome
(Kawasaki disease). Oral Surg Oral Med Oral Pathol 67:569–572
Pinder SE, Colville A 1992 Mycobacterial cervical lymphadenitis in
children: can histological assessment help differentiate infections
by nontuberculous mycobacteria from *Mycobacterium tuberculosis*.
Histopathology 22:117–119
Ruef C 1999 Tuberculosis in Europe at the end of the second
millennium. Infection 27:311–312
Sakai O, Curtin HD, Romo LV et al 2000 Lymph node pathology. Benign
proliferative, lymphoma and metastatic disease. Radiol Clin N Am
38:979–998

Stansfeld AG, d'Ardenne AJ, eds 1992 Lymph node biopsy
interpretation, 2nd edn. Churchill Livingstone, Edinburgh
Steiner M, Gould A, Wilkie W, Porter K 1994 Cat-scratch disease in
the submandibular region: report of a case. J Oral Maxillofac Surg
52:614–618
Terezhalmy GT 1979 Mucocutaneous lymph node syndrome. Oral Surg
Oral Med Oral Pathol 47:26–30

Cardiovascular disease

Cardiovascular disease is common and many patients with heart disease require dental treatment. Heart disease becomes more frequent and severe in later life and is the most frequent single cause of death in Britain. Younger patients can also be affected. Infective endocarditis is one of the few ways in which dental treatment can lead to death of a patient, but only very rarely. As mentioned earlier (Ch. 5), surveys have suggested that dental disease may possibly also contribute to the development of atherosclerosis and myocardial infarction, but though evidence is still being produced, the hypothesis is not widely accepted.

Acute angina and myocardial infarction are causes of major emergencies in the dental surgery and prompt measures by the dental surgeon may be life-saving (Ch. 36).

In terms of dental management, patients fall into two main groups (Box 27.1), but a few may fall into both; drug treatment may create additional problems (Table 27.1). It must be appreciated, therefore, that the following management suggestions are generalisations and each case must be considered on its own merits.

Box 27.1   Dental management in major types of heart disease

Valvular or related defects (congenital or due to past rheumatic fever) or who have a prosthetic replacement
- Prophylactic antibiotic cover, particularly before extractions, is mandatory

Ischaemic heart disease with or without severe hypertension and cardiac failure
- Routine dentistry presents little hazard, but the risk of dangerous arrhythmias must be minimised
- Local anaesthetics in normal dosage have only theoretical dangers, but pain and anxiety must be minimised
- The main risk is from general anaesthesia

GENERAL ASPECTS OF MANAGEMENT

Patients chiefly at risk are severe hypertensives and those who have angina or have had a myocardial infarct due to ischaemic heart disease. Anxiety or pain can cause outpouring of

---

Table 27.1   Some dental implications or side-effects of drugs used for heart disease

Drugs	Implications for dental management
Diuretics	Dry mouth sometimes
Angiotensin-converting enzyme (ACE) inhibitors, captopril, perindopril, etc.	Burning mouth symptoms, lichenoid reactions
Angiotensin II receptor blockers, losartan, dysopyramide, etc.	Taste disturbance, dry mouth
Calcium channel blockers, amlodipine, diltiazem, etc.	Gingival hyperplasia (especially with diltiazem and nifedipine – Fig. 27.1)
Beta-adrenergic blockers, lobetalol, propranolol, etc.	Dry mouth, lichenoid reactions, theoretical interaction with epinephrine
Antihypertensives (as above)	Potentiated by general anaesthetics with reactions
Anticoagulants	Risk of prolonged postoperative bleeding
Warfarin	Risk of prolonged postoperative bleeding

Antianginal drugs
    Nicorandil
    Digoxin
	Aphthous-like stomatitis
	Enhanced risk of dysrhythmias with halothane

epinephrine which can both greatly increase the load on the heart and also precipitate dangerous dysrhythmias.

To die of fright is not a figure of speech but it can sometimes result from severe dysrhythmia. The first essential for these patients is therefore to ensure painless dentistry and to alleviate anxiety.

Patients should be asked whether routine dental treatment under local anaesthesia is acceptable and in any session of treatment as little or as much may be done as they feel able to tolerate.

Oral temazepam may be helpful (5 mg on the preceding night and again half an hour before treatment, and the patient accompanied by a responsible adult). If sedation is required, inhalational sedation is safer because nitrous oxide has no cardiorespiratory depressant effects and is more controllable, but it should be administered by an expert and not given within three months of a heart attack or recent angina.

Patients with severe or longstanding hypertension are at risk from ischaemic heart disease. Medical advice should be sought before treating those with blood pressures of 160–179/95–109. If considered at low risk from dental treatment, the same precautions should be taken for those with ischaemic heart disease.

Local anaesthesia for patients with cardiac disease

For local anaesthesia, an effective surface anaesthestic should be applied and the injection given very slowly to minimise pain. The most effective agent is 2% lidocaine with epinephrine and, after half a century of use, no local anaesthetic has been shown to be safer. The epinephrine content can *theoretically* cause a hypertensive reaction in patients receiving beta-blocker antihypertensives, because of an unopposed alpha-adrenergic effect. However, it is relevant that when an elderly woman receiving beta-blockers was given 16 cartridges (yes, really) of local anaesthetic with fatal results, the post-mortem conclusion

was that she had died from lidocaine overdosage rather than exacerbated hypertension. This interaction is only likely if doses of epinephrine are considerably larger than normally used in dentistry.

Though patients with cardiovascular disease need to be treated with care, the risks of routine dental treatment under local anaesthesia (despite many statements to the contrary) and of significant adverse reactions are very low indeed.

In Britain, all three deaths associated with dental local anaesthesia during the 10 years 1980–1989 were related to the use of prilocaine. This does not, of course, mean that prilocaine is necessarily dangerous, but it hardly suggests that it is safer than the more widely used lidocaine with epinephrine.

Local anaesthetics can undoubtedly cause mild dysrhythmias, but it is not always appreciated that more severe dysrhythmias can be triggered by anxiety before they have been given, or later during the operation. However, doses of local anaesthetics should be kept to a minimum and no more than 2 or 3 cartridges should be given (or be necessary) for an acceptable session of treatment. If larger doses have to be given, for example for multiple extractions, then continuous cardiac monitoring is necessary.

If general anaesthesia is unavoidable, it must be given by a specialist anaesthetist in hospital, especially as some of the drugs used for cardiovascular disease increase the risks. Cardiovascular disease is the chief cause of sudden death under anaesthesia.

PATIENTS WITH VALVE OR OTHER HEART DEFECTS AT RISK FROM INFECTIVE ENDOCARDITIS

Patients at risk are mainly those with congenital anomalies, such as valve or septal defects, or who have prosthetic heart valve replacements (Appendix 27.1). The majority of these patients have no symptoms and some valve defects, such as a bicuspid aortic valve, do not limit athletic activities.

Normally, bacteria entering the bloodstream are rapidly cleared by circulating leucocytes but, if there is a cardiac defect which can be colonised, infective endocarditis can develop.

There are many sources of bacteraemias, such as cardiac surgery, intravenous catheterisation and intravenous drug addiction. Bacteraemias can also be detected in over 80% of persons after extractions and even after toothbrushing, but the numbers of bacteria released are often very small. Even in a patient with a heart lesion, infective endocarditis does not necessarily follow.

Relatively few bacteria inhabit the oral mucosa and most are being constantly washed away by the saliva. By contrast, vast numbers of bacteria inhabit the gingival margins when oral hygiene is poor and even greater numbers occupy periodontal pockets. These bacteria are in close contact with dilated, thin-walled blood vessels (Fig. 27.2). Movement of teeth in their sockets repeatedly compresses and stretches or ruptures these vessels, so that bacteria can be pumped into the bloodstream.

Fig. 27.1 Drug-induced gingival hyperplasia resulting from treatment of hypertension with nifedipine. These swellings are centred on the interdental papillae.

Fig. 27.2 **Subgingival plaque.** The area of pocket wall in contact with plaque is large and the tissue contains numerous thin-walled blood vessels near the surface. This illustration serves to remind how easily microorganisms may be transferred into the circulation.

Fig. 27.3 Poor oral hygiene and severe pocketing such as this constitutes a risk to life, particularly in an elderly patient with a cardiac valve defect.

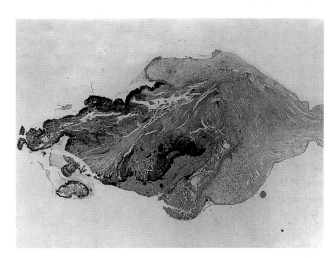

Fig. 27.4 **Heart valve in subacute infective endocarditis.** The free edge of the valve lies to the left of the picture and is covered by vegetations; centrally the valve is inflamed and thickened; and to the right the normal thickness of the valve is seen, at its attachment to the heart.

Fewer than 15% of cases of infective endocarditis can be related to (but not necessarily caused by) dental operations but, in these cases, extractions have been preceded by the infection in over 95%. Viridans streptococci, such as those which colonise the teeth, are of low virulence, but may be able to colonise heart valves because of attachment mechanisms (Ch. 3) which also enable them to cause dental disease.

Factors determining susceptibility to infective endocarditis are unclear. For example, children with Down's syndrome – who are prone to severe periodontal disease, have multiple immune defects and, frequently, congenital cardiac defects – are not particularly susceptible to infective endocarditis.

Currently, advanced age, especially if there is periodontal sepsis, is the main risk factor (Fig. 27.3). Infective endocarditis is rare in children and the peak incidence and mortality is after the age of 60 years. For cardiac transplantation, patients are deeply immunosuppressed and might be considered to be at high risk of infective endocarditis after dental operations. However, data are limited and there is no agreed protocol for such patients.

Once infective endocarditis develops, vegetations of bacteria and fibrin form on the valves, which are progressively destroyed (Fig. 27.4). Cardiac failure is the main cause of death, but emboli and bacteria released into the bloodstream can also cause renal or cerebral damage.

Prevention is all important. Patients in high-risk categories should receive preventive advice and, if treatment becomes necessary, antibiotic prophylaxis (see below and Appendix 27.1) before treatment that disturbs the gingival margin. This is likely to release significant numbers of bacteria from the gingivae or, particularly, periodontal pockets. Other dental procedures, such as fitting metal bands which extend deep to the gingival margins, though they may cause bacteraemias, have rarely been followed by infective endocarditis and antibiotic cover has not been officially recommended in the past. However, if the clinician considers the patient to fall into a high-risk group, then it may be prudent to give cover. Otherwise, orthodontic procedures in general are not recommended for antibiotic cover, particularly because most of these patients are children in whom infective endocarditis is rare. Endodontic treatment rarely, if ever, leads to infective endocarditis and the risks of antibiotic prophylaxis exceed any benefits.

Infective endocarditis does not appear to be a risk after myocardial infarction or coronary artery bypasses, or for wearers of cardiac pacemakers, and antibiotic cover is not recommended for them.

It is important to appreciate that the onset of infective endocarditis is typically very insidious. Even when antibiotic cover has been given, patients must be made to understand that they should report any mild, unexplained, febrile illness within 3 months of the dental treatment. Delay in diagnosis is the main factor affecting survival in infective endocarditis.

While prevention of infective endocarditis is clearly mandatory, there is growing doubt how best this can be achieved. Several surveys have shown that few cases of infective endocarditis can be reliably related to dental operations. Also, because spontaneous bacteraemias, due for example to mastication, are common, it is by no means certain that when infective endocarditis has followed a dental procedure, that the procedure was the actual cause. Moreover, it cannot be proved that the recommended prophylactic measures are effective or that the risks outweigh the benefits. One survey calculated that, in the UK, in a year, no fewer than 670 000 at-risk patients may be undergoing high-risk dental procedures without antibiotic prophylaxis. Yet, there are fewer than 2500 cases of infective endocarditis, of which only a minority are related to dentistry, in the same period. Sceptics also point out the incidence of infective endocarditis has not fallen, despite the introduction of scientifically-based prophylactic measures.

On the one hand, therefore, it cannot be denied that endocarditis can occasionally follow dental treatment. On the other hand, there is growing doubt whether this happens so frequently as to justify antibiotic prophylaxis or even whether the risks of antibiotic prophylaxis outweigh the benefits. Nevertheless, until these questions are answered, it is necessary to follow the current recommendations for at-risk patients (Appendix 27.1). Also, by doing so, the risk of medicolegal claims (of which there have been many) may be minimised.

ANTIBIOTIC PROPHYLAXIS REGIMENS FOR ENDOCARDITIS

It was found long ago that oral bacteria entered the bloodstream after dental operations. It was later shown that these bacteria could infect a damaged heart and cause potentially fatal infective endocarditis.

Eventually, formal recommendations for appropriate antibiotic prophylaxis have been adopted, even though their basis could not be entirely scientific. As a result, these regimens have become so controversial that it may be helpful to explain some of the problems. Nevertheless, it remains mandatory to follow the published recommendations, both medical and medicolegal, whenever an 'at-risk' patient is going to have certain types of dental procedure.

Recommendations for antibiotic prophylaxis against infective endocarditis are made by many groups including the British Society for Antimicrobial Chemotherapy, European Cardiac Society and the American Heart Association. In the UK, the definitive guidance is that of the Endocarditis Working Party of the British Society for Antimicrobial Chemotherapy, which is published in the British National Formulary. At the time of writing, the formulary contains the 1992 revision of the guidelines.

It has always been accepted that there is little evidence that prophylaxis is effective and, in recent years, there has been an opinion that the guidance requires a major overhaul. Reasons for this view include:

- Lack of evidence that prophylaxis is effective. The guidance is poorly supported by evidence and what evidence there is has been largely anecdotal or inadequately controlled
- Clear evidence that infective endocarditis may develop despite appropriate prophylaxis
- Recent case-control studies have failed to show a link between endocarditis and dental treatment
- Bacteraemia results from chewing, tooth brushing and similar activity. Although the absolute counts of bacteria in the blood are low, cumulatively this is greater bacterial challenge than tooth extraction and may account for many cases of endocarditis
- Recognition that animal data supporting previous guidance were obtained in models in which the risk of endocarditis was abnormally high
- If the benefit is small, the risk of anaphylaxis and antibiotic resistance become more significant. It has been estimated that death from anaphylaxis to penicillin cover is approximately 5 times more likely than death from endocarditis. (It is true severe anaphylaxis may follow a high oral dose of penicillin, but this should be largely preventable by careful history taking.)
- A feeling that endocarditis prophylaxis has become dominated by the principles of defensive medicine.

New guidance from the British Society for Antimicrobial Chemotherapy has been published and it proposes dramatic changes that have generated controversy. The Working Party recommend retaining prophylaxis for only the highest-risk patients. Others feel that the new guidance goes too far and risks deaths from endocarditis and its treatment. They point out that a lack of evidence of effectiveness does not mean that prophylaxis is ineffective. The differences between the two sets of guidance are highlighted in Table 27.2. Under these new recommendations fewer patients would require antibiotic cover, but the range of dental procedures requiring cover is increased.

The new guidance was reviewed by the National Institute for Clinical Excellence and their initial assessment of the evidence is similar but even more radical. They conclude that there is no evidence to support antibiotic prophylaxis in dentistry and recommend that it should cease. Prevention of endocarditis should rely on a high standard of oral health, the responsibility of both patient and professionals. It is expected that this guidance will be published in the National Formulary in March 2008. Prophylaxis is still recommended for gastrointestinal and urological procedures.

Table 27.2 Key differences between current and proposed endocarditis prophylaxis regimens

British Society for Antimicrobial Chemotherapy 1992 and British National Formulary current in 2007	British Society for Antimicrobial Chemotherapy 2006	National Institute for Clinical Excellence Provisional Guidance 2007
All risk patients covered	Cover for only the highest-risk patients or where mortality would be high	All at risk patients considered to be at equal risk
Based on the precautionary principle	Based on a risk/benefit calculation	Based on a risk/benefit/cost calculation
Intravenous dosing only for specific indications and antibiotics	Intravenous administration may be used as alternative to oral dosing if expedient	No cover required for dental procedures
No repeat doses of penicillin within 3–4 months	Sequential procedures should be a minimum of 14 days apart, repeat doses may be given, alternating amoxicillin and clindamycin	Reliance on improved oral health
	Less emphasis on data from animal models	
	Increased emphasis on oral hygiene and local measures	

CARDIAC PACEMAKERS

Pacemakers provide a stimulus to cardiac contraction when the normal rhythm is disturbed by disease of the sinoatrial node or conducting tissues as a result, for example, of myocardial infarction.

Any ultrasonic scaler or electrosurgical equipment that interferes with pacemaker function should be avoided, but pulp testers are safe and there is no indication for antibiotic prophylaxis.

DYSRHYTHMIAS

Disorders of heart rhythm are a complex variety of disorders some of which may be precipitated by anxiety, alcohol, epinephrine, cocaine and other influences. Patients with treated or untreated ischaemic heart disease are particularly susceptible. Dysrhythmias are usually symptomless but can also underlie acute symptoms by lowering cardiac output to cause breathlessness, palpitations, syncope or even left ventricular failure. By contrast, atrial fibrillation can, in other cases, be symptomless and can be resistant to treatment, while ventricular fibrillation can be fatal within a few minutes of its onset.

Pacemakers are implanted electronic devices which detect and control excessively high or low heart rates. Implantable cardioverter defibrillators are highly effective in controlling life-threatening dysrhythmias. A variety of electromagnetic and electronic devices, including MRI, can interfere with the function of these devices, particularly if these devices are powerful and the patient is in close proximity to them. Drug treatment of dysrhythmias is complex as suggested by the many drugs available for this purpose. In some cases treatment is little more than by trial and error.

KAWASAKI'S DISEASE (MUCOCUTANEOUS LYMPH NODE SYNDROME)

Now that rheumatic carditis has become rare in the West, congenital heart disease and Kawasaki's disease are the most important cardiac diseases of infancy.

As noted earlier (Ch. 12), Kawasaki's disease is also the only form of serious heart disease with specific orofacial manifestations, namely mucositis and cervical lymphadenopathy. Cardiac damage is the result of vasculitis which may result in coronary artery aneurysm formation, myocardial infarction and a mortality of over 5%.

Aspirin (80–100 mg/kg daily) has been the standby of treatment, but more effective if supplemented with intravenous gammaglobulin.

Before certain types of dental surgery (Appendix 27.1), antibiotic prophylaxis should be given when there is any evidence of congenital or a history of Kawasaki's disease.

SUGGESTED FURTHER READING

Aitken C, Cannell H, Sefton AM et al 1995 Comparative efficacy of oral doses of clindamycin and erythromycin in the prevention of bacteraemia. Br Dent J 178:418–422
Blinder D, Shemesh J, Taicher S 1996 Electrocardiographic changes in cardiac patients undergoing dental extractions under local anaesthesia. J Oral Maxillofac Surg 54:162–165

Campbell JH, Huizinga PJ, Rodriguez JP et al 1996 Incidence and significance of cardiac arrythmia in geriatric oral surgery patients. Oral Surg Oral Med Oral Pathol Oral Radiol Endod 82:42–46
Durack DT 1995 Prevention of infective endocarditis. N Engl J Med 332:38–45

Findler M, Galili D, Meidan Z et al 1993 Dental treatment in very high risk patients with active ischaemic heart disease. Oral Surg Oral Med Oral Pathol 76:298–300

Findler M, Mazor Z, Galili D, Garfunkel AA 1993 Dental treatment in a patient with malignant pheochromocytoma and severe uncontrolled high blood pressure. Oral Surg Oral Med Oral Pathol 75:290–291

Glick M 1995 Intravenous drug abusers: a consideration for infective endocarditis in dentistry? Oral Surg Oral Med Oral Pathol 80:125

Gould FK, Elliot TSJ, Foweraker J et al 2006 Guidelines for the prevention of endocarditis: report of the Working Party of the British Society for Antimicrobial Chemotherapy. J Antimicrob Chemother 57:1035–1042

Lockhart PB 1996 An analysis of bacteremias during dental extractions. Arch Int Med 156:513–520

Mattila KJ, Valtonen VV, Neiminen M, Huttunen JK 1995 Dental infection and the risk of new coronary events: prospective study of patients with documented coronary artery disease. Clin Infect Dis 20:588–592

Rahn R, Schneider S, Diehl O et al 1995 Preventing post-treatment bacteremia. JADA 126:1145–1148

Smith AJ, Adams D 1993 The dental status and attitudes of patients at risk from infective endocarditis. Br Dent J 174:59–64

Strom BL, Abrutyn E, Berlin JA et al 1998 Dental and cardiac risk factors for infective endocarditis. Ann Intern Med 729:761–769

Uyemura MC 1995 Antibiotic prophylaxis for medical and dental procedures. Postgrad Med 98:137–152

Van der Meer JTM, van Wilk W, Thompson J et al 1992 Awareness of need and actual use of prophylaxis: lack of patient compliance in the prevention of bacterial endocarditis. J Antimicrob Chemother 29:187–194

Working Party of the British Society for Antimicrobial Chemotherapy 1992 Antibiotic prophylaxis of infective endocarditis. Lancet 339:1292–1293

APPENDIX 27.1

Antibiotic prophylaxis of infective endocarditis for dental patients

Recommendations from the British Society for Antimicrobial Chemotherapy (1992) and British National Formulary 2007

Prophylaxis is recommended for dental extractions, scaling or periodontal surgery. Prophylaxis is not considered necessary for other procedures, such as orthodontic manipulations, unless there is likely to be significant damage to the gingival margins.

Under local or no anaesthesia	Under general anaesthesia
• Patients not allergic to the penicillins and who have not received penicillin more than once in the previous month • Patient not allergic to the penicillins, who have not received penicillin more than once in the previous month and who are not special risk patients (see below)	• Patients not allergic to penicillins or who have not received penicillin more than once in the previous month
Amoxycillin	**Amoxycillin**
Adults 3g single oral dose taken under supervision, 1 hour before dental procedure	*Adults* 1g intravenously *or* 1g in 2.5ml 1% lidocaine hydrochloride intramuscularly *or* 3g orally 4 hours before induction then 3g orally as soon as possible after recovery
Children 5–10 years Half adult dose	*Children 5–10 years* Half adult dose
Children under 5 years Quarter adult dose	*Children under 5 years* Quarter adult dose *or* 3g orally plus oral probenicid 1g, 4 hours before procedure
Patients allergic to penicillin or who have received more than a single dose of penicillin in the previous month	Patients allergic to penicillin or who have received more than a single dose of penicillin in the previous month
Clindamycin	See special risk below
Adults 600mg single oral dose taken under supervision, 1 hour before dental procedure	
Children 5–10 years Half adult dose	
Children under 5 years Quarter adult dose	

Antibiotic prophylaxis may be supplemented with chlorhexidine gluconate gel 1% applied to the gingival margins.

Special risk patients who should be referred to hospital

1. Patients who have had a previous attack of infective endocarditis (whether or not general anaesthesia is to be given) and patients with prosthetic valves requiring a general anaesthetic but not allergic to penicillin.
   Adult amoxycillin 1 g i/v or i/m plus gentamicin 120 mg i/v or i/m at induction + 500 mg 6 hours later
   Children 5–10 years amoxycillin half adult dose plus gentamicin 2 mg/kg
   Children under 5 years amoxycillin quarter adult dose plus gentamicin 2 mg/kg
2. Similar patients who are allergic to penicillins or who have received penicillins in the last month
   either vancomycin i/v, 1 g given over at least 100 minutes, then i/v *gentamicin* 120 mg at induction or 15 minutes before dental procedure
   Children under 10 years vancomycin i/v 20 mg/kg, gentamicin 2 mg/kg
   or teicoplanin i/v, 400 mg plus *gentamicin* 120 mg at induction or 15 minutes before dental procedure.
   Children under 14 years teicoplanin 6 mg/kg, gentamicin 2 mg/kg
   or clindamycin i/v, 300 mg given over at least 10 minutes, at induction or 15 minutes before dental procedure, then oral or i/v *clindamycin* 150 mg, 6 hours later
   Children 5–10 years Half adult dose
   Children under 5 years Quarter adult dose
3. When general anaesthesia is required for a patient allergic to penicillin or when more than two doses of penicillin have been received in the last month.

Precautions	
1. When clindamycin is used, periodontal or other multistage procedures should not be repeated at intervals of less than 2 weeks.	2. Whatever antibiotic cover has been given, patients must be instructed to report to the dentist any mild, unexplained, febrile illness developing within 3 months of the dental treatment.

Provisional Recommendations from the National Institute for Clinical Excellence (NICE, 2007)

Antibiotic prophylaxis against infective endocarditis (IE) is not recommended for patients at risk of endocarditis undergoing:

- dental procedures.
- ear, nose and throat procedures
- upper respiratory tract procedures

Chlorhexidine mouthwash for prophylaxis against IE is not recommended for patients at risk of endocarditis undergoing dental procedures.

Patients at risk of endocarditis should achieve high standards of oral health, this requires:

- patient's responsibility
- professional facilitation
- preventive intervention.

Patients at risk of IE should receive clear and consistent information about infective endocarditis including the likely benefits and risks of antibiotic prophylaxis and the specific symptoms that may indicate a diagnosis of endocarditis.

Patients at risk should receive information about the importance of maintaining good oral health.

Patients at risk should be informed of potential risks of undergoing medical and non medical invasive procedures (such as body piercing or tattooing).

The most up to date guidance may be found at http://www.nice.org.uk/

Recommendations from the British Society for Antimicrobial Chemotherapy (2006)

It is recommended that the current practice of giving patients antibiotics before dental treatment be stopped for all patients with cardiac abnormalities, except those who have:

High-risk cardiac factors requiring prophylaxis

- Previous infective endocarditis
- Cardiac valve replacement surgery (mechanical or biological replacement valves)
- Surgically constructed systemic or pulmonary shunt or conduit

Dental procedures requiring antibiotic prophylaxis

- All dental procedures involving dento-gingival manipulation or endodontics

Prophylaxis regimen

Patients should concentrate on achieving and maintaining a high standard of oral and dental health. When possible dental treatment should be performed at least 14 days before cardiac surgery. If this is not possible, delay treatment at least 3 months post-surgery.

When cover is required:

Population	Age			Timing of dose before procedure
	>10 years	≤5 to >10 years	<5 years	
General	amoxicillin 3 g oral	amoxicillin 1.5 g oral	amoxicillin 750 mg oral	1 hour
Allergic to penicillin	clindamycin 600 mg oral	clindamycin 300 mg oral	clindamycin 150 mg oral	1 hour
Allergic to penicillin and unable to swallow capsules	azithromycin 500 mg oral	azithromycin 300 mg oral	azithromycin 200 mg oral	1 hour
Intravenous regimen expedient	amoxicillin 1 g i/v	amoxicillin 500 mg i/v	amoxicillin 250 mg i/v	Just before procedure or at induction of anaesthesia
Intravenous regimen expedient and allergic to penicillin	clindamycin 300 mg i/v[a]	clindamycin 150 mg i/v[a]	clindamycin 75 mg i/v[a]	

[a]Given over at least 10 minutes
Where a course of treatment involves several visits, the procedures should be performed at least 14 days apart. If this is not possible, the antibiotic regimen should alternate between amoxicillin and clindamycin. Expert advice should be sought if the patient is allergic to penicillin.
Preoperative mouthrinse with chlorhexidine gluconate 0.2% (10 ml for 1 minute)

Respiratory tract disease

ACUTE SINUSITIS → Summary p. 448

Maxillary sinusitis is a very common condition that often presents with pain suggesting a dental cause. However, almost all acute sinusitis is a sequela of viral infection, or rarely allergic inflammation, in the nasal passages and antra. Inflammation inhibits mucociliary clearance and oedema restricts sinus drainage by narrowing the ostium, raising the internal pressure.

Clinical features

There is sudden onset of pain from the sinus, often poorly localized, with tenderness of the overlying skin. Teeth with roots in or close to the antrum are painful on pressure. There is also nasal congestion, weakened sense of smell and sometimes referred pain to the ear. Fluid will often discharge into the nose on tilting the head or lying down and movement of the head worsens pain. Involvement of ethmoid or sphenoid sinuses is often perceived by patients as headache.

Management

Radiography of the sinuses provides little additional information in acute sinusitis. The diagnosis may usually be made on the history and examination. Computerised tomography is the method of choice if radiographs are required (Fig. 28.1).

Fig. 28.1 Acute sinusitis involving maxillary antrum and ethmoid sinuses, which are completely filled by oedematous sinus lining mucosa and inflammatory exudate. Courtesy Mr EJ Whaites.

Acute sinusitis is self-limiting. No active treatment may be required but nasal decongestants aid drainage, speed recovery and provide symptomatic relief. Many patients manage well with non-prescription steam inhalations containing menthol or eucalyptus oils. More severe cases benefit from ephedrine or oxymetazoline nose drops, but these should not be continued for more than 7 days.

Bacterial infection is uncommon and antibiotic treatment is not indicated, at least initially. Persistence or worsening of symptoms after 10 days or presence of pus suggest bacterial infection and development of chronic sinusitis. The usual organisms are aerobes such as *Strep. pneumoniae*, *H. influenzae* and beta-haemolytic streptococci. *Staph. aureus* is a more frequent isolate from the sphenoid sinus. These pathogens frequently show antimicrobial resistance and either high-dose amoxicillin or amoxicillin with clavulanic acid are appropriate empirical first-line drugs. If these fail, a pus sample for sensitivity testing must be obtained by puncture of the sinus.

Dental causes need to be excluded, but are present in only 5% of cases and are much more likely to be identified in chronic sinusitis (see below).

Though most cases resolve, sinusitis may become recurrent or chronic.

CHRONIC SINUSITIS → Summary p. 448

Chronic sinusitis may develop with or without a preceding acute sinusitis.

Fig. 28.2 Chronic sinusitis with an antral polyp, a localised area of mucosal oedema and thickening. Mucosal thickening or polyps on the floor of the antrum indicate a need to exclude dental and periodontal causes. Courtesy Dr S Connor. See also Fig. 28.3.

The clinical features are those of the acute disease but milder and without the generalised symptoms of upper respiratory tract viral infection. When pain is poorly localised, radiographic examination of the sinuses may reveal mucosal thickening or a fluid level. Computerised tomography is the examination of choice (Fig. 28.2), but the maxillary antrum is well visualised on panoramic tomography or occiptomental view.

Management

Dental causes are relatively frequent. The roots of the maxillary molar teeth lie close to or within the antrum. In some patients, the root apex perforates the cortex so that only mucous membrane covers it. The commonest dental causes of sinus inflammation are therefore periapical periodontitis from a non-vital molar, extraction, root treatment or severe periodontal disease. Non-dental causes include fractures. These are best identified by vitality testing, clinical examination and dental radiography.

When no dental cause is present, the bacteria are initially those found in acute sinusitis, but the flora gradually shift to an anaerobic population after 3 months. When dental infection is a factor, additional anaerobic oral bacteria such as *Prevotella* spp. and *Fusobacterium* spp. are found. Antibiotic treatment is only effective in conjunction with removal of the cause. Appropriate regimens are amoxicillin with clavulanic acid or a penicillin with metronidazole or as guided by culture and sensitivity.

If dental and other local causes are confidently excluded or treated and treatment fails, the patient should be referred to investigate the possibility of nasal predisposing causes such as polyps, allergic or fungal sinusitis.

Fungal sinusitis

Sinusitis results from inhalation of air-borne fungal spores. These would normally be cleared by mucociliary transport but become trapped if the transport is compromised by inflammation or if the spores germinate or trigger an allergic reaction. The causative fungi grow in soil and their spores are widespread in the enviroment.

The commonest type is a 'fungus ball' or mycetoma, a tangled mass of fungal hyphae bound together with mucous and inflammatory exudate. The ball may grow to fill the sinus and is commonly *Aspergillus* spp. Radiographic diagnosis is aided by the frequent presence of spotty mineralisation in the fungus ball.

Mycetoma formation has been associated with particles of zinc-containing root filling material. These presumably enter the sinus after root treatment and may sometimes be seen on radiographs. Inflammation from apical periodontitis would favour retention of spores and zinc encourages fungal growth.

In those mounting a florid allergic reaction to the fungus, the sinuses fill with thick secretions containing numerous eosinophils but fewer fungal hyphae. Some studies have suggested that almost all cases of chronic sinusitis refractory to treatment

are caused by these fungi, usually black pigmented species such as *Bipolaris* spp.

Mycetomas and allergic fungal sinusitis are treated by surgical removal of the fungus followed by topical or systemic antifungal treatment.

In the immunocompromised, the fungi may invade the sinus wall, cause rapid extensive destruction and often a fatal outcome. Such cases are caused by more virulent environmental fungi such as *Mucor* spp. and require aggressive surgical and antifungal treatment.

SURGICAL DAMAGE TO THE MAXILLARY ANTRUM

The floor of the antrum may be damaged during dental extractions which cause an oroantral communication. If the antrum is opened during an extraction, a displaced root or bacteria from the mouth can introduce infection. There is also damage to the ciliated lining and loss of normal mucociliary transport which carries foreign material out of the cavity. If sinusitis becomes established and the fistula has not been closed, the walls of the passage may become epithelialised and the opening becomes a permanent fistula.

Displacement of a root or tooth into the maxillary antrum

A whole tooth can be driven into the antrum if the tooth is conical and considerable upward force has been used. More frequently, a root is driven into the antrum when an attempt is made to dig it out via the socket, particularly when a thin antral floor extends down into the alveolar ridge.

Clinical features

Displacement of a tooth or root into the antrum can give rise to signs (Box 28.1), partly depending on the size of the opening.

Box 28.1   Signs suggesting a tooth or root displaced into the antrum

- The root or tooth suddenly disappears during the extraction
- Blowing the nose may force air into the mouth or cause frothing of blood from the socket
- The patient may notice air entering the mouth during swallowing, or fluid from the mouth escapes into the nose
- Bleeding from the nose on the affected side, occasionally
- Later, a salty taste or unpleasant discharge
- Facial pain if acute sinusitis develops
- Rarely, antral lining may prolapse into the mouth

Management

The position of the root or tooth should be confirmed. Sometimes it is still within the alveolar process or outside the antrum and between its lining and bony floor.

A periapical radiograph should be supplemented with occlusal intraoral views. If the root has been displaced far, antral views should be taken with the head in two different positions to determine whether the tooth is mobile.

A root displaced into the antrum usually causes sinusitis, but it may cause no more than mucosal thickening. Severe sinusitis is less common. The root should be removed from the antrum and any oroantral opening closed. Several measures are important (Box 28.2).

Box 28.2 Principles of management of a root displaced into the antrum

- Explain to the patient how the accident has happened and give the necessary reassurance
- Do not to try to retrieve the lost root immediately by digging through the socket opening and damaging the antral floor and lining further
- If a root or tooth has been displaced into the antrum, it should be removed by elective surgery (see below)
- If the tip of a root causes a minimal antral reaction or lies between the bony floor and the mucosal lining, removal may not be essential but there is a risk of infection later

---

After any acute sinusitis has been treated, the surgical approach depends on the position of the root and whether there is a wide oroantral opening. The usual method is to reflect a mucoperiosteal flap in the labiobuccal sulcus, open the antrum in the canine fossa (Caldwell–Luc approach) and find the root by endoscopy. The tooth or fragment may then be removable on a sucker nozzle small enough to prevent it from disappearing into the suction apparatus and being lost before confirmation of its removal.

Oroantral fistula

Rarely, the antrum may be accidentally opened during extractions if the antral floor is damaged. If the communication is not obvious, its presence may be verified by telling the patient to blow gently while blocking the nose by pinching the nostrils together. Air (detectable with a tuft of cotton wool held in tweezers), blood, pus, or mucus will then be expelled from the opening into the mouth. Occasionally, an opening may be blocked by prolapsed lining or antral polyp which is purplish red (Fig. 28.3) and, if the opening is large enough, it may sometimes be pushed gently back into the antrum, thus confirming its origin. Alternatively, a silver probe can be gently insinuated beside the mass into the antral cavity to detect the opening.

Epithelialisation of the communication forms a fistula, which is thereby prevented from healing spontaneously. Usually, a large oroantral fistula gives adequate drainage, but a pinhole fistula blocks drainage and is often associated with recurrent attacks of sinusitis. If the patient is not seen until late after the accident, there is typically chronic antral infection, persistent discharge and proliferation of granulation tissue.

Fig. 28.3 Antral polyp. A polyp of inflamed antral mucosa has prolapsed through an oroantral fistula left untreated after the extraction of an upper first permanent molar.

The inflamed antral lining is usually much thickened and polyps may fill part of the cavity.

Principles of management are summarised in Box 28.3.

Box 28.3 Principles of management of an oroantral communication

The communication (non-epithelialised)

- Reflect a mucoperiosteal flap and suture it to give an air-tight seal over the opening

The established fistula (epithelialised communication) with infection

- Control chronic sinusitis by removal of any polyps, usually via a Caldwell–Luc approach, or through the oral opening if the fistula is sufficiently large
- Excise the entire epithelialised fistula
- Close the opening by reflecting a mucoperiosteal flap over it

Postoperatively

- Give penicillin for 5 days and a 10-day course of decongestant nose drops and inhalations
- Warn the patient against blowing the nose

Aspiration of a tooth, root or instrument

A tooth or root can rarely slip from extraction forceps but is more frequently swallowed than inhaled. The patient should be reassured but should be sent for a chest radiograph and, if necessary, bronchoscopy. Small instruments such as reamers can also occasionally be inhaled (Fig. 28.4).

If left, a tooth in a bronchus can cause collapse of the related lobe and a lung abscess.

COMMON VIRAL UPPER RESPIRATORY TRACT INFECTIONS ('COLDS')

Colds often precede sinusitis. They are a contraindication to general anaesthesia. Transmission to the dentist is also a hazard.

Fig. 28.4 Radiograph of the chest used to localise an inhaled reamer.

Fig. 28.5 **Sarcoidosis.** Microscopically, the granulomas are compact with heavy peripheral lymphocytic infiltrate. However, they are not distinguishable by microscopy alone from other granulomatous diseases such as tuberculosis.

TUBERCULOSIS

Dentists and dental personnel in the UK should all have received a BCG vaccination and be immune to tuberculosis, though occasional individuals respond poorly. A non-immune dentist is at significant risk from acquiring tuberculosis from such patients, in some of whom the infection is unsuspected or dismissed as 'smokers' cough'. This can be particularly dangerous if the mycobacteria are multiply drug-resistant.

Rigorous infection control must therefore be maintained, particularly now that the incidence of tuberculosis is rising.

Dental aspects

Tuberculous cervical lymphadenopathy is frequently due to non-tuberculous mycobacteria and can affect otherwise healthy children; it is discussed in Chapter 26. Rarely, tuberculous infection of extraction sockets and tuberculous lymphadenopathy have been transmitted to patients by an infected dentist. In the USA, HIV-positive dental staff have acquired the infection from patients and some have died as a consequence.

Open pulmonary tuberculosis can occasionally cause lingual ulceration as a result of coughed-up mycobacteria in the sputum and, rarely, the diagnosis of pulmonary tuberculosis has been made as a result of a biopsy of such a lesion (Ch. 12). Tuberculous parotitis is uncommon but can rarely be seen in immunocompetent persons. After treatment of a tuberculous patient, equipment must be rigorously disinfected.

SARCOIDOSIS → Summaries pp. 316, 324, 409

Sarcoidosis is a chronic disease of unknown cause, in which granulomas form, particularly in the the hilar nodes of the lungs, but also in many other sites. The HSP(+2437)-C allele appears to confer susceptibility.

The mean age of patients is about 40 years. Many minor abnormalities of immune responses, such as anergy to some antigens such as tuberculin and, frequently, hypergammaglobulinaemia, are detectable, but patients are not unusually susceptible to infection. Almost any tissue can be affected. Common effects include fever, loss of weight, fatigue, breathlessness, cough and arthralgia. Eye lesions can lead to blindness. Erythema nodosum is the most common skin lesion. Hypercaldaemia can lead to nephrocalcinosis. The mortality rate is 10–12%.

Pathology

Sarcoid granulomas are non-caseating, contain multinucleate giant cells and are surrounded by lymphocytes (Fig. 28.5). Th1 and Th2 cytokines are released in the lungs and may be important in production of the granulomas. In an oral biopsy, sarcoid granulomas have to be distinguished from other granulomatous diseases (Box 28.4). Sarcoidosis can develop as a consequence of restored immunological function after treatment of HIV infection with HAART and appears to result from the proliferation of CD4 lymphocytes. Sarcoidosis can also develop after treatment with interferon-alpha.

> **Box 28.4   Important granulomatous diseases**
>
> **Infections**
> - Tuberculosis and non-tuberculous mycobacterioses
> - Syphilis
> - Systemic mycoses
> - Cat-scratch disease
> - Toxoplasmosis
>
> **Reactive**
> - Foreign body reactions
>
> **Unknown causes**
> - Sarcoidosis
> - Crohn's disease
> - Melkersson–Rosenthal syndrome
> - Cheilitis glandularis
> - Orofacial granulomatosis
> - Wegener's granulomatosis

Management

Diagnosis depends on chest radiograpy (Fig. 28.6) with combined clinical and laboratory findings, particularly signs of pulmonary involvement and biopsy of affected tissue. Labial gland biopsy showing granulomas may greatly facilitate diagnosis. In the active stages of the disease, plasma levels of angiotensin converting enzyme (ACE) are frequently raised. Also, as mentioned above, there is typically anergy to tuberculin. A strongly positive Mantoux reaction therefore virtually excludes sarcoidosis.

Treatment with systemic corticosteroids is indicated for pulmonary fibrosis, cerebral lesions or hypercalcaemia, but is not indicated for mild symptoms. Infliximab, a TNF-alpha-inhibitor, is reportedly effective for severe sarcoidosis and sarcoid uveitis. Lung transplantation is required for end-stage pulmonary sarcoidosis, but the disease recurs in the transplants in about 50%.

Dental aspects

Oral lesions, usually painless swellings, are a recognised manifestation. The most frequently affected sites are the gingivae (Fig. 28.7), lips, palate and buccal mucosa. Oral lesions, usually

Fig. 28.7   Sarcoidosis. Gingival swelling is not clinically distinguishable from several other possible causes, but biopsy showed granuloma formation.

Fig. 28.8   Sarcoidosis of a salivary gland. There is a scattered lymphoplasmacytic infiltrate and granulomas are scattered through the tissue. The granuloma contains several large, multinucleate giant cells (arrowed).

Fig. 28.6   Sarcoidosis. Prominent hilar lymphadenopathy is the main radiological finding, though granuloma formation may be widespread.

painless swellings, may be seen. In over 50% of patients with bilateral hilar lymphadenopathy, biopsy of a labial salivary gland shows typical granulomas and is a valuable, minimally invasive diagnostic aid (Fig. 28.8). Gingival swelling showing granulomas on biopsy occasionally precedes other manifestations of sarcoidosis. In other cases, no systemic granulomatous disease develops and the diagnosis is then 'orofacial granulomatosis', as discussed in the next chapter.

Clinical involvement of major salivary glands is uncommon but can cause tumour-like swellings. Parotid swelling due to sarcoidosis, with xerostomia, uveitis and, often, facial palsy is known as *Heerfordt's syndrome*. Enlargement of major salivary glands is occasionally the first manifestation of sarcoidosis; Mikulicz disease is a term that has been given to bilateral swelling of the salivary and lacrimal glands that can be a rare manifestation of sarcoidosis (Fig. 28.9), but in the first patient in whom it was described, the cause appears to have been a MALT lymphoma (Ch. 22).

CHRONIC OBSTRUCTIVE AIRWAYS DISEASE (COAD)

Chronic obstructive airways disease is typically caused by smoking and recurrent respiratory infections. Patients are

Fig. 28.9 Bilateral parotid swelling in a case of sarcoidosis.

hypoxic and may be cyanotic. COAD is a contraindication to intravenous sedation because of its respiratory depressant effect and to general anaesthesia except in hospital.

ASTHMA

Asthma is a common respiratory disease characterised by paroxysmal wheezing on expiration due to intermittent bronchospasm. Cough and variable degrees of dyspnoea may be associated. Many cases are mild with only minor wheezing but, at the opposite extreme, it can be a potentially lethal disease which accounts for at least 2500 deaths a year.

Asthma is the main type of atopic disease (Ch. 25), but only so-called extrinsic asthma is a response to allergens such as house-dust mites, feathers or animal dander and is IgE mediated. Intrinsic asthma is non-allergic and is a result of mast cell degranulation and a hyperresponsive airway. Attacks of either types of asthma can be triggered by inhaled irritants such as tobacco smoke, respiratory infections, exercise and food additives. Emotional stress can also precipitate episodes; nevertheless, such stress by causing catecholamine release can sometimes provide a relief. A famous phsician at the turn of the century was temporarily cured of his asthma when the brakes of his car failed and it went out of control.

Management is by identification and avoidance of allergens and respiratory irritants. Many patients respond well to beta-2 agonists such as salbutamol. Leukotriene receptor antagonists may also be helpful. For more severe cases, inhaled or systemic corticosteroids may be required. The monoclonal antibody, omalizumab, lowers total IgE serum levels and lessens symptoms of extrinsic asthma.

The mortality from asthma is mainly due to undertreatment such as reluctance to give corticosteroids

Dental aspects

Inhaled corticosteroids can precipitate oropharyngeal thrush and systemic cortisteroid therapy can bring its well-recognised problems, particularly abnormal susceptibility to infection, to dental management (Ch. 31).

Rarely, acute severe asthma can precipitate an emergency in the dental surgery and calls for immediate attention. It can progress to the potentially lethal condition of *status asthmaticus* (Ch. 36). Sensitivity to a variety of drugs is another possible problem.

MIDLINE GRANULOMA SYNDROMES

These formerly ill-defined diseases can cause variable degrees of destruction of the central facial tissues and a fatal outcome as their main features.

They start in the upper respiratory tract and are not clinically distinguishable in their early stages. They are now recognised to result from either Wegener's granulomatosis or a peripheral (nasopharyngeal) T- or NK-cell lymphoma (Ch. 22).

Wegener's granulomatosis → Summary p. 324

Wegener's granulomatosis is a potentially lethal but uncommon systemic vasculitis of unknown cause with features summarised in Box 28.5. It is possible that the vasculitis is an anomalous immune reaction to an infection or environmental agent (such as organic solvents and other toxic industrial waste) but, in most cases, no cause is identifiable. There is a strong genetic association with major histocompatibility genes that modulate immune responses.

Box 28.5 Wegener's granulomatosis: key features

- Granulomatous inflammation of nasal tract
- Cavitation of the lungs
- Potentially fatal glomerulonephritis
- Proliferative gingivitis occasionally
- Oral mucosal ulceration occasionally
- Antineutrophil cytoplasmic antibodies (ANCAs) typically present
- Histologically, granulomatous inflammation with giant cells and vasculitis

---

The pathogenesis is now better understood. Circulating antibodies ('antineutrophil cytoplasmic antibodies' or ANCA) to the neutrophil granule proteinase, proteinase 3, bind to the enzyme when it is secreted onto the surface of neutrophils in an inflammatory focus or during emigration through vessel walls. The antibody activates the neutrophil and triggers a positive feedback loop of acute inflammation. ANCA-producing autoreactive B cells migrate into granulomas in the lesion and produce the antibody locally to further sustain the inflammation.

Clinically, granulomatous inflammation of the nasal tissues and discharge is typically the first sign and can result in destruction of the nasal septum and a saddle nose deformity. A retrospective examination of his medical records suggests that Heinrich Hertz[1] died from this disease.

Pathology

Biopsy of affected gingivae typically shows a finely nodular surface, epithelial proliferation, a dense inflammatory infiltrate and collections of giant cells (Figs 28.10 and 28.11). In deeper tissues, vasculitis with destruction of small arteries is seen, but granulomas are frequently inconspicuous.

Management

The diagnosis must be established by biopsy at the earliest possible moment and may be possible as a result of the gingival

---

[1]Hertz, by discovering electromagnetic (radio) waves and the photoelectric effect in the 1880s, made possible the development of radio, radar and television and, as a result, has had as much influence on the present-day world as any other single person.

Fig. 28.10 **Wegener's granulomatosis.** There is epithelial hyperplasia with deeply penetrating irregular broad rete processes. In the connective tissue, there is a dense mixed, inflammatory infiltrate in which eosinophils are prominent and there are occasional scattered giant cells.

Fig. 28.11 **Wegener's granulomatosis.** Gingival biopsy showing clusters of giant cells.

changes. Detection of antineutrophil cytoplasmic antibodies (ANCA) is valuable and these are present in approximately 85% of cases. Detection of antibodies directed against proteinase 3 (PR3) is highly specific. These autoantibodies are valuable for distinguishing Wegener's granulomatosis from nasopharyngeal lymphoma when it presents a similar clinical picture and, frequently, arteritis-like changes histologically.

Examination of the nasopharynx, chest radiographs and renal function tests should also be carried out. Haematuria suggests glomerulonephritis and a poor prognosis. Treatment is frequently with cyclophosphamide and corticosteroids; if given early this may be life-saving. Rituximab is probably more effective and less toxic for control of severe treatment-refractory

Fig. 28.12 **Wegener's granulomatosis.** There is irregular gingival hyperplasia affecting a few teeth and redness extending the full depth of the attached gingiva. The distribution is not related to plaque.

disease, but there have also been reports of lack of efficacy. Also under consideration are etanercept and infliximab to achieve tumour necrosis factor alpha blockade.

Dental aspects

Occasionally, a characteristic proliferative gingivitis is the first sign. The changes initially resemble pregnancy gingivitis, but the gingivae become swollen with a granular surface and dusky or bright red ('strawberry gums' – Fig. 28.12). Biopsy of such lesions can occasionally lead to exceptionally early diagnosis with the chance of a cure. The changes can be widespread or patchy. Alternatively, superficial mucosal ulceration can be widespread but appears at a later stage. Parotitis is an uncommon early manifestation of Wegener's granulomatosis.

Nasopharyngeal T- and NK-cell lymphomas

These are rare causes of midline granuloma syndrome but also start in the upper respiratory tract. They are discussed here because, in their early stages, they can be indistinguishable clinically from Wegener's granulomatosis. However, they are ANCA negative.

Key features are shown in Box 28.6.

Box 28.6 **Nasopharyneal T-cell lymphoma: key features**

- Onset typically indistinguishable from Wegener's granulomatosis
- Downward extension may cause central ulceration or necrosis of the palate enabling early diagnosis
- Histologically, the cellular picture is pleomorphic and pseudo-inflammatory, but damage to blood vessels mimics vasculitis
- T-cell or NK-cell markers help to confirm the diagnosis
- Spread of disease is similar to that of other lymphomas and, usually, a fatal outcome
- Spread may be limited or delayed by radiotherapy

If neglected, nasopharyngeal lymphomas can cause extensive destruction of the centre of the face to the extent that, in the past particularly, the cranial cavity could be opened to the exterior.

Histological diagnosis is difficult as these lymphomas are cellularly pleomorphic and show pseudo-inflammatory changes. The tumour lymphocytes attack blood vessels and thus simulate vasculitis, but T- or NK-cell markers can facilitate diagnosis. Secondary inflammation may also obscure the lymphoma cells, so that several biopsies may be required. Granulomas are not a feature.

In the past, death could result from infection secondary to massive facial necrosis. Usually now, death results from dissemination of the lymphoma, but this may be delayed by radiotherapy.

Some of these tumours have a slow and remittent course but eventually disseminate. The main principles of treatment are radiotherapy, usually with combination chemotherapy.

Dental aspects

Extension of the disease through the palate can cause swelling and ulceration as a presenting feature. A small central palatal ulcer can extend until the whole of the palate becomes necrotic and the anterior teeth can rarely become loosened. A deep biopsy is necessary to obtain lesional tissue not obscured by necrosis.

CARCINOMA OF THE ANTRUM

Carcinoma of the antrum is rare. As with cancer of the mouth, pain is not an early symptom. Later, anaesthesia in the distribution of any sensory nerves involved is almost as common as pain.

Oral and dental symptoms from carcinoma of the antrum result from involvement of its floor. This may cause pain in the teeth or under a denture. As the disease advances, teeth may become loose and a swelling becomes obvious (Fig. 28.13).

Radiographs should be taken for signs of destruction of the bony antral walls. It is a general rule that an opaque maxillary antrum in a person over 40 years of age without obvious underlying dental or nasal disease should have the antrum explored. If a mass is found, biopsy must be carried out.

MYCOPLASMAL (PRIMARY ATYPICAL) PNEUMONIA

Mycoplasmal pneumonia occasionally triggers bullous erythema multiforme (Ch. 13).

CYSTIC FIBROSIS (MUCOVISCIDOSIS)

In this disease, obstruction of the airways by the viscid sputum causes recurrent respiratory infections in childhood.

Fig. 28.13 Antral carcinoma. Occasionally, an antral carcinoma will present intraorally, either after eroding the maxilla or through an extraction socket.

Development and eruption of the teeth may be delayed and hypoplastic defects may be seen. Salivary gland swelling is another possible effect. Administration of tetracycline, for recurrent chest infections, during dental development may cause staining of teeth.

SLEEP APNOEA SYNDROME

In sleep apnoea syndrome, there is recurrent spontaneous obstruction of the airway during sleep. In the middle-aged population approximately 2–4% are affected. Obese males, in particular, are affected and suffer daytime drowsiness and difficulty in concentrating (with a consequently raised risk of road traffic accidents) and impaired work performance. Depression and irritability may be associated. In the longer term, there is a significantly raised risk of hypertension, ischaemic heart disease and stroke.

During sleep there are snoring and breathing pauses. The cause is recurrent occlusion at the back of the throat, partly due to relaxation of the palatoglossus and genioglossus which, during wakefulness, maintain the patency of the airway. Because of the apnoea there is lowered oxygen saturation and risk of dysrhythmias.

Management

Medical treatment involves weight loss and avoiding evening alcohol and sedatives. Intraoral appliances that hold the mandible 2–5 mm anteriorly can be worn at night. These increase the size of the airway by pulling the soft palate forward; long-term compliance is good and they are highly effective in mild obstructive sleep apnoea. Trials have found that oral appliances

are as effective for improving oxygenation as continuous positive airways pressure, delivered by a nasal mask, but only the latter has been shown to improve mortality in the long term. An intraoral appliance to provide mandibular protrusion is probably as effective as drastic surgical intervention.

In the event that the mandible cannot be held sufficiently forward with an appliance and pressure ventilation fails, surgery may be required. Orthognathic surgery may help by advancing the facial skeleton and hyoid bone to expand the airway. This may need to be combined with uvulopalatopharyngoplasty if there is both oro- and hypopharyngeal obstruction. This may seem drastic, but failure to control symptoms may necessitate a tracheostomy, which can bring other complications.

BRONCHOGENIC CARCINOMA

Carcinoma of the lung is the most common cancer in the Western world. The causative role of cigarette smoking was confirmed statistically in a well-designed study in Nazi Germany in the 1940s and later, in Britain, by Doll and Bradford Hill.

Carcinoma of the lung was predominantly a disease of men but, as a result of more smoking by women, in the USA, the mortality rate for women has almost equalled that of men ('unwanted equality').

Clinically, recurrent cough is the most common feature and often ignored as 'smoker's cough'. Later manifestaions include haemoptysis, chest pain and dyspnoea. Loss of weight and anorexia may also develop. The diagnosis is confirmed by radiography, CT and MRI, sputum cytology, bronchoscopy and endoscopic biopsy.

Only about 25% of patients are suitable for surgery. Treatment is frequently therefore by radiotherapy; chemotherapy is usually ineffective. The 5-year survival rate for early cases treated by surgery is 24%. The overall 5-year survival rate is 8%.

Dental aspects

Management depends greatly upon the stage of the cancer when the patient is seen. In the early stages, dental treatment can be carried out as usual but conscious sedation should preferably be avoided. Abnormal sensitivity to muscle relaxants may make general anaesthesia hazardous. Time should not be spent on elaborate restorations intended to last for years. In the later stages, minimal 'rescue' dental treatment is all that can be done.

Metastases to the jaw or cervical lymph nodes are usually a late manifestation and an uncommon manifestation is diffuse pigmentation of the soft palate.

Lung cancer is incidentally relatively common in dental technicians, probably as a result of smoking or dust inhalation.

SUGGESTED FURTHER READING

Abrahams JJ, Glassberg RM 1996 Dental disease: a frequently unrecognised cause of dental sinus abnormalities? AJR 166:1219–1223

Bartlett JGA 1996 Antibiotic selection in sinusitis. Arch Otolaryngol Head Neck Surg 122:422–423

Benatar SR 1994 Sarcoidosis. Medicine Int 22:43–50

Brook I 2005 Microbiology and antimicrobial management of sinusitis. J Laryngol Otol 119:251–258

Brook I, Frazier EH, Gher ME 1996 Microbiology of periapical abscesses and associated maxillary sinusitis. J Periodontol 67:608–610

Calverley PMA 1995 Management of COPD. Medicine UK 23:308–312

Cawson RA 1965 Gingival changes in Wegener's granulomatosis. Br Dent J 118:30–32

Davies KJ, Herbert A-M, Westmoreland D, Bagg J 1994 Seroepidemiological study of respiratory virus infections among dental surgeons. Br Dent J 176:262–263

Davies PDO 1995 Tuberculosis. Medicine UK 23:325–332

Devaney KO, Travis WD, Hoffman G, Leavitt R, Lebovics R, Fauci AS 1990 Interpretation of head and neck biopsies in Wegener's granulomatosis. A pathologic study of 126 biopsies in 70 patients. Am J Surg Pathol 14:555–564

Eufinger H, Machtens E, Akuamoa-Boateng E 1992 Oral manifestations of Wegener's granulomatosis. Int J Oral Maxillofac Surg 21:50–53

Fernald GW, Roberts MW, Boat TF 1990 Cystic fibrosis: a current review. Pediatr Dent 12:72–78

Friedlander AH, Friedlander IK, Pogrel MA 2000 Dentistry's role in the diagnosis and co-management of patients with sleep apnoea/hypopnoea syndrome. Br Dent J 189:76-80

Harrison B 1995 Acute severe asthma in adults. Medicine UK 23:298–301

Hoffman GS, Kerr GS, Leavitt RY et al 1992 Wegener granulomatosis: an analysis of 158 patients. Ann Intern Med 116:488–498

John CJ 1995 Pulmonary sarcoidosis. Medicine UK 23:405–408

Kretzschmar DP, Kretzschmar JL 2003 Rhinosinusitis: review from a dental perspective. Oral Surg 96:128–135

Landau L 1995 Cystic fibrosis. Medicine UK 23:400–404

Mahaney MC 1986 Delayed dental development and pulmonary disease in children with cystic fibrosis. Arch Oral Biol 31:363–367

Nachbar FN, Classen V, Nachbar T et al 1996 Orificial tuberculosis detection by polymerase chain reaction. Br J Dermatol 135:106–109

Parsons E, Seymour RA, Macleod RI et al 1992 Wegener's granulomatosis. A distinct gingival lesion. J Clin Periodontol 19:64–66

Gastrointestinal and liver disease

Though the mouth is the entry to the gastrointestinal tract, few gastrointestinal diseases directly affect the oral cavity.

GASTRO-OESOPHAGEAL REFLUX AND GASTRIC REGURGITATION

Gastro-oesophageal reflux ('heart burn') is a common type of dyspepsia. Smoking, excessive alcohol consumption, obesity, frequent stooping and over-large meals are frequent precipitating factors. If allowed to persist, damage to the oesophageal lining can result, but protein pump inhibitors, such as omeprazole, are highly effective in controlling it. Since there is no significant regurgitation of gastric acid there are no adverse dental effects. By contrast, chronic vomiting of gastric acid contents, due to such causes as hypertrophic pyloric stenosis, can lead to erosion of the palatal aspect of the anterior teeth particularly (Fig. 29.1). This type of dental erosion is an important diagnostic sign of self-induced vomiting in bulimia.

Fig. 29.1 Erosion of the palatal surfaces of the upper teeth due to repeated vomiting.

COELIAC DISEASE

Coeliac disease is one of the most common genetic disorders and is an important cause of malabsorption. It is due to a form of hypersensitivity to gluten in flour. The disease is frequently asymptomatic and it may not be recognised until adult life as a result of its complications. It can also have a great variety of effects. In addition to malabsorption, stunting of growth, fatty diarrhoea and abdominal pain or discomfort are typical consequences. The malabsorption can lead to vitamin and mineral deficiencies resulting in anaemia or bleeding tendencies, as discussed below.

Dental aspects

Anaemia can have a variety of oral effects such as glossitis or recurrent aphthae as discussed in Chapter 22. Up to 5% of patients with coeliac disease may have recurrent aphthae, even in the absence of anaemia.

CROHN'S DISEASE → Summaries pp. 324, 409

Crohn's disease and ulcerative colitis are types of inflammatory bowel disease which may have common symptoms but which are otherwise distinct entities. Crohn's disease is of unknown aetiology. It most frequently affects the ileocaecal region, causing thickening and ulceration. Symptoms vary with the severity of the disease, but effects can include abdominal pain, variable constipation or diarrhoea and, sometimes, obstruction and malabsorption. Repeated bowel resections may ultimately be needed. Joint pain can also be troublesome.

Dental aspects

Cobblestone mucosal swelling and ulceration (Figs 29.2–29.4), particularly when associated with abdominal symptoms, can lead to the diagnosis of Crohn's disease (Box 29.1). Occasionally, oral lesions precede gastrointestinal symptoms by a long period.

Fig. 29.2 Crohn's disease. Soft nodular hyperplasia of the oral mucosa is a typical feature and, in this case, was associated with facial swelling and intermittent diarrhoea.

Fig. 29.3 Crohn's disease. Gross labial swelling and intraoral mucosal proliferation with typical histological changes led to the finding of extensive intestinal involvement.

Fig. 29.4 Crohn's disease. The gingivae are hyperplastic and irregular and erythematous. These changes are obvious, but more subtle signs are easily missed. The appearances are identical to those in sarcoidosis in the gingivae.

Fig. 29.5 Crohn's disease. The granulomas are frequently isolated and loose in texture with scanty peripheral lymphocytic infiltrate, as here.

Box 29.1   Typical orofacial features of Crohn's disease

- Diffuse soft or tense swelling of the lips, or mucosal thickening
- Cobblestone thickening of the buccal mucosa, with fissuring and hyperplastic folds
- Gingivae may be erythematous and swollen
- Sometimes, painful mucosal ulcers, linear or resembling aphthae
- Mucosal tags in sulcuses sometimes present
- Glossitis due to iron, folate or vitamin B_{12} deficiency can result from malabsorption

---

Histologically, there is formation of non-caseating granulomas resembling those in the intestine. The granulomas are typically small, loose and with few multinucleate giant cells. They are often deep in the corium and may be difficult to find. A biopsy may need to extend unusually deeply (Figs 29.5–29.7). In the absence of symptoms, sigmoidoscopy and colonoscopy will show the degree of bowel involvement. However, in the absence of symptoms, many gastroenterologists prefer to leave patients in peace until they should develop because of the

Fig. 29.6 Crohn's disease. The granulomas are frequently deep in the mucosa and widely dispersed. Here granulomas are present in muscle, showing the importance of adequate biopsy depth.

Fig. 29.8 Orofacial granulomatosis. There is conspicuous swelling of the upper lip with eversion of the vermilion border. The lip is thickened and tense.

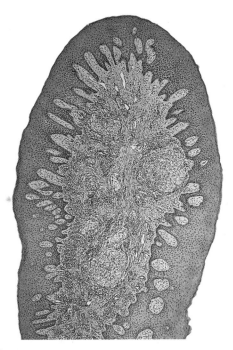

Fig. 29.7 Crohn's disease. A hyperplastic tag of gingiva contains several large round granulomas.

Fig. 29.9 Orofacial granulomatosis. Below the epithelium is a patchy inflammatory infiltrate and scattered granulomas containing large multinucleate giant cells.

lack of entirely satisfactory treatment even when symptoms develop. Under such circumstances, mucosal Crohn-type granulomas may be mistaken, for a time at least, for orofacial granulomatosis (see below).

Management

Oral symptoms may resolve when intestinal Crohn's disease is controlled with, for example corticosteroids, sulfasalazine or mesalazine. Alternatively, oral lesions may respond to oral sulfasalazine or to intralesional injections of a corticosteroid.

OROFACIAL GRANULOMATOSIS → Summaries pp. 324, 409

The term orofacial granulomatosis applies to swellings of such sites as the gingivae or lips (Fig. 29.8) due to granulomatous inflammation (Fig. 29.9), but not caused by any of the recognised diseases. Some of these patients develop Crohn's disease or sarcoidosis later, but many others remain otherwise healthy or have subclinical bowel disease.

In some, the granulomatous reaction appears to result from common food additives such as cinnamon or tartrazine. Such causes can only be confirmed by an exclusion diet which, if faithfully maintained, may greatly lessen the swellings. Otherwise, intralesional corticosteroids may help.

When no cause can be found, regular follow-up should be maintained to ensure that any underlying condition, such as Crohn's disease or sarcoidosis, is recognised at an early stage.

The term 'orofacial granulomatosis' should not incidentally be confused with midfacial granulomas which are lethal diseases (Ch. 28).

MALABSORPTION SYNDROMES

Malabsorption syndromes (Box 29.2) can cause haematological deficiencies which can contribute to development or exacerbation of recurrent aphthae, glossitis or other symptoms.

Box 29.2   Important causes of malabsorption syndrome

- Coeliac disease
- Crohn's disease
- Resection of stomach or ileum
- Pancreatic insufficiency
- Liver disease (failure of bile secretion into the gut)
- Some parasitic and other chronic gut infections

ULCERATIVE COLITIS

Ulcerative colitis is a disease of the large intestine causing inflammation and ulceration. Patients are typically between 15 and 50 years. The main effect of the bowel lesions is intractable diarrhoea with blood, mucus and pus in the stools. Abdominal pain, fever, anorexia and weight loss are seen in severe cases. Development of psychiatric symptoms is a not surprising feature of this distressing and disabling disease.

Serious complications are dilatation and perforation of the bowel (toxic megacolon) and, in longstanding cases, carcinoma of the bowel. Resection of the bowel will eliminate this risk and is curative.

Dental aspects

Anaemia can have its usual effects on the oral mucosa. Rarely, chronic ulceration (pyostomatitis gangrenosum) or multiple intraepithelial microabscesses (pyostomatitis vegetans) develop. As a result of such ulceration and complications such as skin lesions and arthralgia, there may be confusion with Behçet's disease.

FAMILIAL POLYPOSIS COLI

Polyposis of the of colon is a feature of Gardner's syndrome comprising multiple osteomas of the jaws, polyposis coli with a high malignant potential and, often, other abnormalities such as dental defects and epidermal cysts. It is inherited as an autosomal dominant trait.

The osteomas of the jaws are typically multiple and may be ranged along the alveolar ridge, along the borders of the mandible or form endosteal radiopacities. However, the importance of this syndrome is that most of those affected die of bowel cancer by the age of 50. Though some members of the family do not have polyposis coli, the finding of multiple osteomas of the jaws should prompt examination for bowel disease.

PEUTZ–JEGHERS SYNDROME

In this disorder, pigmented macules, particularly oral, are markers for intestinal polyposis (see Fig. 21.5). Polyps may develop throughout the gastrointestinal tract and, in the small bowel, can cause recurrent abdominal pain and minor intestinal obstruction. Follow-up of the original family for 38 years and other cases has shown that cancer of the colon is an important complication, but the risk for breast and gynaecological cancers is also high.

PSEUDOMEMBRANOUS COLITIS

Diarrhoea with passage of blood and mucus in the stools and sometimes fragments of necrotic bowel mucosa (pseudomembrane) is typically a complication of usually prolonged antibiotic therapy particularly with clindamycin or lincomycin. It is due to proliferation of *Clostridium difficile* resistant to these antibiotics. Pseudomembranous colitis particularly affects the elderly and debilitated, some of whom have died as a result. Treatment with metronidazole or oral vancomycin is usually effective.

It does not appear that this disease can follow a single dose of clindamycin given for the prevention of infective endocarditis.

LIVER DISEASE

Common types of liver disease are infections (particularly viral hepatitis), obstructive jaundice, cirrhosis (often due to alcohol) and tumours. Rarely, liver disease has followed dental treatment when halothane or other hepatoxic drugs have been given; transmission of viral hepatitis is a greater problem. There are various aspects of liver disease that are relevant to dentistry (Box 29.3).

Box 29.3   Important aspects of liver disease relevant to dentistry

- Haemorrhagic tendencies (Ch. 26)
- Impaired drug metabolism
- Transmission of hepatitis B, particularly
- Drug-dependent patients are frequently viral hepatitis carriers
- Rarely (mainly in the past), a toxic reaction to halothane
- Cutaneous manifestations (purpura, telangiectasia, finger clubbing)
- Sialadenosis
- Sjögren's syndrome (in primary biliary cirrhosis)

Impaired drug metabolism

Most drugs are metabolised in the liver and no drugs should be given to patients with liver disease without first consulting the British National Formulary. Causes of parenchymal liver disease and liver failure are shown in Box 29.4. Cirrhosis is frequently the result of alcoholism but often of unknown cause. Halothane is a rare cause of severe liver damage and its use in dentistry has greatly declined.

> **Box 29.4**   **Important causes of liver failure**
>
> - Idiopathic cirrhosis
> - Alcoholic cirrhosis
> - Viral hepatitis (particularly C)
> - Drugs, including halothane

VIRAL HEPATITIS

The main types of hepatitis, relevant here, are B, C and D. Hepatitis B is the chief risk to dental personnel, but hepatitis C can also be transmitted during dentistry. The hepatitis B virus can also carry within it the delta agent which can cause a particularly virulent infection (hepatitis D).

Hepatitis A

Hepatitis A is the common form of infectious hepatitis. It is frequently acquired from contaminated food during a holiday abroad in the sun. There is little evidence that hepatitis A is transmitted during dentistry and long-term complications are extremely rare. A vaccine is available.

Hepatitis B

Hepatitis B can be readily transmitted during dentistry and, despite the outbreak of AIDS, is currently the greatest infective hazard to dental staff (Box 29.5).

> **Box 29.5**   **Special hazards to dental staff from hepatitis B**
>
> - The virus is widespread
> - A chronic infective carrier state is common
> - Minute traces of body fluids can transmit infection
> - The virus survives well outside the body
> - The virus is relatively resistant to disinfection
> - Hepatitis B infection can cause serious complications (Box 29.6)

The risk of transmission of hepatitis B is emphasised by its previous name 'syringe jaundice'. In the past particularly, countless patients were infected via imperfectly sterilised syringes and needles. The effects of hepatitis B infection vary widely (Box 29.6).

> **Box 29.6**   **Possible results of hepatitis B infection**
>
> - Complete resolution
> - Asymptomatic carrier state
> - Acute hepatitis (rarely fatal)
> - Chronic active hepatitis
> - Cirrhosis
> - Liver failure
> - Liver cancer

Clinical aspects

The incubation period is at least 2–6 months. The majority of infections are subclinical (anicteric) but 5–10% of patients, particularly those who have had no overt illness, become persistent carriers and can transmit the infection. A minority develop acute hepatitis with loss of appetite, muscle pains, fever, jaundice and often a swollen, painful liver. The illness is often severe and debilitating but usually followed by complete recovery and long-lasting immunity. Overall mortality from clinical infection is probably about 1%. Occasionally, it has been as high as 30%, probably as a result of co-infection by the delta agent.

Biochemical markers of infection are raised serum levels of liver transaminases, such as alanine aminotransferase (ALT), aspartate aminotransferase (AST) and gamma glutamyl transpeptidase (GGT), along with raised levels of bilirubin and often of alkaline phosphatase. However, confirmation of the diagnosis is by serology (Table 29.1).

Serological markers of hepatitis B

The hepatitis B virus (HBV) is a DNA virus termed the Dane particle. The Dane particle consists of a central core and an outer shell. The core contains DNA, an enzyme (DNA polymerase – DNA-P) and the hepatitis B core antigen (HBcAg). The protein shell contains the hepatitis B surface antigen (HBsAg).

The carrier state and complications

Most patients with acute hepatitis B recover completely within a few weeks. Approximately 5–10% fail to clear the virus within 6–9 months and become chronic carriers.

Chronic carriage of HBsAg but not HBeAg has a low risk of severe liver damage. Persistent carriage of both HBsAg and HBeAg is associated with chronic active (aggressive) hepatitis. These patients have biochemical evidence of liver damage. They are chronically ill and at special risk from cirrhosis and, possibly, carcinoma of the liver.

Chronic active hepatitis with persistent malaise, and sometimes mild jaundice, is particularly likely to develop in the very young or old and HIV-positive patients. Cirrhosis can result and lead to liver failure or hepatocellular carcinoma. It is possible that the risk of liver cancer is enhanced by genetic factors; of these, many c-myc-regulated genes appear to be involved.

CHAPTER
29

Table 29.1 Serological markers of hepatitis B and their significance

Serological marker	Relation to infection	Significance
The surface antigen (HBsAg)	HBsAg particles detectable in late incubation period and during acute and chronic infections	HBsAg carriage indicates past infection, but confers little risk of transmitting infection, unless HBeAg is also present
Antibody to HB surface antigen (HBsAb)	Begins to appear when recovery starts but HBsAg may briefly disappear before anti-HBs becomes detectable. Both serological tests then become negative	During recovery, anti-HBs usually appears and rises in titre; it usually implies persistent immunity. Anti-HBs also appears after hepatitis B immunisation
Hepatitis B core antigen (HBcAg)	Found only in liver cells, not serum	
Antibody to HB core antigen (HBcAb)	Anti-HBc appears at onset of disease Quickly rises in titre and persists for many years	One of the most sensitive indicators of past infection
Hepatitis B e antigen (HBeAg)	Appears in the serum simultaneously with HBsAg but disappears earlier if there is full recovery	Indicator of high infectivity
Antibody to e antigen (anti-HBe, HBeAb)*	Usually appears in the serum soon after the e antigen and heralds recovery	Failure of development of anti-HBe indicates high infectivity
DNA polymerase (DNA-P)		Indicates high infectivity

*Carriers of both HBsAg and HBeAg but who lack anti-HBe are more likely to develop chronic active hepatitis and serious complications, and to transmit the infection.

Risks to dental staff

The carriage rate of hepatitis B virus in the general population of Britain is 0.1–0.2%. The rate in British dentists is probably double that in the general population, though this should fall now that dentists are vaccinated.

In hot climates such as Asia and Africa, it may be 5–40% and dental staff there are at high risk. There are also high-risk groups (Box 29.7) and the hazard of infection is highest in inner urban areas, particularly for oral surgeons and periodontists. In the USA, 20% of American oral surgeons have serological evidence of previous infection and one of the highest infection rates of all health workers.

Box 29.7 Patients with higher risk of being hepatitis B carriers

- Male homosexuals and STD (VD) clinic patients
- Intravenous drug addicts
- Patients and staff of dialysis and transplant units
- Patients (especially with Down's syndrome) and staff of institutions for the handicapped
- Immunosuppressed or immunodeficient patients
- Patients who have received unscreened blood or blood products
- Patients who have had acupuncture or tattooing, especially in tropical countries
- Consorts of patients with hepatitis B or of any of the above
- Certain associated diseases, particularly AIDS, some chronic liver diseases and polyarteritis nodosa
- Immigrants or travellers from high-risk areas, particularly tropical or subtropical countries

Transmission of HBV

Blood and blood products are most dangerous and can transmit infection in as little as 0.0000001 ml fluid, particularly when containing the e antigen. Many cases have followed needlestick injuries, injections and blood transfusions. Saliva can also contain hepatitis B antigens and, experimentally, can transmit the virus. Saliva is frequently also contaminated with blood and, when splashed on to the conjunctiva, might transmit infection to a dentist. Hepatitis B can also be transmitted heterosexually, but more readily by male homosexual activity. Men who have sex with men, particularly in the USA, are frequently also HIV positive and, in London, 30% of male prostitutes (many of them teenagers) are estimated to be HBV carriers and 20% of them to be HIV positive.

As discussed earlier, the risk of infection is indicated by the serological markers. Infective carriers can only be suspected if they have a history of jaundice or are in a high-risk group. Nevertheless, it must be emphasised that only 1 in 4 carriers gives a positive medical history. In statistical terms, therefore, if a dentist treats 20 patients a day, one hepatitis B carrier will be encountered every 7 working days. Many infectious patients, as in the case of HIV carriers, will therefore be treated unknowingly.

Dental staff who are carriers of or incubating hepatitis B can also transmit infection to patients, some of whom have died as a consequence. The dangers to dentists have been emphasised by the death from hepatitis B of an unvaccinated male nurse, after being bitten by a mentally handicapped carrier.

Prevention and management of hepatitis B

It is *essential* for dentists to have active immunisation. It is effective, safe and protects against both hepatitis B and delta infection. Three injections should be given at intervals into the deltoid muscle, but adequate protection may not develop until after 6 months. Side-effects are mild and rare, but a few (particularly the obese) do not produce adequate antibody levels after a normal course of vaccination and may need it to be repeated. Booster doses are needed at 3–5-year intervals, or more frequently in persons in whom the half-life of the response is brief. In the past antibody levels were checked repeatedly. Levels are now considered to be a poor reflection of longstanding immunity and repeated testing and re-vaccination should be avoided, provided an adequate response has been observed immediately after vaccination. Those who have not been immunised, but are wounded while treating a high-risk patient or known carrier, should have immediate active immunisation. Passive immunisation with hepatitis B immunoglobulin as well has also been advised. Treatment of chronic active hepatitis is with alpha-interferon which may prevent cirrhosis or other complications.

In addition to vaccination, strict infection control procedures should be maintained.

The delta agent: hepatitis D virus (HDV)

The delta agent is a defective RNA virus that can only replicate in the presence of HBsAg. Delta infection is mainly transmitted by blood or blood products. It is widespread among intravenous drug abusers and in endemic areas such as the Mediterranean region. Delta infection causes acute hepatitis. This usually resolves, but fulminant liver disease can follow and the mortality rate is high. A few dental patients have acquired delta hepatitis and some have died. Immunisation against hepatitis B also protects against the delta agent and this strengthens the need for immunisation.

Chronic delta hepatitis is currently treated with interferon-alpha-2b which gives a 5-year survival rate of 65%. This may be improved to 85% by the addition of lamivudine.

Hepatitis C

It is important to understand the scale of the problem of hepatitis C infection. The hepatitis C virus (HCV) was the most common cause of post-transfusion hepatitis after hepatitis B, but donors are now screened for both hepatitis C and B. Before hepatitis C screening was available and blood products were inactivated, almost 100% of haemophiliacs became infected and remain carriers. However, hepatitis C has become the most common chronic blood-borne infection in the USA; the estimated prevalence of anti-HCV in 2006 was 4.1 million persons; the number of cases of chronic HCV infection was 3.2 million. Nearly 50% of anti-HCV positive individuals had a history of intravenous drug use. Infection rates and adverse consequences are more frequent in males aged between 35 and 64. Worldwide, it is estimated that over 170 million are infected.

> **Box 29.8** **Important differences between hepatitis C and B**
>
> **Hepatitis C:**
> - is less widespread
> - is less readily transmitted by needle-stick injuries
> - is more vulnerable to antiseptics
> - is rarely transmitted during dentistry
> - acute hepatitis is uncommon and usually mild
>
> **But**
> - no protective vaccine is as yet available
> - infections persists in 80%
> - infection more frequently leads to chronic active hepatitis
> - there is a higher risk of cirrhosis and liver cancer

Hepatitis C and B are similar in most respects but have some important differences (Box 29.8).

In the USA, 2% of oral surgeons and 0.7% of general dentists were found to be anti-HCV positive in 1996. This compares with 21% of oral surgeons and 8% of general dentists who were anti-HBV positive in the same group.

As shown in Box 29.8, the risk for cirrhosis and hepatocellular carcinoma is greater than for HBV infection. It appears that smoking worsens the risk of fibrosis in patients with chronic HBC infection. Other serious effects are that hepatitis C cirrhosis has become the main indication for liver transplantation worldwide, but it is also the most common cause of rejection of liver transplants. The prognosis of liver transplantation has, as a result, failed to improve since 1992. It has also recently been shown to cause myocarditis and heart failure.

Management

HCV can be detected serologically. Most of those who are seropositive by immunoassay are viraemic and, despite the presence of antibodies, are infective. Diagnosis of chronic hepatitis C liver damage can be confirmed by biopsy.

Hepatitis C, particularly in its chronic active stage, is treated with pegylated interferon plus ribavirin which provides a sustained virological response in 55%. It is also effective in dialysis patients who have a high prevalence of this infection. It has been reported that the addition of thalidomide in six patients non-responsive to ribavirin and pegylated interferon produced negative RNA PCR findings and complete resolution.

Co-infection with both HCV and HIV may affect over 10 500 persons in the USA. However, HCV does not appear to enhance the risk of death from AIDS or affect the initial immunological and virological response to initial HAART. Early treatment with ribavirin and pegylated interferon-alpha 2a is also effective in acute HCV infection associated with HIV.

The HCV NS3 protease is essential for viral replication so that newer drugs include HCV NS3 protease inhibitors. Cirrhosis develops in approximately 20% of patients, 10% of whom may develop liver cancer over a mean of 20–30 years. In one series of 131 patients with post-transfusion hepatitis C,

14.5% died from cirrhosis or hepatocellular carcinoma and the risk of the latter is 20–30 times greater than in the uninfected population. The risk of advanced hepatic fibrosis due to hepatitic C may be, partly at least, genetically determined and persons carrying DDX5 minor allele or DDXG-POLG2 haplotypes are reportedly at greater risk. There is also a small but significant risk of development of immunoproliferative (mainly lymphomas) malignancies.

Control of transmission of viral hepatitis

Because of the ease of transmission of hepatitis, the basic precautions are summarised in Box 29.9.

> **Box 29.9   Basic precautions against transmission of viral hepatitis**
>
> - Treat all patients as infectious ('universal precautions')
> - Wear gloves for all clinical dental work
> - Take special care to avoid needle-stick injuries
> - Wear goggles for eye protection
> - Use disposable instruments and autoclave all others
> - Be immunised against hepatitis B

Gloves, masks and eye shields provide only partial protection. Double gloving is necessary for surgeons at high risk from acquiring or transmitting these infections. Immunisation is therefore the single most important protective measure as it is virtually impossible completely to prevent transmission of hepatitis B by other means.

There is as yet no vaccine against hepatitis C and there are some strains of hepatitis B against which the current vaccine apparently confers no protection. Though the hazard from these is statistically small, the risk from them emphasises the need to maintain rigorous infection control.

Dental aspects of hepatitis B and C infection

The main differences between these infections which affect dental management are summarised in Box 29.8. Hepatitis B can be present in saliva and has been transmitted by bites. Hepatitis C has also been transmitted in healthcare facilities. About 1 in 1000 of the population of the UK are HBsAg-positive, but this prevalence has probably risen with the inrush of immigrants from high-risk countries. About 75% of HBsAg carriers are probably non-infective, but HBeAg carriers should preferably be identified as presenting a high risk of transmitting hepatitis B. HCV has been detected in saliva and has been transmitted in a human bite. In the past particularly, hepatitis B has been acquired by surgeons and dental staff, but the risk has declined since the introduction of an effective vaccine and the application of universal infection control. The risks of transmitting HCV are small in the dental environment compared with hepatitis B, but the same precautions should be taken against both viruses. In some countries, particularly in Italy, an association between hepatitis C infection and sicca syndrome, non-Hodgkin lymphoma, lichen planus and sarcoidosis following antiviral treatment has been reported, but this has not been confirmed in Britain.

Hepatitis E

Hepatitis E transmission is by the faecal–oral route. Infection is endemic in the Far East and in some countries there has been a significant mortality. The risk to travellers abroad is small. No vaccine is available.

Sterilisation and disinfection for viral hepatitis

Hepatitis B virus is tougher than HCV, but sterilisation and disinfection measures (Box 29.10) apply to both.

> **Box 29.10   Sterilisation and disinfection for hepatitis B and C**
>
> **Sterilisation**
> - Autoclaving at 134°C for 3 minutes or
> - Hot air at 160°C for 1 hour (effective but automatic control necessary; not used in UK)
>
> **Disinfectants**
> - Sodium hypochlorite, 1% of freshly diluted stock solution (0.1% + detergent for surface disinfection) (HCV is also susceptible to solvent detergents)

Dentists must ensure that infection control procedures are up to standard for their own protection. They are also legal obligations under the Health and Safety at Work Act. Acquisition of viral hepatitis as a consequence of dental treatment could result in substantial claims for compensation. Restrictions on dentists who are viral hepatitis carriers have been summarised in Appendix 29.1.

SUGGESTED FURTHER READING

Bowden DS, Moaven LD, Locarnini SA 1996 New hepatitis viruses: are there enough letters in the alphabet? Med J Aust 164:87–89
De Mitri MS, Poussin K, Baccarini P et al 1995 HCV liver cancer without cirrhosis. Lancet 345:413–415
Gross JB, Persing DH 1995 Hepatitis C: advances in diagnosis. Mayo Clin Proc 70:296–297
Hosey MT, Gordon G, Kelly DA et al 1995 Oral findings in children with liver transplants. Int J Paediatr Dent 5:29–34
Porter SR, Lodi G 1996 Hepatitis C virus (HCV) – an occupational hazard to dentists. Br Dent J 180:473–474
Sanchez-Tapias JM, Rodes J 1995 Interferon in chronic hepatitis C. Lancet 346:s11
Shahara AI, Hunt CM, Hamilton JD 1996 Update. Hepatitis C. Ann Intern Med 125:658–668
Thomas DL, Gruninger SE, Siew C et al 1996 Occupational risk of hepatitis C infections among general dentists and oral surgeons in North America. Am J Med 100:41–45

APPENDIX
29.1

SUMMARY OF HEALTH SERVICE RESTRICTIONS ON HEPATITIS B-INFECTED HEALTHCARE WORKERS

The following are restricted from performing exposure-prone procedures:

- Those carrying the e antigen (HBeAg positive)
- Those who are HBeAg negative but with a viral load (HBV DNA) exceeding 10^3 genome equivalents/ml

HBeAg-negative healthcare workers or those who have an HBV DNA level not exceeding 10^3 genome equivalents/ml are not restricted from performing exposure-prone procedures

SUMMARY OF HEALTH SERVICE RESTRICTIONS ON HEPATITIS C-INFECTED HEALTHCARE WORKERS

The following are restricted from performing exposure-prone procedures:

- Those who are hepatitis C viraemic (Virus RNA positive)

Healthcare workers (including students entering dental school), embarking on a career performing exposure-prone procedures should be tested for hepatitis C antibodies and, if positive, for HCV DNA.

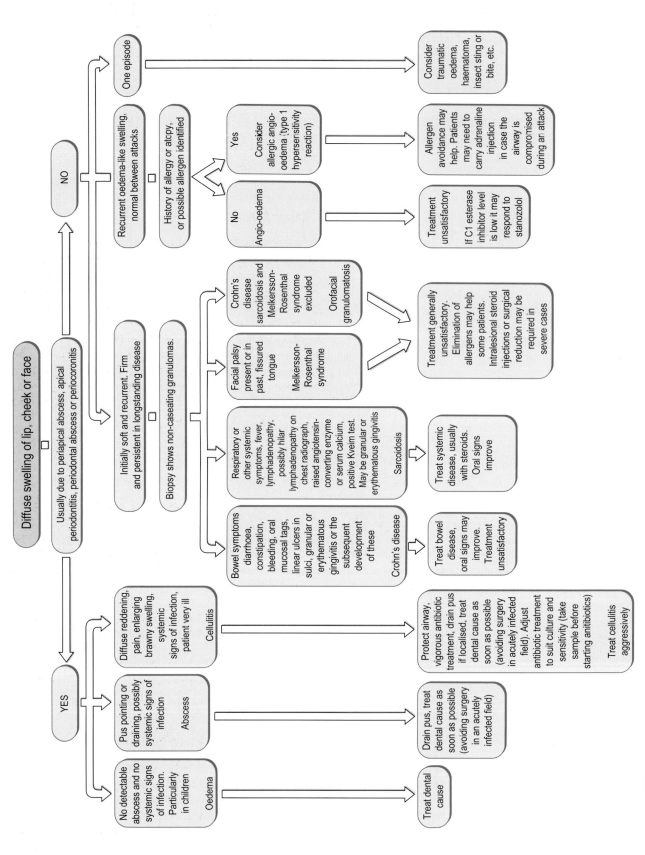

Diffuse swelling of lip, cheek or face

YES

- Usually due to periapical abscess, apical periodontitis, periodontal abscess or periocoronitis

  - No detectable abscess and no systemic signs of infection. Particularly in children — **Oedema** → Treat dental cause

  - Pus pointing or draining, possibly systemic signs of infection — **Abscess** → Drain pus, treat dental cause as soon as possible (avoiding surgery in an acutely infected field)

  - Diffuse reddening, pain, enlarging brawny swelling, systemic signs of infection, patient very ill — **Cellulitis** → Protect airway, vigorous antibiotic treatment, drain pus if localised, treat dental cause as soon as possible (avoiding surgery in acutely infected field). Adjust antibiotic treatment to suit culture and sensitivity (take sample before starting antibiotics)

    Treat cellulitis aggressively

NO

- Initially soft and recurrent. Firm and persistent in longstanding disease

  Biopsy shows non-caseating granulomas.

  - Bowel symptoms diarrhoea, constipation, bleeding, oral mucosal tags, linear ulcers in sulci, granular or erythematous gingivitis or the subsequent development of these — **Crohn's disease** → Treat bowel disease, oral signs may improve. Treatment unsatisfactory

  - Respiratory or other systemic symptoms, fever, lymphadenopathy, possibly hilar lymphadenopathy on chest radiograph, raised angiotensin-converting enzyme or serum calcium, positive Kveim test. May be granular or erythematous gingivitis — **Sarcoidosis** → Treat systemic disease, usually with steroids. Oral signs improve

  - Facial palsy present or in past, fissured tongue — **Melkersson-Rosenthal syndrome** → Treatment generally unsatisfactory. Elimination of allergens may help some patients. Intralesional steroid injections or surgical reduction may be required in severe cases

  - Crohn's disease, sarcoidosis and Melkersson-Rosenthal syndrome excluded — **Orofacial granulomatosis**

- Recurrent oedema-like swelling, normal between attacks

  History of allergy or atopy, or possible allergen identified

  - **Yes** → Consider allergic angio-oedema (type 1 hypersensitivity reaction) → Allergen avoidance may help. Patients may need to carry adrenaline injection in case the airway is compromised during an attack

  - **No** → Angio-oedema → Treatment unsatisfactory. If C1 esterase inhibitor level is low it may respond to stanozolol

- One episode → Consider traumatic oedema, haematoma, insect sting or bite, etc.

Summary chart 29.1 Causes and treatment of diffuse swelling of the lips and mucosa.

Nutritional deficiencies

Patients with nutritional deficiencies are rarely seen in Britain. Susceptible patients are the elderly living on a scanty diet, food cranks and severe alcoholics living on a grossly unbalanced diet. Malabsorption syndromes (Ch. 29) are another cause.

Several oral conditions of doubtful cause, such as periodontal disease or glossitis, have been ascribed to vitamin deficiencies, though patients have been otherwise healthy and well-fed. In such cases, giving vitamin preparations brings benefit only to the multibillion pound vitamin industry. Vitamin deficiencies are not a contributory cause of dental caries.

VITAMIN DEFICIENCIES

The effects of specific deficiencies are summarised in Table 30.1.

Table 30.1 Effects of specific vitamin deficiencies

Deficiency	Systemic effects	Oral effects
Vitamin A	Night-blindness, xerophthalmia	Unconfirmed contribution to leukoplakia and cancer
Thiamin (B$_1$)	Neuritis and cardiac failure	None
Riboflavin (B$_2$)	Dermatitis	Angular stomatitis and glossitis
Nicotinamide	Dermatitis, CNS disease, diarrhoea	Glossitis, stomatitis and gingivitis
Vitamin B$_{12}$	Pernicious anaemia	Glossitis, aphthae
Folic acid	Macrocytic anaemia	Glossitis, aphthae
Vitamin C	Scurvy (purpura, delayed wound healing, bone lesions in children)	Gingival swelling and bleeding
Vitamin D	Rickets	Hypocalcification of teeth (severe rickets only)

Vitamin A deficiency

In rats, vitamin A deficiency has severe effects on secretory epithelium. Columnar cells become squamous in type and keratinised. Dental development is severely affected and secretory cells of salivary glands also become squamous and keratinised. However, there is no evidence that vitamin A deficiency causes such changes in humans.

Successful treatment of keratotic plaques (leukoplakias) with retinoids (vitamin A derivatives) has been claimed but not confirmed. The toxic effects of these drugs are severe and they are teratogenic. Epidemiological studies have suggested an association between low vitamin A intake and oral and other cancers, but there is growing doubt whether beta-carotene is beneficial or harmful.

Riboflavin (B$_2$) deficiency

Riboflavin deficiency can occasionally result from a malabsorption syndrome. In severe cases, there is typically angular stomatitis, with painful red fissures at the angles of the mouth, and shiny redness of the mucous membranes. The tongue is commonly sore. A peculiar form of glossitis in which the tongue becomes magenta in colour and granular or pebbly in appearance, due to flattening and mushrooming of the papillae, may be seen but is uncommon. The gingivae are not affected. Resolution follows within days when riboflavin (5 mg three times a day) is given.

Riboflavin is ineffective for the commonly seen cases of glossitis and angular stomatitis, which are rarely due to vitamin deficiency.

Nicotinamide deficiency (pellagra)

Pellagra, which affects the skin, gastrointestinal tract and nervous system, is rare in Britain but may occasionally result from malabsorption or alcoholism. Weakness, loss of appetite and changes in mood or personality are followed by glossitis or stomatitis and dermatitis. The tip and lateral margins of the tongue become red, swollen and, in severe cases, deeply ulcerated. The dorsum of the tongue becomes coated with a thick, greyish fur which is often

Fig. 30.1 **Scurvy.** There is gross periodontal destruction with deep pocketing and mobility of several teeth resulting from the combination of poor oral hygiene and deficiency of vitamin C. (See also Ch. 10.)

Fig. 30.2 Gross dental caries of the anterior teeth due to over-indulgence in sugar-rich vitamin C syrup.

heavily infected. The gingival margins also become red, swollen and ulcerated and generalised stomatitis may develop.

Vitamin B$_{12}$ deficiency

This disease, unlike the others described in this section, is primarily a defect of absorption (Ch. 29). It is exceptionally rare for it to be caused by dietary deficiencies (veganism).

Folic acid deficiency

Deficiency can result from malnutrition but is more often seen in pregnancy, or as a result of malabsorption or drug treatment (particularly with phenytoin) (Ch. 35). Women are advised to take folic acid supplements preconceptually with the aim of reducing the risk of neural tube defects. It also appears that multivitamin preparations containing folic acid may reduce the risk of orofacial clefts.

Vitamin C deficiency

Scurvy, once common among crews of sailing ships, is now exceedingly rare. In Britain, scurvy may very occasionally be seen among elderly people with an inadequate income, or in those devoted to eccentric diets. The main features of scurvy are dermatitis and purpura and, in advanced cases, anaemia, delayed healing of wounds and swollen bleeding gums may develop (Fig. 30.1). In children, bone formation may be disturbed.

There is no evidence that deficiency of vitamin C plays any part in periodontal disease except in frank scurvy and there is no correlation between low plasma ascorbic acid levels and gingivitis. There is no justification for giving ascorbic acid to healthy patients with periodontal disease.

Though it may be thought that scurvy is of historical interest only, a 24-year-old engineer was reported in 1983 to have the

disease in classical form including swollen, bleeding gums. He had lived largely on peanut butter sandwiches, recalled having eaten an apple 4 years previously but could not recall ever having eaten an orange.

It has been suggested that massive doses of ascorbic acid prevent or ameliorate the common cold. This is unproven and the effect, if any, is marginal. Moreover, cessation of mega-dose intake of ascorbic acid can lead to rebound deficiency and scurvy. In one bizarre case, intravenous injection of no less than 80 g of ascorbic acid proved to be lethal. This really does seem to be carrying prevention too far.

Nevertheless, giving children vitamin C-rich fruit syrups is common. An incidental effect of this can be gross caries of the anterior teeth (Fig. 30.2).

Vitamin D deficiency

Deficiency of vitamin D during skeletal development causes rickets (Ch. 10).

A rich source of vitamin D is fish liver oils, but small amounts are also present in eggs and butter. In strong sunlight, vitamin D can be synthesised in the skin. In Britain, margarine is fortified with vitamins A and D, but requirements are small except during bone growth and pregnancy.

Rickets is now rare, but immigrants in the North of Britain are at risk. Contributory factors are lack of sunlight, a high-carbohydrate diet and possibly also the use of wholemeal flour (as in chupattis) containing factors which impair calcium absorption. However, there is no basis for the idea that dental caries is due to poor calcification of the teeth and giving vitamin D and calcium for dental caries is valueless. There are also dangers associated with raising children's intake of vitamin D. Some are sensitive to this potent drug and hypervitaminosis D causes hypercalcaemia and renal calcinosis. Dental defects (hypocalcification) are a feature only of exceptionally severe rickets (Ch. 2).

ANOREXIA NERVOSA AND BULIMIA

Anorexia nervosa is, in simple terms, an eating disorder particularly affecting young females, in which there is determined and persistent avoidance of food leading to emaciation and occasionally death. It is typically ascribed to fear of obesity and a distorted body image.

Bulimia is the term given to binge eating alternating with self-induced vomiting or purging to control excessive obesity, but emaciation is not usually achieved. In a single eating binge up to 20 000 calories may be consumed and there may be addiction to drugs or alcohol also.

Oral and perioral effects of anorexia and bulimia are parotid swelling (sialadenosis) and dental erosion due to vomiting. Dentists may be able to identify such signs before medical intervention becomes imperative.

SUGGESTED FURTHER READING

Nowak R 1994 Beta-carotene: helpful or harmful? Science 294:500–501
Robb ND, Smith BGN 1996 Anorexia and bulimia nervosa (the eating disorders): conditions of interest to the dental practitioner. J Dentistry 24:7–16

Endocrine disorders and pregnancy

Endocrine disorders, apart from diabetes mellitus and thyroid disease, are uncommon. They are rare causes of oral disease but, occasionally, oral changes can lead to their diagnosis. Patients with Addison's disease, diabetes mellitus and thyrotoxicosis, in particular, may also need special care for dental surgery.

ANTERIOR PITUITARY HYPERFUNCTION – GIGANTISM AND ACROMEGALY

Overproduction of growth hormone by the anterior pituitary during the period of skeletal growth causes gigantism. Overgrowth of the skeleton and soft tissues causes the patient to become a giant. Acromegaly usually develops later.

After the epiphyses have fused, an adenoma of growth hormone cells causes acromegaly. There is renewed growth, particularly of the jaws, hands and feet. The condylar growth centre becomes active and the mandible becomes enlarged and protrusive (Fig. 31.1). Radiographically, the whole jaw is lengthened and the angle becomes more oblique (Fig. 31.2). The jaw and other bones are also made thicker by subperiosteal bone deposition. The teeth become spaced or, if the patient is edentulous, dentures cease to fit the growing jaw. The hands and feet become spade-like (Fig. 31.3). Overgrowth of soft tissues causes thickening and enlargement of the facial features, particularly the lips and nose.

Headaches and visual disturbances due to the pituitary tumour are common. Later, weakness and often diabetes mellitus develop. Blindness due to pressure of the tumour on the optic chiasma may develop. Hypertension is common and may be associated with cardiomyopathy and dysrhythmias. Irradiation or trans-sphenoidal resection of the pituitary tumour may relieve the symptoms.

Fig. 31.1 Acromegaly. The typical facial appearance, resulting from excessive mandibular growth.

Fig. 31.2 Acromegaly. The mandible is enlarged with an elongated ramus and increased obliquity of the angle. The pituitary fossa is also enlarged due to the tumour causing the disease.

Rarely, a growth hormone-producing pituitary tumour is part of type 1 multiple endocrine neoplasia syndrome (MEN1) as described below. In such patients, gingival papules have also been described.

Dental considerations

Orthognathic surgery may be considered to improve the appearance. There is a risk of postoperative airways obstruction, particularly because the glottis is narrowed and the large tongue may press back on to the pharynx. Close observation is therefore needed to release the dental ligatures in emergency or asphyxia will result. Systemic complications as described above can also affect dental management. Otherwise, there is no special risk from local analgesia or sedation.

THYROID DISEASE

Hyperthyroidism

Hyperthyroidism (Box 31.1) is most common in young adults, particularly women. There is usually a diffuse goitre and the disease is typically autoimmune with thyroid-stimulating autoantibodies. Less frequently, the cause is a toxic (hyperthyroid) goitre due to hormone-producing adenomas.

Box 31.1 Important features of hyperthyroidism
• Irritability and anxiety
• Loss of weight
• Exophthalmos (Fig. 31.4)
• Tachycardia
• Cardiovascular disease, particularly in untreated hyperthyroidism in older patients

Dental considerations

Treatment of hyperthyroid patients may be affected by several factors (Box 31.2) and, in particular, may be made difficult because of excitability and anxiety. Excessive cardiac excitability is only a theoretical contraindication to lidocaine with epinephrine and no other local anaesthetic has been shown to be safer. Conscious sedation (nitrous oxide and oxygen) is frequently helpful, but benzodiazepines may potentiate antithyroid drugs.

Box 31.2 Dental management of hyperthyroid patients
• Control of nervousness and excitability
• If clinical signs are seen but the patient is not under treatment, refer to a physician
• Avoid general anaesthesia in patients with longstanding thyrotoxicosis, particularly older patients

Fig. 31.3 Acromegaly. The jaw is enlarged and protrusive, the features thickened and the hands broad and spade-like. (Taken before the advent of colour photography.)

Fig. 31.4 Thyrotoxicosis. Exophthalmos is typical but the enlarged thyroid is not conspicuous. The patient had not then started to lose weight. (Taken before the advent of colour photography.)

Treatment of hyperthyroidism is by surgical removal of part of the gland, or by means of drugs such as thiouracil or carbimazole. Iodine[131] can effect a permanent cure, but may also cause hypothyroidism. There appears to be risk of neoplastic change due to treatment with this isotope.

Hypothyroidism

Cretinism

Cretinism results from deficient thyroid activity at birth (Fig. 31.5). It is most common in areas of endemic goitre, but rare now that goitre is controlled with iodine. A cretin is occasionally the offspring of a normal mother. The main features are particularly short stature and intellectual impairment, but dental abnormalities are frequently associated (Box 31.3). In the untreated patient, sedatives and tranquillisers such as benzodiazepines can precipitate myxoedemic coma and should generally be avoided. Conscious sedation with nitrous oxide and oxygen can be given.

> **Box 31.3 Typical features of cretinism**
>
> - Skeletal development and dental eruption greatly delayed
> - Impaired mental development
> - Broad, rather flat face partly due to defective growth of the skull and facial bones
> - Overlarge, protrusive tongue
> - Dull facial expression, dry thick skin
> - Short stocky build and, often, umbilical hernia

Treatment with thyroid hormone must be begun early to provide normal physical development and improvement in the mental defect.

Fig. 31.5 Cretinism in a child. The facial expression, excessive broadening of the features and the protruding tongue are characteristic. (Taken before the advent of colour photography.)

Adult hypothyroidism

Hypothyroidism (Box 31.4) is frequently autoimmune, but can follow radioiodine treatment or excessive surgical removal of thyroid tissue for hyperthyroidism.

> **Box 31.4 Typical features of adult hypothyroidism**
>
> - Weight gain
> - Slowed activity and thought
> - Dry skin and hair loss
> - Intolerance of cold
> - Susceptibility to ischaemic heart disease

Aspects of dental management of hypothyroidism are summarised in Box 31.5.

> **Box 31.5 Dental management of hypothyroidism**
>
> - Avoid sedatives including diazepam, opioid analgesics and general anaesthetics because of the risk of myxoedemic coma
> - Anaemia or ischaemic heart disease may require modification of dental treatment
> - Local anaesthesia always preferable
> - Nitrous oxide/oxygen sedation acceptable
> - Sjögren's syndrome occasionally associated and requires treatment

Lingual thyroid

Thyroid tissue is occasionally present in the tongue as a result of imperfect descent of the anlage into the neck. Females are mainly affected. Clinically, it usually causes an asymptomatic midline, purplish soft swelling, but may cause dysphagia. It may not be recognised for thyroid tissue until after biopsy which may cause considerable bleeding. Otherwise, the nature of the swelling may be determined by I[131] or technetium scanning, or by CT or MRI. Scanning of the neck to ensure the presence of a thyroid gland is therefore essential before the lingual thyroid is removed. However, this may have to be done anyway if it is causing significant obstruction. If no normally positioned thyroid tissue is present, life-long thyroxine supplementation is then given. Malignant change in ectopic thyroid is rare.

PARATHYROID DISEASE → Summary p. 173

Hyperparathyroidism

This uncommon disease is usually caused by an adenoma of the parathyroids. Secondary hyperparathyroidism is a reaction to low serum calcium levels caused by chronic renal failure or prolonged dialysis. Parathormone overproduction can cause decalcification of the skeleton and cyst-like areas of bone resorption (osteitis fibrosa cystica). These lesions are giant cell 'tumours', but are rarely seen now that hyperparathyroidism is recognised earlier by its non-specific symptoms (Ch. 10). As discussed below, hyperparathyroidism is the presenting sign of the uncommon disease, type 1 multiple endocrine neoplasia syndrome (see below).

Typical features of hyperparathyroidism are summarised in Box 31.6

> **Box 31.6** Typical features of hyperparathyroidism
>
> - General malaise
> - Peptic ulceration
> - Bone resorption
> - Renal stones or nephrocalcinosis
> - Polyuria

Hyperparathyroidism-jaw tumour syndrome

Hyperparathyroidism-jaw tumor syndrome is a rare autosomal dominant disease. Its gene location is 1q21-q32 whose function is a tumor-suppressor gene whose product is parafibromin. The features include parathyroid adenomas or carcinomas, renal cysts and fibro-osseous jaw lesions. Renal, mixed and uterine tumours may be associated.

Jaw lesions are typically multiple and can involve both mandible and maxilla. Unlike sporadic hyperparathyroidism, giant cells are not the main feature. The lesions are fibro-osseous and may resemble ossifying or cementifying fibroma, non-ossifying fibroma, or even fibrous dysplasia. However, their essential features are a cellular fibrous stroma, sometimes with a suggestion of a storiform pattern containing trabeculae of bone or cementicle-like particles. Only a few giant cells may be seen among bone trabeculae. The lesions are typically sharply demarcated.

In terms of management, the main problem is that of the parathyroid and other tumours. Parathyroid adenomas usually respond to surgery, but management of parathyoid carcinoma is more difficult. The prognosis is also affected by the behaviour of associated tumours of the kidneys or uterus. Jaw lesions usually shell out quite readily but some have recurred. Otherwise, they may regress spontaneously after removal of the parathyroid tumour, though this may take months or even years.

Hypoparathyroidism

Post-surgical hypoparathyroidism

The most common cause of hypoparathyroidism is thyroidectomy. The resulting hypocalcaemia causes heightened neuromuscular excitability and tetany. These are controlled by giving the vitamin D analogue 1,25-dihydrocholecalciferol (DHCC) orally. Later, any residual parathyroid tissue undergoes compensatory hyperplasia.

Tetany

In mild cases, tetany is latent but can be triggered by tapping on the skin over the facial nerve; this causes the facial muscles to contract. In more severe cases, muscle cramps and tonic contractions of the muscles may progress to generalised convulsions. An early symptom of tetany is paraesthesiae of the lip and extremities. Tetany more frequently results from overbreathing, often neurotic in origin (hyperventilation syndrome).

Idiopathic hypoparathyroidism

Early-onset hypoparathyroidism is rare. It sometimes forms part of the polyendocrinopathy syndrome with autoantibodies to a variety of glandular tissues and deficiency states (particularly Addison's disease) and, frequently, mucocutaneous candidosis (see below). Otherwise, the disease and its treatment are similar to post-surgical hypoparathyroidism.

Effects on calcified tissues are summarised in Box 31.7.

> **Box 31.7** Effects of hypoparathyroidism on calcified tissues
>
> - Retarded new bone formation and diminished resorption are usually in equilibrium so that skeletal changes are rare
> - Aplasia or hypoplasia of developing enamel*, which becomes deeply grooved
> - Dentine may be incompletely mineralised but lamina dura may be thickened
> - Short roots to teeth (Ch. 2)
>
> *Results from associated ectodermal defects.

ADRENOCORTICAL DISEASES – HYPOFUNCTION

Adrenocortical insufficiency is rarely primary (Addison's disease) and more frequently secondary to corticosteroid therapy.

Addison's disease

Addison's disease results from atrophy of the adrenal cortices and failure of secretion of cortisol and aldosterone. The result is a severe disorder of electrolyte and fluid balance and serious clinical effects (Box 31.8). The disease is usually autoimmune with organ-specific circulating autoantibodies. Tuberculous or

> **Box 31.8** Typical clinical features of Addison's disease
>
> - Lassitude, anorexia, weakness and fatigue
> - Abnormal oral and cutaneous pigmentation
> - Gastrointestinal disturbances
> - Loss of weight
> - Low blood pressure
> - Susceptibility to hypotensive crises
> - Associated with chronic mucocutaneous candidosis in polyendocrinopathy syndrome (p. 419)

Fig. 31.6 **Addison's disease.** A close-up shows the characteristic distribution of pigment rather patchily along the attached gingivae. It is a brownish-black in colour.

Fig. 31.7 **Addison's disease.** Deep pigmentation of the buccal mucosa.

fungal adrenal destruction are rare causes but can be secondary to HIV infection. Addison's disease is also the most frequent feature of the rare polyglandular autoimmune syndromes and is then associated with chronic mucocutaneous candidosis as described below.

Pigmentation is often an early sign and, in the mouth, is patchily distributed on gingivae, buccal mucosa and lips (Figs 31.6 and 31.7). It is brown or almost black. However, Addison's disease is an exceptionally uncommon cause of oral pigmentation. The skin pigmentation looks similar to suntan but with a sallow appearance due to underlying pallor. Exposed and normally pigmented areas are most severely affected.

Though Addison's disease is rare, it should be considered in a patient, other than a black individual, with pigmentation of the oral mucous membrane. A weak voice caused by general weakness and lassitude is also suggestive.

In an Addisonian crisis, there is a rapid fall in blood pressure, circulatory collapse (shock) and vomiting. These crises, which may be fatal, are often precipitated by such causes as infections, injuries, surgery or anaesthesia. Immediate treatment

with intravenous hydrocortisone (several 100 mg) and fluid replacement may be life-saving.

Long-term treatment of Addison's disease is usually by oral hydrocortisone which allows patients to live almost normal lives but with complications described below.

Corticosteroid treatment

Corticosteroids have a wide variety of uses in medicine and some uses for oral diseases (Box 31.9). Topical corticosteroids are sometimes given for aphthous stomatitis.

Box 31.9 **Uses of systemic corticosteroids**

Adrenal insufficiency
- Addison's disease
- Hypopituitarism

Post-transplantation

Allergic disorders, particularly asthma

Connective tissue diseases
- Systemic lupus erythematosus
- Rheumatoid arthritis
- Others

Gastrointestinal disorders
- Crohn's disease
- Ulcerative colitis

Blood dyscrasias
- Idiopathic thrombocytopenic purpura
- Lymphocytic leukaemia
- Some lymphomas

Renal disease
- Nephrotic syndrome
- Renal transplants

Mucocutaneous diseases
- Pemphigus
- Mucous membrane pemphigoid (sometimes)

Corticosteroids can have physiological effects resembling those of Cushing's disease (Box 31.10). Thus, there may be sodium and water retention, a raised blood sugar and impaired protein metabolism. Hypertension and diabetes are possible complications and a characteristic moon-face appearance is produced.

Box 31.10 **Important side-effects of long-term use of corticosteroids**

- Depression of adrenocortical function and risk of circulatory collapse
- Depression of inflammatory and immune responses
- Opportunistic infections
- Depressed protein metabolism
- Impaired wound healing
- Moon face
- Raised blood sugar
- Sodium and water retention
- Mood changes

Fig. 31.8 Steroid collapse. This patient, taking only 5 mg prednisolone daily, was given brief sedation for an extraction. Adrenal suppression resulted in collapse and despite considerable doses of corticosteroid and fluid supplementation the patient did not recover fully for 48 hours.

Table 31.1 Polyendocrinopathy syndromes. Percentage of patients affected by the different syndrome components.		
	Type 1	Type 2
Addison's disease	100	100
Hypoparathyroidism	76	–
Chronic mucocutaneous candidosis	73	–
Pernicious anaemia	13	0.5
Alopecia	32	0.5
Malabsorption syndromes	22	–
Gonadal failure	17	3.6
Chronic active hepatitis	13	–
Insulin-dependent diabetes	4	52
Autoimmune thyroiditis	11	69
Female:male ratio	1.5:1	1.8:1

Rarely, the moon-face of Cushing's disease has been mistaken for inflammatory swelling due to a dental infection.

Corticosteroids can also mask serious disease. A patient, for a time at least, can appear to be in perfect health with plump rosy cheeks and often a sense of well-being to match. Thus, a young patient suffering from acute lymphocytic leukaemia taking corticosteroids can appear and feel well. However well a patient appears, the medical and drug history must therefore be carefully evaluated.

However, most important is the risk of circulatory collapse secondary to dental surgery or general anaesthesia (Fig. 31.8; Ch. 36).

Adrenocortical hyperfunction (Cushing's disease)

Cushing's disease is usually due to an adrenocorticotrophic hormone-secreting pituitary adenoma which causes adrenocortical hyperplasia. The effects (Box 31.11) are rarely dentally important.

Box 31.11   Important features of Cushing's disease
• Obesity of trunk and face
• Bruisability and haematomas after venepuncture
• Hirsutism
• Headaches
• Hypertension
• Osteoporosis, especially of the skull
• Glycosuria

POLYGLANDULAR AUTOIMMUNE ENDOCRINOPATHY SYNDROMES (POLYGLANDULAR AUTOIMMUNE DISEASE): TYPES 1 AND 2

Addison's disease is an invariable feature of type 1 polyglandular endocrinopathy syndrome. This uncommon disease features autoantibodies to a variety of glands (Table 31.1) as well as chronic mucocutaneous candidosis. The latter is not a feature of type 2 disease. In type 2 disease, Addison's disease is also an invariable feature, but not hypoparathyroidism. As discussed in Chapter 2, dental defects can also result from hypoparathyroidism in type 1 polyglandular endocrinopathy syndrome.

DISEASES OF THE ADRENAL MEDULLA

Phaeochromocytoma

Phaeochromocytoma is a catecholamine-producing tumour of the adrenal medulla. The main effect is potentially lethal hypertension and dysrhythmias. Occasionally, it is seen as part of the multiple endocrine adenoma syndrome type III, when it is associated with oral mucosal neurofibromas (Box 31.12) Alternatively, it may be associated with neurofibromatosis.

When an oral neurofibroma is found, the possibility of a phaeochromocytoma should be considered, especially if the patient is hypertensive. Other considerations in dentistry are the management of patients with severe hypertension and dysrhythmias but, in such cases, treatment should be delayed until they can be controlled by adminstration of an alpha-adrenergic blocker such as phenoxybenzamine which, after it has taken effect, may be followed by a beta-blocker.

411

Box 31.12 Important features of multiple endocrine neoplasia (MEN) syndromes

MEN 1
- Adenomas of pituitary, adrenals, sometimes thyroid. Insulinoma, gastrinoma. Parathyroid hyperplasia
- Zollinger–Ellison syndrome and peptic ulceration

MEN 2a
- Thyroid medullary cell carcinoma in all patients
- Parathyroid hyperplasia
- Phaeochromocytoma in 33% of patients
- Cutaneous neurofibromas

MEN 2b
- Thyroid medullary cell carcinoma in 80–100% of patients
- Parathyroid hyperplasia
- Phaeochromocytoma in 70% of patients
- Marfanoid skeletal features
- Oral mucosal neurofibromas

MULTIPLE ENDOCRINE NEOPLASIA SYNDROME

Multiple endocrine neoplasia (multiple endocrine adenomatosis) syndromes (MEN) are autosomal dominant disorders with a prevalence of about 1 in 20 000 that cause gland hyperplasia and benign and malignant neoplasms.

The gene for MEN1 is on chromosome 11q13 and encodes a nuclear transcription factor whose function remains unclear. Parathyroid, pancreas and pituitary are affected with presentation in the second and third decades. Hyperparathyroidism develops in 95%. Enteropancreatic tumours develop in over 40% and pituitary tumours in over 30%. Also described are gingival papules and nodular lesions on the vermilion border.

In MEN2, the mutated gene is the RET proto-oncogene, located on chromosome 11q12, a growth factor receptor that affects cell cycle and also the development of autonomic nerves. In this disease, medullary carcinoma of the thyroid is present in 95%, phaeochromocytoma in 50% and hyperparathyroidism in 15%. Two forms are recognised, 2a and 2b. A striking oral feature of MEN2b is mucosal neurofibromas, particularly along the lateral borders of the tongue. As already mentioned, oral neurofibromas are in any case rare and, when found, the possibility of MEN should be considered, particularly if hypertension is associated.

Screening for MEN2 is relatively readily carried out by identifying the RET mutation.

Features of multiple endocrine neoplasia syndrome are summarised in Box 31.12.

DIABETES MELLITUS

Diabetes mellitus is a common and important endocrine disease and results from relative or absolute deficiency of insulin, causing a persistently raised blood glucose. Approximately 2% of the population are affected, but probably at least 50% of diabetics with mild or early disease pass unrecognised. There are two main clinical types.

Juvenile onset (insulin-dependent) diabetes. Symptoms typically appear before the age of 25 and the disease is usually severe with thirst, polyuria, hunger, loss of weight and susceptibility to infection.

Maturity onset diabetes. Patients are typically over middle-age and obese. The onset is insidious, often with deterioration of vision or pruritus or, sometimes, thirst, polyuria and fatigue. However, many cases are asymptomatic. The disease can be controlled by dietary restriction and, if necessary, oral hypoglycaemic drugs. The current epidemic of childhood obesity seems likely to lead to the onset of this variety of diabetes early in life.

In terms of dental management, it is usually said that the greatest problems are with 'uncontrolled' diabetes. However, 'uncontrolled' applies to several diabetic states. At one extreme, there is the mild, unrecognised and therefore untreated, diabetic. At the other, there is the treated diabetic whose disease is difficult to control ('brittle diabetes') or has been mismanaged. This last group is the one most likely to have oral complications and present difficulties in dental management (Box 31.13).

Box 31.13 Complications of diabetes mellitus that can affect dental management

- Susceptibility to infection, particularly candidosis
- Hypoglycaemic coma
- Diabetic coma
- Ischaemic heart disease
- Acceleration of periodontal disease if control is poor
- Dry mouth secondary to polyuria and dehydration
- Oral lichenoid reactions due to oral hypoglycaemic drugs
- Sialadenosis

Dental aspects

The main oral manifestations of diabetes are usually due to the lowered resistance to infection. Oral signs can occasionally lead to the diagnosis of unsuspected diabetes.

Rapidly destructive periodontal disease can result from severe untreated diabetes mellitus, but is rarely seen now. However, even treated diabetic children have slightly poorer periodontal health than controls. Diabetics also have higher DMFT levels (despite the sugar-free diet) and earlier loss of teeth than controls. Susceptibility to candidosis is another complication. The principles of dental management are summarised in Box 31.14.

Hypoglycaemic coma may be precipitated by dental treatment which delays a normal meal and can cause an emergency in the dental surgery (Ch. 36). Treatment should therefore be so timed as to avoid these risks – ideally, soon after the patient's breakfast.

Diabetic coma is a complication of poorly-controlled diabetes mellitus and much less likely to be seen.

PREGNANCY

Pregnancy (apart from other problems) can cause significant oral effects and can affect dental management (Boxes 31.15 and 31.16).

The main risks of fetal abnormalities are from drugs and radiation: the hazard is greatest during organogenesis in the first trimester. Few drugs are known to be teratogenic for humans and, in many cases, the risk is no more than theoretical or results only from prolonged high dosage. For example, no teratogenic risk from metronidazole for humans has ever been substantiated though effects in animals have led to the avoidance of metronidazole in pregnancy. In the case of antiepileptic drugs, for example, any theoretical risks causing the drug to be witheld must be weighed against that of damage to the fetus by uncontrolled fits.

Dental considerations

The chief oral effects are aggravation of gingivitis (Fig. 31.9) and possible development of a pregnancy epulis (Fig. 31.10; Ch. 5). Initiation of a high standard of dental care and dental education at the earliest opportunity is essential. However, prenatal fluorides are not indicated as they have no useful effect on tooth germs. Anticaries measures (avoidance of sugar) may instead be necessary.

Occasionally, recurrent aphthae remit during pregnancy, but may worsen due to any iron or folate deficiency.

Fig. 31.9   **Pregnancy gingivitis.** Marginal gingivitis despite relatively good oral hygiene during the first trimester of pregnancy.

Fig. 31.10   **Pregnancy epulis.** When these lesions are not inflamed their vascular nature becomes obvious, as shown here.

A few women in late pregnancy become hypotensive when laid supine, when the swollen uterus impedes venous return. They should be treated in a sitting position. Respiratory reserve is diminished and there is a risk of fetal hypoxia. Neonatal respiration is further depressed by drugs such as general anaesthetics and sedatives, especially barbiturates, diazepam and opioids, all of which cross the placenta. Non-steroidal anti-inflammatory drugs in high dosage may cause premature closure of the ductus arteriosus and fetal pulmonary hypertension. Aspirin may also increase the risk of neonatal haemorrhage and paracetamol is the preferred analgesic. Systemic corticosteroids can cause fetal adrenosuppression. However, the only drugs known to be teratogenic are thalidomide (used occasionally for major aphthae), etretinate (used experimentally for leukoplakia) and possibly azathioprine (used occasionally for Behçet's syndrome and sometimes for autoimmune diseases). For details of drug usage in pregnancy, see the current British National Formulary.

The risks from dental radiography are small, but only essential radiographs should be taken, the minimal radiation exposure should be given and the patient should wear a lead apron.

There is no evidence of risks from local anaesthesia and its use is desirable rather than submit the pregnant woman to operative pain. As noted above, the risks from benzodiazepines such as midozalam for sedation are such that intravenous sedation is contraindicated. Nitrous oxide sedation carries with it a risk of interference with B_{12} and folate metabolism after prolonged administration[1], but there is no evidence that it is teratogenic. The main precautions are to give it only after the first trimester and for less than 30 minutes: 50% oxygen should, of course, be given.

---

[1]This effect was first noticed in patients in intensive care who had been given continuous nitrous oxide and oxygen for periods of 3 weeks.

SUGGESTED FURTHER READING

Cawson RA, Spector RG, Skelly AM 1995 Basic pharmacology and clinical drug use in dentistry, 6th edn. Churchill Livingstone, Edinburgh

Darling TN, Skarulis MC, Steinberg SM, Marx SJ, Spiegel AM, Turner M 1997 Multiple facial angiofibromas and collagenomas in patients with multiple endocrine neoplasia type 1. Arch Derm 133:853-857

Franklyn JA 1993 Hypothyroidism. Medicine (UK) 21:161–163

Franklyn JA 1993 Hyperthyroidism. Medicine (UK) 21:164–169

Learoyd DL, Delbridge LW, Robinson BG 2000 Multiple endocrine neoplasia. Aust NZ Med 30:675–682

Nathan DM 1993 Long-term complications of diabetes mellitus. N Engl J Med 328:1676–1685

Stephenson E, Haug RH, Murphy TA 1995 Management of the diabetic oral and maxillofacial surgery patient. J Oral Maxillofac Surg 53:175–182

Trainer PJ, Howlett T, Besser EM 1993 Cushing's syndrome. Medicine Int 21:178–183

Trainer PJ, Howlett T, Besser EM1993 Addison's disease. Medicine Int 21:184–188

Williams JD, Slupchinsku O, Sclafani AP et al 1996 Evaluation and management of the lingual thyroid gland. Ann Otol Rhinol Laryngol 105:312–316

Renal disease

Renal disease has become important in dentistry because of the growing number of patients who, as a result of renal dialysis or transplantation, survive renal failure. Aspects of renal disease relevant to dentistry are summarised in Box 32.1.

Box 32.1 **Aspects of renal disease affecting dental management**

- Heparinisation before dialysis
- Possible hepatitis B or C carriage after chronic dialysis
- Permanent venous fistulae susceptible to infection
- Secondary hyperparathyroidism
- Immunosuppressive treatment for nephrotic syndrome or transplant patients
- Oral lesions due to drugs, particularly for immunosuppression
- Lower doses or withholding of many drugs: e.g. some cephalosporins and tetracyclines
- Oral lesions of chronic renal failure (Box 32.2)

CHRONIC RENAL FAILURE

Some patients are unsuitable for, or unable to obtain, dialysis or a transplant. They can suffer a variety of oral effects (Box 32.2).

Box 32.2 **Oral changes in renal failure**

- Mucosal pallor (anaemia)
- Xerostomia
- Purpura
- Mucosal ulceration
- Thrush or bacterial plaques
- White epithelial plaques (Ch. 15)
- Giant-cell lesions of the jaws (secondary hyperparathyroidism)

Dental management of patients with renal disease, but particularly chronic renal failure, may be affected by many factors (Box 32.3).

RENAL OSTEODYSTROPHY AND SECONDARY HYPERPARATHYROIDISM

Prolonged dialysis or renal failure are now more common causes of giant-cell lesions of bone than primary hyperparathyroidism. The jaws may be first affected (Ch. 10).

Box 32.3 **Factors potentially affecting dental management of patients with renal disease**

- Corticosteroid and other immunosuppressive treatment
- Haemorrhagic tendencies
- Anaemia
- Impaired drug excretion
- Hypertension
- Hepatitis B or C carriage
- Underlying causes (e.g. diabetes mellitus, hypertension, or connective tissue disease)

RENAL TRANSPLANTATION

Patients in renal failure may receive regular dialysis while awaiting a transplant, but remain otherwise in reasonably good general health. About 70% can return to full-time work. However, they are heparinised before dialysis and haemostasis is impaired for 6 to 12 hours.

These patients' permanent venous fistula for the dialysis lines is susceptible to infection and antibiotic cover may be considered for dental surgical procedures. Drugs, including sedation, should not be given intravenously, because of the risk of damage to superficial veins which are patients' lifelines. Dialysis patients also have an greater incidence of cardiovascular and cerebrovascular disease.

Normal renal function and health can be restored by transplantation, but it is associated with the complications of prolonged immunosuppressive treatment, particularly susceptibility to infections or lymphomas.

Ciclosporin, which is widely used to help control graft rejection, can cause persistent gingival hyperplasia with false pocketing which readily progesses to periodontal destruction in some patients. If a calcium channel blocker, such as nifedipine, is also being given for hypertension, gingival hyperplasia is virtually inevitable and uncontrollable unless oral hygiene is meticulous. Unfortunately, patients on dialysis may develop increased calculus.

Hairy leukoplakia can rarely develop in HIV-negative renal transplant patients as a complication of immunosuppression.

Complications of graft rejection, such as bone lesions due to secondary hyperparathyroidism, may be seen (see Fig. 10.21).

Graft rejection is frequently due to patients' non-compliance with immunosuppressive regimens because of their adverse effects.

Children with renal failure may have enamel hypoplasia and dysplastic dentine with delayed eruption of teeth.

SUGGESTED FURTHER READING

Cove-Smith R 1995 Drugs and the kidney. Medicine Int 23:165–173
King GN, Fullinfaw R, Higgins TJ et al 1993 Gingival hyperplasia in renal allograft patients receiving cyclosporin A and calcium antagonists. J Clin Periodontol 20:286–293
King GN, Healy CM, Glover MT et al 1994 Prevalence and risk factors associated with leukoplakia, hairy leukoplakia, erythematous candidiasis and gingival hyperplasia in renal transplant recipients. Oral Surg Oral Med Oral Pathol 78:718–726

Mallick NP 1995 Presenting features of renal disease. Medicine Int 23:91–96
Mallick NP 1995 Renal transplantation. Medicine Int 23:156–158
Proctor R, Kumar N, Stein A et al 2005 Oral and dental aspects of chronic renal failure. J Dent Res 84:199–208
Ziccardi VB, Siani J, Demas PN, Braun TW 1992 Management of the oral and maxillofacial surgery patient with end-stage renal disease. J Oral Maxillofac Surg 50:1207–1212

Intellectual and physical disability and psychiatric disorders

The terminology for disability is confusing, evolving and subject to the forces of political correctness. Healthcare professionals often demand clear-cut definitions of degrees of disability that can be used to plan dental services. Unfortunately, this approach over-simplifies the problems. People with disability see their needs in social terms rather than just the sum of their medical problems and, rightly, demand individualised care. The dentist must consider what each patient is prevented from doing, rather than concentrating on the physical or mental impairments themselves. This way of thinking illustrates the social and environmental aspects of disability, and highlights ways in which the individual's environment can be adapted to limit, or even abolish, handicap. Current terminology for disability is shown in Table 33.1.

Table 33.1 Current terminology for disability

Term	Definition
Impairment	Any loss or abnormality of physiological function or anatomical structure
Disability or limitation of activity	Restriction or lack of ability to perform a function considered normal
Handicap	The disadvantage for the individual, resulting from their disability, which prevents them from performing a normal role in society

Nowhere is terminology more difficult than in the case of intellectual impairment. The terms mental retardation, subnormality, deficiency or handicap are considered stigmatising and no longer acceptable. In practice, intellectual impairments cause a wide range of disability. Some patients are intelligent but cannot cooperate (e.g. cerebral palsy), others are intelligent but uncooperative (e.g. hyperactivity), yet others are intellectually impaired but may sometimes be easily treated (e.g. mild Down's syndrome). The specific diagnosis and its severity are much more helpful in planning treatment than non-specific labels such as learning difficulty or intellectual impairment.

The prevalence of inherited disability is estimated at 1.5 to 2 per 1000 live births. Intellectual impairments account for approximately 0.9 per 1000 and major physical impairments for the remainder. The prevalence is rising as a result of better medical care for adults and improved survival for babies with congenital disorders. Approximately 12 000 children with disabilities are registered with dental practitioners. The management of their dental care is affected by both the disability and parents' motivation and attitudes. However, mental or physical disability does not necessarily mean that dental care has to be compromised, though this may sometimes be inevitable.

Children and adults with disability present a wide variety of problems of dental management, but up to 90% of them can probably be managed by conventional means without sedation or general anaesthesia. Nevertheless, people with disability are a dentally neglected group, even though valiant attempts have been made to overcome this deficiency in recent years.

Preconceptions that 'the disabled' are necessarily grimacing, drooling and uncooperative are seriously misplaced. In fact, those who manage children with disability find the work more rewarding than dentistry in normal children. Dental treatment, which involves both relatively prolonged personal attention and a change from routine, can be a pleasure for them. One Down's syndrome child, for instance, though well looked after by affectionate parents, was in a state of mysteriously eager expectation for days at the prospect (it was later found) of having an X-ray. Dental treatment may, therefore, be a real source of pleasure for those so deprived.

There is a welcome concern about the dental care of children with disability, but it should be remembered that disability persists for life. The transition from special school to community care can worsen dental disease because dental care must be provided in a less controlled setting and intensive prevention is more difficult to maintain. The elderly probably suffer more disabilities than children, because of the additional problems of declining health but, unfortunately, are less likely to get sympathetic help.

Difficulties in the provision of dental care for people with disability are summarised in Box 33.1. Unless the disability is severe, most of these difficulties can be overcome with patience, training and experience. It should be remembered that when disability is viewed in its social context, many difficulties become the responsibility of the dentist rather than being a problem associated with the patient.

Box 33.1   **Typical difficulties with dental care of patients with disability**

- Poor cooperation with routine dental treatment
- Difficulties in performing routine home oral hygiene
- Associated systemic disease
- Difficulties with transport and access to the surgery
- Need for sedation or general anaesthesia
- Medications or diets promoting caries
- Dysphagia, drooling, bruxism
- Oral effects of medication
- Competence to give consent
- Financial problems for patients
- Discrimination or prejudice in health care

Mental illness often manifests itself as challenging behaviour and patients suffer many problems in common with people with disability, particularly discrimination and poor access to dental care. Those with personality defects can sometimes be totally uncooperative and their dental treatment may be severely compromised.

Epilepsy is often associated with other disabilities but, with modern treatment, should present no special difficulties. There may be problems with phenytoin-induced fibrous gingival hyperplasia (Ch. 5). It is also important to be able to recognise and manage a major fit should it happen in the dental surgery (Ch. 36).

The importance of good prevention cannot be overemphasised. Many of the problems arising from treatment of people with disability would be solved by good preventive regimens.

Disabilities relevant to dentistry are summarised in Box 33.2.

Box 33.2   **Common medical disabilities affecting dental management**

Intellectual impairment
- Learning difficulty
- Down's syndrome
- Microcephaly and hydrocephalus
- Metabolic disorders
- Hypoxia at birth
- Some syndromes

Behavioural disorders
- Autism
- Attention deficit hyperactivity disorder

Physical impairment
- Cerebral palsy
- Severe defects of the hands or arms
- Muscular dystrophies
- Spina bifida
- Epilepsy
- Some syndromes
- Communication problems: visual and hearing impairment
- Cleft palate (Ch. 2)

Physical and intellectual impairment are frequently combined, as in Down's syndrome and some cases of cerebral palsy. Intellectual impairment (often associated with physical impairment) affects by far the largest group of children with disability needing dental care. All patients with Down's syndrome, many

with cerebral palsy and some with epilepsy are also intellectually impaired. These four groups account for approximately 70–75% of children with disability. Conversely, many patients with cerebral palsy have normal intelligence but may be mislabelled as mentally impaired because of communication difficulties.

Heart disease, haemorrhagic disease (particularly haemophilia), diabetes mellitus and other systemic diseases are discussed in Chapters 26 to 32.

DISCRIMINATION LEGISLATION

The UK Disability Discrimination Act 2005 is intended to abolish discrimination and applies to all employers and service providers including dentists.

The Act defines disability as a physical or mental impairment which has a substantial and long-term adverse effect on an individual's ability to carry out normal day-to-day activities. The definition is broad and applies equally to conditions such as colour blindness, visual or hearing impairment and severe learning difficulty.

Under the Act, service providers must not use any reason related to patients' disability as an excuse to treat disabled people less favourably than other people. Dentists must make 'reasonable adjustments' so that disabled people can access and use their services. This means more than providing wheelchair ramps. All aspects of the clinical practice and business of dentistry must comply. Some examples of the measures expected under the Act are shown in Box 33.3. Which are reasonable in any particular setting depends on guidance from the Disability Rights Commission and will change over time and with legal precedents.

Box 33.3   **Some factors to ameliorate disability in dental practice**

Access	Level access, ramps, easy-grip door handles, doors hold open easily, wide corridors and aisles, obstructions clearly marked, if necessary provide off-site or domiciliary visits. Provide for guide dogs
Design and structure of buildings	Colour schemes contrast floors and walls, well lit, alarms in toilets (visible and audible)
Signs and practice leaflets and paperwork	Large type, succinct, good colour contrast, easy to read, use symbols as well as words, use sans serif fonts, no justification of right hand margins, simple page layouts. Consider Braille and audio versions
Websites	Should meet British Standard Specification for accessible websites
Staff and policies	Provide disability awareness training for staff, record and survey needs of disabled users and consult local disability groups. Each practice should have a disability policy

---

Practices that are 'disability-friendly' will also be more suitable for the elderly and many other groups of normal patients.

LEARNING DIFFICULTY

Learning difficulty is an all-inclusive term to describe those with intellectual impairment whether caused by a specific disorder or of unknown cause. Down's syndrome, fragile X syndrome and hypoxia at birth are the more common causes and the specific features of these conditions are dealt with below. Learning difficulties may be unrelated to any physical disorder, or physical defects may be severe, as in some cases of cerebral palsy. A minority of patients with genetic syndromes have craniofacial anomalies associated with intellectual impairment.

Intellectual impairment is classified according to the level of learning difficulty and children are taught either in mainstream schools or special schools, according to the degree of impairment. Institutional care is avoided if possible. Unfortunately, the learning difficulty classification gives no more than a broad indication of probable problems with dental care because patients vary so widely.

Children with mild learning difficulty can usually be coaxed into accepting regular treatment and (if the parents are supportive) to maintain acceptable standards of oral hygiene. However, oral hygiene is usually suboptimal or poor when it depends on parents or carers. At the other extreme, all that may be possible, particularly for children with uncontrollable muscular activity such as jaw clenching, is first-aid dentistry under general anaesthesia. All intermediate grades exist, but the level of dental health that can be achieved depends greatly upon the level of the dentist's skill and devotion to the task (Fig. 33.1) and prevention by carers.

Down's syndrome

Down's syndrome is the most common clinically recognisable syndrome with severe learning difficulty. It is caused by trisomy of chromosome 21 giving a total complement of 47 chromosomes instead of 46. This is usually caused by failure of the chromosomes to separate during meiosis in the ovum, a defect closely linked to maternal age. The overall incidence is 1 in 700 live births, but the risk rises to 1 in 25 in mothers aged 45 years or over. Because the defect arises in the ovum, both parents are normal and the condition is not inherited.

In contrast, about 4% of Down's patients have the additional chromosome 21 genetic material translocated to another chromosome. The translocation is transmitted in a familial pattern, but the parents are normal and the risk of an affected child is relatively low.

The rarest form is mosaic Down's syndrome in which the trisomy arises during early development and the patients have a mosaic of cells with and without trisomy 21. In this type of Down's syndrome, the features are very variable and intelligence may be normal despite the typical appearance.

General features

Down's children have a characteristic facial appearance (Fig. 33.2), abnormalities of the skull and frequently of the dentition, abnormal susceptibility to infection (particularly viral) due to multiple immune defects and congenital cardiovascular disease in up to 50%.

The prominent medial epicanthic skin fold gives the eyes their readily recognisable appearance. There is hypoplasia of the mid-face, poorly developed paranasal sinuses and a malformed upper respiratory tract. Upper respiratory tract infections are common and breathing is often partially obstructed. Underdevelopment of the maxillae is usually associated with a protrusive mandible and class III malocclusion, with anterior open bite (Fig. 33.3, Box 33.4). The ears are often malformed and there is excess skin on the neck.

Fig. 33.1 Traumatic ulceration. This child with learning difficulties produced this deep and extensive ulcer after a local anaesthetic for dental treatment.

Fig. 33.2 Down's syndrome. This shows both the characteristic facial appearance and a cyanotic flush caused by associated congenital heart disease.

Box 33.4   Down's syndrome: features relevant to dentistry

- Class III malocclusion with hypoplastic maxilla
- Protrusive, fissured and apparently enlarged hypotonic tongue (Fig. 33.4)
- Lip hypotonia, mouth breathing and drooling
- Everted, thick, dry and crusted lips
- Oligodontia
- Delayed eruption of permanent teeth
- Hypoplastic dental defects and short roots
- Low caries activity
- Gross plaque accumulation
- Rapidly progressive periodontal disease
- Bruxism
- Short stature with short limbs
- Poor muscle tone
- Generalised susceptibility to infection
- Visual or hearing impairment in 50%
- Cardiac anomalies in 40%
- Weakness of atlantoaxial joint
- Susceptibility to leukaemia
- Alzheimer-like dementia in later life

Upper lateral incisors are often absent and the teeth have short roots. Despite a higher than normal incidence of enamel

hypoplasia, caries risk is low. The low caries activity has been ascribed to the form and spacing of the teeth and to the high bicarbonate content and pH of the saliva. Despite the relative resistance, use of a sweetened dummy, poor diet or medications with sucrose can readily lead to caries.

Plaque accumulation and poor oral hygiene, due to the patient's disabilities and made worse by mouth breathing, together with the systemic predisposition to infection, contribute to the early onset of periodontal disease and early tooth loss (Fig. 33.5). Acute ulcerative gingivitis is also common and often recurs.

Management

All Down's children have learning difficulties, some severe, but they continue to learn throughout life and may develop many skills if supported by good educational programmes and occupational therapy. Some can maintain an independent life. Patients with Down's syndrome are often, but not invariably, good-natured, cooperative within their ability and affectionate and receptive to dental care. However, this stereotype fails to

Fig. 33.3   Down's syndrome. This shows the characteristic anterior open bite together with gross gingival hyperplasia caused by phenytoin treatment for concomitant epilepsy.

Fig. 33.4   Down's syndrome. As is frequently the case there are many missing teeth and, in the gaps between them, the hypotonic tongue is protruding.

Fig. 33.5   Down's syndrome. Poor oral hygiene, periodontal destruction and malocclusion. (By kind permission of Professor C Scully.)

recognise many who are frightened or more severely affected and completely uncooperative. The success of dental treatment depends mainly on the level of care provided. Those with milder learning disability can be treated normally in the dental chair, while the more severely affected may require general anaesthesia.

Control of periodontal disease is usually difficult and success depends almost entirely on prevention by good oral hygiene. Teeth may be lost relatively early because of their short roots. Retention of teeth is important because dentures are usually poorly tolerated and retained because of the large protrusive tongue, poor muscle tone and poor comprehension. The apparently large tongue results from muscle hypotonia and forward posture, which also cause problems with mastication and swallowing.

Other features of the syndrome may affect dental treatment. The unstable atlanto-occipital joint is at risk of dislocation with severe consequences if the head is manipulated, particularly during general anaesthesia or sedation. All Down's syndrome patients should have been screened for this anomaly during early childhood. Deafness and visual problems are common. With improved medical care, life expectancy in Down's syndrome has lengthened and patients often live into their sixth decade. Unfortunately, almost half of older Down's patients suffer an Alzheimer-like dementia, which further compromises their independence.

Cardiac defects are present in 40% and half of these are severe enough to warrant surgical intervention. Atrial and ventricular septal defects, mitral and tricuspid valve defects, Fallot's tetralogy and patent ductus are common. These are repaired in childhood but, in later life, valvular regurgitation and prolapse may develop. Despite many contributory factors, the incidence of infective endocarditis does not appear to be particularly high, but prophylactic antibiotic cover must be given as for normal patients (Ch. 27).

Fragile X syndrome

Fragile X syndrome is the next most common chromosomal defect with learning disability after Down's syndrome; it affects at least 1 in 1000 of the population.

In this syndrome, the tip of the X chromosome appears as a thin thread of chromatin that is weakly attached and may break off.

Clinical features include learning disability, hyperactivity and behaviour similar to that of autism. Open bite and crossbite are frequent.

Hydrocephalus

Hydrocephalus is caused by failure of drainage of cerebrospinal fluid and may be seen in isolation or associated with spina bifida. Compression of the cerebral tissue can cause severe intellectual impairment. Treatment is to relieve the intracranial pressure by insertion of a catheter and, in the past, this

released the cerebrospinal fluid directly into the right atrium (Spitz–Holzer valve). This shunt is susceptible to infection, causing blockage rather than endocarditis. Although antibiotic prophylaxis is not of proven effectiveness, antibiotics are usually given as a precaution, using the same regimen for infective endocarditis. Younger patients are more likely to have a shunt into the peritoneal cavity and this type does not require antibiotic prophylaxis. Severe hydrocephalus can also cause the skull to be so distended and heavy that the head has to be supported during treatment.

BEHAVIOURAL DISORDERS

Autism

Autism is a specific defect of mental development in which there is lack of emotional development, disordered use of language, defective communication and extreme 'aloneness'. The cause is unknown and both environmental and genetic causes are suspected. The condition is much more common in males. At one extreme, there is severe learning disorder and repetitive behaviour so that it may be impossible to communicate with, or manage, autistic children without general anaesthesia. At the other, sympathy and patience may achieve all that is needed. Asperger's syndrome is the mildest form of autism. Typical features are summarised in Box 33.5.

Box 33.5   Autism: typical features

- 'Aloneness'
- Lack of social interaction
- Lack of eye contact with others
- Communication problems
- Apparent unawareness of others
- Fixation on a single object or toy
- Persistent hand-slapping or other repetitive activity
- Rarely, extreme mathematical or artistic talents
- Learning difficulties in 70%

Vey rarely, autistic persons possess bizarre, incomprehensible skills, often mathematical. If, for example, one of these 'autistic savant' is asked what day of the week March 7th 2025 will be, an immediate accurate answer is provided.

Hyperactivity/attention deficit disorder

These conditions are often grouped together despite their different presentations. Attention deficit is characterised by daydreaming, limited ability to concentrate and perform complex tasks. Hyperactivity is characterised by excessive movement, inability to concentrate on one task and, sometimes, repetitive movements. The number of children diagnosed with these conditions has risen dramatically since the advent of the drug methylphenidate (Ritalin), but there is no agreed dividing line between this disorder and normal child behaviour. Some cases seem to respond to dietary modification. It has been suggested that some children labelled as suffering hyperactivity/attention deficit are no more than mildly disruptive underachieving children. Such cases might be difficult dental patients but can be expected to respond to good behaviour management. Conversely, severe hyperactivity is profoundly disturbing and may be associated with self-mutilation. Extreme cases may require sedation or anaesthesia.

PHYSICAL IMPAIRMENT

Cerebral palsy

Cerebral palsy is common, with an incidence of 1:1000 and can be one of the most severe disabilities. These children, in the past loosely referred to as spastics, suffer various types of neuromuscular dysfunction (Box 33.6).

Box 33.6 **Types of cerebral palsy**

- Spastic
  - Monoplegic
  - Paraplegic
  - Diplegic
  - Quadriplegic
- Athetotic
- Ataxic
- Hypotonic
- Mixed types

Neuromuscular dysfunction

Neuromuscular dysfunction can be so severe as to make speech unintelligible (dysarthria) and cause the children to appear intellectually impaired. Communication can sometimes be possible if dentists are prepared to spend time learning to comprehend them. Many cerebral palsy patients have visual speech-aids or computerised devices to help them communicate.

Spasticity affects half the patients and causes fixed contraction of affected muscles and general stiffness. This may be so great that it may not even be possible to move an affected limb passively. Hemiplegia is the most common type: in such cases intellectual impairment is uncommon but other neurological disorders, such as epilepsy, are frequent. Quadriplegics, by contrast, are frequently intellectually impaired but less often epileptic. Athetosis refers to involuntary jerking movements, often of a wriggling character, sometimes accompanied by grimacing, and is seen in almost half the patients.

Ataxia is least common and characterised by lack of balance, an unsteady gait and poor control over voluntary movements. In addition to variants of these three main types of disease, different parts of the body may be affected to a greater degree than others.

Dental aspects

Access to dental care for their wheelchairs is frequently difficult for those with cerebral palsy. Many have severe caries and often periodontal disease due to inability to maintain oral hygiene and their dental care is difficult, however willing they may be.

The first consideration is full assessment of the patient's capabilities. The child's ability to deal with dental disease can then be judged. If the child is uncontrollably anxious, sedation may help. If disabilities are not too severe, many of these children can be treated satisfactorily in the dental chair. The chief difficulty with athetotic children is their irregular movements. These may make it impossible to carry out good restorative work and also make it easy for the child to be injured with sharp dental instruments. The mildest cases may respond well to relaxation with inhalation sedation, but some will need full sedation or general anaesthesia. It is always essential to use a mouth prop with conscious athetotic patients, as the jaws may suddenly clench. Epilepsy, falls and sudden uncontrolled movements also render them prone to dental injury. Bruxism and masseteric hypertrophy are frequent and drooling may result from the open mouth posture and defective swallowing. These latter complaints often most trouble these patients.

Many cerebral palsy patients suffer epilepsy and drug-induced gingival overgrowth.

Key features are summarised in Box 33.7.

Box 33.7 **Cerebral palsy: key dental features**

- Usually class II malocclusion and anterior open bite
- Muscle hypotonia
- Frequently severe caries and periodontal disease
- Bruxism and masseteric hypertrophy
- Impaired swallowing reflex but exaggerated gag reflex
- Dental erosion and gastric reflux
- Enamel hypoplasia
- Mouth breathing
- Dental trauma
- Delayed eruption
- Drooling

Multiple sclerosis

This distressing and potentially disabling disease is one of the most common causes of long-term disability. Symptoms are disseminated in both site and time and the onset is typically in early adulthood. Common initial features include optic neuritis with transient blindness of one eye, remittent sensory symptoms, subacute loss of function of an arm and palsy of the VIth cranial nerve. Effects of the latter include convergent squint and diplopia. The outcome is highly variable; in the great majority there are short acute attacks of disability but, in about 10%, there is progressive deterioration culminating in widespread paralysis and incontinence.

In the absence of a cure, symptomatic treatment is mainly needed. Interferon beta-1a and -1b may cause there to be fewer relapses. Intravenous immunoglobulin, plasma exchange and the monoclonal antibody, natalizumab, are as yet of unconfirmed benefit.

Dental aspects

The majority of minor cases can be treated normally, but there are the usual problems associated with the severely disabled. Oral hygiene can deteriorate and preventive dental care is necessary. For severely disabled patients, treatment under local anaesthesia is acceptable, but they should not be put in the supine position because of possible respiratory difficulties. Trigeminal neuralgia-like pain may respond to carbamazepine or gabapentin, but less reliably than the more common variety. Facial palsy can be another complication. The (unjustified) concern that amalgam restorations can cause or worsen the disease is discussed in Chapter 25.

Key features of multiple sclerosis are summarised in Box 33.8.

> **Box 33.8 Multiple sclerosis: key features**
>
> - Onset before age 60
> - Neurological deficits in several sites
> - CNS involvement can consist of:
>   Several remittent episodes lasting 24 or more hours, or
>   Progressive slow progression over 6 or more months
> - Absence of other cause of symptoms
> - Occasionally trigeminal neuralgia-like pain

Epilepsy

Epilepsy is a common brain disorder causing fits (seizures) and disturbances of consciousness; it is most frequently idiopathic. The main types of epilepsy are summarised in Box 33.9. Epilepsy is most common in adolescence or young adulthood and is then usually idiopathic, but may be due to alcohol or drug abuse or HIV infection. The onset of epilepsy in the middle-aged or elderly is likely to be a sign of a brain lesion such as a cerebral tumour, cerebrovascular disease or senile or Alzheimer's dementia.

> **Box 33.9 Types of epilepsy**
>
> **Generalised seizures**
> - Tonic-clonic (grand mal)
> - Absence seizures (petit mal)
>
> **Partial seizures**
> - Simple (Jacksonian epilepsy)
> - Complex (temporal lobe epilepsy)

Clinically, grand mal epilepsy comprises loss of consciousness, typically preceded by an aura (a warning hallucination), a momentary tonic phase (rigidity) followed by clonic convulsions (repetitive jerking movements of the whole body) and a flaccid phase of semi-coma. Respiratory muscle spasm in the tonic phase can cause a brief cry and cyanosis. The patient falls to the ground and is at risk of injury. The main features are usually complete within five minutes. The recovery period is often characterised by headache and confusion, sleep for 12 or more hours. In susceptible subjects, fits can be precipitated by fatigue, starvation, acute anxiety, infections, menstruation or rapidly flickering lights.

Petit mal attacks ('absence seizures') are most common in children. The features are little or no movement apart from blinking, sudden but brief loss of awareness or activity, without significant loss of postural or muscular control and lasting a few seconds. Consciousness is regained without recollection of the episode. Most patients with petit mal have or develop grand mal epilepsy.

Temporal lobe epilepsy is characterised by impaired consciousness and, typically, delusions. Paranoid or schizophrenic features are often associated. For the literary-minded, Henry James' *The Turn of the Screw* is regarded as a vivid description of temporal lobe epilepsy.

Management

The diagnosis must be confirmed: a history of recurrent fits, a physical examination including blood chemistry and an electroencephalogram are usually adequate. The main anticonvulsant drugs for major fits are sodium valproate, carbamazepine, lamotrigine or gabapentin. Phenytoin, which causes troublesome drowsiness and many other adverse effects, is largely obsolete. Ethosuximide is the drug of choice for petit mal.

Dental aspects

The risk of a fit in the dental surgery is so disturbing that all precautions should be taken to minimise this hazard. The key is to identify triggers for attacks in the patient history. Flashing lights are the best-known trigger but this is relatively rare. Alcohol, tiredness, menstruation and hypoglycaemia are often blamed by individual patients and relatively easily avoided. Unfortunately, stress is a common trigger.

Treatment should be arranged for 'good phases' when attacks are infrequent. During treatment, a mouth prop must be kept in place to prevent the patient from biting the tongue or the dentist's fingers if an attack develops and management of the fit itself and its most dangerous complication, status epilepticus, is discussed in Chapter 36. As much equipment as possible should be kept out of reach of the patient. Gingival hyperplasia, folate deficiency and lymphadenopathy due to phenytoin are less likely to be seen now. Although large doses of intravenous lidocaine given for severe dysrhythmias can occasionally precipitate fits, there is no evidence of any risk from lidocaine in local anaesthetics. Injuries from a major fit can include lacerations of the tongue or lips, and injuries due to falling such as maxillofacial damage and fractures to vertebrae or limbs.

Spina bifida

Spina bifida is failure of fusion of the vertebral arches and may be inherited or environmental in aetiology. Approximately

1:1000 children are affected. The mildest form (spina bifida occulta) is common but no more than a radiographic finding, sometimes with a tuft of hair overlying the defect. In the severe form (spina bifida cystica), there is a gross defect in the lower vertebral canal. The meninges and, often, nerve tissue protrude through it as a sac, which may be covered by skin. The consequences are paralysis and deformities of the lower limbs with loss of sensation and reflexes, incontinence and other complications. Meningitis is an obvious hazard and epilepsy is frequently associated. Hydrocephalus is associated in almost all cases.

Since the upper part of the body is normal, the main difficulty in dental management is getting a chair adapted to the child's disability. Associated epilepsy may also affect dental management.

Severe limb defects

These are rare but have been brought to public notice by the thalidomide tragedy. One of the striking effects of this drug is absence of the proximal part of a limb (phocomelia). Thus, the hands, often also defective, are attached close to the shoulder.

These children can receive normal dental care, but are totally dependent on physical aids, parents or carers for tooth brushing. Again, preventive measures to minimise caries activity are important.

The muscular dystrophies

Muscular dystrophies, of which the Duchenne type is the most common (approximately 1 in 5000 male births), are the main crippling diseases of childhood. Weakness of the muscles leads to progressively severe disability and is frequently associated with cardiomyopathy and respiratory impairment.

There appear to be no specific dental problems other than that of stabilising a severely affected child in the chair. General anaesthesia is dangerous in the presence of cardiac disease or respiratory impairment.

Myasthenia gravis

Myasthenia gravis is a disabling autoimmune disease causing weakness and rapid fatigue of voluntary muscles. Women between 20 and 30 are mainly affected. Circulating autoantibodies to the nicotinic, acetylcholinergic receptor of the neuromuscular end-plates weakens the response to acetylcholine.

Clinically, there is rapidly developing, severe fatigue. Disability is worsened by cold, emotional stress and overexertion. Involvement of the respiratory muscles is potentially lethal and is most likely to affect the elderly.

Dental aspects

Weakness of the masticatory muscles causes the 'hanging jaw sign' for which patients characteristically support the jaw with a hand. Other effects include difficulties with speech, mastication

and swallowing. Paresis or atrophy of the tongue are occasional complications. In the rare syndrome of thymoma, myasthenia gravis and depressed cell-mediated immunity are associated with chronic mucocutaneous candidosis. Other rare associations are pemphigus vulgaris and Sjögren's syndrome. Use of anticholinesterases can cause excessive salivation.

Intravenous sedation is contraindicated because of the risk of respiratory involvement. Many drugs used in anaesthesia, particularly muscle relaxants, can severely aggravate myasthenic manifestations.

Management

Diagnosis is confirmed by exposure to an anticholinesterase, such as edrophonium, which raises the concentration of acetylcholine at the motor end-plates and improves muscular activity. Serum antibodies to acetylcholine receptors are detectable in about 85%. Anticholinesterases, such as pyridostigmine, are the mainstay but cholinergic effects such as nausea, diarrhoea and bradycardia may be troublesome. Alternatives are corticosteroids in combination with azathioprine or ciclosporin.

THE ELDERLY

While the problems of looking after handicapped children centre largely on their physical and mental limitations, these are compounded in the elderly by the lack of parents or, often, carers to help them. Mobility and access to care are often severely compromised. Also, there is a great variety of oral complaints that they may suffer. In extreme cases, for example, an elderly patient may be so intellectually impaired, deaf and depressed as to make communication excessively difficult but may also have oral cancer.

Communication is often the key problem in the management of the elderly. Factors which may disable the elderly are summarised in Box 33.10.

Box 33.10   Causes of disabilities in the elderly

Neurological and psychological disorders
- Intellectual deterioration
- Depression
- Dementia (particularly Alzheimer's disease)
- Confusional states
- Paranoia
- Dependence on hypnotics
- Parkinson's disease
- Strokes
- Deafness
- Impaired sight
- Trigeminal neuralgia (Ch. 34)

Mental deterioration is a common consequence of ageing and can affect all aspects of mental activity, such as intelligence, memory, emotional state and personality. These different functions tend to be affected to a variable and unpredictable extent. Thus, the patient may seem bright enough but may immediately forget instructions, for example, about how to look after dentures. Other patients become confused, querulous, or even aggressive, behave in an irresponsible fashion, have delusions of persecution and are generally 'difficult'. Alzheimer's disease, the most common cause of dementia after middle age, can present in any of these ways.

In general, the older the patients, the less adaptable they are likely to be. While preservation of teeth for as long as possible may be desirable, it may create greater problems if extractions have to be postponed until late in life. The wearing of full dentures demands a remarkable feat of adaptation at any age and older patients face greater difficulties. Also, some older patients may no longer care about appearance, may have few social contacts and may prefer a soft diet. Motivation, which plays so large a part in adaptation to denture wearing, may also therefore be diminished.

Difficulties with and complaints about dentures by elderly patients may therefore be as much due to mental deterioration as physical problems. Poor communication, often due to deafness, makes matters worse. Exasperating though such complaints may become, they must be treated with understanding and sympathy. This mental deterioration is something we all have to suffer if we live long enough; in the words of a physician *'insightless atrophy and ultimate obliteration of normal mental life … is a remorseless enemy of the natural dignity of man'.*

Limitations on mobility

Conditions which may make it difficult for the elderly to attend for dental treatment are summarised in Box 33.11.

Box 33.11 Some causes of limitation of mobility in the elderly

- Ataxia
- Strokes
- Arthritis
- Heart disease
- Late Alzheimer's disease
- Blindness
- Poor balance

Systemic disease in the elderly

Systemic diseases which particularly affect the elderly are shown in Box 33.12.

A variety of drugs used for cardiovascular disease can also cause oral reactions (Ch. 27). As noted earlier, the elderly with heart lesions are at the highest risk for infective endocarditis and form the peak age group for this disease.

Malnutrition is particularly likely to affect the elderly. Poverty, poor mobility (which interferes with both cooking and shopping) and mental deterioration are some of the contributory

---

Box 33.12 Important systemic diseases more common in the elderly

Cardiovascular
- Hypertension and ischaemic heart disease (Ch. 27)
- Cardiac failure (any cause) (Ch. 27)
- Giant-cell (temporal) arteritis and polymyalgia rheumatica (Ch. 11)

Respiratory
- Chronic bronchitis and emphysema
- Pneumonia

Haematological
- Anaemia (especially pernicious anaemia) (Ch. 22)
- Chronic leukaemia (Ch. 22)
- Myeloma (Ch. 9)

Neurological
- Parkinson's disease
- Trigeminal neuralgia
- Post-herpetic neuralgia
- Dementia

Carcinomas (all sites)

---

factors. Poorly functioning dentures and impairment of taste sensation may make matters worse.

However, deficiency states, particularly scurvy and vitamin B group deficiencies, are remarkably rare nowadays, even in old age. It is important, nevertheless, that denture function should be the best possible in order not to worsen nutritional problems in older patients.

Pernicious anaemia due to impaired absorption of vitamin B_{12} is mainly seen after middle age. Iron deficiency often persists into later life or may be made worse by defects of absorption.

These conditions can cause oral signs and symptoms, particularly sore tongue (Ch. 14). Sore tongue or signs of atrophy of the mucosa should be investigated by haematological examination.

Parkinson's disease

This common disease is characterised by rigidity, often most obvious as a mask-like fixity of facial expression, tremor sometimes affecting the lower jaw, and often dribbling as a result of impaired neuromuscular function. Important features are summarised in Box 33.13.

Parkinson's disease, which affects the basal ganglia, may be associated (because of the age of affected patients) with, but is not a cause of, intellectual deterioration.

Dental aspects

Sympathetic management is essential. It is particularly important that the poverty of facial expression is not mistaken for incomprehension and the defective speech be not thought to be due to impaired mental function. It is essential to take care, therefore, not to offend a patient with Parkinson's disease by making such assumptions. Drooling may be particularly

---

Box 33.13   Parkinson's disease: key features

General
- Expressionless face
- Soft indistinct speech
- Stooping posture
- Slowness in starting or repeating movements
- Impaired fine movements especially of fingers

Gait
- Slow to start
- Rapid small steps and tendency to run
- Impaired balance on turning

Tremor
- Usually first in fingers and thumb
- Can affect limbs, jaw and tongue
- Present at rest
- Diminished by activity

Rigidity
- 'Cogwheel' type particularly in the arms
- 'Lead-pipe' type particularly in the legs

Box 33.14   Age changes in the mouth and jaws

- Attrition and toothwear
- Root caries
- Periodontal disease, recession and bone loss
- Possibly diminished salivary function
- Pain or difficulties with dentures
- Mucosal disease

---

troublesome, but antimuscarinic drugs, such as benzhexol or orphenadrine, can cause dry mouth. Involuntary orofacial movements, due to levodopa or bromocriptine, may make use of rotating dental instruments hazardous. Epinephrine may, theoretically at least, interact with catechol-O-methyl transferase (COMT) inhibitors such as entacapone, so that epinephrine-free local anaesthetics may be preferable. Parkinson's disease can cause difficulties with the management of dentures because of the loss of fine control of muscular movement. If there is associated intellectual deterioration, the difficulties are proportionately worsened.

The effects of Parkinson's disease can be diminished by giving anticholinergic drugs such as benzohexol (Artane). But more effective are dopaminic agents such as levodopa. Other drugs which may be helpful include monoamine oxidase B inhibitors such as selegeline and dopamine receptor agonists such as amantadine. However, complete success is rarely achieved and virtually all the drugs have significant side-effects, particularly in long-term use. Different types of neurosurgery have been devised but all have significant limitations.

Cardiovascular disease

It may be worthwhile to emphasise that the elderly are overall at the highest risk from infective endocarditis. A possible contribution to this is periodontal sepsis. In addition, drugs given for cardiovascular disease can be a cause of oral lesions (Ch. 27).

Oral disease in the elderly

To a much greater extent than in the handicapped child, oral disease is likely to require considerably more attention. It comprises the categories in Box 33.14.

All of these are important in varying degree, but the main dental need of most elderly patients is the provision of effective and comfortable dentures. Elderly patients tend to become even more infrequent visitors to the dentist than they once were, especially when dentures have been provided. As a consequence, cancer of the mouth, which both becomes more common as age advances and is insidious in development, is particularly likely to be missed in its earlier stages. The majority of cases of cancer of the mouth are at an advanced stage by the time they come for treatment.

The teeth

The teeth can undergo attrition, abrasion and, frequently, continued destruction by caries (Chs 3 and 4). The roots gradually also become hypercalcified by progressive obliteration of the dentinal tubules. The roots may as a consequence become completely calcified and more brittle, so that they are more likely to fracture during extraction.

The periodontal tissues and jaws

In the edentulous elderly, progressive loss of denture-bearing bone brings with it the well-known difficulties, particularly retention and stabilisation of dentures. Later, as excessive amounts of bone become resorbed, pain can be caused by the dentures pressing upon anatomical structures, such as the mylohyoid ridge or genial tubercles, which become prominent after loss of overlying bone.

The temporomandibular joints

Though osteoarthritis of weight-bearing joints is a common and often disabling disease as age advances, osteoarthritis of the temporomandibular joints is not a significant problem. The condition is uncommon and only likely to be an incidental finding in radiographs and rarely causes pain (Ch. 11).

Pain or other symptoms from the temporomandibular joints in the elderly are remarkably uncommon. However, pain on mastication may be due to temporal arteritis and, if so, requires urgent treatment, because of the risk of loss of sight (Ch. 11).

Salivary function

Evidence that salivary secretion diminishes with age has not been confirmed in all studies. However, depressed salivary flow is overall more common in the elderly as a result of such causes as Sjögren's syndrome or the use of drugs with antimuscarinic activity (Ch. 19).

Elderly patients who have a dry mouth must therefore be investigated accordingly.

Problems affecting denture-wearers

Between the ages of 55 and 64, the proportion of the population who are edentulous in the UK as a whole is 20%, but it is almost 50% in those aged over 65, in northern England and in lower socio-economic groups.

Though mastication with dentures is less efficient than with healthy teeth, this seems to matter little and most denture wearers suffer no more than discomfort or social embarrassment from time to time. Dietary deficiencies in the elderly are likely to be due to poverty or to inability to prepare an adequate diet.

Other troubles affecting the denture wearer may be due to faults in the denture itself or to some condition underlying it. Causes of discomfort or pain relating to dentures are summarised in Box 33.15, but cancer, in particular, must be excluded as it becomes increasingly common as age advances.

Box 33.15   Important causes of pain and other lesions under dentures

- Traumatic ulcers
- Denture hyperplasia
- Denture stomatitis
- Angular stomatitis
- Papillary palatal hyperplasia
- Frictional keratosis and other hyperkeratotic lesions
- Buried teeth, roots, or (rarely) odontomas
- Cysts, particularly residual and, less often, keratocysts
- Carcinoma
- Paget's disease
- Fracture of the jaws (uncommon but a possibility with a heavily resorbed mandible)

It must be emphasised therefore that the cause of progressive complaints about dentures must be looked for and not simply evaded by repeated 'eases' (see Ch. 34).

Mucosal diseases in the elderly

Some changes in the oral mucosa are directly related to age. Examples include Fordyce's granules, lingual varicosities and enlarged foliate papillae (Ch. 2). These are often causes of anxiety in the elderly, who need to be reassured.

Mucosal diseases that may affect the elderly are summarised in Box 33.16 and discussed in more detail in Chapter 15.

It must be emphasised that recurrent aphthae are uncommon in older persons but, when seen, it is important to look for some underlying cause such as pernicious anaemia.

Box 33.16   Mucosal diseases in the elderly

- Lichen planus
- Mucous membrane pemphigoid
- Pemphigus vulgaris
- Herpes zoster
- Glossitis
- Burning mouth syndrome
- Leukoplakia
- Carcinoma

Radiation injury

Because of the rising frequency of carcinoma with advancing age, the elderly are more likely than the young to have had radiotherapy. They may therefore suffer from xerostomia or be at risk from osteoradionecrosis. Denture trauma can occasionally precipitate this complication, and experts in this field may not permit patients to wear lower dentures after radiotherapy (Ch. 22).

Factors affecting dental care of the elderly

Many factors limit the mobility of elderly patients who are frequently arthritic, may be unsteady on their feet, unwell for a variety of reasons or simply be unable to afford the cost of dental care or transportation. Arthritis of the hands may also make oral hygiene difficult or defective.

Illustrative of the dental problems of the elderly have been the findings in a survey of inhabitants of a residential home; 12% had denture stomatitis, 3% had oral ulcers, 19 of 1041 had red or white lesions, 250 had difficulty with eating, 206 had impaired taste and 241 had difficulty caring for their mouths. Only 4% of dentate and 20% of edentulous persons had seen a dentist in the past 2 years. No systematic dental care was provided, or dental assessments made before admission. Domiciliary dental care of the elderly is even more inadequate.

PSYCHIATRIC DISORDERS

Psychiatric disorders are common and frequently unrecognised if manifestations are mild and regarded merely as eccentricity. The main psychiatric disorders are summarised in Box 33.17.

Box 33.17   Important psychiatric disorders

- Anxiety states
- Obsessive-compulsive disorder
- Disturbances of affect (mood)
  - Depression and manic-depressive psychosis
  - Chronic fatigue syndrome
- Psychoses
  - Schizophrenia

General aspects of psychiatric disorders that can affect dental management are summarised in Box 33.18.

Box 33.18   Aspects of psychiatric disease that may affect dental management

- Erratic attendance
- Oral neglect
- Inability to cooperate
- Psychosomatic disorders
- Munchausen's syndrome
- Uncontrollable fear of dental treatment (phobia)
- Associated alcoholism
- Violence
- Drug therapy

Psychiatric disorders can also be secondary to organic brain disease or damage as a result of head injury or use of drugs.

Anxiety disorders

Anxiety is fear or uncertainty anticipating a real or imagined threat, often with physical manifestations sufficient to impair normal activity. Fear at the close proximity of a cobra is a normal and healthy response. Fear at the sight of a pigeon is clearly abnormal. Anxiety disorders therefore comprise several conditions summarised in Box 13.19.

Box 33.19   Anxiety states

- Phobias
  - Dental
  - Social
  - Others
- Panic disorder
- Post-traumatic stress disorder

It is perfectly normal to feel anxiety at the prospect of dental treatment, but the normal person can overcome these fears, because there is genuine desire for dental care. Active hostility to treatment is usually a manifestation of anxiety. Signs of anxiety include muscle tension (gripping the arms of the dental chair hard), rapid breathing and heart beat, sweating, pallor and excessive chattering. The 'uncooperative patient' is in a moderate anxiety state and can be managed by sympathetic discussion, the use of sedatives, particularly a benzodiazepine, and the use of conscious sedation. However, the latter may not make the next appointment any easier because of the complete amnesia for the treatment. Nitrous oxide sedation is likely to be more satisfactory, though it is frequently difficult for the patient to accept the mask over the face.

Dental phobia is an extreme manifestation of anxiety and may sometimes result from painfully traumatic dental experiences or be of unknown origin. It is sometimes manageable as above but may require referral to specialist care.

Social phobia is the term given to uncontrollable anxiety in normal social situations. Persistent and chronic fear of being watched or judged by others, and fear of being humiliated by their behaviour or appearance, are typical features. Cognitive therapy may be indicated. Alternatively, medication with beta-blockers, benzodiazepines or antidepressants may be required.

Depression

Depression is a serious illness whose impact on life is frequently underestimated. It is common and may sometimes underlie oral symptoms. Typical manifestations of depression are summarised in Box 33.20.

Box 33.20   Typical manifestations of depression

- Feeling 'low' or miserable
- Uncontrollable pessimism
- Inability to sleep or early wakening
- Disturbance, usually loss, of appetite
- Loss of libido
- Tiredness
- Irritability
- Inability to look forward to any pleasurable activity
- Resorting to alcohol or drugs
- Thoughts of suicide

Sometimes depression is triggered by unpleasant experiences such as bereavement or financial difficulties, but is abnormal if symptoms are excessively prolonged. Serious, particularly life-threatening illnesses, can also be triggering factors. Thus, it can be important in the treatment of patients with terminal cancer to give antidepressants as well as analgesics. Suppression of depression by alcohol is common. Alternatively, suppression of depression by an act of will can be revealed by breakdown triggered by alcohol, graphically described as 'crying into his beer'.

Unfortunately, depression is widely regarded as 'weakness', particularly in Britain where it is essential to keep a stiff upper lip and not to make a 'fuss'. Weeping is totally unacceptable. In other countries, screaming and crying as a result of depression is regarded as normal and, indeed, outward expression of grief is therapeutic.

Dental aspects of depression

Depression can manifest itself as burning mouth, ill-defined but severe facial pain (Ch. 34) or TMJ pain dysfunction syndrome.

Occasionally, such patients can insist on not being depressed despite the fact that they are weeping uncontrollably or having histories of such events as multiple suicides in the family. Inevitably, therefore, treatment is difficult so that it is important to make it clear to patients that depression is a real illness which is common and frequently disabling. It is nothing to be ashamed of. However, it is unwise to suggest that the patient may need psychiatric help; rather it should be suggested that the help of a pain specialist would be valuable. A significant number of patients with 'atypical facial pain' are depressed and respond to antidepressants.

Depressed patients may sometimes be 'difficult' or even aggressive and need to be treated particularly tactfully and sympathetically, but the main problem with those already under treatment is that of the oral effects of antidepressant drugs. Tricyclic antidepressants, in particular, can cause severe xerostomia and, rarely, ascending parotitis has developed as a consequence. However, no antidepressant is probably free of this side-effect.

Factitious oral injuries These can have their origin in depression as discussed earlier (Ch. 13). In one such case, a teenager, who had inflicted oral injuries on himself, later hanged himself, and any form of self-harm requires further investigation.

Chronic fatigue syndrome This widely publicised disorder is of uncertain nature. A feature suggesting that it is a psychological disorder is that the symptoms are non-specific and usually comprise tiredness, emotional lability, joint or muscle pains, poor memory and often other symptoms. Despite the fact that such symptoms are typical of depression, patients insist (often angrily) that they are not depressed and refuse even to try antidepressant drugs. Many patients complain that they have not had a 'proper' diagnosis (depression is often not regarded by patients as a diagnosis) and insist that they have a viral infection. Though post-influenzal depression is well recognised and chronic Epstein–Barr virus infection can cause similar symptoms, these rarely apply to the great majority of patients. Even if a virus were the cause, no treatment is available. However, if an antidepressant is given without revealing its nature but suggesting that it is a medicine which, for example 'stimulates the immune system', recovery may sometimes be dramatic. Surprisingly, despite the complaints of various pains without any clinical basis for them, 'atypical facial pain' does not appear to have been reported as a feature of chronic fatigue syndrome. The only oral symptom that has been reported is dry mouth.

Obsessive-compulsive disorder

It is common to worry whether the front door has been locked or that the gas has been turned off when leaving the house. Obsessive-compulsive disorder is an extreme manifestation of this type of anxiety in which patients have uncontrollable ritualistic thoughts or behaviour that interfere with normal life. Thus, an affected patient can ring the dental surgeon repeatedly to confirm the date of the appointment. Obsessive-compulsive states can lead to depression and are sometimes secondary to schizophrenia.

Antidepressants are likely to be effective when depression is associated. If anxiety is conspicuous, an anxiolytic such as diazepam can be helpful.

Obsessions affecting dental management may include compulsive toothbrushing, possibly causing dental abrasion,

excessive use of antiseptic mouthwashes, or fear of oral infections, of cancer or of halitosis, and refusal to be reassured.

Post-traumatic stress disorder

Post-traumatic stress disorder is a response to a terrifying experience in which severe injury is threatened or suffered. The ordeal is frequently re-experienced as flashbacks or nightmares particularly triggered by events or references reminding the patient of the trauma.

Physical symptoms can include headaches, chest pain, dizziness or gastrointestinal complaints. Mood changes include anxiety, irritability or depression. Alcohol abuse is a typical reaction.

Dental aspects

The fear of dental treatment is not such as to precipitate post-traumatic stress disorder, but it could follow a severe maxillofacial injury.

Schizophrenia

Schizophrenia is the commonest form of severe mental illness; it can be chronic and severely disabling and affects 1% of the population, usually with onset between 20 and 30 years of age.

A great range of symptoms and abnormal behaviour is possible. In particular, mood, thoughts and behaviour become abnormal and disorganised. Hallucinations and delusions are typical. An hallucination might be that of seeing a flock of elephants flying past. A delusion would be to believe yourself to be Adolf Hitler and to expect appropriate respect. More often in these days of electronic marvels, patients receive, via mysterious rays and other unlikely routes, orders or messages that may torment them.

Imaginary voices may tell patients that they are being poisoned or, rarely, order them to carry out violent acts that may even be murderous.

Confusion and inappropriate behaviour, and blunted or flattened mood are, however, more common. Patients may not follow or be able to construct a logical chain of thoughts. Intelligence is unimpaired and insight may even be retained. A dental student who developed schizophrenia and delusions that he was being influenced by messages coming through the gas pipes recovered with treatment and then, touchingly, apologised for telling such strange stories.

General management can be difficult. Normal persons can sometimes behave in a schizoid manner, while schizophrenics do not necessarily behave abnormally all the time. Patients are likely to be taking newer generation or atypical neuroleptic drugs such as risperidone. However, many patients remain on phenothiazines and some patients require medication only for a short period. Expert psychiatric treatment is required.

Dental aspects

Mild schizophrenia may appear merely to be stupidity or result in inappropriate behaviour. Responses to questions may indicate a failure to get through or elicit entirely inappropriate answers. There is a risk that some patients will become violent.

Provided that the patient is cooperative, there are no major restrictions on the form of dental treatment that can be provided. Any reaction between epinephrine in local anaesthetics and phenothiazines appears to be no more than theoretical.

Phenothiazines and some other neuroleptics can cause severe xerostomia, particularly in long-term use. Phenothiazines can also cause involuntary facial movements (dyskinesias) or parkinsonism. These can respond to anticholinergics, but levodopa is contraindicated. *Tardive dyskinesia* can develop in about 30% of patients treated long-term with phenothiazines. Involuntary movements particularly involve the face and are irreversible. Repeated grimacing and chewing movements may be violent and result in scarring and deformities of the tongue. Newer antipsychotics may be partially or completely free from these types of adverse effects.

Munchausen's syndrome

This is a bizarre form of abnormal behaviour in which patients exaggerate, invent or induce signs and symptoms for the 'pleasure' of receiving treatment. In extreme cases, patients have moved from one area to another area to achieve this objective as soon as their disability is recognised at one hospital. Munchausen's syndrome rarely appears to affect the maxillofacial area.

SUGGESTED FURTHER READING

Cumming CG, Wight C, Blackwell CL et al 1989 Denture stomatitis in the elderly. Oral Microbiol Immunol 5:82–85

Fiske J, Shafik HH 2001 Down's syndrome and oral care. Dental Update 28:148–156

Flint S, Scully C 1988 Orofacial age changes and related disease. Dental Update 15:337–341

Hammond J 1996 Cerebral palsy. Medicine UK 24:82–84

Hildebolt OF 1997 Osteoporosis and oral bone loss. Dentomaxillofacial Radiol 26:3–15

Hollins S, Howlin P 1996 Learning disability and autism. Medicine UK 24:47–48

Ibbetson RJ, Setchell DJ 1989 Treatment of the worn dentition: 1 & 2. Dental Update 16:247–252, 300–304

Moore RS, Hobson P 1989 A classification of medically handicapping conditions and the health risks they present in the dental care of children. Part I – Cardiovascular, haematological and respiratory disorders. J Paediatr Dent 5:73–83

Moore RS, Hobson P 1989 A classification of medically handicapping conditions and the health risks they present in the dental care of children. Part II – Neoplastic, renal, endocrine, metabolic, hepatic, musculoskeletal, neuromuscular, central nervous system and skin disorders. J Paediatr Dent 6:1–14

Mouradian WE, Wehr E, Crall JJ 2000 Disparities in children's oral health care and access to dental care. JAMA 284:2625–2631

Nunn J 2000 Disability and oral care. International Association for Disability and Oral Health/FDI World Dental Press, London

Sheiham A 1990 Dentistry for an ageing population: responsibilities and future trends. Dental Update 17:70–75

Simons D, Kidd EAM, Beighton D 2000 Oral health of elderly occupants in residential homes. Lancet 353:1761

Smith DG, Seymour RA 1988 Periodontal disease and treatment in the elderly. Dental Update 15:18–22

Walls AWG, Barnes IE 1988 Gerodontology: the problem? Dental Update 15:186–190

Walls AWG, Barnes IE 1989 Treatment planning for the ageing patient. Dental Update 16:438–443

Ward-Booth P 1988 Oral surgery for the older patient. Dental Update 15:410–414

Pain, anxiety, neurological and psychogenic disorders

> '…within my private knowledge, two persons who had suffered alike from toothache and cancer, have pronounced the former to be on the scale of torture, by many degrees to be the worse' *Confessions of an English Opium Eater Thomas de Quincey 1821*

Pain is the most common symptom for which patients seek help. Approximately 40% of the British population only visit a dentist for pain relief. Toothache can be so agonisingly severe that De Quincey, as well as quoting the opinions shown above, also claimed that it had made him dependent on opium. In the lay mind, dentistry and pain are inseparable and there is the persistent belief that dental treatment is necessarily painful. This belief emphasises the important point that pain has strong emotional associations which, in turn, may be determined to a varying degree by patients' preconceptions. Emotional disturbance itself can also produce the symptom of physical pain.

There are many causes of oral or maxillofacial pain (Box 34.1). Pulpitis and periapical periodontitis as sequels of dental caries are by far the most common causes. The source of such pain is usually obvious on examination, but some sources of dental pain can be exceedingly difficult to identify (Box 34.2).

Box 34.1   Causes of pain felt in the oral tissues

- Disease of teeth and/or supporting tissues
- Oral mucosal diseases
- Diseases of the jaw
- Pain in the edentulous patient
- Postoperative pain
- Pain triggered by mastication
- Referred pain
- Neurological diseases
- Psychogenic (atypical) facial pain

These account for most causes of pain in this area. Disease of the teeth (usually the result of dental caries) and adjacent tissues must always be excluded in the investigation of pain.

Box 34.2   Causes of pain from the teeth or supporting tissues

- Pulpitis
- Dentine hypersensitivity, cracked tooth or cracked cusp syndrome
- Periapical periodontitis
- Lateral (periodontal) abscess
- Acute necrotising ulcerative gingivitis
- HIV-associated periodontitis
- Pericoronitis

PULPITIS

Pulpitis is usually the cause when hot or cold food or drinks trigger the pain. It is also the main cause of spasmodic, poorly localised attacks of pain which may be mistaken for a variety of other possible causes. The pain of acute pulpitis is of a sharp lancinating character peculiar to itself, impossible to describe but unforgettable once experienced. Recurrent attacks of less severe, subacute or chronic pain, often apparently spontaneous, suggest a diseased or dying pulp.

Investigation of pulpitis has been discussed earlier (Ch. 4). The only non-dental condition that is indistinguishable from pulp pain by the patient is the pain of herpes zoster (Ch. 12). If no local cause can be found after the most careful search, it is important to look for early signs of the characteristic rash. Herpes zoster is an uncommon cause of toothache-like pain, but countless teeth have been extracted in patients with prodromal zoster under the mistaken impression that the pain was dental.

ACUTE PERIODONTITIS → Summary p. 448

Pain from acute periapical periodontitis should be readily identifiable as there is precisely localised tenderness of the tooth in its socket. Radiographs are of little value in the early stages but useful after sufficient destruction shows itself as loss of definition of the periapical lamina dura. In other cases, acute inflammation may supervene on chronic and a rounded area of radiolucency is seen.

Acute maxillary sinusitis can rarely cause similar tenderness of a group of teeth, particularly upper molars, as discussed later.

LATERAL PERIODONTAL ABSCESS

The tooth is tender in its socket, but is usually vital and there is deep localised pocketing (Ch. 6). Occasionally, both a periodontal and periapical abscess may form together on a non-vital tooth with severe periodontal disease, or a periodontal abscess may be precipitated by endodontic treatment when a reamer perforates the side of the root.

ACUTE NECROTISING ULCERATIVE GINGIVITIS AND HIV-ASSOCIATED NECROTISING PERIODONTITIS

Acute ulcerative gingivitis usually causes soreness, but when it extends deeply and rapidly, destroying the underlying bone, there may be severe aching pain. In such cases, the diagnosis is usually obvious clinically. HIV-associated periodontitis presents a somewhat similar picture and is acutely painful.

ACUTE PERICORONITIS

Pericoronitis usually produces a characteristic clinical picture (Ch. 6).

PAINFUL MUCOSAL LESIONS

Ulcers generally cause soreness rather than pain, but deep ulceration may cause severe aching pain. Carcinoma, in particular, causes severe pain once nerve fibres become involved. It is important to emphasise again that early carcinoma is painless; pain is a late symptom. By the time that pain becomes troublesome the tumour is usually easily seen unless it is far back in the mouth.

As mentioned above, Herpes zoster causes severe aching pain, sometimes indistinguishable from toothache, because of involvement of cervical ganglia (Ch. 12).

PAINFUL JAW DISEASES

The important feature of these conditions (Box 34.3) is that, as well as the history and clinical presentation, the provisional

---

Box 34.3 **Painful jaw diseases**

- Fractures
- Osteomyelitis
- Infected cysts
- Malignant neoplasms
- Sickle cell infarcts

---

diagnosis depends on the radiographic findings. Fractures and osteomyelitis should be recognisable by such means. Other lesions of the jaws, by contrast, sometimes have less clear-cut clinical and radiographic features and the differentiation of (say) an infected cyst from a malignant tumour may be difficult.

With the exception of fractures and osteomyelitis, diagnosis depends on biopsy and histological examination.

PAIN IN EDENTULOUS PATIENTS

These conditions (Box 34.4) differ from most others because dental causes can be excluded. The chief difficulty is to decide whether the pain is due to the dentures themselves, or to some condition of the mucosa or jaws on which a denture is pressing.

Box 34.4 **Important causes of pain in edentulous patients**

- Denture trauma
- Excessive vertical dimension
- Diseases (enumerated earlier) of the denture-bearing mucosa
- Diseases of the jaws (Box 34.3)
- Teeth or roots erupting under a denture

Traumatic ulcers, usually the consequence of over-extension, often cause trouble with a new denture. After the denture has been relieved, these ulcers heal within 24–48 hours. Persistent ulceration after adequate relief of the denture is likely to be due to some more serious cause, particularly a neoplasm. Biopsy is then essential. Later, dentures cause traumatic pain when the bone has become severely resorbed, allowing the denture to bear on the mylohyoid ridge or genial tubercles. These result from the patients having worn the denture too long, and a well-designed replacement is necessary.

Lack of freeway space due to excessive vertical dimension of the dentures prevents the mandible and masticatory muscles from reaching their natural rest position. This causes the teeth to be held permanently in contact. Aching pain is usually felt in the fatigued masticatory muscles, but the excessive stress imposed on the denture-bearing area sometimes causes pain in this region. Very occasionally, patients seem unable to tolerate dentures however carefully they are constructed and complain of such symptoms as gripping, burning, or 'drawing' pain, particularly under the upper denture. These symptoms are not associated with any physical changes and are psychogenic.

It is usually straightforward to decide whether pain is caused by the dentures themselves or by some lesion under the dentures. Denture stomatitis is painless, but surprisingly few other mucosal diseases affect the denture-bearing area itself. Lichen planus can extend to the sulcus and impinge on the margin of the denture-bearing area. The most important condition to be excluded is carcinoma, either affecting the alveolar margin or in the labial or buccal sulcus, or floor of the mouth. Persistent lesions, whether ulcerated or not, developing beneath or at the margins of dentures, must be biopsied without hesitation, as it is in the edentulous age group that the incidence of carcinoma is highest. A carcinoma can persist for a long time with minimal symptoms and the patient may notice no more than the fact that the fit of the denture has deteriorated.

Jaw lesions causing pain in the edentulous patient may be associated with a swelling or an area of radiolucency and have been discussed above. A painful swelling of the jaw in the edentulous patient is probably most often due to an infected residual cyst. Malignant tumours are very much less common but must be considered, as they cannot be reliably distinguished from cysts and other benign conditions by radiography alone. Histological examination is therefore essential. Osteomyelitis of the jaws in edentulous patients must be considered virtually only in those who have had radiotherapy to this region. In such patients, denture ulceration can allow infection to penetrate and set up persistent painful chronic osteomyelitis of the ischaemic bone.

Retained roots or, rarely, late eruption of buried teeth beneath a denture become painful as they reach the surface, causing the mucosa to be pinched between them and the denture. This trouble will be obvious on clinical or radiographic examination, as are the late effects of a healed malaligned fracture.

POSTOPERATIVE PAIN

Important causes are summarised in Box 34.5. By far the most common cause of pain after dental extractions is alveolar osteitis (dry socket), which can usually be recognised on clinical examination (Ch. 6). Fracture of the jaw following operative

---

Box 34.5   Postoperative pain

- Alveolar osteitis (dry socket)
- Fracture of the jaw
- Damage to the temporomandibular joint
- Osteomyelitis
- Damage to the nerve trunks or involvement of nerves in scar tissue

---

treatment is rare but can also be recognised from the history and by clinical and radiographic examination. Forcible opening of the mouth under general anaesthesia, particularly for removing wisdom teeth, can damage the temporomandibular joint and lead to persistent pain on opening or during mastication. Postoperative osteomyelitis should be a thing of the past, but could develop in an immunodeficient patient with, for example, unrecognised leukaemia.

Persistent postoperative pain is sometimes ascribed to damage to nerve fibres, either as a result of operative trauma or by involvement in scar tissue. However, if there is no objective evidence of disturbed sensation, there is little or nothing abnormal to be found. Operative intervention in the attempt to relieve such pain may do more harm than good. In some such cases, there is complaint of persistent pain unresponsive to treatment but without any organic cause.

Rarely, damaged nerve tissue may proliferate to form a traumatic neuroma which is tender to pressure. Its excision should lead to relief of the pain. However, meticulous investigation of postoperative pain is important as it is a major cause of medicolegal claims.

PAIN INDUCED BY MASTICATION

The common dental cause for pain on mastication is apical periodontitis, but any condition which causes the tooth to be tender in its socket, whether it be a lateral periodontal abscess or, occasionally, maxillary sinusitis, can cause this symptom (Box 34.6).

Box 34.6   Pain induced by mastication

- Disease of teeth and supporting tissues
- Pain dysfunction syndrome
- Diseases of the temporomandibular joint
- Temporal arteritis
- Trigeminal neuralgia (rarely)
- Salivary calculi

The *least* common cause of pain during eating is organic disease of the temporomandibular joint. Pain during eating comes much more frequently from the many other structures involved. Fractures and dislocations of the temporomandibular joint are usually obvious from the history, their effects on the occlusion and the radiographic changes (Ch. 11).

Pain dysfunction syndrome

Dull, aching pain, often associated with clicking sounds from the joint, episodes of locking and some limitation of opening, in varying combinations are characteristic. Young women are predominantly affected and there is typically a strong neurotic element (Ch. 11).

Cranial arteritis → Summary p. 448

The typical manifestation of cranial (giant-cell) arteritis is headache, but though uncommon, is a particularly important cause of masticatory pain because of the high risk of blindness. It should be considered particularly in patients over middle age with this symptom. The pain is due to ischaemia of the masticatory muscles, caused by the arteritis and is comparable to intermittent claudication (Ch. 11). Corticosteroids are effective in controlling the disease and relieving symptoms. They should be given when there is headache or masticatory pain associated with a tender scalp vessel and a high ESR.

Trigeminal neuralgia

The characteristic pain is very occasionally triggered by mastication. Trigeminal neuralgia may then be misdiagnosed as dental or due to pain dysfunction syndrome. However, the quality of these types of pain is quite different, as discussed later.

Calculi

Particularly when obstructing the parotid duct, these can cause pain when salivation is triggered by eating. Hence, the history of the relationship of the pain to stimulation of salivation rather than to mastication itself is distinctive.

PAIN FROM EXTRAORAL DISEASE

Extraoral causes of pain are summarised in Box 34.7. Antral disease can cause pain felt in the upper teeth, but a sinus radiograph should provide the diagnosis. Salivary gland and ear diseases typically cause preauricular pain. They may simulate temporomandibular joint symptoms, but are rarely mistaken for dental problems.

Box 34.7   Causes of facial and oral pain from extraoral disease

Diseases of the maxillary antrum
- Acute sinusitis
- Carcinoma, particularly when it involves the antral floor

Diseases of the salivary glands
- Acute parotitis
- Salivary calculi (see above)
- Sjögren's syndrome
- Malignant neoplasms

Disease of the ears
- Otitis media
- Neoplasms in this region

Myocardial infarction

Acute sinusitis is the most common paranasal disease that causes facial pain but antral carcinoma is rare (Ch. 28).

Mumps is a common cause of pain from, and swelling of, the parotid glands. In children, the diagnosis is usually quickly made on clinical grounds. In adults, the diagnosis may not be immediately suspected and, occasionally, these patients think they have dental disease.

Suppurative parotitis is uncommon but can be a complication of dry mouth. Acute parotitis may therefore be seen as a complication of Sjögren's syndrome or irradiation damage to the glands. Sjögren's syndrome itself can occasionally cause parotid pain and swelling of the glands (Ch. 18).

Swelling rather than pain is usually the first symptom of malignant tumours of salivary glands. Parotid gland tumours can also cause facial palsy and, finally, ulceration and fungation.

Myocardial infarction usually causes constricting or crushing pain substernally, but pain may radiate down the inside of the left arm or up into the neck or jaw. Rarely, cardiac pain is felt in the jaw alone. There is even a case on record where a dentist recognised the cardiac cause of jaw pain to the dismay of his patient, who was a cardiologist. This pain can come on at any time, at rest or during exercise. The clinical picture is variable but, in typical cases, the patient is obviously anxious, pale and sweating with a rapid pulse and low blood pressure.

INTRACRANIAL AND PSYCHOLOGICAL DISORDERS

Trigeminal neuralgia is one of the most important of these conditions (Box 34.8).

Box 34.8   Painful intracranial and psychological disorders

- Trigeminal neuralgia
- Multiple sclerosis
- Herpes zoster
- Postherpetic neuralgia
- Migrainous neuralgia
- Intracranial tumours
- Bell's palsy
- Psychogenic pain (atypical facial pain)

Trigeminal neuralgia → Summary p. 448

Typical features are summarised in Box 34.9. Elderly patients are affected, and though the pain is excruciatingly severe, there is complete, or almost complete, relief between spasms. During an attack the patient's face is often distorted with anguish, while between attacks the patient may appear apprehensive at the thought of recurrence. The severity of the pain may also make the patient depressed.

Box 34.9   Typical features of trigeminal neuralgia

- Pain confined to the distribution of one or more divisions of the trigeminal nerve
- Pain is paroxysmal and very severe
- Trigger zones in the area
- Absence of objective sensory loss
- Absence of detectable organic cause

The pain is paroxysmal, severe, sharp and stabbing in character, but lasts only seconds or minutes. It may be described as 'like lightning'. However, attacks may sometimes be quickly recurrent at short intervals. Stimuli to an area (trigger zone) within the distribution of the trigeminal nerve can provoke an attack. Common triggers are touching, draughts of cold air, or toothbrushing. Occasionally, masticatory effort induces the pain.

There are no objective signs. Either the second or third division of the trigeminal nerve is usually first affected, but pain soon involves both. The first division is rarely affected and pain does not spread to the opposite side. Less typical features of trigeminal neuralgia, which make diagnosis difficult, are more continuous, long-lasting, burning or aching pain, absence of trigger zones and extension of the pain beyond the margins of the trigeminal area, though not to the opposite side.

Typically, the disease undergoes spontaneous remissions, with freedom from pain for weeks or months. These remissions may make it difficult to decide whether treatment has been effective.

Diagnosis

In typical cases, the diagnosis should be readily made from the features described. In some patients, multiple sclerosis should be excluded. A careful search should be made for diseased teeth, though pain of this severity is unlikely to be due to dental disease. An inflamed pulp can cause stabs of severe pain in its early stages, but the pain changes in character and soon becomes more prolonged. Pulpitis can usually also be identified as toothache by most patients and is felt to be different in character from pain in the face due to neuralgia. Any diseased teeth should of course be treated, though this does not affect the neuralgia. In the absence of disease, teeth should not be arbitrarily extracted, as this only adds to the patient's misfortunes. Pulp stones in particular, seen on a radiograph, are not a reason for extracting teeth.

Treatment

The most effective drugs are anticonvulsants, particularly carbamazepine and gabapentin, and to a lesser extent phenytoin. Carbamazepine, with or without phenytoin, will usually relieve the pain, at least for a time. The action seems specific and other types of pain are not relieved. Abolition of the pain of trigeminal neuralgia by giving an anticonvulsant, such as carbamazepine, also helps to confirm the diagnosis. Carbamazepine (100 mg/day gradually raised if necessary to 800 mg/day) must be given long term (essentially prophylactically) to reduce the frequency and severity of attacks. If a patient has trigeminal neuralgia which appears unresponsive to carbamazepine, it sometimes transpires that instructions about continuous use have either not been given or not understood so that the drug has been used as if it were an analgesic. Up to 80% of patients are relieved of pain partly or completely by carbamazepine, but minor side-effects are common. Drowsiness, dryness of the mouth, giddiness, diarrhoea and nausea are all to some extent dose-related. A small initial dose should therefore be given and gradually raised as necessary. In some patients, tolerance to the side-effects may develop. Leucopenia is a rare toxic effect.

Surgical treatment A few patients are unresponsive to carbamazepine or cannot tolerate the side-effects. If drug treatment fails, the final resort is surgery. The simplest option is cryotherapy to the trigeminal nerve or, if this fails, cryotherapy at the base of the skull. If these fail, microvascular decompression of the trigeminal ganglion may be required. This operation requires great skill and a mortality of 1% has been noted in some studies. In a series of over 1000 patients treated in this way in the USA, the mortality was 0.2%, 30% had recurrences of pain and 11% underwent a second operation. Overall, it has been claimed that 70% of patients were pain-free without medication 10 years postoperatively. A newer treatment with minimal morbidity is gamma knife ablation, in which the nerve is destroyed using a fine focused beam of radiation.

Trigeminal neuropathy

Trigeminal neuropathy is the term given to disturbances of sensation that particularly follows severe and irreparable damage to the trigeminal nerve by such causes as surgical trauma. Other possible causes include neoplasms and metabolic or inflammatory disorders. Anaesthesia or hypoaesthesia may develop between attacks of pain. The latter is typically burning or stabbing in character, or there may be persistent unilateral pain with sensory loss. In the most severe type, there is continuous pain associated with complete anaesthesia and it can follow surgical treatment for trigeminal neuralgia. Detailed examination of trigeminal neuropathy is needed, particularly to exclude a neoplastic cause. Gabapentin or a tricyclic antidepressant may provide some relief.

Benign trigeminal neuropathy consists of transient sensory loss in one or more divisions of the trigeminal nerve. It is sometimes associated with a connective tissue disorder.

Glossopharyngeal neuralgia

This rare condition is characterised by pain similar to that of trigeminal neuralgia but felt in the base of the tongue and fauces on one side. It may also radiate deeply into the ear. The pain, which is sharp, lancinating and transient, is typically triggered by swallowing, chewing, or coughing. It may be so severe that patients may be terrified to swallow their saliva and try to keep the mouth and tongue as completely immobile as possible. Glossopharyngeal neuralgia sometimes responds to carbamazepine, but less often than trigeminal neuralgia. Once an organic cause has been excluded, surgical treatment may be needed. However, like trigeminal neuralgia, there can be spontaneous remissions, sometimes for years.

Postherpetic neuralgia → Summary p. 448

Up to 14% of patients who have had trigeminal herpes zoster develop persistent neuralgia and pain that persists more than one month after healing. Most cases resolve slowly and only 3% have pain after 1 year. Neuralgia is particularly likely in the elderly and when the infection is severe.

The pain is more variable in character and severity than trigeminal neuralgia. It is typically persistent rather than paroxysmal, but limited to the dermatome affected by the zoster attack. The skin in the affected area may have reduced sensitivity to touch. The diagnosis is straightforward if there is a history of facial zoster or if scars from the rash are present.

Unfortunately, postherpetic neuralgia is remarkably resistant to treatment. Nerve or root section are ineffective and the response to drugs of any type, including carbamazepine, is poor. When pain is severe, large doses of analgesics can be given and may give relief. Alternative drugs include amitriptiline and gabapentin. Application of transcutaneous electrical stimulation to the affected area by the patient himself is sometimes effective. The instrument is applied hourly for 5–10 minutes every day, and persistent bombardment of the sensory pathways by the stimulator may prevent perception of pain centrally.

Longstanding postherpetic neuralgia carries a significant risk of depression.

Multiple sclerosis

A minority of patients with multiple sclerosis have pain indistinguishable from trigeminal neuralgia, usually as a late symptom. Between 2 and 3% of patients with 'classical' symptoms of trigeminal neuralgia may have multiple sclerosis, but this unusual presentation is usually in younger persons (under 50). In about 30%, pain, unlike trigeminal neuralgia, may be persistent and lack trigger zones, or may spread beyond the trigeminal area. Disturbances of sensation are capriciously distributed according to the sites of lesions in the brain. The lip may be affected and symptoms may range from paraesthesia to extreme hypersensitivity, whereby the patient will literally jump or scream with pain if the lip is touched.

The diagnosis usually depends on the presence of multiple deficits, particularly defects of vision, weakness of the limbs and sensory losses. Disturbed sensation in the trigeminal area is likely only to be seen in patients with advanced disease and multiple paralyses. There is unlikely to be any doubt about the diagnosis as a consequence.

Carbamazepine or gabapentin is sometimes effective, otherwise surgical treatment as for trigeminal neuralgia may be required.

Migraine

Migraine is a common cause of headache but not of facial pain. It affects up to 10% of the population, most only occasionally, but a few, daily.

Key features are summarised in Box 34.10.

Box 34.10 **Typical features of migraine**

- Intense throbbing headache, usually unilateral
- Visual disturbances (aura) in classic migraine, not in common migraine
- Photophobia
- Sometimes nausea and vomiting
- Triggers: stress, hunger, certain foods, caffeine, cheese and red wine, menstruation, which vary between patients
- Usually a good response to 5HT agonists such as sumatriptan

---

Migrainous neuralgia (cluster headache) →
Summary p. 448

Migrainous neuralgia may occasionally be mistaken for trigeminal neuralgia. It is rarely seen in dental practice. Migrainous neuralgia is thought to be caused by oedema or dilatation of the wall of the internal carotid and probably also the external carotid arteries. It causes severe pain in the region of the eye and maxilla, associated with facial flushing, nasal congestion and lacrimation.

Key features are summarised in Box 34.11.

Box 34.11 **Typical features of migrainous neuralgia**

- Commonest in young adult and middle-aged men
- Piercing intense unilateral orbital, retro-orbital or temporal pain
- Conjunctival vessel dilatation and eyelid oedema
- Lacrimation
- Nasal congestion and rhinorrhoea
- Attacks often at the same time each night (or day, 'alarm clock headache')
- Usually attacks recur for several days then remit for many weeks or months
- Triggers: stress, alcohol, organic solvent inhalation
- Early in acute attack oxygen or sumatriptan highly effective
- Established attack can be treated with intranasal dihydroergotamine or intranasal lidocaine or subcutaneous sumatriptan
- Prophylaxis possible with verapamil or ergotamine

An uncommon variant of cluster headache is a chronic variety with attacks confined to the cheek or lower jaw, known as lower half headache.

Management

MRI may be needed to confirm the diagnosis. Relief of the pain by oxygen inhalations is virtually diagnostic. Otherwise, ipsilateral instillation of 4% intranasal lidocaine can also be effective. Some patients respond to simple analgesics or to ergotamine. Ergotamine should be given an hour before the expected attack and is most effective by subcutaneous injection or by suppository. Alternatively, ergotamine powder can be inhaled from a spinhaler. Success depends on an accurate idea of the timing of the attacks, and two or three doses a day for the duration of the cluster of attacks may be necessary. Treatment should preferably be stopped for one day each week to see whether there has been spontaneous remission.

Intracranial tumours

Pain resembling trigeminal neuralgia can rarely be caused by intracranial tumours. Features suggesting an intracranial lesion are associated sensory loss, especially if associated with cranial nerve palsies. Frequently, anatomically related nerves (especially III, IV and VI, causing disordered oculomotor function) are affected. Pain associated with neurological deficits in the area is known as trigeminal neuropathy.

Bell's palsy

As discussed later, facial paralysis is the predominant and most troublesome feature. In about 50%, pain, usually in or near the ear but sometimes spreading down the jaw, either precedes or develops at the same time as the facial palsy. Rarely, a patient with early Bell's palsy seeks a dental opinion for the pain felt in the jaw, since this may precede paralysis by several days.

Psychogenic (atypical) facial pain → Summary p. 448

Pain is not a simple sensation, but has been described as the unpleasant experience felt 'when hurt in body or mind'. The psychological aspects of pain are often overwhelmingly important and the patient's reaction is affected by such factors as mood, emotional characteristics, personality and cultural background. At one extreme, a footballer may receive a relatively severe injury in the middle of a game without feeling it. At the other extreme, there are patients who complain bitterly and persistently about trivial lesions. Pain causes emotional disturbance and prolonged severe pain, as in rheumatoid arthritis, can cause depression. There are many patients whose facial pain is psychogenic rather than organic in nature.

It must be emphasised that the diagnosis of psychogenic facial pain is a diagnosis by exclusion, but it is important to try to recognise the condition however limited diagnostic methods may be. The symptoms (Box 34.12) cause real enough suffering to the patient and should, if possible, be relieved. It is also important to avoid unnecessary surgery.

> **Box 34.12** **Features suggestive of psychogenic (atypical) facial pain**
>
> - Women of middle age or older mainly affected
> - Absence of organic signs
> - Pain often poorly localised
> - Description of pain may be bizarre
> - Delusional symptoms occasionally associated
> - Lack of response to analgesics
> - Unchanging pain persisting for many years
> - Lack of any triggering factors
> - Sometimes good response to antidepressive treatment

A common site for the pain is the maxillary region or in relation to the upper teeth, but localisation may not be precise or in a recognisable anatomical pattern. The description of the pain may be vague, bizarre ('drawing' or 'gripping') or exaggerated ('unbearable'), but without obvious effect on the patient's health. It is often described as having been continuous, even unremitting and unchanging for several years.

Pain is usually not provoked by any recognisable stimulus such as hot or cold foods or by mastication. Despite the fact that the pain may be said to be continuous and unbearable, the patient's sleeping or even eating may be unaffected. Analgesics are often said to be completely ineffective, but some patients have not even tried them, despite the stated severity of the pain. Objective signs of disease are absent. Although teeth have

often been extracted and diseased teeth may be present, none of these can be related to the pain. As a consequence, treatment of diseased teeth does not relieve the symptoms.

Other signs of emotional disturbance are highly variable. Some patients are more or less obviously depressed; some of them mention, in passing, difficulties they have had, for instance, at work with their colleagues. Others may complain how miserable the pain makes them. Others may complain of bizarre (delusional) symptoms such as 'slime' in the mouth or 'powder' coming out of the jaw.

Pain can be a symptom of depression. Since mental illness, even now, carries with it a stigma, patients frequently suppress the overt misery of depression. The patient may also fear (often rightly) that doctors or dentists are intolerant of what is regarded as their weakness in being unable to cope with their life situation. This pain can be regarded as their cry for help. This is occasionally strikingly evident in a patient who appears emotionally in control but who, when given a chance to describe the complaint at length, suddenly loses control and starts to weep uncontrollably. At the other extreme, there are patients who so aggressively reject the idea of mental illness that they insist from the start that the pain is not 'due to their nerves' and typically refuse psychiatric help. Occasionally, anxiety such as cancerophobia can give rise to atypical facial pain and may respond to reassurance.

Burning mouth syndrome

In this distressing and troublesome condition, symptoms may affect the whole mouth or only the tongue may be sore. This complaint has many features in common with atypical facial pain and may be a variant of it. Clinical features (Box 34.13) may suggest psychogenic factors.

> **Box 34.13** **Features suggestive of 'burning mouth syndrome'**
>
> - Middle-aged or older women are mainly affected
> - No visible abnormality or evidence of organic disease
> - No haematological abnormality
> - Pain typically described as 'burning'
> - Persistent and unremitting soreness without aggravating or relieving factors, often of months or years duration; no response to analgesics
> - Bizarre patterns of pain radiation inconsistent with neurological or vascular anatomy
> - Sometimes, bitter or metallic taste associated
> - Associated depression, anxiety or stressful life situation
> - Obsession with symptoms may rule the patient's life
> - Constant search for reassurance and treatment by different practitioners
> - Occasionally, dramatic improvement with antidepressive treatment

---

These symptoms are seen in varying combination, but psychological disturbance is frequently well disguised or suppressed. In practice, as with atypical facial pain, there are many patients who complain bitterly and persistently of sore tongue, in whom no organic disease can be found and who show no response to psychoactive drugs or any other form of treatment.

Similar symptoms have been ascribed to the angiotensin converting enzyme inhibitors lisinopril and captopril.

Management

The first essential is to exclude organic disease by a careful search for all possible sources of pain. Any potential sources of pain must be dealt with, but there should not be too much expectation of benefit.

If no organic cause can be found and if sympathetic discussion suggests psychogenic factors, then it may help to explain to the patient, in simple terms, that depression and other emotional disturbances are just as much illnesses and cause as much suffering as physical diseases. It is also important to explain that emotional disturbances affect almost everyone to some degree. It may also help to point out that more common symptoms, particularly headache, are rarely due to organic disease. Patients should also be reassured that there is no dangerous disease and that frightening possibilities such as cancer can be confidently excluded. Such reassurance is sometimes remarkably effective.

While it is obviously reasonable gently to recommend psychiatric help, patients are often resentful of the idea and it is more tactful to refer to the psychiatrist as a 'pain expert'. Sometimes, antidepressant treatment with dothiepin, or one of the newer generation antidepressive drugs, is strikingly effective.

Unfortunately, there is a hard core of patients who complain of persistent facial pain, have gone the round of specialists (including psychiatrists), have been treated with a wide range of drugs, but still continue to complain of severe pain. This problem may be a reflection of the limited range of treatment available, or perhaps such patients 'need' their pain for obscure emotional reasons.

It is essential also to appreciate that a few patients thought to have atypical facial pain are found later to have some disease such as an occult adenoid cystic carcinoma infiltrating nerve fibres. If there is any suggestion that the pain has a neurological distribution, imaging is mandatory.

Psychogenic dental pain (atypical odontalgia) →
Summary p. 448

This is a less common variant of atypical facial pain. Pain is often precisely localised in one tooth or in a row of teeth, which are said either to ache or to be exquisitely sensitive to heat, cold or pressure. If dental disease is found, treatment has no effect, or if, as a last resort, the tooth is removed, the pain moves to an adjacent tooth. Again, if no organic cause can be found and treatment is ineffective, psychiatric assessment is needed. Early diagnosis is essential to avoid overtreatment and serious dental morbidity.

Factitious ulceration (self-inflicted oral lesions)

Factitious ulcers in the mouth are traumatic but considerably less common than the usual type. They are typically a consequence

of a disturbed mental state ('a call for attention'). Rarely, factitious oral ulceration has been a prelude to suicide.

The most common type of self-inflicted oral injuries has been so-called self-extraction of teeth. The diagnosis of self-inflicted injuries may be difficult, but suspicious features are shown in Box 34.14.

> **Box 34.14 Features suggestive of factitious oral lesions**
> - Lack of correspondence with any recognisable disease
> - Bizarre configuration with sharp outlines
> - Usually in an otherwise healthy mouth
> - Clinical features inconsistent with the history
> - In areas accessible to the patient

Investigation may be needed to exclude organic disease. Underlying emotional disturbance is typically well concealed. Frequently, the diagnosis can be confirmed only by discreet observation after admission to hospital. The patient's family doctor should be told of the need for specialist psychiatric assessment.

Important causes of facial pain are summarised in Summary chart 34.1.

PARAESTHESIA AND ANAESTHESIA OF THE LIP

Paraesthesia of the lip can be caused by osteomyelitis or fracture of the jaw. Very occasionally, it results from neurological disease. The main causes of anaesthesia or paraesthesia of the lip are summarised in Box 34.15.

> **Box 34.15 Important causes of paraesthesia or anaesthesia of the lip**
> - Inferior dental blocks
> - Trauma (fracture or operative damage)
> - Acute osteomyelitis
> - Malignant tumours of the mandible
> - Exposed mental foramen
> - Herpes zoster
> - Multiple sclerosis
> - Tetany

Interestingly, though of little relevance to dental practice, paraesthesia of the lips is a striking feature, with diarrhoea and vomiting, from tropical reef fish poisoning by tetrodoxin and ciguatera toxins.

Prolonged anaesthesia or paraesthesia of the lip can occasionally follow inferior dental blocks, possibly as a result of damage to the nerve by the needle. Spontaneous recovery usually takes place.

Paraesthesia of the lip can be a complication of fractures of the mandible where the nerve has become stretched, particularly over the sharp edge of the canal. The effect is temporary, but complete recovery may take some months. The inferior

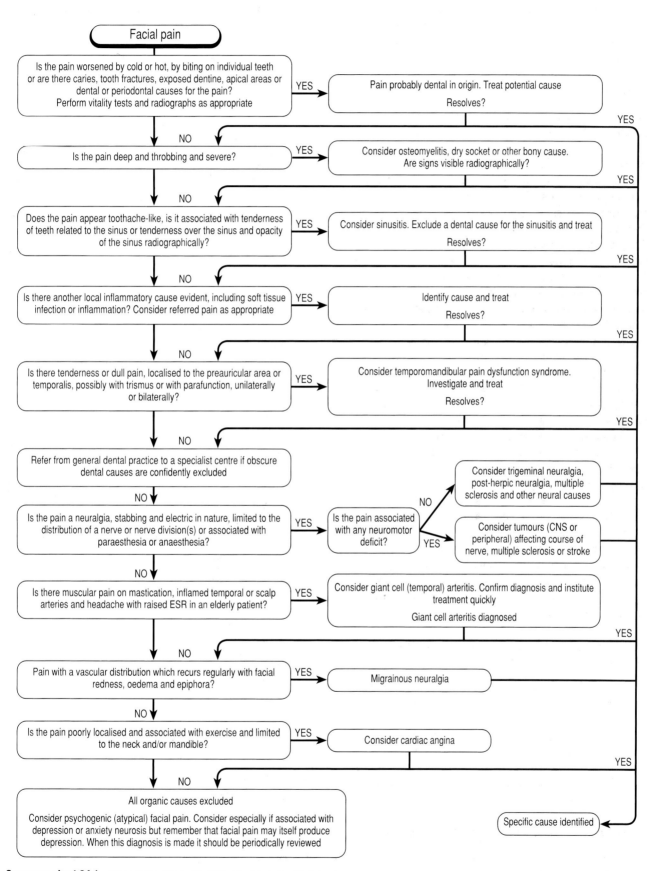

Summary chart 34.1   Steps in the diagnosis of important causes of facial pain.

dental nerve may occasionally be damaged in operations on the mandible and there may be anaesthesia or paraesthesia lasting for many months. Complete loss of sensation is unusual, but recovery may take a year or more.

The inferior dental nerve is rarely involved in osteomyelitis but, with effective treatment, recovery is the rule. Alternatively, it may be compressed by a neoplasm or a tumour may infiltrate the nerve sheath. A jaw tumour causing pain or paraesthesia strongly suggests malignancy. In such cases, the prognosis is poor, either because the tumour may be a secondary carcinoma or a primary, but highly malignant tumour, such as an osteosarcoma.

The mental foramen can become exposed by excessive resorption of mandibular bone in an edentulous patient. The denture can then press upon the nerve as it leaves the foramen. Though these changes are common, they rarely cause paraesthesia of the lip.

Herpes zoster affecting the trigeminal nerve can leave residual disturbances of sensation. The most severe and troublesome is postherpetic neuralgia but, in other patients, there may be persistent paraesthesia in the nerve distribution affected.

Disturbances of sensation of the face and other regions can be caused by multiple sclerosis as discussed earlier.

Tetany is the result of hypocalcaemic states and causes heightened neuromuscular excitability together with minor disorders of sensation such as paraesthesia of the lip. A significant cause of tetany is overbreathing, usually due to anxiety (hyperventilation syndrome).

FACIAL PALSY

Important causes of facial palsy, which include both upper and lower motor neurone lesions, are summarised in Box 34.16.

Box 34.16   Causes of facial palsy

Extracranial causes
- Bell's palsy
- Malignant parotid neoplasms
- Parotid surgery
- Sarcoidosis (Heerfordt's syndrome)
- Misplaced local anaesthetic
- Melkersson–Rosenthal syndrome

Intracranial causes
- Strokes
- Cerebral tumours and other neurological diseases
- Multiple sclerosis
- HIV infection
- Lyme disease
- Ramsay–Hunt syndrome
- Trauma to the base of the skull

In upper motor neurone lesions, the lower part of the face is mainly affected and spontaneous emotional facial reactions may be retained. They are typically due to intracranial causes. In lower motor neurone lesions, such as Bell's palsy, emotional movements of the face, the blink reflex and ability to wrinkle the forehead are lost, the tongue deviates to the affected side on protrusion and drooling from the affected side is common.

Bell's palsy

Bell's palsy is a common cause of facial paralysis. It probably results from compression of the facial nerve in its canal as a result of inflammation and swelling. A viral infection, particularly herpes simplex, is suspected as the cause. Either sex may be affected, usually between the ages of 20 and 50. As mentioned earlier, pain in the jaw sometimes precedes the paralysis

(A)

(B)

Fig 34.1   Bell's palsy. (A) When trying to shut the eyes, that on the affected (right) side fails to close completely but the eyeball rolls up normally. (B) When trying to smile, the mouth fails to move on the affected side, which remains expressionless, having lost all natural skin folds. The difference is made more striking by covering each side of the picture in turn. This patient, incidentally, complained primarily of facial pain, though was increasingly aware of the facial disability. The severely disfiguring effect of this disorder and the need for early treatment is obvious. In this case, response was complete. (By kind permission of the patient.)

or there may be numbness in the side of the tongue. Though this disease is uncommon in dental practice, its recognition is important as early treatment may prevent permanent disability and disfigurement.

Function of the facial nerve is tested by asking the patient to perform facial movements. When asked to close the eyes, the lids on the affected side cannot be brought together, but the eyeball rolls up normally, since the oculomotor nerves are unaffected. When the patient is asked to smile, the corner of the mouth on the affected side is not pulled upwards and the normal lines of expression are absent (Fig. 34.1). The wrinkling round the eyes which accompanies smiling is also not seen on the affected side and the eye remains staring. This is a lower motor neurone lesion unlike the upper motor neurone lesion seen, for example, after a stroke, as discussed below.

The majority of patients recover fully or partially without treatment. At least 10% of patients with Bell's palsy are unhappy about the final outcome because of permanent disfigurement or other complications. A guide to the need for treatment is the severity of the paralysis when first seen. Full recovery is usual in patients with an incomplete palsy seen within a week of onset, but more than half of those with a complete lesion fail to recover completely. Electromyography and other electrodiagnostic techniques can be used to measure the degree of functional impairment as a guide to the need for treatment. Prednisolone, by mouth (20 mg four times a day) may be given for 5–10 days and then tapered off over the following 4 days, and may be effective if given within 24 hours of the onset. The addition of aciclovir appears to produce more reliable results and also suggests a role for a herpes virus.

If treatment fails or is not given, persistent facial weakness is disfiguring. The affected part of the face sometimes also contracts involuntarily in association with movement of another part. There may, for example, be twitching of the mouth when the patient blinks. More uncommon is unilateral lacrimation (crocodile tears) when eating. The majority of patients with persistent denervation develop contracture of the affected side of the face. Watering of the eye (epiphora) due to impaired drainage of tears, or occasionally to excessive and erratic lacrimal secretion, may remain particularly troublesome.

Dental aspects

Rarely, as mentioned earlier, pain felt in the jaw may precede paralysis. If persistent, oral cleaning can deteriorate and food debris can accumulate in the vestibule on the affected side. If treatment fails, sagging of the affected side of the face may be limited by an intraoral prosthesis.

Melkersson–Rosenthal syndrome → Summary p. 409

Melkersson–Rosenthal syndrome in its rare complete form comprises unilateral recurrent facial paralysis, which may become permanent, labial or facial swelling and fissured tongue. Not all these features are present in all patients. Recurrent, soft, painless facial swelling is more common, but may become persistent due to progressive fibrosis. The buccal mucosa may develop a cobblestone pattern like that in Crohn's disease and, histologically, granulomas are found. Variants of this disorder include oedema of the eyelids, bilateral facial or rarely multiple cranial nerve palsies, oedema of the lip and there is a rare familial type. There is possibly an immunological basis for this disease and there is sometimes a response to intralesional corticosteroids, either temporary or, rarely, permanent. Successful treatment with thalidomide has been claimed but not confirmed. Overall, therefore, there is no specific or uniformly reliable form of treatment.

Other causes of facial palsy

Cerebrovascular accidents (thrombosis or haemorrhage) are a common complication of hypertension in the elderly. Unilateral paralysis (hemiplegia) and often loss of speech (aphasia) are frequent in survivors of the acute episode. Unilateral facial palsy is common, but differs from Bell's palsy in that the lower part of the face is mainly affected and spontaneous emotional facial reactions may be retained. As in the case of persistent paralysis in Bell's palsy, an intraoral prosthesis may limit sagging of the face. A stroke is occasionally the cause of an emergency in the dental surgery (Ch. 36).

Facial palsy is an uncommon but characteristic manifestation of a *malignant parotid tumour*. Alternatively, a facial nerve may have been sacrificed during resection of a malignant parotid tumour, or is accidentally damaged during a parotidectomy. The variable course of the facial nerve within the parotid gland makes it particularly vulnerable to surgical injury and great skill is needed to trace its course.

Ramsay–Hunt syndrome is severe facial palsy with pain, usually felt in the throat. Vesicles of herpes zoster may be seen in the external auditory meatus or throat.

Lyme disease is caused by *Borrelia burgdorferi* and transmitted by animal ticks. It is common in the USA but now seen in many other countries. Facial palsy or cervical lymphadenopathy are sometimes prominent, but arthritis is the chief effect.

Heerfordt's syndrome is the rare combination of facial palsy, uveitis and parotid swelling caused by sarcoidosis of cranial nerves and salivary glands.

DISTURBANCES OF TASTE AND SMELL

Loss of taste is a distressing symptom for many patients, but it is poorly understood and difficult to investigate. The sensation of taste depends heavily on smell and the two must be considered together. A complaint of loss of taste is frequently explained by loss of smell.

A few patients have a psychogenic complaint of altered taste or smell. The abnormal taste may appear bizarre or limited to a part of the mouth. A complaint of an unremitting bitter taste often accompanies burning mouth syndrome.

Table 34.1   Some drugs causing taste disturbance

Drug	Effect
Metronidazole	Bitter metallic taste
Tetracycline	Bitter metallic taste
Tegretol	Taste loss
Biguanide anti-diabetic drugs	Bitter metallic taste
Allopurinol	Bitter metallic taste
Penicillamine	Bitter metallic taste and taste loss
Terbinafine	Taste loss
Many chemotherapy drugs	Abnormal taste and taste loss
Sodium lauryl sulphate (toothpaste detergent)	Loss of subsequent salt and sweet taste
Angiotensin-converting enzyme inhibitors	Weakened taste
Nifedipine	Abnormal taste
Beta blockers	Loss of smell

Some drugs that have been associated with taste disturbance are listed in Table 34.1; many more have been reported. Some appear to interfere with detection, while others have a strong taste and are secreted into saliva, such as metronidazole. In most cases, the alterations are reversible, but some drugs can cause permanent taste loss.

The commonest cause of taste loss is probably ageing (Box 34.17). This may be compounded by complete dentures that

Box 34.17   Causes of weakened taste sensation

- Ageing (affects smell and taste)
- Loss of smell through nasal disease
- Dry mouth and nose, Sjögren's syndrome
- Parkinson's disease
- Diabetes mellitus
- Liver disease
- HIV infection
- Halitosis
- Trauma and surgery to nerves, particularly the olfactory nerve
- Radiotherapy

cover taste buds on the palate. Dry mouth prevents transport of soluble taste molecules to the receptors. Infection may produce a bad taste, particularly when pus is present or in acute ulcerative gingivitis. Taste is rarely disturbed by sensory nerve lesions because of the large number of nerves that supply taste sensation. Conversely, smell depends on a small area of the nasal mucosa and a single cranial nerve.

Testing for taste disturbance is complex and best performed in a specialised centre. There is no scientific basis for 'taste maps' suggesting that specific tastes are sensed in different anatomical areas. They cannot be used to investigate taste clinically.

SUGGESTED FURTHER READING

Adour KK, Rubioyianes JM, von Doerstein PG et al 1996 Bell's palsy treatment with acyclovir and prednisone compared with prednisone alone: a double-blind, randomized, controlled trial. Ann Otol Rhinol Laryngol 105:371–378

Baringer JR 1996 Herpes simplex virus and Bell's palsy. Ann Intern Med 124:63–65

Barker FG, Jannetta PJ, Bissonett DJ et al 1996 The long term outcome of microvascular decompression for trigeminal neuralgia. N Engl J Med 334:1077–1083

Bergdahl J, Anneroth G, Perris H 1995 Cognitive therapy in the treatment of patients with resistant burning mouth syndrome: a controlled study. J Oral Pathol Med 24:213–215

Devlen J 1994 Anxiety and depression in migraine. J Roy Soc Med 87:338–341

Fields HL 1996 Treatment of trigeminal neuralgia (editorial). N Engl J Med 334:1125–1126

Huong W, Rothe MJ, Grant-Kels JM 1996 The burning mouth syndrome. J Am Acad Dermatol 34:91–98

Kost RG, Straus SE 1996 Postherpetic neuralgia – pathogenesis, treatment and prevention. N Engl J Med 335:32–42

Maizels M, Scott B, Cohen W, Chen W 1996 Intranasal lidocaine for treatment of migraine. J Am Med Assoc 276:319–321

Morgan M, Nathwain D 1992 Facial palsy and infection: the unfolding story. Clin Infect Dis 14:263–271

Shafshak TS, Essa AY, Bakey FA 1994 The possible contributing factors for the success of steroid therapy in Bell's palsy: a clinical and electrophysiological study. J Larngol Otol 108:940–943

Spielman AI 1998 Chemosensory function and dysfunction. Crit Rev Oral Biol Med 9:267–291

Whitley RJ, Weiss H, Gnann JW 1996 Acyclovir with and without prednisone for the treatment of herpes zoster. A randomized, placebo-controlled trial. Ann Intern Med 125:376–383

Zakrzewska JM 1996 Assessment of a patient with orofacial pain. Primary Dent Care 3:57–60

Complications of systemic drug treatment

About 10% of ambulant outpatients may be having systemic drug treatment. Though not a common source of difficulties, some drugs can complicate dental management, occasionally catastrophically (Table 35.1). Drugs abusers are also a growing clinical problem. The effects of systemically administered drugs on dental management are varied (Box 35.1).

Box 35.1   Significance of (conventional) drug treatment to dental management

- Drugs may complicate dental treatment itself (Table 35.1)
- Drugs may react with drugs given for dental purposes
- Drugs may cause stomatitis (Ch. 13) or have other oral effects

---

ORAL REACTIONS TO DRUGS

Many drugs can occasionally cause oral reactions. They are varied in type, but frequently lichenoid or ulcerative (Figs 35.3 and 35.4).

The mechanisms of reactions to drugs are often obscure, but the various types are shown in Box 35.2.

Box 35.2   Important types of oral drug reactions

I. Local reactions to drugs
- Chemical irritation
- Interference with the oral flora

II. Systematically mediated reactions
- Depression of marrow function
- Depression of cell-mediated immunity
- Lichenoid reactions
- Erythema multiforme (Stevens–Johnson syndrome)
- Fixed drug eruptions
- Toxic epidermal necrolysis

III. Other effects
- Gingival hyperplasia
- Pigmentation
- Dry mouth

LOCAL REACTION TO DRUGS

Chemical burns

The best-known example is that of aspirin tablets held against the mucosa close to an aching tooth. This causes superficial necrosis and a white patch. When the irritant is removed, dead epithelium is shed and the mucosa heals. Other irritant chemicals are acid etchants, or phenols dropped on the mucosa.

Interference with the oral flora: superinfection

Prolonged topical use of antibiotics (particularly tetracycline) in the mouth kills off sensitive organisms and allows resistant ones, particularly *Candida albicans*, to proliferate, causing thrush. In susceptible patients, use of a topical antibiotic may precipitate candidal infection within 48 hours.

SYSTEMICALLY MEDIATED REACTIONS

Depression of marrow function

Few drugs significantly depress red cell production alone, though any drug which causes anaemia might give rise to oral signs. The main example is prolonged use of phenytoin (for epilepsy) which, in susceptible patients, can occasionally cause folate deficiency and macrocytic anaemia. This, in turn, can cause severe aphthous stomatitis. Response promptly follows administration of folate and the blood picture returns to normal.

White cell production is depressed by a variety of drugs. Leucopenia may be severe enough to produce the clinical picture of agranulocytosis, with necrotising ulceration of the gingivae and throat which can go on to a severe prostrating illness and septicaemia if untreated. Drugs which may have this effect include antibacterials, particularly co-trimoxazole, chloramphenicol, analgesics, particularly amidopyrine (obsolete in the UK), phenothiazines and antithyroid agents. When the main effect is on granulocytes, low-grade oral pathogens, particularly of the gingival margins, are able to overcome local resistance and produce necrotising ulceration (Ch. 22).

Other drugs may cause haemostasis and cause oral purpura (Ch. 23). Drug-induced purpura is often also an early sign of

443

Table 35.1 Examples of prescribed drugs having dentally relevant adverse effects

Type of drug	Dentally relevant adverse effects
Antibiotics	Superinfection (usually candidosis) Allergy (mainly penicillin) (Figs 35.1 and 35.2)
Anticoagulants	Risk of postoperative haemorrhage
Calcium channel blocker antihypertensives (e.g. nifedipine) and diltiazem (an antidysrhythmic)	Gingival hyperplasia
Phenytoin	Gingival hyperplasia Lymphadenopathy occasionally Folate deficiency occasionally
Aspirin	Potentiation of any haemorrhagic tendencies Avoid in children because of risk of Reye's syndrome
Other non-steroidal anti-inflammatory analgesics	Oral lichenoid reactions rarely
Hypnotics and sedatives[a]	Potentiation of general anaesthetics and other sedating drugs
Barbiturates	Risk of erythema multiforme
Phenothiazine antipsychotics ('major tranquillisers')	Dry mouth Tardive dyskinesia (uncontrollable facial movements) Parkinsonian tremor Postural hypotension Oral mucosal pigmentation
Metoclopramide	Clenching of jaw muscles
Tricyclic antidepressants (e.g. amitriptyline)[b]	Dry mouth
Monoamine oxidase inhibitors[b]	Dry mouth Dangerous interactions with opioids, particularly pethidine
Insulin	Risk of hypoglycaemic coma
Antihistamines	Dry mouth Drowsiness Potentiate sedatives
Corticosteroids	Opportunistic infections Risk of circulatory collapse (see also Box 31.10)
Other immunosuppressive and cytotoxic drugs	Oral ulceration (especially methotrexate) Opportunistic infections Cisplatin can cause grey gingival line Vincristine can cause jaw pain and weakness of the facial muscles
Ciclosporin	Gingival hyperplasia
Bisphosphonates	Necrosis of mandible and maxilla (see Ch. 6)

[a]Benzodiazepines ('minor tranquillisers') have few adverse effects apart from sedation, additive effects with other CNS depressants, and slight respiratory depression which is not significant in normal persons. However, they are addictive.
[b]*Do not* cause significant interactions with adrenaline (epinephrine) in local anaesthetics.

aplastic anaemia caused by drugs such as chloramphenicol, which depress marrow function, as indicated above. Purpura can produce severe spontaneous gingival bleeding or blood blisters and widespread submucosal ecchymoses.

Depression of cell-mediated immunity

Immunosuppression by such drugs as corticosteroids is induced in patients having organ transplants or with immunologically-mediated diseases (see Fig. 24.1). Viral and fungal infections

of the mouth are common in immunosuppressed patients and can be severe. Recurrences of childhood viral infections, such as measles and chickenpox, are also possible.

Lichenoid reactions

Several drugs, notably gold and antimalarials (both used in the treatment of rheumatoid arthritis or other collagen diseases), and the antihypertensive agent methyldopa can cause disease indistinguishable from lichen planus, both clinically and

Fig. 35.1 Collapse caused by type I hypersensitivity to penicillin.

Fig. 35.2 **Hypersensitivity to penicillin.** There is a generalised slight oedema of the face, pallor and a macular rash.

Fig. 35.3 **Lichenoid reaction to captopril.** In this milder reaction, there are several small ulcers, but the main effect is the production of striae covering the whole ventral surface of the tongue.

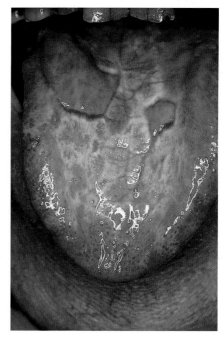

Fig. 35.4 **Lichenoid reaction to gold treatment for rheumatoid arthritis.** There is extensive ulceration of the dorsal tongue, atrophy and keratosis. Biopsy showed changes very similar to lichen planus.

histologically (Ch. 13). The mechanism of such reactions is unknown.

Acute erythema multiforme → Summary p. 221

As discussed earlier, sulphonamides, barbiturates or other drugs are occasionally implicated, but the mechanisms are unknown and more frequently there is no evidence of a drug reaction.

Toxic epidermal necrolysis

This, which probably represents the extreme end of the spectrum of erythema multiforme, is one of the most dangerous and severe types of drug reaction. Mucosal involvement is common and causes widespread erosions due to epithelial

destructions. Oral ulceration may precede the dermal changes and cause the patient to seek treatment for the extreme soreness of the mouth. Early diagnosis and treatment is important as the reaction can be lethal. Metals such as gold salts are important causes, but phenylbutazone, barbiturates and other drugs have also been implicated. Healing of oral lesions may leave a pattern of lichen planus.

Fixed drug eruptions

These consist of sharply circumscribed skin lesions recurring in the same site or sites each time the drug is given. Many drugs are capable of causing this reaction, but phenolphthalein, a widely use component of purgatives, is one of the more common causes. Involvement of the oral mucous membrane has been described but is exceedingly rare.

Angio-oedema

Angio-oedema of the face, tongue and airway may result from angiotensin converting enzyme inhibitors, which activate bradykinin. These drugs can also cause symptoms of *burning mouth*.

Osteonecrosis

Caused by high-potency bisphosphonate drugs (Ch. 6).

Taste and smell

These can be disturbed by many medications (Ch. 34).

OTHER DRUG EFFECTS (BOX 35.2)

Gingival hyperplasia

Phenytoin and other drugs (Ch. 5) can cause fibrous hyperplasias, particularly concentrated at the interdental papillae.

Oral pigmentation

Heavy metals such as mercury, bismuth and lead can cause black or brown deposits in the gingival sulcus by interaction with bacterial products to form sulphides. The blue lead line may be particularly sharply defined and indicate the level of the floor of the pocket. These effects are rarely seen now that mercury and bismuth are no longer used in medicine and lead is no longer a major industrial hazard. However, cisplatin, a cytotoxic drug, can cause a blue line. Topical antibiotics and antiseptics may cause dark pigmentation, particularly of the dorsum of the tongue, due to overgrowth of pigment-forming bacteria.

Dry mouth

This is a relatively common side-effect of drugs, particularly those with an atropine-like action, such as the tricyclic antidepressants which are widely used (Ch. 18).

Oral ulcers

Oral ulcers similar to major aphthae develop in patients taking Nicorandil.

MANAGEMENT CONSIDERATIONS

Oral reactions to drugs are not overall common; nevertheless, they may be important as an early sign of a dangerous or lethal reaction.

However, a drug being taken by a patient is not necessarily the cause of any oral symptoms. Coincidence is often difficult to exclude, particularly with common oral diseases such as lichen planus. The problem is made more difficult by multiple drug treatment. However, it is essential to get a detailed history of drug treatment as this may affect other aspects of dental treatment.

Precautions

Though drugs only occasionally cause clinical difficulties, patients must always be asked whether they are under medical treatment. In such enquiries, the word 'drugs' should be avoided as inevitably leading to misinterpretation. Patients should be asked whether they are taking 'medicines, tablets, injections, or any sort of medical treatment for *any* purpose' or have received any medications recently, or whether they have been given any sort of hospital card.

CHEMICAL DEPENDENCE

Drug dependence, particularly addiction to intravenous drugs, is a major social problem, particularly in large cities, but has now spread to rural areas.

Alcohol remains the most widely abused drug but, of the illegal drugs, crack cocaine and heroin are currently the most frequently misused. The changes in illegal drug habits depend to a large extent on their cost. This in turn, and cocaine and heroin in particular, results from changes in the world situation.

There are few direct oral effects of drug dependence apart from maxillofacial injuries secondary to alcohol abuse particularly, but difficulties in management are more common (Box 35.3). Methamphetamine (speed etc), in particular, is likely to cause considerable oral damage in long-term use. It is acidic and also causes dry mouth. Great thirst, which tends to be relieved by almost continuous consumption of carbonated drinks, some of which have a high sugar content, is a common response. Together with oral neglect, gross caries and periodontal disease can result.

Box 35.3 Implications of drug dependence for dental management

- Stealing prescription pads
- Attempts to manipulate dentists into prescribing drugs
- Carriage of hepatitis viruses or HIV by intravenous addicts
- Maxillofacial injuries, particularly among alcoholics
- Impaired liver function secondary to alcoholism or hepatitis
- Lymphadenopathy secondary to drug injection in unusual sites
- Infective endocarditis secondary to dirty injections
- Severe infections such as osteomyelitis among alcoholics
- Increased risks from general anaesthesia
- Gross oral neglect and sometimes enhanced sensitivity to pain
- Rarely, ulceration of the palate secondary to cocaine-induced ischaemia of the nasal cavity
- Occasionally, parotid swelling in alcoholics
- Interactions with other drugs

Other problems are that addicts may manipulate dentists into prescribing drugs, particularly opioids, by complaining of pain. Multiple drug abuse is also common and attempts may be made to obtain any drugs, such as benzodiazepines or antihistamines, which are mood-altering or sedative. Because of the risk of dependence, benzodiazepines should only be prescribed for short periods. Codeine or dextropropoxyphene (in co-proxamol) are opioids and occasionally a cause of dependence.

Liver function damaged by alcoholism or hepatitis impairs drug metabolism. This makes general anaesthesia, in particular, hazardous, as does respiratory disease or covert use of the drug of abuse preoperatively. Once infective endocarditis has resulted from dirty injections, the damaged heart becomes vulnerable to endocarditis after some types of dental procedures (Ch. 27).

SUGGESTED FURTHER READING

Cawson RA, Spector RG, Skelly AM 1995 Basic pharmacology and clinical drug use in dentistry, 6th edn. Churchill Livingstone, Edinburgh

Passeri LA, Ellis E, Sinn DP 1993 Relationship of substance abuse to complications with mandibular fractures. J Oral Maxillofac Surg 51:22–25

Robb ND, Smith BGN 1996 Chronic alcoholism: an important condition in the dentist–patient relationship. J Dentistry 24:17–24

Strang J 1995 Substance abuse: the size of the problem. Medicine Int 23:41–44

Vale A 1995 Alcohol intoxication and alcohol–drug interactions. Medicine Int 23:51–53

Emergencies in dental practice

Dentists must know how to recognise and manage medical emergencies, rare though they may be. Their professional skills and equipment should enable them occasionally to save patients' lives. Patients suffering life-threatening emergencies should be quickly transferred to hospital, but city traffic and the load on ambulance services are so heavy that the delay can be considerable. Under such circumstances, measures taken by the dentist may be critical.

Dentists are also required to ensure that all members of their staff are able to provide practical assistance in these circumstances.

Many types of emergencies may have to be faced (Box 36.1).

Box 36.1   Emergencies that may arise during dental procedures

Sudden loss of consciousness (collapse)
- Fainting
- Acute hypoglycaemia
- Circulatory collapse secondary to corticosteroid therapy
- Anaphylactic shock
- Myocardial infarction
- Cardiac arrest
- Strokes

Acute chest pain
- Angina
- Myocardial infarction

Difficulty in breathing
- Asthma
- Anaphylactic shock
- Left ventricular failure

Convulsions
- Epilepsy
- Any other cause of loss of consciousness, including fainting

Other emergencies
- Haemorrhage
- Drug reactions and interactions
- Major maxillofacial injuries

---

in the dental surgery. There are several predisposing factors (Box 36.2), but some patients are particularly prone to faint and frequently do so. Signs and symptoms are usually readily recognisable (Box 36.3).

Box 36.2   Factors predisposing to fainting

- Anxiety
- Pain
- Injections
- Fatigue
- Hunger

Box 36.3   Fainting: signs and symptoms

- Premonitory dizziness, weakness or nausea
- Pale, cold moist skin
- Initially slow and weak pulse becoming full and bounding
- Loss of consciousness

Sometimes consciousness is lost almost instantaneously. Minor convulsions or incontinence are occasionally associated. Principles of management are summarised in Box 36.4.

Box 36.4   Management of a fainting attack

- Lower the head, preferably by laying the patient flat*
- Loosen any tight clothing round the neck
- Give a sweetened drink when consciousness has been recovered
- If no recovery within a few minutes, consider other causes of loss of consciousness

* To keep the patient upright worsens cerebral hypoxia and is harmful.

SUDDEN LOSS OF CONSCIOUSNESS

Fainting

Fainting, caused by transient hypotension and cerebral ischaemia, is the most common cause of sudden loss of consciousness

Prevention

Regular fainters are frequently helped by an anxiolytic, such as temazepam 5 mg orally, on the night before and again an hour before treatment, but must be accompanied by a responsible adult.

Acute hypoglycaemia

Hypoglycaemia affects diabetic patients after an overdose of insulin or if prevented from eating at the expected time by dental treatment (Box 36.5).

Box 36.5 Signs and symptoms of acute hypoglycaemia

- Premonitory signs are similar to those of a faint, but little response to laying the patient flat
- Unconsciousness steadily deepens

Management of hypoglycaemia is important (Box 36.6). If there is any doubt about the cause of loss of consciousness, insulin must never be given as it can be fatal to a hypoglycaemic patient.

Box 36.6 Management of hypoglycaemia

- Patients often aware of what is happening and able to warn the dentist
- Before consciousness is lost, give glucose tablets or powder, or sugar (at least four lumps) as a sweetened drink, repeated if symptoms not completely relieved
- If consciousness is lost, give sterile intravenous glucose (up to 50 ml of a 50% solution). This is difficult to administer and, in dental practice, the next steps may be easier in an emergency situation while venous access is obtained
- If sterile glucose not available give subcutaneous glucagon (1 mg) then give sugar by mouth during the brief recovery period
- Hypostop, a gel containing glucose, may provide sufficient glucose absorbed through the oral mucosa to combat declining consciousness

---

Circulatory collapse in patients on corticosteroid treatment

The response of patients on long-term corticosteroid treatment to surgery is unpredictable, but near-fatal circulatory collapse can follow minor dental extractions under anaesthesia in a patient taking as little as 5 mg of prednisone a day. All patients who are taking or have been taking systemic corticosteroids are at risk. Adrenocortical function may possibly take up to 2 years to recover. Corticosteroid skin preparations used liberally, particularly for widespread eczema, can also lead to stress-related collapse.

Since large doses of corticosteroids given for a short period are safe and can be life-saving, management (Box 36.7) should lean towards being over-protective. Prevention is all important.

Causes and clinical features of corticosteroid-related collapse

General anaesthesia, surgical or other trauma, infections or other stress are the main causes (see Fig. 31.8).

Box 36.7 Signs and management of corticosteroid-related collapse

Signs
- Pallor
- Rapid, weak or impalpable pulse
- Loss of consciousness
- Rapidly falling blood pressure

Management
- Lay the patient flat and raise the legs
- Give at least 200 mg hydrocortisone sodium succinate intravenously*
- Call an ambulance for immediate transfer to hospital
- Give oxygen and, if necessary, artificial ventilation
- Consider other possible reasons for loss of consciousness

*The intramuscular route can be used if a vein cannot be found but absorption is slower.

Myocardial infarction

A patient typically has severe chest pain, but may suddenly lose consciousness as a result of a myocardial infarct (see below).

Anaphylactic reactions

Penicillin is the most common cause of these type I hypersensitivity reactions. Similar reactions due to direct histamine release by morphine or intravenous barbiturate anaesthetics are rare. Anaphylactic reactions can also be precipitated by insect stings, foods (nuts or shellfish particularly) and, exceptionally rarely, by aspirin.

In general, the quicker the onset the more severe the reaction. A severe reaction to penicillin may start within a minute of an injection, but immediate loss of consciousness is more likely to be due to fainting. A reaction starting 30 minutes after an injection is unlikely to be dangerous. Acute reactions to oral penicillins are rare but can develop after half an hour or more because of slower absorption from the gut.

Collapse is due to widespread vasodilatation and increased capillary permeability causing potentially fatal hypotension (see Figs 35.1 and 35.2).

Signs and symptoms

The clinical picture is variable (Box 36.8).

Box 36.8 Typical features of acute anaphylaxis

- Initial facial flushing, itching, paraesthesiae or cold extremities
- Facial oedema or urticaria
- Bronchospasm (wheezing)
- Loss of consciousness
- Pallor going on to cyanosis
- Cold clammy skin
- Rapid weak or impalpable pulse
- Deep fall in blood pressure
- Death if treatment is delayed or inappropriate

Management

Epinephrine is the mainstay of treatment (Box 36.9) and the live-saving element. It raises cardiac output, combats excessive capillary permeability and bronchospasm, and also inhibits release of mediators from mast cells.

Box 36.9   Management of anaphylactic collapse

- Lay the patient flat. Raise the legs to improve cerebral blood flow
- Give 0.5–1 ml of 1:1000 epinephrine (adrenaline) by intramuscular injection. Repeat every 15 minutes if necessary, until the patient responds
- Give 10–20 mg chlorpheniramine (diluted in the syringe with 10 ml of blood) slowly intravenously
- Give 200 mg of hydrocortisone sodium succinate intravenously
- Give oxygen and, if necessary, assisted ventilation
- Call an ambulance

Circulatory collapse is probably largely due to histamine release which is combated by parenteral chlorpheniramine. Hydrocortisone is slow to take effect but maintains the blood pressure for some hours and combats the continued effect of the antigen–antibody reaction.

Rapid transfer to hospital is necessary to provide circulatory support by intravenous fluids and other measures. The patient must also be given a card warning against the use of the causative drug.

Minor anaphylactic reactions, such as urticaria, can be treated with oral or intramuscular chlorpheniramine.

Cardiac arrest

Cardiac arrest can follow myocardial infarction, or the acute hypotension of an anaphylactic reaction or of corticosteroid insufficiency. Otherwise, it may be the result of an anaesthetic accident and due to hypoxia, anaesthetic overdose or severe hypotension.

Dentists should be aware of and alert to the possibility of cardiac arrest and be able to recognise it (Box 36.10) and manage it (Box 36.11) when it happens. Speed of response is essential and there is a legal obligation that the dental team should be trained in cardiopulmonary resuscitation and be able to carry it out immediately. Basic life support requires a firm surface, ideally the floor. If the patient is too heavy to lift out of a dental chair but can be laid supine there, resuscitation can be carried out by the operator and assistant standing beside the chair. An operator's stool can be placed under the headrest to stabilise the chair.

Box 36.10   Signs and symptoms of cardiac arrest

- Sudden loss of consciousness
- Absence of arterial pulses (the carotid artery, anterior to sternomastoid should be felt)
- Absence of breathing follows shortly

Box 36.11   Basic Life Support (BLS)

- Start BLS immediately because of
  Absence of breathing in a non-responsive patient
  Abnormal breathing (infrequent noisy 'agonal' gasps)
- Check area for danger
- Assess responsiveness by shaking shoulders and shouting
- Shout for help (do not call 999 – yet)
- Open the airway (head tilt and chin lift or jaw thrust)
- Check mouth for vomit/debris and remove with finger scoops
- Assess breathing – listen and feel for breathing whilst observing chest movements. Take no more than 10 seconds
- If breathing is abnormal (infrequent, noisy gasps) call the emergency services '999'. (You may have to leave the victim to do this). Then:
- Perform 30 chest compressions of 4–5 cm each, over the centre of the sternum at a rate of 100 per minute. Then:
- Give 2 ventilations. If available, use oxygen and a self-inflating bag
- Continue compressions and ventilations until help arrives or the victim shows signs of life or until you are physically exhausted and unable to carry on

Resuscitation of children
- Sequence includes 5 initial rescue breaths before the start of chest compressions
- Start CPR (30 compressions to 2 breath cycles) for 1 minute before going to call the emergency services (may be able to take a small child with you if distance to telephone is great)
- Compressions:
  Compress the chest by one third of its depth
  Prepubertal – one hand (centre of chest)
  <1 year – 2 fingers (centre of line between the nipples)
  Single rescuer 30:2 breaths   Dual rescuer 15:2 breaths

Guidelines of the Resuscitation Council UK 2005

Respiratory arrest and eventual cyanosis, pupil dilatation and loss of reaction to light, and absence of measurable blood pressure are other signs, but resuscitation must be started before they develop. Guidelines were recently simplified (2005) and recognise only two situations in which basic life support is indicated, unconsciousness and 'agonal' gasps, sharp gasping breaths in the first minutes after arrest.

The optimal pressure for chest compression is about 40 or 50 kg (the weight of the upper part of the body applied through stiffly extended arms). External cardiac massage is tiring and another person should preferably take over as soon as the first operator becomes fatigued.

Signs of restoration of blood pressure are disappearance of facial pallor and a good spontaneous pulse, contraction of the pupils, return of reflex activity such as the blink reflex and reaction of the pupils to light, lightening of unconsciousness and purposeful spontaneous movements – not twitching or convulsions. If no signs of life appear within 15 minutes (timed by the clock) recovery is unlikely, but chest compressions and ventilation must be continued for as long as possible.

Unless the operator is skilled in its use, time should not be wasted in trying to pass an endotracheal tube. However, a self-inflating bag with an oxygen supply should be available to provide positive pressure ventilation. A plastic airway should be put in the patient's mouth and the mask applied firmly over the nose and mouth with the resuscitation bag attached. The patient's lungs should be inflated with oxygen by squeezing the bag, so that the chest is visibly expanded at each respiration. Passive recoil of the chest wall causes spontaneous expiration as soon as the pressure is removed.

If a self-inflating bag is not available, mouth-to-mouth ventilation can be given, preferably with an intervening Laerdal-type pocket mask.

During artificial ventilation the patient's nose must be closed. Deep inflations are given by the operator and time allowed for passive recoil of the chest. If there is no airway adjunct available, direct mouth-to-mouth resuscitation, with the nose occluded, must be given. Causes of failure are summarised in Box 36.12.

Box 36.12 Causes of failure of cardiopulmonary resuscitation

- Giving artificial ventilation without cardiac compression (current guidance emphasises compression over ventilation)
- Failing to clear the airway or to keep it open by failing to hyperextend the head adequately
- Failing to close the nose during mouth-to-mouth ventilation
- Failing to fit the mask closely onto the patient's face when using an inflating bag
- Failing to make sure that ventilation is adequate, as shown by movement of the chest
- Timidity in applying external cardiac compression, and using insufficient force to compress the heart. The risk of cracking a rib should be disregarded
- Failing to release pressure on the chest completely between compressions and thus preventing cardiac filling
- Compressing the chest too rapidly to allow the heart to fill between compressions
- Putting the hands in incorrect positions
- Failing to act sufficiently quickly and fretting about details rather than getting on with the essentials of external cardiac compression and artificial ventilation

---

Strokes

Patients are usually hypertensive and middle-aged or elderly. The clinical picture varies with the size and site of brain damage (Box 36.13). Subarachnoid haemorrhage from a ruptured berry aneurysm on the circle of Willis is the main cause of stroke in a younger person. It typically causes intense headache followed by coma without localising signs.

Box 36.13 Signs and management of a stroke

Signs
- Loss of consciousness
- Weakness of an arm and leg on one side
- Drooping of the side of the face
- Often stertorous breathing

Management
- Maintain the airway
- Call an ambulance for transfer to hospital

CHEST PAIN

Angina pectoris

Acute chest pain due to myocardial ischaemia is the only symptom. A first anginal attack may come as a consequence of an emotional response to dental treatment. Intensity of pain may dictate stopping treatment. Glyceryl trinitrate should be given sublingually (Box 36.14).

Box 36.14 Management of angina

- Give the patient his anti-anginal drug (usually 0.5 mg of glyceryl trinitrate sublingually) *or*
- Glyceryl trinitrate spray* (400 mg) gives rapid relief
- If there is no relief within 3 minutes the patient has probably had a myocardial infarct (see below)

*Glyceryl trinitrate spray has a better shelf-life for the emergency kit.

Many patients have already had attacks and carry medication, but may need nitrates and sedation pre-operatively.

Myocardial infarction

Myocardial infarction is a common cause of death and must be recognised (Box 36.15), as the patient's fate may be decided by the first few minutes' treatment. Several aspects of dentistry, particularly apprehension, pain or the effect of drugs, might contribute to make this accident more likely in a susceptible patient.

Box 36.15 Typical signs and symptoms of myocardial infarction

- Severe crushing retrosternal pain
- Shallow breathing
- Vomiting
- Weak or irregular pulse

Some patients die within a few minutes after the start of the attack and it is rash to try over-ambitious treatment. Drugs, apart from those described below, should not be used as, without continuous monitoring, they may do more harm than good.

Pain can radiate to the left shoulder or down the left arm but, very occasionally, is felt only in the left jaw. Vomiting is common and there is sometimes shock or loss of consciousness. Principles of management are summarised in Box 36.16.

Aspirin is a valuable antiplatelet drug, but it is only feasible to give a fibrinolytic drug, such as streptokinase, in hospital where lidocaine or other antidysrhythmic drugs can be given as appropriate.

There is concern about dentists giving aspirin under these circumstances in case there has been a misdiagnosis and the pain is due to a perforated peptic ulcer or dissecting aneurysm. However, the danger of giving a single tablet of aspirin in such conditions is unlikely to be significant.

Box 36.16   **Management of myocardial infarction**

- Put the patient in a comfortable position that allows easy breathing. Do not lay flat if there is left ventricular failure and pulmonary oedema
- Send an assistant to telephone for an Intensive Care ambulance
- Give 50/50 nitrous oxide and oxygen from a general anaesthetic or relative analgesia machine, to relieve pain and anxiety
- Constantly reassure the patient
- Give oxygen if necessary
- Give aspirin 150 mg by mouth as soon as more urgent measures have been carried out
- Check for possible cardiac arrest

DYSPNOEA

Status asthmaticus

Causes

Loss of or forgetting to bring a salbutamol inhaler, anxiety, infection or exposure to a specific allergen are possible causes.
Features are shown in Box 36.17.

Box 36.17   **Signs and management of status asthmaticus**

Signs
- Breathlessness
- Inability to talk
- Expiratory wheezing (may be disguised as rapid shallow breathing)
- Rapid pulse (usually over 110 per minute). Progress to bradycardia is a danger sign
- Accessory muscles of respiration start to come into action
- Cyanosis

Management
- Call an ambulance for transfer to hospital
- Reassure the patient
- Do *not* lay the patient flat
- Give normally used anti-asthmatic drugs (such as salbutamol) by inhaler or better, by nebuliser
- Give hydrocortisone sodium succinate 200 mg intravenously
- Give oxygen
- If no response within 2–3 minutes, ideally, give salbutamol 250 mg by slow i/v injection
- If i/v salbutamol not available and patient continues to deteriorate, give epinephrine (adrenaline) as for anaphylaxis

---

Left ventricular failure

Extreme breathlessness is the main sign. It may be associated with chest pain if secondary to myocardial infarct. It can occasionally result from a severe dysrhythmia, particularly in a patient who has had a previous myocardial infarct. Apart from measures for an infarct, sitting the patient upright and giving oxygen, little possible can be done in the dental surgery apart from immediately calling an Intensive Care ambulance.

CONVULSIONS

Epilepsy

Hunger, menstruation and some drugs such as methohexitone, tricyclic antidepressants, alcohol or frequently flashing lights (not merely turning the operating lamp on and off) may sometimes precipitate a fit (Box 36.18).

Box 36.18   **Signs and management of a tonic-clonic epileptic attack**

Signs
- Sometimes a brief warning cry as the chest muscles contract and air is forced through a closed larynx
- Consciousness lost immediately
- The body becomes rigid (tonic phase) and cyanosis appears
- Widespread jerking movements start (clonic phase)
- Sometimes incontinence or frothing of the mouth
- Flaccidity sometimes follows after a few minutes
- Consciousness regained after a variable period. Confusion or drowsiness may persist

Management
- Put the patient prone in the coma ('recovery') position as soon as possible
- Prevent patients from injuring themselves
- Do not try to put anything in the mouth in the attempt to prevent the patient biting the tongue
- Make sure the airway is clear after convulsions have subsided
- Do not give any medication but await recovery
- Reassure patients as soon as consciousness returns
- Only allow patients to return home when fully recovered and accompanied by a responsible adult

---

Status epilepticus

If convulsions do not stop within 15 minutes, or are rapidly repeated, the patient is in status epilepticus and can die from anoxia (Box 36.19).

Box 36.19   **Management of status epilepticus**

- Give 10 mg intravenous diazepam to an adult patient
- If venous access cannot be obtained give 5 mg of intramuscular midazolam* (absorption of intramuscular diazepam is slow and erratic)
- Repeat diazepam or midazolam if no recovery within 5 minutes
- Maintain the airway and give oxygen
- Call an ambulance and transfer to hospital

*Not officially approved for this purpose but can be life-saving.

OTHER EMERGENCIES

Haemorrhage

Prolonged bleeding is usually due to traumatic extractions. A major vessel is unlikely to be opened during dental surgery and patients are unlikely to lose any dangerous amount of blood if promptly managed (Box 36.20). Post-extraction bleeding is usually only an emergency in the sense that the dentist may be woken up at 3 o'clock in the morning by a frightened patient.

Occasionally, bleeding is due to unsuspected haemophilia or other haemorrhagic disorders.

> **Box 36.20** **Management of prolonged dental haemorrhage**
>
> - Reassure the patient
> - Coax any excited relatives out of the surgery
> - Clean the mouth with swabs and locate the source of bleeding
> - If there is point bleeding from bone, crush the vessel with a small instrument. Soft tissue bleeding will usually respond to pressure alone
> - Give epinephrine (adrenaline)-containing local anaesthetic, remove ragged tissue, squeeze up the socket edges and suture it. A small piece of oxidized cellulose (Surgicel) may be placed loosely in the socket below the suture to aid haemostasis, but is usually unnecessary
> - When bleeding has been controlled, ask about the history and especially any family history of prolonged bleeding
> - If bleeding continues despite suturing or if the patient is obviously anaemic or debilitated, transfer to hospital for investigation and management of any haemorrhagic defect
> - Meanwhile, limit bleeding as much as possible with a pressure pad over the socket and by supporting the patient's jaw with a firm barrel bandage
> - Ideally, tranexamic acid (500 mg in 5 ml, by slow intravenous injection) should be given and may be effective in a mild haemophilic while awaiting transfer to hospital

Drug reactions and interactions

Apart from anaphylactic reactions discussed earlier, very few other drug reactions or interactions endangering life are likely to be seen in the dental surgery.

Local anaesthetics with vasoconstrictors

Norepinephrine (noradrenaline) (1:20 000), used as a vasoconstrictor in local anaesthetic solutions, has caused deaths from acute hypertension or cerebral haemorrhage. Such reactions can be combatted by an alpha-blocker such as phentolamine. Quite apart from its dangers, noradrenaline (norepinephrine) has no advantages and is no longer available.

Epinephrine (adrenaline). There is no evidence of hypertensive reactions to epinephrine (adrenaline) used in normal concentration and quantity.

Interactions with beta blockers. Epinephrine (adrenaline), in large doses, can interact with drugs such as propranolol to raise the blood pressure. It causes constriction of skin and visceral vessels (alpha effect) but dilatation of muscle arterioles (beta effect).

Dilatation of muscle vessels by epinephrine is opposed by the beta blocker, but the alpha effect on skin and visceral vessels is unopposed. The consequent constriction of both muscle and skin vessels raises the peripheral resistance and blood pressure.

Clinically, occasional cases of hypertensive interactions between epinephrine and propranolol have been reported in patients receiving large amounts of epinephrine in local analgesics for plastic surgery. In 1995, a dentist was convicted of manslaughter after causing the death of a patient on beta blockers by giving her 16 cartridges of lidocaine with epinephrine though it appears overdose of lidocaine was the cause. Though healthy adults can tolerate large amounts of lidocaine with epinephrine, the dose should be limited to 5 cartridges given over the space of an hour unless cardiac monitoring is available.

Otherwise, in all three deaths associated with dental local anaesthetics in the 10-year period 1980–1989, prilocaine had been given.

Monoamine oxidase inhibitors

Monoamine oxidase inhibitors (MAOIs) can cause severe reactions with opioids. The onset can be very sudden and, with pethidine, can be fatal. Monoamine oxidase inhibitors also interact with indirectly-acting sympathomimetic drugs (such as ephedrine used as a nasal decongestant) to cause acute severe hypertension. The treatment is to give an alpha blocker such as phentolamine. Epinephrine or norepinephrine in local anaesthetics do not cause hypertensive reactions with MAOIs.

General anaesthetics

General anaesthetics, particularly intravenous barbiturates, have been the main cause of fatalities in the dental surgery.

Corticosteroids

As already described, patients on long-term corticosteroid treatment when exposed to stress can suffer circulatory collapse as a result of adrenal suppression.

Violence

Violence towards health-providers is steadily growing. Aggressive behaviour can be the result of psychiatric disease (particularly schizophrenia), drug abuse (particularly of alcohol) or brain damage. The risk to dental clinical staff can be significant, especially because of the ready availability of sharp instruments.

The ambulance service is not equipped to deal with such cases so that the police must be called. Patients who abuse NHS staff may have their access to healthcare limited after investigation.

SUGGESTED FURTHER READING

Cawson RA, Spector RG, Skelly M 1995 Basic pharmacology and clinical drug use in dentistry, 6th edn. Churchill Livingstone, Edinburgh

Edmondson HD, Frame JW, Malins AF 1989 Medical emergencies in dental practice: an update on drugs and the management of acute airway obstruction. Dental Uptake August:254–256

Fisher M 1992 Treating anaphylaxis with sympathomimetic drugs. In severe anaphylaxis adrenaline by any route is better than none (editorial). BMJ 305:1107–1108

Gallagher EJ, Lombardi G, Gennis P 1995 Effectiveness of bystander cardiopulmonary resuscitation and survival following out-of-hospital cardiac arrest. JAMA 274:1922–1925

Pennycook A, Makower R, Brewer A et al 1993 The management of dental problems presenting to an accident and emergency department. J Roy Soc Med 86:702–703

Resuscitation Guidelines 2005. Resuscitation Council UK. http://www.resus.org.uk/

Sanders BJ, Weddell JA, Dodge NN 1995 Managing patients who have seizure disorders: dental and medical issues. J Am Dent Assoc 126:1641–1647

Self-assessment questions and learning guides

These self-assessment questions and learning guides are based on the material of the previous section, but may also link to material covered elsewhere. They are not intended to be comprehensive, but give an indication of the understanding and problem solving abilities expected at an undergraduate level. You will not find all the information you require to answer these questions in this textbook of essential facts. Use these questions to guide your additional reading and learning.

CHAPTER 22

- How would you investigate a patient presenting with a sore uniformly-depapillated tongue?
- How would you differentiate the various causes of anaemia using special investigations?
- Which malignant neoplasms may present as gingival swellings or gingival enlargement?
- How might a dentist notice the first signs of lymphoma or leukaemia?
- What are the oral complications of chemotherapy for lymphoma and leukaemia?

CHAPTER 23

- How would you manage a patient presenting with post-extraction haemorrhage?
- How may post-extraction haemorrhage be prevented?

CHAPTER 24

- What systemic complications of HIV infections may impact on the provision of routine dental care?
- Which oral lesions might raise suspicion of immunodeficiency?
- How do the presentations of gingivitis and periodontitis in patients with immunodeficiency differ from those in normal patients?

CHAPTER 25

- How would you investigate and manage a patient with an enlarged upper lip?
- Discuss non-infectious occupational risks of the practice of dentistry. How may they be prevented?

CHAPTER 26

- Which features of an enlarged cervical lymph node would suggest malignancy?
- Which features of an enlarged cervical lymph node would suggest a reactive cause?
- How may tuberculosis present in the head and neck?
- What investigations should be performed to aid diagnosis for a patient with a chronically enlarged cervical lymph node? What is the value of each test?

CHAPTER 27

- Why has the recommended antibiotic prophylaxis for infective endocarditis in dental patients changed over the last few years?
- What local measures should complement systemic antibiotic prophylaxis in the prevention of infective endocarditis in dentistry?
- How and why has the prevalence of the different risk factors for infective endocarditis changed over the last decades?

CHAPTER 28

- When should antibiotics be prescribed for acute or chronic sinusitis?
- How would you diagnose and treat an oroantral communication?
- What are granulomas and why do they form?
- Is there a connection between granulomas, granulation tissue and pyogenic granuloma?

- Which diseases of the head and neck, excluding the oral mucosa, show granulomatous inflammation histologically?
- Discuss the differential diagnosis for a patient with diffuse enlargement of the gingiva.

CHAPTER 29

- How may a patient with hepatitis B or C be identified and their infectivity assessed?
- What are the causes of lip swelling?
- What are the causes of granulomatous inflammation in the oral mucosa?

CHAPTER 31

- How does diabetes mellitus affect the provision of dental treatment?
- What are the causative connections between endocrine disease and gingival enlargement?
- How might a dentist aid diagnosis of thyroid diseases, including neoplasms?

CHAPTERS 32 AND 33

- What features of Down's syndrome might affect provision of dental treatment?
- How might a dentist aid the diagnosis of diseases common in the elderly?
- In which conditions is there an increased risk of trauma to teeth and oral tissues? How may this be managed?
- How may preventive regimens be adapted to suit patients with the conditions in these chapters?
- How may consent for dental treatment be obtained in patients with learning difficulties or mental illness?
- Why are patients with renal disease prone to latex allergy?

CHAPTER 34

- How may dental causes for facial pain be identified?
- What are the features of pain of vascular origin and how do they differ from those of pain of neural origin?
- How may depression present in a dental setting?
- How would you decide whether or not to refer a patient with intractable pain to their medical practitioner?
- For which types of facial pain might a computerised tomogram or magnetic resonance scan be indicated?
- How may atypical facial pain be identified and how should it be treated?
- What analgesics might be prescribed by a dentist to treat orofacial pain?

CHAPTER 35

- Which drugs can cause lichen planus-like reactions?
- Which drugs can cause symptoms of burning mouth?
- Which drugs can cause oral or facial pigmentation?

CHAPTER 36

- How would you differentiate the causes of loss of consciousness?
- How would you treat each of the medical emergencies listed in this chapter?
- In each case, which of the actions should be performed first?
- What adverse effects might ensue if you inadvertently administered the wrong treatment for a medical emergency?
- Where could you check the current Resuscitation Council UK guidelines for basic life support?
- Are you able to use an automatic defibrillator?

Index

457